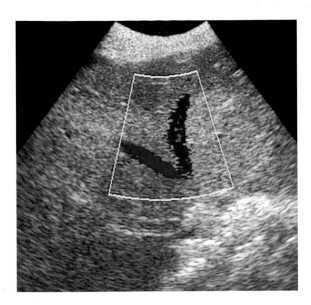

Color Plate 1 Sagittal image of the liver. (See Fig. 7-9, p. 100.)

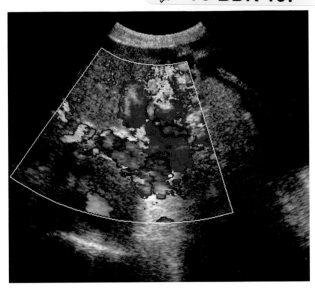

Color Plate 2 Doppler image of the left upper quadrant. (See Fig. 7-10, p. 101.)

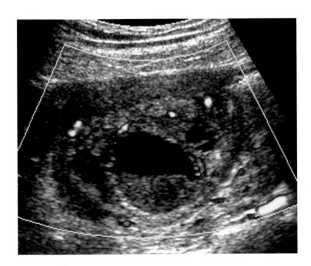

Color Plate 3 Transverse power Doppler image. (See Fig. 8-13, p. 118.)

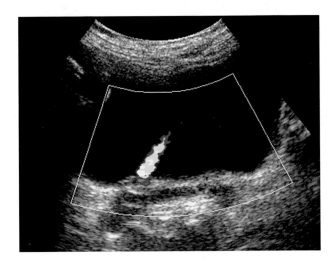

Color Plate 4 Transverse Doppler sonogram. (See Fig. 10-17, p. 153.)

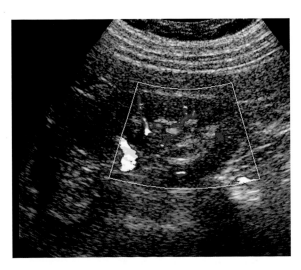

Color Plate 5 Sagittal Doppler image. (See Fig. 10-18, p. 153.)

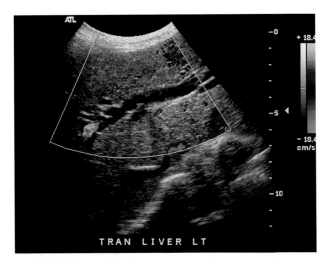

Color Plate 6 Transverse sonogram of the liver. (See Fig. 24, p. 282.)

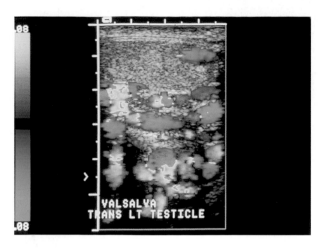

Color Plate 7 Duplex sonogram of the inferior portion of the left scrotum. (See Fig. 36, p. 286.)

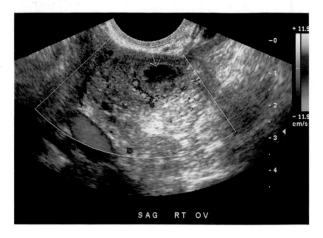

Color Plate 8 Endovaginal sonogram. (See Fig. 20-21, p. 323.)

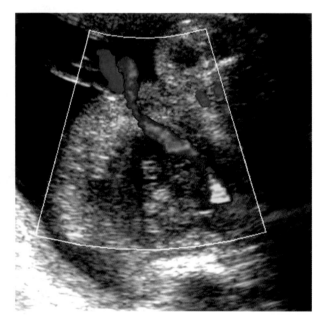

Color Plate 9 (See Fig. 28-6, p. 419.)

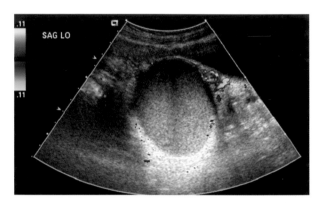

Color Plate 10 Sonogram of the adnexa. (See Fig. 17, p. 443.)

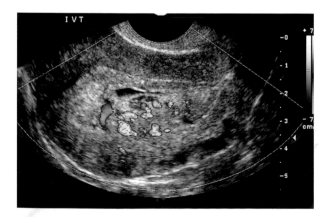

Color Plate 11 (See Fig. 30, p. 450.)

Mosby's Comprehensive Review

for GENERAL SONOGRAPHY EXAMINATIONS

Susanna Ovel, RDMS, RVT, RT(R)

Clinical Instructor and Senior Sonographer
Sonography Consultant
Sacramento, California

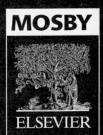

MOSBY

ELSEVIER

11830 Westline Industrial Drive
St. Louis, Missouri 63146

Notice

Knowledge and best practice in this field are constantly changing. As new research and experience broaden our knowledge, changes in practice, treatment and drug therapy may become necessary or appropriate. Readers are advised to check the most current information provided (i) on procedures featured or (ii) by the manufacturer of each product to be administered, to verify the recommended dose or formula, the method and duration of administration, and contraindications. It is the responsibility of the practitioner, relying on their own experience and knowledge of the patient, to make diagnoses, to determine dosages and the best treatment for each individual patient, and to take all appropriate safety precautions. To the fullest extent of the law, neither the Publisher nor the Author assumes any liability for any injury and/or damage to persons or property arising out of or related to any use of the material contained in this book.

The Publisher

Library of Congress Cataloging-in-Publication Data

Ovel, Susanna.
  Mosby's comprehensive review for general sonography examinations / Susanna Ovel. — 1st ed.
    p. ; cm.
  Includes bibliographical references.
  ISBN 978-0-323-05282-5 (pbk. : alk. paper)
1. Ultrasonic imaging—Examinations, questions, etc. 2. Ultrasonic imaging—Examinations—Study guides. I. Title. II. Title: Comprehensive review for general sonography examinations.
  [DNLM: 1. Ultrasonography—Examination Questions. 2. Abdomen—ultrasonography—Examination Questions. 3. Diagnostic Techniques, Obstetrical and Gynecological—Examination Questions. WN 18.2 O96m 2009]
  RC78.7.U4O96 2009
  616.07'543076—dc22

2008042873

Publisher: Jeanne Olson
Senior Developmental Editor: Linda Woodard
Publishing Services Manager: Deborah L. Vogel
Project Manager: Pat Costigan
Book Design: Teresa McBryan

Printed in the United States of America

Last digit is the print number: 9 8 7 6 5 4 3 2 1

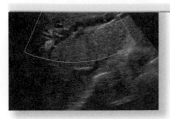

About the Author

Susanna Ovel, RDMS, RVT, RT(R), began her career in 1979 as a radiological technologist at Radiological Science Associates in Sacramento. She became a Registered Diagnostic Medical Sonographer (RDMS) in abdomen and obstetric/gynecology in 1985, a Registered Vascular Technologist (RVT) in 1993, and a Pioneer Breast Sonographer in 2002.

Susanna has lectured in both introductory and advanced courses in obstetrics/gynecology and abdominal sonography as well as sonography physics and instrumentation at Sacramento City Community College. She was the clinical coordinator for a new diagnostic medical sonography program for Kaiser Permanente Richmond Medical Center in Richmond, California.

She is a site visitor for the Joint Review Committee–Diagnostic Medical Sonography (JRC-DMS) and is a consultant for new sonography programs across the country. She has written instructor materials and test bank ancillaries for Elsevier textbooks and continues to lecture on various sonographic subjects while working as a sonographer and clinical instructor at Radiological Science Associates in Sacramento.

To my husband Joe.

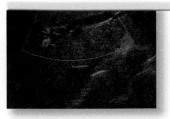

Reviewers

Janice Dolk, MA, RDMS, RT(R)
Lab Instructor, Consultant for Sonography Projects
Palm Beach Community College
Port St. Lucie, Florida

Debbie Henson, AAS, RDMS, RDCS, RVT, RT(R,M)
Clinical Instructor
Tyler Junior College
Tyler, Texas

Harry H. Holdorf, PhD, MPA, RDMS, RT(R)
Director, Diagnostic Medical Sonography Program
Harold B. and Dorothy A. Snyder Schools
Plainfield, New Jersey

Carol Mitchell, PhD, RDMS, RDCS, RVT, RT(R)
Program Director, School of Diagnostic Medical Sonography
University of Wisconsin Hospital and Clinics
Madison, Wisconsin

Anthony E. Swartz, BS, RDMS, RT(R)
Sonographer and Resident Sonography Education Coordinator
University of North Carolina: Specialty Women's Center at Rex
Raleigh, North Carolina

Regina Swearengin, AAS, BS, RDMS
Department Chair, Sonography
Austin Community College
Austin, Texas

Jan Viken, RDMS, RT(R)
Clinical Coordinator, Diagnostic Medical Sonography
Tyler Junior College
Tyler, Texas

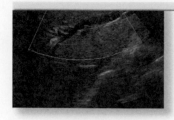

Preface

CONTENT AND ORGANIZATION

Mosby's Comprehensive Review for General Sonography Examinations is designed for students preparing for the American Registry of Diagnostic Medical Sonography (ARDMS) examinations.

The text is divided into three major sections covering these general topics: Sonography Principles and Instrumentation, Abdomen, and Obstetrics and Gynecology. Each section follows and thoroughly covers the ARDMS examination outline.

- **Part One: Sonography Principles and Instrumentation** includes the most recent material covered on the ARDMS examination beginning in spring of 2009. Patient Care and Communications is included along with information on Doppler ultrasound and hemodynamics.
- **Part Two: Abdomen** divides the material into specific organs, vascular structures, and associated areas within the abdominal cavity. Superficial structures and extracranial arteries are also included. Each chapter includes associated laboratory values, congenital anomalies, and normal and pathological sonographic appearance of specific structure(s). Differential considerations are also included.
- **Part Three: Obstetrics and Gynecology** divides the material into smaller sections, enabling the sonography student to review specific areas. Each chapter includes laboratory values, sonographic appearance, and differential considerations.

Individual chapters follow a consistent format utilizing tables whenever possible. Differential considerations and laboratory values are included in the Abdomen and Obstetrics and Gynecology sections, **allowing usage of the text as a reference and study guide.**

FEATURES

REGISTRY-LEVEL QUESTIONS

Fifty multiple choice Registry-level questions follow each chapter. Rationales accompany all questions, pointing out key words within the question and/or reasons why the correct answer is right and the distracters are wrong for this specific question. Rationales increase comprehension and retention of specific material and allow for focus on areas needing more review.

A **mock Registry examination** follows each section to help students in assessing accumulated knowledge in each part. Each exam includes images, rationales, and the exact number of questions in the actual Registry exam.

IMAGES AND ILLUSTRATIONS

More than 350 anatomical illustrations and scans demonstrating normal anatomy and pathologic conditions are utilized in the Abdomen and Obstetrics and Gynecology sections within the text and in the mock examinations. Three-dimensional images are included in the Obstetrics and Gynecology section. These help with recognition of sonographic findings in both normal and abnormal cases. Because color images are now being included on the Registry exams, **color Doppler images** have also been included to help identify blood flow and can be found in a special color insert at the front of the book.

CD-ROM

One of the most valuable features of this review resource is the accompanying CD-ROM, which can run on both Mac and PC and is designed to simulate the computer-based exam administered by the ARDMS. It contains 645 questions—all different from the 1815 questions in the text and all relevant to preparation for the ARDMS examinations. In practice mode, particular topics that need review can be chosen. For example, if the student is preparing for the Abdomen Registry exam and is a bit uncertain of his or her knowledge of anatomy and sonography of the liver and gastrointestinal tract, he or she can choose Practice Mode and answer only questions on these two topics. Rationales provide immediate feedback, and questions can be bookmarked for later reference. In test mode, a virtually unlimited number of randomly generated multiple-choice questions are available in a timed format that replicates the actual time constraints of the Registry exams. More than one third of these mock exam questions include images, some in color.

The CD-ROM also includes two entertaining review games, **Sonography Millionaire and Tournament of Sonography**, which make studying for the Registry exam more fun and less stressful. The games can be played in timed or untimed versions. Timed games and examinations help students practice time-management skills.

The CD-ROM, along with the text, makes this the premier general sonography review book, reference, and study guide, all in one product.

HOW TO USE

The text provides information on the common three general sonography ARDMS examinations and is an effective study guide to use throughout the general sonography program. The content outline may be referenced as a supplement to most courses in the general sonography curriculum.

As a review book, this text provides a logical, well-thought-out approach to preparing for the Registry examinations. The content outline, so effective throughout the educational program, is particularly appreciated at review time. All content that may be tested is presented in a format that is easy to use and understand. Since I have taught these subjects, my approach to the reader is the same as if class were being held each time the book is opened.

Care has been taken to create multiple-choice questions that cover the primary information taught in general diagnostic sonography programs and are therefore relevant to the ARDMS examinations. This philosophy, along with the outline and table formats, helps students make optimal use of study time. All questions in this text and CD-ROM are written in the style of multiple-choice questions used on the Registry examinations. Explanations of answers describe key words and/or reasons why distracters are incorrect. This approach increases comprehension of the subject material.

Information provided in each individual chapter should be reviewed prior to attempting the subject's examination. Tests and files can be dated for later review. Reviewing the answers from previous examinations can demonstrate repetitive problem areas, guiding the student on which subjects or areas are in need of additional review.

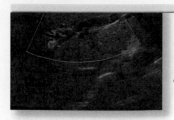

Acknowledgments

I would like to recognize and thank several people for their contributions. My sincere thanks to Jeanne Olson, whose vision and support made this text possible. I extend special recognition and appreciation to Linda Woodard for her expert editing, encouragement, and undying support. My sincere thanks to the Elsevier staff for their professional and prompt contributions to this text. Given the superior talents of the Elsevier staff, any errors or omissions in this book are solely mine.

Very special recognition and thanks go to my husband Joe for his love, understanding, and phenomenal support! "You were right."

I extend special thanks to the late Dr. Thomas K. Bellue for his encouragement and for helping me to progress in my career and life.

Susanna Ovel

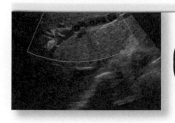

Contents

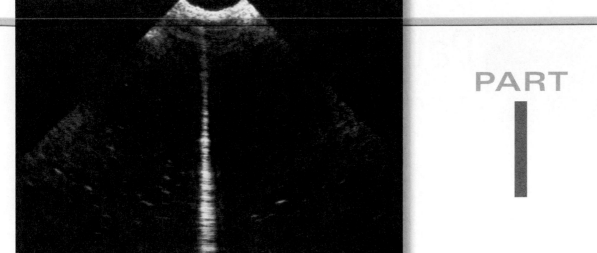

Sonography Principles and Instrumentation

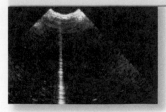

CHAPTER 1

Patient Care, Safety, and Communication

KEY TERMS

acoustic exposure   amount of acoustic energy the patient receives.

ALARA principle   as low as reasonably achievable; used to reduce biological effects in humans and the fetus.

biological effect   effect of ultrasound waves on living organisms, including their composition, function, growth, origin, development, and distribution.

cavitation   interaction of the sound wave with microscopic gas bubbles found in tissues.

epidemiology   studies of various factors determining the frequency and distribution of diseases in the human community.

ex vivo   refers to experimentation done in or on living tissue in an artificial environment outside the organism.

in vitro   refers to the technique of performing a given experiment in a test tube or, generally, in a controlled environment outside a living organism.

in vivo   refers to experimentation done in or on the living tissue of a whole, living organism as opposed to a partial or dead one. Animal testing and clinical trials are forms of in vivo research.

mechanical index (MI)   describes the likelihood of cavitation occurring.

pulse average (PA)   average intensity over the pulse duration.

radiation force   force exerted by the sound beam on an absorber or reflector.

spatial average (SA)   average intensity across the entire sound beam.

spatial peak (SP)   peak intensity found across the sound beam.

standard precautions   suggested program to provide safety to both the patient and caregiver from bloodborne or airborne infections.

temporal average (TA)   average intensity during the pulse repetition period.

temporal peak (TP)   greatest intensity during the pulse.

thermal index (TI)   relates to the heating of tissue.

thermal index for bone (TIB)   relates to the heating of bone.

thermal index for cranium (TIC)   relates to the heating of the cranium.

thermal index for soft tissue (TIS)   relates to the heating in soft tissue.

PATIENT CARE

- Current standards of patient care recommend using standard/universal precautions in all direct patient contact.

STANDARD PRECAUTIONS AND INFECTION CONTROL

- Previously termed universal precautions.
- Precautions compiled by the Centers for Disease Control and Prevention (CDC) and other federal agencies.
- To provide safety to both the patient and caregiver.
- Practiced two ways.
  1. General measures taken to keep health care workers, patients, and the environment clean to prevent the spread of germs.
  2. Isolated precautions that are carried out to confine disease-producing germs.

Standard Precautions (Tier One) for Use with All Patients*

- Standard precautions apply to blood, all body fluids, secretions, excretions, nonintact skin, and mucous membranes.
- Hands are washed if contaminated with blood or body fluid, immediately after gloves are removed, between patient contact, and when indicated to prevent transfer of microorganisms between patients or between patients and environment.
- Gloves are worn when touching blood, body fluid, secretions, excretions, nonintact skin, mucous membranes, or contaminated items. Gloves should be removed and hands washed between patient care.
- Masks, eye protection, or face shields are worn if patient care activities may generate splashes or sprays of blood or body fluid.
- Gowns are worn if soiling of clothing is likely from blood or body fluid. Perform hand hygiene after removing gown.
- Patient care equipment is properly cleaned and reprocessed, and single-use items are discarded.
- Contaminated linen is placed in leakproof bags to prevent skin and mucous membrane exposure.
- All sharp instruments and needles are discarded in a puncture-resistant container. CDC recommends that needles be disposed of uncapped or a mechanical device be used for recapping.

From Perry AG, Potter PA: *Clinical nursing skills and techniques*, ed 5, St Louis, 2002, Mosby. Originally modified from Centers for Disease Control and Prevention, Hospital Infection Control Practice Advisory Committee: Guidelines for isolation precautions in hospitals, *Am J Infect Control* 24:24, 1996.
* Formerly universal precautions and body substance isolation.

Bloodborne Pathogen Precautions

Standard Precautions: Use standard precautions for the care of all patients.

   Airborne Precautions: In addition to standard precautions, use airborne precautions for patients known or suspected to have serious illnesses transmitted by airborne droplet nuclei. Examples of such illnesses include the following:
- Measles
- Varicella (including disseminated zoster)*
- Tuberculosis†

Droplet Precautions: In addition to standard precautions, use droplet precautions for patients known or suspected to have serious illnesses transmitted by large particle droplets. Examples of such illnesses include the following:
- Influenza
- Pneumonia
- Meningitis
- Other serious bacterial respiratory infections spread by droplet transmission, including the following:
  - Diphtheria
  - Mycoplasma pneumonia
  - Pertussis
  - Pneumonic plague
  - Streptococcal pharyngitis or scarlet fever in infants and young children
- Serious viral infections spread by droplet transmission, including the following:
  - Adenovirus*
  - Influenza
  - Mumps
  - Parvovirus B19
  - Rubella

Contact Precautions: In addition to standard precautions, use contact precautions for patients known or suspected to have serious illnesses easily transmitted by direct patient contact or by contact with items in the patient's environment. Examples of such illnesses include the following:

- Gastrointestinal, respiratory, skin, or wound infections or colonization with multidrug-resistant bacteria judged by the infection control program—based on current state, regional, or national recommendations—to be of special clinical and epidemiologic significance
- Enteric infections with a low infection dose or prolonged environmental survival, including the following:
  - *Clostridium difficile*
  - For diapered or incontinent patients: enterohemorrhagic *Escherichia coli* 0157:h7, *Shigella*, hepatitis A, or rotavirus
- Respiratory syncytial virus, parainfluenza virus, or enteroviral infections in infants and young children
- Skin infections that are highly contagious or that may occur on dry skin, including the following:
  - Diphtheria (cutaneous)
  - Herpes simplex virus (neonatal or mucocutaneous)
  - Impetigo
  - Major (noncontained) abscesses, cellulitis, or decubiti
  - Pediculosis
  - Scabies
  - Staphylococcal furunculosis in infants and young children
  - Zoster (disseminated or in the immunocompromised host)*
- Viral hemorrhagic conjunctivitis
- Viral hemorrhagic infections (Ebola, Lassa, or Marburg)

Modified from Perry AG, Potter PA: *Clinical nursing skills and techniques*, ed 5, St Louis, 2002, Mosby. Originally modified from Centers for Disease Control and Prevention, Hospital Infection Control Practice Advisory Committee: Guidelines for isolation precautions in hospitals, *Am J Infect Control* 24:24, 1996.
* Certain infections require more than one type of precaution.
† See CDC Guidelines for Preventing the Transmission of Tuberculosis in Health Care Facilities.

OSHA Standards for Reducing Occupational Exposure to Bloodborne Pathogens

1. Gloves must be worn when there is a reasonable expectation that the employee may contact blood, for example, during venipuncture.
2. Contaminated needles and other sharps must be placed in puncture-resistant containers properly labeled as a biohazard; when the containers are full, they are to be sealed and disposed of properly.
3. Contaminated needles should not be bent, sheared, recapped, or removed from the syringe after use.
4. Reports to Occupational Safety and Health Administration (OSHA) of needle-stick injuries are required, and the health care agency must provide medical evaluation and follow-up.
5. Hepatitis B vaccination is to be made available to all employees who have occupational exposure.
6. Training and education must be offered to high-risk workers concerning precautions for prevention of exposure and use of personal protective equipment.
7. Each facility must have an infection control plan, including methods for the reduction of the health care worker's exposure to biohazardous wastes.
8. Facilities must have engineering and work practice controls to eliminate or minimize employee exposure. Controls may include sharps disposal containers and self-sheathing needles.

Modified from Perry AG, Potter PA: *Clinical nursing skills and techniques*, ed 5, St Louis, 2002, Mosby. Originally modified from Occupational Safety and Health Act: Bloodborne pathogens, *Federal Register* 56(235):64, 175, 1991.

Emergency Situations

SITUATION	CAUSES	TREATMENT
Cardiac distress	• Heart attack • Respiratory arrest • Medication interaction	• Cardiopulmonary resuscitation (CPR) • Automated external defibrillator (AED)
Choking Respiratory distress	• Obstruction • Heart attack • Stroke • Seizures • Fainting	• Abdominal thrusts • Open airway • 1-2 ventilations lasting 1-2 seconds each
Syncope	• Dehydration • Postural hypotension • Medications • Diabetes mellitus • Stroke • Vasovagal reaction	• Lay person supine with legs elevated • If sitting, place head down between knees

PATIENT–SONOGRAPHER INTERACTION

- Sonographer–patient interaction is unique.
- Communication skills are an important aspect of the sonography profession.
- Keeping the patient relaxed and comfortable is the responsibility of the system operator.

Patient–Sonographer Interaction

TIME FRAME	INTERACTION
Prior to examination	• Review medical order • Verify that proper examination is scheduled • Review prior diagnostic studies, if available • Review institution's examination protocol, if needed • Address patient by his or her first and last name • Introduce yourself to the patient and family • Explain examination requested by the physician prior to beginning the scan • Obtain patient history, including possible medication or latex allergies in a private environment • Verify that patient name and identification number is correct on imaging screen • Select the proper transducer frequency limiting acoustic output in compliance with the ALARA principle
During examination	• Maintain patient modesty and privacy • Alleviate and address patient's concerns • Expand on examination protocol as needed
After examination	• Explain expected time frame for the patient's physician to receive a report • Clean transducer(s), equipment, and keyboard • Write technical impression of real-time examination

BIOEFFECTS AND ALARA PRINCIPLE

SAFETY

- Knowledge of bioeffects is important for the safe and prudent use of ultrasound.
- The Food and Drug Administration (FDA) regulates ultrasound instruments according to application, output intensities, and thermal and mechanical indexes.
- The American Institute of Ultrasound in Medicine (AIUM) recommends prudent use of ultrasound in the clinical environment.
- Use ultrasound imaging only when medically indicated.
- Exposure time should be kept at a minimum.

ALARA PRINCIPLE

- *As Low As Reasonably Achievable.*
- Achieve information with the least amount of energy exposure to the patient.
- Prudent and conservative use of ultrasound should be exercised by minimizing exposure time and output intensity.

Acoustic Output Quantities

QUANTITIES	DEFINITION	UNITS	RELATIONSHIP
Acoustic exposure	• Amount of acoustic energy the patient receives	• sec	• Directly related to the intensity of the sound beam and exposure time
Intensity	• Power divided by area	• W/cm^2 • mW/cm^2	• Proportional to acoustic output and amplitude squared • Determined by a hydrophone or force balance system
Power	• Rate at which work is performed	• mW	• Proportional to the amplitude squared • Determined by a hydrophone
Pressure	• Force divided by area	• Pa • MPa • mm Hg	• Areas of compression and rarefaction are measured • Determined by a hydrophone

INTENSITY OF ULTRASOUND

- Intensity varies across the sound beam.
- Intensity is highest in the center of the sound beam and falls off near the periphery.
- Intensity varies with time and is zero between pulses.
- Intensity varies within a pulse starting high, decreasing near the end of the pulse.
- Lowest to highest intensity values for various imaging modalities include:
  - 1-200 mW/cm^2 spatial peak–temporal average (SPTA) for gray-scale imaging
  - 70-130 mW/cm^2 SPTA for M-mode imaging
  - 20-290 mW/cm^2 SPTA for pulsed wave Doppler
  - 10-230 mW/cm^2 SPTA for color Doppler
- Intensity of pulsed wave Doppler is greater than continuous wave Doppler.

SPATIAL PEAK (SP)

- Greatest intensity found across the sound beam.
- Usually located at the center of the sound beam.

SPATIAL AVERAGE (SA)

- The average intensity across the entire sound beam.
- Equal to the total power across the beam divided by the beam area.

TEMPORAL PEAK (TP)

- Greatest intensity during the pulse.

TEMPORAL AVERAGE (TA)

- The average intensity during both the transmitting and receiving times (pulse repetition period).
- Equal to the pulse average (PA) intensity multiplied by the duty factor (DF).

PULSE AVERAGE (PA)

- The average intensity over the entire duration of the pulse (pulse duration).
- For continuous wave, the pulse average is equal to the temporal peak.

INTENSITY VALUES (LOWEST TO HIGHEST)

SPATIAL AVERAGE–TEMPORAL AVERAGE (SATA)

- Averages the spatial and temporal intensities of the sound beam.
- Lowest intensity value for a given sound beam.
- Heat is most dependent on SATA intensity.

SPATIAL PEAK–TEMPORAL AVERAGE (SPTA)

- The average intensity at the center of the beam.
- Used to determine biological effects.
- Typically higher than SATA values by a factor of 2-3 for unfocused and 5-200 for focused transducers.

SPATIAL AVERAGE–PULSE AVERAGE (SAPA)

- Average intensity within the beam over the duration of the pulse.

SPATIAL PEAK–PULSE AVERAGE (SPPA)

- Peak intensity of the sound beam averaged over the duration of the pulse.

SPATIAL AVERAGE–TEMPORAL PEAK (SATP)

- The average intensity within the beam at the highest intensity in time.

SPATIAL PEAK–TEMPORAL PEAK (SPTP)

- Peak intensity of the sound beam in both space and time.
- Highest intensity value for a given sound beam.

INSTRUMENT OUTPUT

- Imaging instruments have the lowest output intensity.
- Pulsed wave Doppler has the highest output intensity.
- Determined by a hydrophone.

BIOLOGICAL EFFECTS

- As a form of energy, ultrasound has a small potential to produce a biological effect.
- Ultrasound is absorbed by tissue, producing heat.
- Adult tissues are more tolerant of temperature increases than fetal or neonatal tissues.
- **No confirmed significant biological effects in mammalian tissue for exposures below 100 mW/cm^2 with an unfocused transducer and 1 W/cm^2 with a focused transducer.**

- Higher intensities are needed to produce bioeffects with a focused transducer.
- Exposure duration up to 50 hours has not demonstrated significant bioeffects.

CAVITATION

- Result of pressure changes in soft tissue causing formation of gas bubbles.
- Can produce severe tissue damage.
- Relevant parameters include pressure, amplitude, and intensity.
- The introduction of bubbles into the tissues and circulation from contrast agents may increase the risk for cavitation.

Stable Cavitation

- Involves microbubbles already present in tissue.
- When pressure is applied, microbubbles will expand and collapse.
- Bubbles can intercept and absorb a large amount of acoustic energy.

Transient Cavitation

- Dependent on the pressure of the ultrasound pulse.
- May occur with short pulses.
- Bubbles expand and collapse violently.
- Pulses with peak intensity greater than 3300 W/cm^2 (10 MPa) can induce cavitation in mammals.

Studies on the Bioeffects of Ultrasound

STUDY	PURPOSE	FINDINGS
Animals	• Determination of the conditions under which thermal and nonthermal bioeffects occur	• Postpartum mortality • Fetal abnormalities and weight reduction • Tissue lesions • Hind limb paralysis • Blood flow stasis • Slow wound healing • Tumor regression
Cells	• Useful for identifying cellular effects	• Ultrasonically induced changes of the cytoskeleton seem to be nonspecific and temporary
Epidemiology	• Long-term studies on the fetus or humans with a history of previous sonograms • Evaluation of birth weight, anomalies, intelligence, and overall health	• No significant biological differences have been detected between exposed and unexposed patients
In vivo	• Observation of living tissue • Ability to explore and evaluate specific tissues or areas	• Focal lesions can occur at spatial peak–temporal average intensities greater than 10 W/cm^2
Plants	• To understand cavitational effects in living tissue	• When tissues contain micrometer-sized, stabilized gas bodies, pulse ultrasound can produce damage

ACOUSTIC OUTPUT LABELING STANDARDS

- Voluntary output display standard.
- Includes two types of indexes: mechanical and thermal.

Acoustic Output Indexes

INDEX	DESCRIPTION	RELATIONSHIP
Mechanical index (MI)	• Indicator of cavitation • Equal to the peak rarefactional pressure divided by the square root of the operating frequency	• Value <1 indicates a low risk of adverse effects or cavitation • Proportional to the output • Inversely proportional to the operating frequency • Relates to temporal resolution
Thermal index (TI)	• Ratio of acoustic power produced by the transducer and the power required to raise tissue temperature 1°C • Relates to attenuation (heat) and the spatial peak–temporal average intensity	• Value <2 indicates a low risk of adverse effects • A rise in temperature exceeding 2°C is significant • Above 39°C biological effects are determined by the temperature and exposure time • In situ, above 41°C is dangerous to the fetus • Proportional to exposure time • Calculated by analyzing acoustic power, beam area, operating frequency, attenuation, and thermal properties of soft tissue
Thermal index for bone	• Relates to the heating of bone	• Increases with focal diameter • Absorption is higher in bone than soft tissue, especially in the fetus
Thermal index for cranium	• Relates to the heating of the cranium	• Exposure must not exceed 33 continuous minutes to avoid thermal damage to the brain surface • Transcranial Doppler (TCD) demonstrates a rapid rise in temperature
Thermal index for soft tissue	• Relates to the heating in soft tissue	• Increases with an increase in frequency

BIOEFFECTS AND SAFETY REVIEW

1. Which of the following are types of cavitation?
   a. stable and thermal
   b. in vivo and in vitro
   c. transient and stable
   d. spatial and transient
   e. mechanical and thermal

2. Which of the following displays the lowest intensity value in pulsed-wave ultrasound?
   a. SPTP
   b. SAPA
   c. SPTA
   d. SATA
   e. SPPA

3. With a focused transducer, there are no confirmed significant biological effects in mammalian tissue for exposures below:
   a. 1 W/cm^2
   b. 1 mW/cm^2
   c. 20 mW/cm^2
   d. 100 W/cm^2
   e. 100 mW/cm^2

4. The acronym SPPA denotes:
   a. spatial pulse–peak average
   b. spatial peak–peak amplitude
   c. spatial peak–pulse average
   d. spatial pulse–pressure average
   e. spatial pulse–pulse amplitude

5. Which of the following imaging modalities demonstrates the highest intensity?
   a. M-mode
   b. color Doppler
   c. real-time imaging
   d. pulsed wave Doppler
   e. continuous wave Doppler

6. Standard precautions apply to all of the following EXCEPT:
   a. hair
   b. blood
   c. excretions
   d. body fluids
   e. mucous membranes

7. Plant studies are useful for understanding:
   a. the effects on wound healing
   b. when focal lesions will occur
   c. the thermal effects on living tissues
   d. the long-term effects on human tissues
   e. the cavitational effects on living tissues

8. Transient cavitation is most dependent on the:
   a. thermal index
   b. ultrasound pulse
   c. size of gas bubble
   d. type of contrast agent used
   e. expansion rate of the microbubble

9. The study of various factors determining the frequency and distribution of diseases in the human community describes:
   a. cavitation
   b. epidemiology
   c. thermal index
   d. mechanical index
   e. biological effects

10. Mechanical index indicates the:
    a. likelihood cavitation will occur
    b. peak intensity of the sound beam
    c. amount of heat absorbed by human tissues
    d. likelihood tissue temperature will rise 2°C
    e. relationship between attenuation and peak temporal intensity

11. When researching the biological effects of diagnostic ultrasound, which intensity is most commonly used?
    a. SATA
    b. SPTA
    c. SPPA
    d. SATP
    e. SPTP

12. Clinical trials are examples of which of the following?
    a. in situ studies
    b. in vivo studies
    c. ex vivo studies
    d. in vitro studies
    e. in utero studies

13. Which intensity is the greatest during the pulse?
    a. spatial peak
    b. pulse average
    c. temporal peak
    d. spatial average
    e. temporal average

14. Pulse average is defined as the average intensity:
    a. of the pulse
    b. over the pulse area
    c. over the duration of a pulse
    d. across the entire sound beam
    e. during the pulse repetition period

15. Cavitation is the interaction of the sound wave with:
    a. bone
    b. living organisms
    c. an acoustic reflector
    d. gas bubbles in the aqueous gel
    e. microscopic gas bubbles found in tissues

16. Which of the following organizations regulates ultrasound equipment?
    a. ACR
    b. FDA
    c. AIUM
    d. ALARA
    e. CAAHEP

17. The American Institute of Ultrasound in Medicine recommends:
    a. ultrasound as a safe obstetrical procedure
    b. a high acoustic output with minimal exposure time
    c. prudent use of ultrasound in the clinical environment
    d. obstetrical examinations for sex determination of a fetus
    e. ultrasound systems to the Food and Drug Administration

18. Cavitation is the result of:
    a. a rise in tissue temperature exceeding $1°C$
    b. using a high-frequency phased-array transducer
    c. the attenuation of the sound wave as it travels through soft tissue
    d. pressure changes in soft tissue causing the formation of gas bubbles
    e. introduction of bubbles into the tissues and circulation from contrast agents

19. Absorption of the sound beam is highest in:
    a. air
    b. bone
    c. fluids
    d. muscle
    e. soft tissue

20. Heating of soft tissue is proportional to the:
    a. tissue thickness
    b. mechanical index
    c. operating frequency
    d. spatial peak intensity
    e. propagation speed of the medium

21. Washing hands before and after an examination are examples of:
    a. reverse isolation
    b. OSHA standards
    c. isolation techniques
    d. respiratory isolation
    e. standard precautions

22. What are the units for power?
    a. mW
    b. MPa
    c. W/cm
    d. W/cm^2
    e. mW/cm^2

23. The mission of the ALARA principle is to:
    a. provide image consistency
    b. reduce the biological effects of ultrasound
    c. explain hemodynamics of arterial blood flow
    d. provide a method of evaluating system accuracy
    e. explain the cavitational effects of sonographic imaging

24. Which of the following denotes the likelihood cavitation will occur?
    a. epidemiology
    b. thermal index
    c. radiation force
    d. SATA intensity
    e. mechanical index

25. Which of the following intensities is greatest across the sound beam?
    a. pulse peak
    b. spatial peak
    c. temporal peak
    d. spatial average
    e. temporal average

26. Research has revealed transcranial Doppler (TCD) imaging results in:
    a. a minimal amount of cavitation
    b. tissue lesions in small mammals
    c. hind limb paralysis in large mammals
    d. a rapid increase in the temperature of the cranium
    e. a minimal increase in the temperature of the cranium

27. Ultrasound has a small potential to produce a biological effect because:
    a. it is a form of energy
    b. of the frequency range employed
    c. contrast agents introduce bubbles into the tissues
    d. of the routine request for sonographic examinations
    e. fetal tissue is less tolerant to temperature increases

28. Biological studies of the cytoskeleton have shown:
    a. ultrasound modifies cancer cells
    b. ultrasound increases the risk of cavitation
    c. ultrasound-induced changes are temporary
    d. ultrasound produces long-term tissue damage
    e. ultrasound increases the risk of tissue hyperplasia

29. The use of contrast agents in diagnostic sonography:
    a. has induced cell changes
    b. may increase the risk of cavitation
    c. does not increase the risk of biological effects
    d. demonstrates a rapid increase in tissue temperature
    e. determines the conditions under which thermal effects occur

30. Limiting the exposure time to a fetus is an example of:
    a. Snell's law
    b. SATA intensity
    c. mechanical index
    d. ALARA principle
    e. Huygens principle

31. Experimentation on living tissue in an artificial environment describes which of the following?
    a. in situ
    b. in vivo
    c. ex situ
    d. ex vivo
    e. in vitro

32. Heat is most dependent on which of the following intensities?
    a. SPPA
    b. SPTP
    c. SATP
    d. SATA
    e. SPTA

33. Pulses can induce cavitation in mammals with a peak intensity exceeding:
    a. 10 MPa
    b. 20 MPa
    c. 10 W/cm^2
    d. 2000 W/cm^2
    e. 2500 mW/cm^2

34. Higher intensities are necessary to produce bioeffects with a(n):
    a. focused transducer
    b. unfocused transducer
    c. linear-array transducer
    d. multifrequency transducer
    e. three-dimensional transducer

35. Which type of cavitation involves the microbubbles already present in tissues?
    a. stable
    b. spatial
    c. thermal
    d. transient
    e. mechanical

36. With an unfocused transducer, there are no confirmed significant biological effects in mammalian tissue for exposures below:
    a. 1 W/cm^2
    b. 1 mW/cm^2
    c. 20 mW/cm^2
    d. 100 W/cm^2
    e. 100 mW/cm^2

37. The average intensity during the pulse repetition period defines:
    a. temporal peak
    b. spatial average
    c. temporal average
    d. spatial average–pulse average
    e. spatial average–temporal average

38. Which of the following reduces occupational injuries?
    a. strict isolation
    b. sterile techniques
    c. OSHA standards
    d. reverse precautions
    e. wound–skin precautions

39. Which of the following techniques is likely performed in a laboratory?
    a. in situ
    b. ex vivo
    c. in vivo
    d. in utero
    e. in vitro

40. Which of the following most accurately defines radiation force?
    a. measurement of acoustic output
    b. ability to identify weak intensities
    c. ability to place echoes in the proper position
    d. force exerted on the sound beam by an absorber
    e. measurement of the likelihood that cavitation will occur

41. The common intensity over the extent of a pulse defines:
    a. duty factor
    b. pulse average
    c. spatial average
    d. acoustic output
    e. temporal average

42. Exposure of a fetus to ultrasound is dangerous above:
    a. $10°\text{C}$
    b. $35°\text{F}$
    c. $39°\text{C}$
    d. $40°\text{F}$
    e. $41°\text{C}$

43. Epidemiology studies on the biological effects of diagnostic ultrasound have determined:
    a. pulse ultrasound damages soft tissue
    b. no significant biological effects
    c. cavitation is proportional to the operating frequency
    d. temperatures above 39°C are dangerous to the fetus
    e. focal lesion can occur at SPTA intensities greater than 10 W/cm²

44. Pressure changes in soft tissue is most likely to result in:
    a. cavitation
    b. tissue lesions
    c. blood flow stasis
    d. fetal abnormalities
    e. postpartum mortality

45. Microbubbles will expand and collapse when:
    a. pressure is applied
    b. disease is encountered
    c. the thermal index reaches 2.0
    d. the temperature of bone increases by 1°C
    e. the temperature of soft tissue increases by 2°C

46. Which of the following is consistent with the ALARA principle?
    a. limited exposure time and high acoustic output
    b. low acoustic output and limited exposure time
    c. low acoustic output and high operating frequency
    d. high operating frequency and limited exposure time
    e. low operating frequency and limited acoustic output

47. Use of ultrasound for entertainment is:
    a. approved by the FDA
    b. recommended by the AIUM
    c. medically approved examination
    d. discouraged by the medical community
    e. an excellent bonding tool for mother and fetus

48. Power is defined as:
    a. resistance to acceleration
    b. energy between two points
    c. rate at which work is performed
    d. rate of motion with respect to time
    e. amount of force over a specific area

49. Animal testing is a form of what type of research?
    a. in situ
    b. in vivo
    c. ex situ
    d. ex vivo
    e. in vitro

50. The intensity of M-mode imaging is greater than the intensity of:
    a. color Doppler
    b. power Doppler
    c. gray-scale imaging
    d. pulsed wave Doppler
    e. continuous wave Doppler

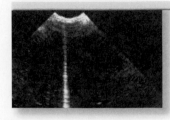

CHAPTER 2

Physics Principles

KEY TERMS

acoustic   having to do with sound.

acoustic impedance   resistance of sound as it propagates through a medium.

acoustic variables   effects on the sound beam caused by the medium; includes pressure, density, and particle motion (distance and temperature).

amplitude   relates to the strength of the compression wave; maximum variation of an acoustic variable.

area   amount of space within a specific boundary.

attenuation   weakening of sound as it propagates through a medium.

attenuation coefficient   attenuation occurring with each centimeter sound travels.

bandwidth   range of frequencies found in pulse ultrasound.

circumference   distance around the perimeter of an object.

compression   region of high pressure or density in a compression wave.

continuous wave   a nonpulsed wave in which cycles repeat indefinitely.

cycle   one complete variation in pressure or other acoustic variable.

decibel   a unit used to compare the ratio of intensities or amplitudes of two sound waves or two points along the wave.

density   concentration of mass, weight, or matter per unit volume.

distance   amount of space from one object to another.

duty factor   fraction of time pulse ultrasound is on.

energy   the capability of doing work.

fractional bandwidth   compares the range of frequencies (bandwidth) with the operating frequency.

frequency   number of cycles in a wave occurring in 1 second.

fundamental frequency   original operating frequency.

half value layer (HVL)   thickness of tissue required to reduce the intensity of the sound beam by one-half; also known as depth of penetration, half boundary layer, or penetration depth.

harmonic frequency   echoes of twice the frequency transmitted into the body reflect back to the transducer, improving image quality.

hertz (Hz)   one cycle per second; unit of frequency.

impedance   determines how much of an incident sound wave is reflected back from the first medium and how much is transmitted into the second medium.

incident angle   direction of incident beam with respect to the media boundary.

incident beam   initial or starting beam.

intensity   rate at which energy transmits over a specific area.

kilohertz (kHz)   one thousand cycles per second.

longitudinal wave   wave traveling in a straight line.

oblique incidence   incident ultrasound traveling at an oblique angle to the media boundary.

period   time to complete one cycle.

perpendicular incidence   incident ultrasound traveling at an angle perpendicular to the media boundary.

pressure   concentration of force.

propagation speed   speed at which a wave moves through a medium.

pulse   a collection of a number of cycles that travel together.

pulse duration   portion of time from the beginning to the end of a pulse; sonography generally uses 2 to 3 cycles while Doppler uses 5 to 30 cycles per pulse.

pulse repetition frequency   number of pulses per second.

pulse repetition period   time between the beginning of one cycle to the beginning of the next cycle.

pulse ultrasound   consists of a few pulses of ultrasound followed by a longer pause of no ultrasound. During this "silence," returning echoes are received and processed.

quality factor (Q factor)   for short pulses, the Q factor is equal to the number of cycles in a pulse; the lower the Q factor, the better the image quality.

rarefaction   regions of low pressure or density in a compression wave.

Rayleigh's scatter   occurs when the reflector is much smaller than the wavelength of the sound beam.

reflected beam   the beam redirected back to the transducer after striking a media boundary.

reflection   redirection (return) of a portion of the sound beam back to the transducer.

reflection angle   angle between the reflected sound and a line perpendicular to the media boundary.

refraction   change in direction of the sound wave after passing from one medium to another.

scattering redirection of sound in several directions on encountering a rough surface; also known as nonspecular reflections.

sound a traveling variation of acoustic variables.

spatial relating to space.

spatial pulse length distance over which a pulse occurs.

speckle multiple echoes received at the same time generating interference in the sound wave, resulting in a grainy appearance of the sonogram.

specular reflections make up the boundaries of organs and reflect sound in only one direction; specular reflections are angle dependent.

stiffness resistance of a material to compression.

temporal relating to time.

transmitted beam the sound beam continuing on to the next media boundary.

volume amount of occupied space of an object in three dimensions.

wavelength distance (length) of one complete cycle.

SOUND CATEGORIES

INFRASOUND

- Below 20 Hz.
- Below human hearing.

AUDIBLE SOUND

- Above 20 Hz and below 20,000 Hz.
- Within human hearing.

ULTRASOUND

- Above 20,000 Hz.
- Above human hearing.

SOUND WAVES

- A traveling variation of acoustic variables (pressure, density, and particle motion).
- Longitudinal, mechanical, pressure waves.
- Matter must be present for sound to travel; it cannot travel through vacuum.
- Sound waves carry **energy**—not matter—from one place to another.
- Vibrations from one molecule **carry** to the next molecule along the same axis. These oscillations continue until friction causes the vibrations to cease.
- Contain regions of compression [high pressure] and rarefaction [low pressure].

Metric Prefixes		
METRIC PREFIX	VALUE	SYMBOL
Giga	10^9 (billion)	G
Nano	10^{-9} (billionth)	n
Mega	10^6 (million)	M
M	10^{-6} (millionth)	μ
Kilo	10^3 (thousand)	k
Milli	10^{-3} (thousandth)	m
Hecto	10^2 (hundred)	h
Centi	10^{-2} (hundredth)	c
Deca	10^1 (ten)	Da
Deci	10^{-1} (tenth)	d

Wave Variables
Wavelength (λ) = Propagation Speed (c)/Frequency (f)

WAVE VARIABLE	DEFINITION	UNITS	DETERMINED BY	RELATIONSHIP
Frequency (f)	• Number of cycles in 1 sec	• Hz • kHz • MHz	• Transducer	• **Proportional** to image quality and attenuation • **Inversely** proportional to the wavelength, period, and penetration depth
Period (T)	• Time for one cycle to occur	• sec • ms • µs	• Transducer	• **Proportional** to the wavelength • **Inversely** proportional to frequency
Propagation speed (c)	• Speed with which a wave travels through a medium	• sec • ms • µs	• Stiffness and density of the medium	• **Proportional** to the stiffness of the medium • **Inversely** proportional to the density of the medium • **Dense** structures or pathologies **decrease** propagation speed • **Stiff** structures **increase** the propagation speed (bone) • **Soft tissue**—propagation speed is equal to 1.54 mm/µs • **13 µs** for sound to travel 1 cm in soft tissue round-trip
Wavelength (λ)	• Length of one complete cycle	• m • mm	• Transducer • Medium	• **Proportional** to the period and penetration depth • **Inversely** proportional to frequency

Properties of Ultrasound

PROPERTY	DEFINITION	UNITS	DETERMINED BY	RELATIONSHIP
Amplitude	• Maximum variation that occurs in an acoustic variable • Relates to sound strength	• Depends on the acoustic variable	• Ultrasound system • Operator-adjustable using output or power control	• **Proportional** to power • **Decreases** as the wave propagates through tissue
Intensity	• Relates to the strength of the sound beam • Rate at which energy passes through unit area • Equal to the total power of the beam divided by the area over which the power is spread	• W/cm^2 • mW/cm^2	• Ultrasound system • Operator-adjustable using output or power control	• **Proportional** to power • **Inversely** proportional to the beam area • **Proportional** to amplitude of the wave squared
Power	• Rate at which energy is transmitted into the body • Rate at which work is done	• W • mW	• Ultrasound system • Operator-controlled using output or power control	• **Proportional** to intensity
Pressure	• Amount of force over a specific area • Acoustic variable	• Pascal (Pa) • MPa	• Operator-adjustable using output or power control	• **Proportional** to amount of force and volume of the sound wave • **Inversely** proportional to the area covered

PULSE ULTRASOUND

- Electrical energy applied to the transducer produces short bursts of acoustic energy
- A pulse must have a beginning and an end
- There are two components to a pulse: transmitting (on) and receiving (off)

Properties of Pulse Ultrasound

PROPERTY	DEFINITION	UNITS	DETERMINED BY	RELATIONSHIP
Bandwidth	• Range of frequencies contained in a pulse	• MHz	• Transducer • Ultrasound system • **Cannot** be adjusted by the operator	• **Inversely** proportional to the length of the pulse (SPL) and Q factor • Portion of the bandwidth used is adjusted with the multi-Hertz or harmonic control
Duty factor (DF)	• Percentage of time pulsed ultrasound is transmitting (on)	• None	• Transducer • Operator-adjustable with depth control	• **Proportional** to PRF and PD • **Inversely** proportional to PRP
Pulse duration (PD)	• Time it takes for one pulse to occur	• μs	• Ultrasound system • Transducer • **Cannot** be adjusted by the operator	• **Proportional** to the duty factor and number of cycles in a pulse • **Inversely** proportional to PRF
Pulse repetition frequency (PRF)	• Number of pulses occurring in 1 sec	• kHz	• Ultrasound system • Operator-adjustable with depth control	• **Proportional** to the duty factor • **Inversely** proportional to imaging depth and PRP
Pulse repetition period (PRP)	• Time from the start of one pulse to the start of the next pulse	• ms	• Ultrasound system • Operator-adjustable with depth control	• **Proportional** to imaging depth • **Inversely** proportional to the PRF
Spatial pulse length (SPL)	• Length of a pulse from start to finish	• mm	• Ultrasound system • Medium • **Cannot** be adjusted by the operator	• **Proportional** to the wavelength and number of cycles in a pulse • **Inversely** proportional to the frequency • **Shorter** pulse lengths improve image quality

PROPAGATION OF ULTRASOUND

- Sound travels through tissues at different speeds depending on the density and stiffness of the medium.
- Impedance determines how much of the wave will transmit to the next medium.

Impedance (rayls) = medium density (kg/m^3) × medium propagation speed (m/s).

Propagation Speeds

MEDIUM	PROPAGATION SPEED
Air	330 m/s
Fat	1459 m/s
Soft tissue	**1540 m/s or 1.54 mm/μsec**
Blood	1570 m/s
Muscle	1580 m/s
Bone	4080 m/s

INCIDENT BEAM = REFLECTED BEAM + TRANSMITTED BEAM

- **Incident beam** is the initial beam transmitting from the transducer.
- **Reflected beam** is the portion of beam returning to the transducer.
- **Transmitted beam** is the portion of the beam that continues to travel.

PERPENDICULAR INCIDENCE

- Perpendicular direction of the incident beam in relation to the boundary between two media.
- Allows reflection of the sound beam.
- Transmitted beam continues to travel along the path of the incident beam.
- Intensity of reflected and transmitted sound is dependent on the impedance difference between the two media.

OBLIQUE INCIDENCE

- Nonperpendicular direction of the incident beam in relation to the boundary between two media.
- Direction of the incident beam with respect to the media boundary is termed the incidence angle.
- Incidence angle is equal to the reflection angle.
- Transmission angle depends on the propagation speeds in the media.

REFLECTION OF ULTRASOUND

- Redirection of a portion of the sound beam back toward the transducer.
- A difference in acoustic impedance between two structures and striking the media boundary at a perpendicular angle MUST take place for reflection to occur.
- The *greater* the impedance difference between the media, the *greater* the reflection.
- The percentage of the incident beam reflected back toward the transducer once the sound beam passes from one tissue to the next is termed the **intensity reflection coefficient (IRC).**
- IRC is determined by the following formula:

$$IRC = \frac{[Z_2 - Z_1]^2}{[Z_2 + Z_1]} = \frac{\text{Reflected intensity (W/cm}^2)}{\text{Incident intensity (W/cm}^2)}$$

Z_1 = impedance of medium 1
Z_2 = impedance of medium 2

Reflection of Sound

INTERFACE	REFLECTION
Fat–muscle	1%
Fat–bone	50%
Tissue–air	100%

SPECULAR REFLECTIONS

- Occur when the wave strikes a large, smooth surface at a 90° angle (i.e., diaphragm).
- Angle dependent.

SCATTER

- A nonspecular reflection allowing the definition of organ parenchyma.
- A reflector smaller, more irregular, or rougher than the incident beam will demonstrate scattering.
- Not angle dependent.
- Proportional to the frequency.

RAYLEIGH'S SCATTER

- Occurs when the reflector is much smaller than the wavelength of the sound beam (i.e., red blood cells).
- Is directed equally in all directions.

CONTRAST AGENTS

- Injected into the body to enhance anatomic structures.
- Types include encapsulated gas bubbles, free gas bubbles, colloidal suspensions, emulsions and aqueous solutions.
- Reflectivity of small particles is dependent on the frequency.
- Microbubbles increase scatter and emit sound waves at harmonic frequencies.
- Contrast agents approved in the United States include Definity (perflutren lipid microsphere), Imagent (perflexane lipid microsphere), and Optison (perflutren protein-type A microsphere).
- Contrast agents approved in Canada, Europe, and Japan include Echovist®, Levovist®, and SonoVue®.

HARMONIC FREQUENCIES

- Even and odd multiples of the fundamental frequency.
- Generated in the body from tissue interaction or contrast media.
- Improves spatial and contrast resolution.
- Beams are narrower with lower side lobes.
- More harmonics are generated with more concentrated acoustic energy.

TRANSMISSION OF ULTRASOUND

- With perpendicular incidence approximately 99% of the incident beam is transmitted.
- The percentage of the incident beam intensity that is transmitted once the beam passes from one tissue to the next is termed the **intensity transmission coefficient (ITC)**.
- ITC is determined by the following formulas:

$$ITC = \frac{\text{Transmitted intensity} \ (W/cm^2)}{\text{Incident intensity} \ (W/cm^2)}$$

OR

$$ITC = 1 - IRC$$

REFRACTION OF ULTRASOUND

- Redirection or bending of the transmitting beam once it passes through one medium to another.
- Oblique incidence and a change of velocity or propagation speed between two media MUST take place for refraction to occur.
- If the propagation speed in the second medium is *greater* than the speed in the first medium, the transmitted beam will bend *away* from the incident beam. The transmission angle is *greater* than the incident angle and vice versa.
- Snell's law is used to determine the amount of refraction at an interface.

DECIBEL (DB)

- Compares the relationship between two values of intensity or amplitude along the sound wave.
- Does not represent an absolute value.
- Based on a logarithmic scale with a wide range of values.
- Positive decibels arise when the final intensity exceeds the initial intensity (i.e., increasing the gain control).
- Negative decibels arise when the final intensity is less than the initial intensity (i.e., attenuation).

Decibel Values

DECIBEL	VALUE
+3 dB	increased by 2×
+6 dB	increased by 4×
+9 dB	increased by 8×
+10 dB	increased by 10×
+20 dB	increased by 100×
+30 dB	increased by 1000×
+40 dB	increased by 10,000×
−3 dB	decreased by ½
−6 dB	decreased by ¼
−9 dB	decreased by ⅛
−10 dB	decreased by 1/10
−20 dB	decreased by 1/100
−30 dB	decreased by 1/1000
−40 dB	decreased by 1/10,000

ATTENUATION

- Progressive weakening of the amplitude or intensity of the sound wave as it propagates through a medium.
- Owing to absorption, reflection, and scattering of the incidental sound beam.

$$\text{Total attenuation (dB)} = \text{Attenuation coefficient (dB/cm/MHz)} \times \text{Path length (cm)}$$

Attenuation Values

TISSUE	ATTENUATION
Fat	0.6 dB/cm/MHz
Liver	0.9 dB/cm/MHz
Kidney	1.0 dB/cm/MHz
Muscle	1.2 dB/cm/MHz
Air	12.0 dB/cm/MHz
Bone	20.0 dB/cm/MHz

ATTENUATION COEFFICIENT

- Amount of attenuation in the sound beam for every centimeter traveled.

$$\text{Attenuation coefficient (dB/cm)} = \frac{1}{2}\text{Frequency (MHz)}$$

HALF VALUE LAYER

- Thickness of tissue required to reduce the intensity of the sound beam by one half.
- Also known as depth of penetration, half boundary layer, penetration depth.

$$\text{Half value layer (cm)} = \frac{3}{\text{Attenuation coefficient (dB/cm)}}$$

OR

$$\text{Half value layer (cm)} = \frac{6}{\text{Frequency (MHz)}}$$

RANGE EQUATION

- Distance to the reflector.
- Time (μs) is equal to distance (cm).
- Must know the direction of the echo and the distance traveled.
- Proportional to the round-trip time.

$$\text{Distance (mm)} = \frac{1}{2}\text{propagation speed (mm/}\mu\text{s)} \times \text{round-trip time (}\mu\text{s)}.$$

OR

$$\text{Distance (cm)} = \frac{\text{Round-trip time (}\mu\text{s)}}{13\ (\mu\text{s/cm})}$$

Propagation of Sound

PROPERTY	DEFINITION	UNITS	RELATIONSHIP
Attenuation	• Progressive weakening in the intensity of the sound wave as it propagates in the human body	• dB	• **Proportional** to the frequency and penetration depth
	RESULT OF: • **Absorption***: conversion of sound to heat • **Reflection:** redirection of the sound beam back toward the transducer • **Scattering:** redirection of sound in multiple directions		
Attenuation coefficient	• Amount of attenuation per centimeter traveled • In soft tissue, equal to half of the transducer frequency (MHz)	• dB/cm	• **Proportional** to the frequency and penetration depth
Density	• Concentration of mass per unit volume • Weight of 1 cm^3 of material	• kg/m^3	• **Proportional** to impedance and propagation speed
Half value layer	• Thickness of tissue required to reduce the intensity of the sound beam by one half • Equal to an intensity reduction of −3 dB	• cm	• **Inversely** proportional to the frequency
Impedance (Z)	• Equal to the density of the medium multiplied by its propagation speed	• rayls	• **Proportional** to the density and propagation speed of the medium

*Most common cause.

Sonographic Terminology

Anechoic—without internal echoes.

Echogenic—producing echoes of varying intensity.

Heterogeneous—term used to describe a mixed echo texture.

Homogeneous—term used to describe a uniform echo texture.

Hyperechoic—comparative term used to describe an increase in echogenicity when compared to another structure or the normal expected echo pattern of a structure.

Hypoechoic—comparative term used to describe a decrease in echogenicity when compared to another structure or the normal expected echo pattern of a structure.

Isoechoic—echo texture equal to the surrounding structures.

Chapter Formulas

Attenuation (dB) = Attenuation coefficient (dB/cm) × path length (cm)

$$\text{Attenuation coefficient (dB)} = \frac{1}{2}\text{Frequency (MHz)}$$

$$\text{Duty factor (unitless)} = \frac{\text{Pulse duration } (\mu s)}{\text{Pulse repetition period } (\mu s)}$$

$$\text{Fractional bandwidth (unitless)} = \frac{\text{Bandwidth (MHz)}}{\text{Operating frequency (MHz)}}$$

$$\text{Frequency (MHz)} = \frac{1}{\text{Period } (\mu s)}$$

$$\text{Half value layer (cm)} = \frac{3}{\text{Attenuation coefficient (dB/cm)}}$$

Impedance (rayls) = Medium density (kg/m³) × Pr opagation speed (m/s)

$$\text{Intensity (mW/cm}^2) = \frac{\text{Power (mW)}}{\text{Area (cm}^2)}$$

$$\text{Intensity reflection coefficient (IRC)} = \frac{[Z_2 - Z_1]^2}{[Z_2 + Z_1]} = \frac{\text{Reflected intensity (W/cm}^2)}{\text{Incident intensity (W/cm}^2)}$$

$$\text{Period } (\mu s) = \frac{1}{\text{Frequency (MHz)}}$$

$$\text{Pulse repetition period (ms)} = \frac{1}{\text{Pulse repetition frequency (kHz)}}$$

Range equation:

$$\text{Distance (mm)} = \frac{1}{2}[\text{Propagation speed (mm/}\mu s) \times \text{Round-trip time } (\mu s)]$$

$$\text{Distance (cm)} = \frac{\text{Round-trip time } (\mu s)}{13 \, (\mu s/cm)}$$

Spatial pulse length (mm) = Number of cycles in a pulse × Wavelength (cm)

$$\text{Wavelength (mm)} = \frac{\text{Propagation speed (mm/}\mu s)}{\text{Frequency (MHZ)}}$$

PHYSICS PRINCIPLES REVIEW

1. In soft tissue, if the frequency of a wave increases, the propagation speed will:
   a. double
   b. increase
   c. decrease
   d. quadruple
   e. remain the same

2. The range of frequencies found within a pulse describes which of the following terms?
   a. duty factor
   b. bandwidth
   c. harmonics
   d. compression
   e. pulse repetition frequency

3. In gray-scale imaging, how many cycles per pulse are generally used?
   a. 2-3
   b. 4-5
   c. 5-10
   d. 10-15
   e. 10-30

4. Which of the following frequencies is within the audible range?
   a. 15 Hz
   b. 15 kHz
   c. 25 kHz
   d. 5.0 MHz
   e. 25,000 Hz

5. Propagation speed through a medium is determined by the:
   a. pulse repetition period
   b. intensity and amplitude of the wave
   c. density and stiffness of the medium
   d. impedance difference between the media
   e. compressions and rarefactions in the sound beam

6. Which of the following is an acoustic variable?
   a. power
   b. intensity
   c. wavelength
   d. particle motion
   e. propagation speed

7. In soft tissue, a 7.5-MHz transducer with a two-cycle pulse will generate a spatial pulse length of:
   a. 0.2 mm
   b. 0.4 mm
   c. 0.8 mm
   d. 1.5 mm
   e. 0.02 mm

8. If the stiffness of a medium increases, the propagation speed will:
   a. double
   b. increase
   c. decrease
   d. quadruple
   e. remain the same

9. The length of a pulse from beginning to end is termed the:
   a. wavelength
   b. frequency
   c. pulse duration
   d. spatial pulse length
   e. pulse repetition period

10. In which of the following media does sound propagate the fastest?
    a. air
    b. fat
    c. bone
    d. muscle
    e. soft tissue

11. What is the frequency of a sound wave in soft tissue demonstrating a wavelength of 0.1 mm?
    a. 2.0 MHz
    b. 5.0 MHz
    c. 7.5 MHz
    d. 10.0 MHz
    e. 15.0 MHz

12. If the amplitude of a wave doubles, the intensity will:
    a. double
    b. quadruple
    c. remain the same
    d. decrease by one half
    e. decrease by one quarter

13. The time for one pulse to occur defines:
    a. bandwidth
    b. duty factor
    c. pulse duration
    d. spatial pulse length
    e. pulse repetition period

14. Which of the following is associated with a broader bandwidth?
    a. a lower Q-factor
    b. an increase in amplitude
    c. a longer spatial pulse length
    d. an increase in echo scattering
    e. a decrease in the number of frequencies within the pulse

15. Regions of low density in a compression wave are termed:
    a. cycles
    b. bandwidth
    c. frequencies
    d. rarefactions
    e. compressions

16. Which of the following formulas calculates the duty factor?
    a. power of the source divided by the area
    b. pulse duration divided by the pulse repetition period
    c. pulse repetition frequency divided by the pulse duration
    d. frequency of the source multiplied by the propagation speed
    e. number of cycles in a pulse multiplied by the wavelength of the pulse

17. Resistance to the propagation of sound through a medium defines:
    a. speckle
    b. reflection
    c. attenuation
    d. acoustic impedance
    e. Rayleigh's scatter

18. How long will it take sound to travel 5 cm round-trip in soft tissue?
    a. 26 μs
    b. 30 μs
    c. 45 μs
    d. 65 μs
    e. 75 μs

19. Overall compensation gain is set at 36 dB. If the gain is reduced by one half, the new gain setting will be:
    a. 15 dB
    b. 18 dB
    c. 25 dB
    d. 30 dB
    e. 33 dB

20. Attenuation occurring as sound propagates through each centimeter of soft tissue is equal to:
    a. ½ operating frequency
    b. attenuation coefficient × path length
    c. medium density × propagation speed
    d. ½ (propagation speed × round-trip time)
    e. number of cycles in a pulse × path length

21. *Spatial* is a term used to describe:
    a. time
    b. speed
    c. space
    d. density
    e. distance

22. Which of the following units measures the attenuation of sound in soft tissue?
    a. μs
    b. dB
    c. rayls
    d. dB/cm
    e. mW/cm^2

23. If the frequency is increased, pulse duration will:
    a. double
    b. increase
    c. decrease
    d. remain unchanged
    e. decrease by one half

24. Which of the following metric prefixes denotes 1 billion?
    a. deca
    b. mega
    c. kilo
    d. giga
    e. hecto

25. Which of the following units of measurement represents the number of pulses occurring in 1 second?
    a. μs
    b. kHz
    c. mW
    d. W/cm^2
    e. dB/cm^2

26. Which of the following formulas determines the impedance of a medium?
    a. attenuation multiplied by the propagation speed of the medium
    b. propagation speed of the medium multiplied by the round-trip time
    c. density of the medium multiplied by the attenuation coefficient
    d. number of pulses in a cycle multiplied by the operating frequency
    e. density of the medium multiplied by the propagation speed of the medium

27. Weakening of a sound wave as it travels through a medium defines:
    a. scattering
    b. reflection
    c. harmonics
    d. attenuation
    e. acoustic impedance

28. Which of the following occurs when a sound wave strikes a large, smooth surface at a 90° angle?
    a. refraction
    b. reverberation
    c. specular reflection
    d. Rayleigh's scatter
    e. nonspecular reflection

29. With perpendicular incidence, what percentage of the incident beam continues to the next medium?
    a. 33%
    b. 50%
    c. 85%
    d. 99%
    e. 100%

30. The unit of measurement used to describe the amplitude of a pressure wave is:
    a. rayl
    b. watt
    c. meter
    d. joule
    e. variable

31. Which of the following properties is proportional to the pulse repetition frequency?
    a. period
    b. duty factor
    c. penetration depth
    d. spatial pulse length
    e. pulse repetition period

32. Which of the following will most likely decrease the propagation speed of a wave?
    a. increasing the penetration depth
    b. increasing the stiffness of the medium
    c. decreasing the transducer frequency
    d. increasing the density of the medium
    e. increasing the pulse repetition frequency

33. For short pulses, the quality (Q) factor is equal to:
    a. the distance of one pulse
    b. one half of the frequency
    c. the number of cycles in a pulse
    d. the intensity of the sound beam
    e. the propagation speed of the medium

34. The positive half of a pressure wave corresponds to:
    a. amplitude
    b. intensity
    c. rarefaction
    d. attenuation
    e. compression

35. In perpendicular incidence, what percentage of the sound wave will reflect at a boundary if the impedance of medium 1 is 40 rayls and the impedance medium 2 is 50 rayls?
    a. 1%
    b. 10%
    c. 45%
    d. 75%
    e. 99%

36. Bending of a transmitting sound beam once it passes through one medium to another describes:
    a. reflection
    b. scattering
    c. refraction
    d. harmonics
    e. reverberation

37. Attenuation is most commonly a result of:
    a. reflection
    b. scattering
    c. impedance
    d. absorption
    e. transmission

38. Half-value layer is equal to an intensity reduction of:
    a. 3 dB
    b. 6 dB
    c. 10 dB
    d. 25 dB
    e. 50 dB

39. *Homogeneous* is a term used to describe which of the following echo textures?
    a. dense
    b. variable
    c. uniform
    d. striated
    e. irregular

40. Which of the following is proportional to the impedance of a medium?
    a. frequency
    b. wavelength
    c. propagation speed
    d. stiffness of the medium
    e. attenuation coefficient

41. Which of the following units compares the ratio of amplitudes along two points of a sound wave?
    a. W
    b. dB
    c. rayl
    d. kg/m^2
    e. dB/cm

42. Attenuation of the sound beam is proportional to the:
    a. frequency of the sound wave
    b. direction of the incident beam
    c. propagation speed of the medium
    d. reflected intensity of the sound wave
    e. transmitted intensity of the sound wave

43. Which of the following is responsible for determining the amount of reflection and transmission of the sound wave?
    a. density
    b. stiffness
    c. attenuation
    d. impedance
    e. propagation speed

44. Attenuation of the sound wave is a result of all of the following EXCEPT:
    a. heat
    b. reflection
    c. scattering
    d. absorption
    e. transmission

45. At what depth will a 3.0-MHz frequency demonstrate an attenuation of 9 dB?
    a. 2 cm
    b. 3 cm
    c. 6 cm
    d. 9 cm
    e. 12 cm

46. Snell's law determines the amount of:
    a. reflection at an interface
    b. intensity at the spatial peak
    c. refraction at an interface
    d. transmission through a medium
    e. scattering distal to a dense medium

47. Direction of the incident beam with respect to the media boundary is termed the:
    a. specular angle
    b. reflection angle
    c. attenuation angle
    d. propagating angle
    e. transmission angle

48. Demonstration of boundaries between organs is a result of:
    a. refraction
    b. transmission
    c. specular reflection
    d. Rayleigh scattering
    e. harmonic frequencies

49. What is the penetration depth of a 3.5-MHz frequency when imaging the abdominal aorta?
    a. 0.86 cm
    b. 1.71 cm
    c. 3.42 cm
    d. 0.86 mm
    e. 1.75 mm

50. With perpendicular incidence, the larger the impedance difference between the media, the greater the:
    a. refraction
    b. scattering
    c. reflection
    d. absorption
    e. transmission

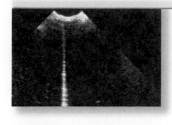

CHAPTER 3

Ultrasound Transducers

KEY TERMS

angle of divergence   refers to the widening of the sound beam in the far field.

aperture   size of the transducer element(s).

apodization   nonuniform driving (excitation) of elements in an array to reduce grating lobes.

array   collection of active elements connected to individual electronic currents in one transducer assembly.

axial resolution   the ability to distinguish two structures along a path parallel to the sound beam.

channels   multiple transducer elements with individual wiring and system electronics.

constructive interference   occurs when two waves in phase with each other create a new wave with an amplitude greater than the original two waves.

convex array   curved linear transducer containing multiple piezoelectric elements.

crystal   piezoelectric element.

Curie point   temperature to which a material is raised, while in the presence of a strong electrical field, to yield piezoelectric properties. If the temperature exceeds the Curie point, the piezoelectric properties will be lost.

damping   material attached to the rear of the transducer element to reduce the pulse duration.

destructive interference   occurs when two waves out of phase with each other create a new wave with an amplitude less than the two original waves.

detail resolution   includes both axial and lateral resolution.

diffraction   deviation in the direction of the sound wave that is NOT a result of reflection, scattering, or refraction.

dynamic aperture   aperture that increases as the focal length increases; minimizes change in the width of the sound beam.

dynamic focusing   a variable receiving focus that follows the changing position of the pulse as it propagates through tissue; the electrical output of the elements can be timed to "listen" in a particular direction and depth.

element   the piezoelectric component of the transducer assembly.

elevation resolution   detail resolution located perpendicular to the scan plane; it is equal to the section thickness and is the source of the section thickness artifact.

far zone   region of the sound beam in which the diameter increases as the distance from the transducer increases.

focal length   distance from a focused transducer to the center of the focal zone; distance from a focused transducer to the spatial peak intensity.

focal point   concentration of the sound beam into a smaller area.

focal zone   area or region of the focus.

Fraunhofer zone   far zone.

Fresnel zone   near zone.

grating lobes   additional weak beams emitted from a multielement transducer that propagate in directions different from the primary beam.

Huygens principle   all points on a wave front or at a source are point sources for the production of spherical secondary wavelets.

interference phenomenon   interference occurring when two waves interact or overlap, resulting in the creation of a new wave.

lateral resolution   the ability to distinguish two structures lying perpendicular to the sound path.

lead zirconate titanate (PZT)   a ceramic piezoelectric material.

matching layer   material attached to the front face of the transducer element to reduce reflections at the transducer surface.

near zone   region of the beam between the transducer and focal point, which decreases in size as it approaches the focus.

operating frequency   natural frequency of the transducer; it is determined by the propagation speed and thickness of the element in pulse ultrasound and by the electrical frequency in continuous wave.

piezoelectricity   conversion of pressure to electric voltage.

phased   applying voltage pulses to all elements in the assembly as a group, but with minor time differences. Phased pulses allow multiple focal zones, beam steering, and beam focusing.

resonance frequency   operating frequency.

sequenced array   operated by applying voltage pulses to a group of elements in succession.

side lobes   additional weak beams traveling from a single-element transducer in directions different from the primary beam.

subdicing   dividing each element into small pieces to reduce grating lobes.

transducer   a device that converts energy from one form to another.

transducer assembly   transducer element, damping, matching layers, and housing; also known as probe, scan head, or transducer.

DIAGNOSTIC ULTRASOUND TRANSDUCERS

- Convert electrical energy into acoustic energy during transmission and acoustic energy into electrical energy for reception.
- Operate on the principle of piezoelectricity.
- Driven typically by one cycle of alternating voltage.
- Diagnostic frequencies range between 2.0 and 15 MHz.

PIEZOELECTRICITY (PIEZOELECTRIC EFFECT)

- Piezoelectric principle states that some materials produce a voltage when deformed by an applied pressure.
- Various forms of ceramics and quartz are naturally piezoelectric.
- Lead zirconate titanate (PZT) is the most common manufactured piezoelectric element.
- PZT placed in a strong electric field while at a high temperature acts as an element with piezoelectric properties **(Curie point).**
- If the material exceeds the Curie point, the element will lose its piezoelectric properties (i.e., autoclave sterilization).

Transducer Assembly

COMPONENT	FUNCTION	DESCRIPTION	RELATIONSHIP
Piezoelectric element, also called • Crystal • Active element • Transducer element	• Converts electrical voltage into ultrasound pulses and the returning echoes back to electric voltage • Electrical energy is applied to the element, increasing or decreasing the thickness according to the polarity of the voltage	• **Thickness** of the element ranges between 0.2 and 1.0 mm • **Propagation speed** of the element ranges between 4 and 6 mm/μs • **Natural materials:** Rochelle salt, quartz, and tourmaline • **Manufactured materials:** Lead zirconate titanate (PZT), barium titanate, lead metaniobate, and polyvinylidene diflouride • Single elements are in the form of a disk • Array transducers contain numerous elements with separate electrical wiring • Contain a bandwidth of frequencies • Impedance is much greater than soft tissue	• Propagation speed of the element is **directly** related to the operating frequency • Thickness of the element is **inversely** related to the operating frequency • Thickness is equal to half of the wavelength • Impedance is 20× greater than that of the skin
Damping, also called • Backing	• Reduces the number of cycles in each pulse • Reduces pulse duration and spatial pulse length	• Attached to the rear face of the element • Made of metal powder and a plastic or epoxy	• **Increases** the bandwidth and axial resolution • **Reduces** sensitivity and Q-Factor Impedance is similar to that of the element
Matching layers	• Reduce the impedance difference between the element and skin • Improve sound transmission across the element–tissue boundary	• Typically two layers are used • Aqueous gel is a matching layer between the transducer face and the skin	• **Increases** the transmission of sound into the body • Thickness equal to one fourth of the wavelength • Impedance of matching layer is in between those of the element and the skin
Transducer housing	• Protects the components of the transducer • Protects the operator and patient from electrical shock • Prevents the transducer from outside interference	• Covering for transducer components • Made of metal or plastic	• Damage to the housing can increase risk of electrical shock and decrease image quality

TYPES OF TRANSDUCERS

CONTINUOUS WAVE

- Produce a continuous wave of sound.
- Are composed of a separate transmit and receiver elements housed in a single transducer assembly.
- Frequency of the sound wave is determined by the electrical frequency of the ultrasound system.
- Demonstrate a narrow bandwidth.

PULSE WAVE

- Transmit pulses of sound and receive returning echoes.
- Classified by the thickness and propagation speed of the element.
- Demonstrate a wide bandwidth and short pulse length.
- Linear, convex, and annular are types of transducer **construction.**
- Sequenced, phased, and vector are types of transducer **operation.**
- Produce a 2- to 3-cycle pulse for gray-scale imaging and 5- to 30-cycle pulse for Doppler techniques.
- Minor or secondary beams traveling in directions different from the primary beam are termed side or grating lobes.
- Frequency of the sound pulse is equal to the operating frequency.

Operating frequency (MHz) =
Propagation speed of the element (mm/μs) × Element thickness (mm)

Pulse Wave Transducers

TYPE	DESCRIPTION	FOCUSING	BEAM STEERING
Annular array	• Multiple elements arranged in rings with a common center • Smaller rings have a shallow focus • Larger rings have a deep focal length • Produces a sector-type image	• Electronic	• Mechanical
Convex sequenced array	• Multiple elements arranged in a curved line • Operated by applying voltage pulses to groups of elements in succession • Pulses travel in different directions, producing a sector-shaped image • Also called: curved array, convex array, curvilinear array	• Electronic	• Electronic
Linear sequenced array	• Straight line of rectangular elements about one wavelength wide • Operated by applying voltage pulses to groups of elements in succession • Pulses travel in straight parallel lines producing a rectangular image. • Also called: linear array	• Electronic	• Electronic
Linear phased array	• Contains a compact line of elements about one-quarter-wavelength wide • Operated by applying voltage pulses to most or all of the elements using minor time differences • Resulting pulses can be shaped and steered • Received echoes follow the changing position of the pulse • Permits multiple focal zones	• Electronic	• Electronic
Mechanical	• Uses a single element with a fixed focal depth • Produces a sector image	• Mechanical	• Fixed
Sector	• Each pulse originates from the same starting point	• Electronic	• Electronic
Vector array	• Emits pulses from different starting points and in different directions • Combines linear sequential and linear phased array technologies • Converts the format of a linear array into a trapezoidal image	• Electronic	• Electronic

UNFOCUSED SOUND BEAM (Figs. 3-1 and 3-2)

- Some beam narrowing will occur.
- The near-zone length is equal to one-half of the beam diameter.
- Two near-zone lengths is equal to the transducer diameter.

Beam Focus Characteristics

CHARACTERISTIC	DESCRIPTION
Far field	• Region distal to the focal point where the sound beam diverges • Intensity of the beam is more uniform • Inversely related to the operating frequency and diameter of the element (increasing the frequency decreases the angle of divergence) • Also called Fraunhofer zone, far zone
Focal length	• Also called near-zone length • Distance from the transducer to the narrowest portion of the beam • Determined by the operating frequency and the diameter of the element • FL (mm) = [crystal diameter (mm^2)] × frequency (MHz) • $\text{FL (mm)} = \dfrac{(\text{crystal diameter})^2}{4 \times \text{wavelength}}$ • Directly related to the operating frequency and diameter of the element • Inversely related to the divergence of the beam in the far field
Focal point	• Narrowest portion of the beam • Width at the focal point is equal to half of the transducer width • Area of maximum intensity in the beam • Also called focus
Focal zone	• Region or area of focus • One half of the focal zone is located in the near field, and the other half is located in the far field • Also called focal area, focal region
Near field	• Region between the transducer and focus • Conical in shape • Intensity variations are the greatest • Length of the near field is directly related to the frequency of the transducer and diameter of the element • Additional focusing can be added in this region • Also called Fresnel zone, near zone

FOCUSING OF THE SOUND BEAM (Fig. 3-3)

- Improves lateral resolution.
- Only accomplished within the near field.
- Creates a narrower sound beam over a specified area.
- Beam diameter in the near field decreases in size toward the focal point.
- Beam diameter in the far field (angle of divergence) increases in size after the focal point.
- Increasing the frequency or diameter of the element will produce a narrower beam, longer focal length, and less divergence in the far field.

TYPES OF FOCUSING

Acoustic Mirrors

- Predetermined focus.
- The sound beam is directed toward a curved acoustic mirror, which reflects the beam into the body.

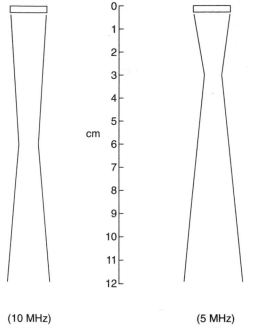

(10 MHz)   (5 MHz)

FIG. 3-1 Beams for disk transducers have a diameter of 6 mm at two frequencies. Higher frequencies produce smaller beam diameters (at a distance greater than 4 cm in this case) and longer near-zone lengths.

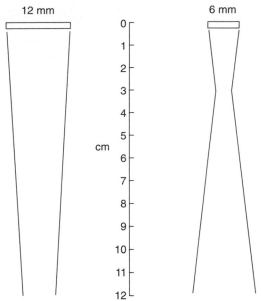

FIG. 3-2 Beams for 5-MHz disk transducers of two diameters. The larger transducer *(left)* produces the longer near-zone length. A smaller transducer *(right)* can produce a larger-diameter beam in the far zone. In this example, the beam diameters are equal at a distance of 8 cm.

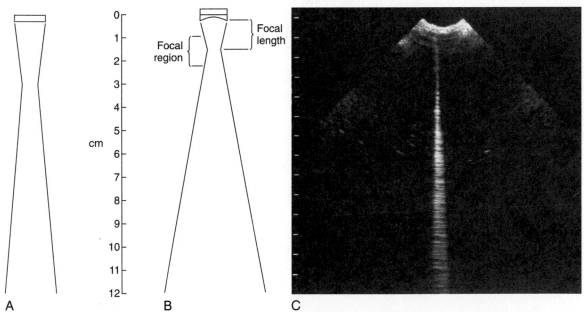

A   B   C

FIG. 3-3 Beam diameter for a 6-mm, 5-MHz transducer without **(A)** and with **(B)** focusing. Focusing reduces the minimum beam width compared with that produced without focusing. However, well beyond the focal region, the width of the focused beam is greater than that of the unfocused beam. **C,** A focused beam. This is an ultrasound image of a beam profile test object containing a thin vertical scattering layer down the center. Scanning this object generates a picture of the beam (the pulse width at all depths). In this case, the focus occurs at a depth of about 4 cm (this image has a total depth of 15 cm). Depth markers (in 1-cm increments) are indicated on the left edge of the figure.

Electronic

- Operator controlled.
- Allows multiple focal zones.
- Utilizes the interference phenomenon to focus the sound beam.
- Pulses are delayed to each element, causing the wavelets to join at variable focal points.
- Applied to individual beams to improve slice thickness and lateral resolution.
- Improves spatial resolution within the focal point.

External

- Predetermined focal range.
- An acoustic lens is placed in front of the crystal to focus the sound beam.

Internal

- Predetermined focal range.
- Piezoelectric element(s) are shaped concavely to focus the sound beam.
- Beam diameter is reduced in the focal point.

STEERING OF THE SOUND BEAM (Fig. 3-4)

- Created by the beam former.
- Electronic steering is operator adjustable.
- Used to sweep the sound wave over a specific area.
- System alters the electronic excitation of the elements, steering the beam in various directions.
- The returning echoes are also delayed.

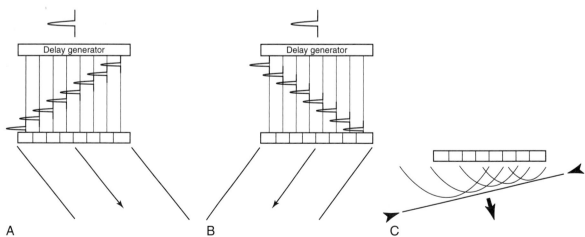

FIG. 3-4 A linear phased array (side view). **A,** When voltage pulses are applied in rapid progression from left to right, one ultrasound pulse is produced that is directed to the right. **B,** Similarly, when voltage pulses are applied in rapid progression from right to left, one ultrasound pulse is produced that is directed to the left. **C,** The delays in **A** produce a pulse whose combined pressure wavefront (arrowheads) is angled from the lower left to the upper right. A wave always travels perpendicular to its wavefront, as indicated by the arrow.

RESOLUTION

- The ability to distinguish two adjacent reflectors as two separate structures.

Types of Resolution

RESOLUTION	DESCRIPTION	DETERMINED BY	RELATIONSHIP
Axial Also called • **Longitudinal** • **Range** • **Depth** • **Spatial**	• Ability to distinguish two structures in a path parallel to the sound beam • Does not vary with distance • Always better than lateral resolution • Diagnostic values: 0.05-0.5 mm	• Transducer • Medium	• Equal to ½ SPL • **Directly** related to the operating frequency • **Inversely** related to the spatial pulse length and penetration depth • Smaller is better
Contrast	• Ability to differentiate similar and dissimilar tissues	• Ultrasound system	• **Directly** related to axial and lateral resolution
Elevation Also called • **Z-axis** • **Slice or section thickness**	• Thickness of the scanned tissue perpendicular to the scan plane	• Transducer	• Related to the beam width • Thinner the slice thickness, the better the image quality
Lateral Also called • **Angular** • **Transverse** • **Azimuthal**	• Ability to distinguish two structures in a path perpendicular to the sound beam • Varies with distance • Improves with focusing	• Beam width	• Equal to beam diameter • **Directly** related to beam diameter, frequency, focusing, and distance
Temporal	• Ability to separate two points in time	• Frame rate	• **Directly** related to the frame rate

TRANSDUCER CARE

- Do not heat-sterilize.
- Do not drop transducer or run over transducer cables.
- Use cleaning agents recommended by the transducer manufacturer.
- Routinely check for damage to the transducer assembly.

Chapter Formulas

$$\text{Axial resolution (mm)} = \frac{1}{2}[\text{Spatial pulse length (mm)}]$$

$$\text{Axial resolution (mm)} = 0.77 \times \text{no. of cycles in a pulse in soft tissue frequency (MHz)}$$

$$\text{Focus diameter (mm)} = \frac{1}{2}\text{Transducer diameter}$$

$$\text{Lateral resolution (mm)} = \text{Beam diameter (mm)}$$

$$\text{Near-zone length (mm)} = \frac{[\text{Crystal diameter (mm)}]^2 \times \text{Frequency (MHz)}}{6}$$

$$\text{Near-zone length (mm)} = \frac{[\text{Crystal diameter (mm)}]^2}{4 \times \text{Wavelength (mm)}}$$

$$\text{Operating frequency (MHz)} = \frac{\text{Propagation speed of the element (mm/}\mu\text{s)}}{2 \times \text{Element thickness (mm)}}$$

TRANSDUCER REVIEW

1. Widening of the sound beam is demonstrated in the:
   a. focal point
   b. focal zone
   c. Fresnel zone
   d. focal length
   e. Fraunhofer zone

2. Weak beams emitted from a linear sequenced array transducer are termed:
   a. side lobes
   b. transverse waves
   c. grating lobes
   d. Huygens waves
   e. mechanical waves

3. The resonant frequency of a pulse wave is determined by the:
   a. diameter of the beam
   b. impedance of the matching layer
   c. output power of the ultrasound system
   d. electrical frequency of the ultrasound system
   e. thickness and propagation speed of the element

4. Heat sterilization is not recommended for diagnostic transducers because:
   a. apodization will occur
   b. the housing may be damaged
   c. the epoxy in the backing will melt
   d. the piezoelectric properties will be lost
   e. moisture will cause the electrical wiring to short

5. Which of the following components is unnecessary in the construction of a continuous wave transducer?
   a. matching layer
   b. damping layer
   c. electrical wiring
   d. exterior housing
   e. two active elements

6. Lateral resolution is determined by the:
   a. beam width
   b. near-zone length
   c. spatial pulse length
   d. thickness of the active element
   e. propagation speed of the medium

7. What is the axial resolution in soft tissue when using a 5.0-MHz frequency with a two-cycle pulse, and an element thickness of 0.5 mm?
   a. 0.3 mm
   b. 0.5 mm
   c. 0.6 mm
   d. 0.8 mm
   e. 1.0 mm

8. What is the operating frequency of a two-cycle pulse with an element thickness of 0.2 mm and a propagation speed of 4 mm/μs?
   a. 1.0 MHz
   b. 3.5 MHz
   c. 5.0 MHz
   d. 7.5 MHz
   e. 10.0 MHz

9. On which of the following principles do diagnostic ultrasound transducers operate?
   a. Snell's law
   b. ALARA principle
   c. Huygens principle
   d. piezoelectric effect
   e. phased array technology

10. If the width of the transducer is 5.0 cm, what is the width at the focal point?
    a. 1.0 cm
    b. 2.5 cm
    c. 5.0 cm
    d. 7.5 cm
    e. 10.0 cm

11. Constructive interference will create a wave with amplitude:
    a. equal to the original waves
    b. less than the original waves
    c. shorter than the original waves
    d. longer than the original waves
    e. greater than the original waves

12. Reducing the impedance difference between the crystal and the skin is the primary function of which of the following transducer components?
    a. aqueous gel
    b. beam former
    c. damping layer
    d. matching layer
    e. backing layer

13. A sound beam demonstrates the most uniform intensity in the:
    a. far field
    b. near field
    c. focal zone
    d. focal length
    e. Fresnel zone

14. What is the near-zone length of a 6-mm, 5-MHz transducer?
    a. 5 mm
    b. 10 mm
    c. 15 mm
    d. 30 mm
    e. 50 mm

15. All of the following are examples of proper transducer care EXCEPT:
    a. Do not use heat sterilization.
    b. Do not drop transducer assembly.
    c. Routinely check the transducer assembly for damage.
    d. Take care not to damage transducer cables when moving the system.
    e. Use cleaning agents recommended by the infectious control department.

16. The near-zone length of a 3-mm, 10-MHz transducer is:
    a. 3 mm
    b. 5 mm
    c. 7 mm
    d. 10 mm
    e. 15 mm

17. Which of the following transducer elements has the longest focal length?
    a. 2 mm, 2.5 MHz
    b. 7 mm, 2.5 MHz
    c. 2 mm, 7.5 MHz
    d. 5 mm, 10.0 MHz
    e. 3 mm, 15.0 MHz

18. The distance from the face of a focused transducer to the point of spatial peak intensity is termed the:
    a. focal region
    b. pulse duration
    c. focal length
    d. spatial pulse length
    e. pulse repetition frequency

19. The narrowest diameter of a sound beam is termed the focal:
    a. zone
    b. area
    c. point
    d. length
    e. region

20. Which of the following best describes apodization?
    a. focusing of the sound beam
    b. widening of the sound beam in the near zone
    c. scattering of the sound beam distal to the focal point
    d. irregular excitation of the elements in an array to reduce grating lobes
    e. creation of a new sound wave with a greater amplitude than the original wave

21. Which of the following determines the diameter of the focus?
    a. spatial pulse length
    b. thickness of the element
    c. diameter of the transducer
    d. propagation speed of the medium
    e. propagation speed of the element

22. The impedance of the damping layer is:
    a. unknown
    b. less than the element's
    c. similar to the element's
    d. greater than the element's
    e. twice that of the element's

23. The purpose of backing material in the transducer assembly is to:
    a. decrease the bandwidth
    b. increase the pulse duration
    c. increase the spatial pulse length
    d. protect the components from moisture
    e. reduce the number of cycles in a pulse

24. Vector array is a type of transducer:
    a. assembly
    b. operation
    c. frequency
    d. construction
    e. composition

25. Focusing of the sound beam is directly related to:
    a. axial resolution
    b. lateral resolution
    c. contrast resolution
    d. temporal resolution
    e. elevation resolution

26. Steering of the sound beam is accomplished by:
    a. constructive interference
    b. focusing of the sound beam
    c. increasing the resonant frequency
    d. using the harmonic frequencies
    e. altering the excitation of the active elements

27. Exceeding the Curie point of a transducer element will result in:
    a. a thinner element
    b. a broader bandwidth
    c. a higher propagation speed
    d. a higher operating frequency
    e. the loss of all piezoelectric properties

28. An active element with a thickness of 0.8 mm and a propagation speed of 4 mm/µs will have an operating frequency of:
    a. 2.5 MHz
    b. 3.5 MHz
    c. 4.0 MHz
    d. 5.0 MHz
    e. 7.5 MHz

29. What is the thickness of the crystal with an operating frequency of 5.0 MHz and a propagation speed of 4 mm/µs?
    a. 0.1 mm
    b. 0.2 mm
    c. 0.3 mm
    d. 0.4 mm
    e. 0.5 mm

30. Temporal resolution is determined by the:
    a. medium
    b. frame rate
    c. beam width
    d. element thickness
    e. operating frequency

31. What is the axial resolution in soft tissue when using a 15-MHz frequency with a two-cycle pulse?
    a. 1 mm
    b. 3 mm
    c. 4 mm
    d. 5 mm
    e. 6 mm

32. Which of the following transducers operates by applying voltage pulses to groups of linear elements in succession?
    a. vector array
    b. annular array
    c. linear phased array
    d. convex phased array
    e. linear sequenced array

33. Focusing of the sound beam is only accomplished within the:
    a. far field
    b. focal area
    c. focal zone
    d. near field
    e. focal region

34. What is the diameter of the sound beam at one near-zone length when using a 6-mm, 2.5-MHz transducer?
    a. 3 mm
    b. 6 mm
    c. 9 mm
    d. 12 mm
    e. 15 mm

35. The ability to distinguish two structures in a path perpendicular to the sound beam describes:
    a. the z-axis
    b. spatial resolution
    c. contrast resolution
    d. temporal resolution
    e. azimuthal resolution

36. The most common piezoelectric material used in diagnostic ultrasound transducers is:
    a. quartz
    b. tourmaline
    c. barium titanate
    d. lead metaniobate
    e. lead zirconate titanate

37. Subdicing the elements in diagnostic ultrasound transducers is used to:
    a. reduce grating lobes
    b. narrow the bandwidth
    c. increase temporal resolution
    d. decrease operating frequency
    e. increase the near-zone length

38. Diagnostic frequencies range between:
    a. 1.0 and 10.0 MHz
    b. 2.0 and 12.0 MHz
    c. 2.0 and 15.0 MHz
    d. 3.5 and 10.0 MHz
    e. 3.5 and 12.0 MHz

39. Detail resolution includes both:
    a. spatial and lateral resolution
    b. elevation and axial resolution
    c. lateral and contrast resolution
    d. temporal and spatial resolution
    e. contrast and temporal resolution

40. During transmission, diagnostic ultrasound transducers convert:
    a. kinetic energy into thermal energy
    b. acoustic energy into electrical energy
    c. electrical energy into thermal energy
    d. electrical energy into acoustic energy
    e. kinetic energy into acoustic energy

41. Which of the following states, "Some materials produce a voltage when distorted by an applied pressure"?
    a. Snell's law
    b. ALARA principle
    c. Huygens principle
    d. Ohm's acoustic law
    e. piezoelectric principle

42. Which of the following is a negative effect of using a damping material in the transducer assembly?
    a. low quality factor
    b. reduced sensitivity
    c. narrow bandwidth
    d. increase pulse duration
    e. reduced contrast resolution

43. How many cycles per pulse are typically used in Doppler imaging?
    a. 2-20
    b. 3-15
    c. 5-30
    d. 6-40
    e. 10-20

44. The sonographer can determine the depth of the focal zone when using a transducer with a(n):
    a. internal focus
    b. external focus
    c. electronic focus
    d. acoustic mirror
    e. mechanical focus

45. The impedance of the matching layer is:
    a. less than the impedance of the skin
    b. greater than the impedance of the crystal
    c. equal to the impedance of the skin
    d. less than the impedance of the crystal
    e. equal to the impedance of the crystal

46. Which of the following transducers displays a trapezoidal image?
    a. convex array
    b. vector array
    c. annular array
    d. curvilinear array
    e. linear phased array

47. Which of the following differentiates similar or dissimilar tissues?
    a. axial resolution
    b. lateral resolution
    c. contrast resolution
    d. temporal resolution
    e. elevation resolution

48. Section thickness is related to the:
    a. frame rate
    b. beam width
    c. penetration depth
    d. operating frequency
    e. propagation speed of the medium

49. Operating frequency of a transducer is directly related to the:
    a. thickness of the element
    b. diameter of the element
    c. impedance of the element
    d. attenuation of the element
    e. propagation speed of the element

50. A focused 10-mm, 15-MHz transducer will demonstrate a focal diameter of:
    a. 2.5 mm
    b. 3.0 mm
    c. 5.0 mm
    d. 7.5 mm
    e. 10.0 mm

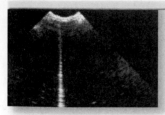

CHAPTER 4

Pulse-Echo Instrumentation

KEY TERMS

artifact   anything not properly indicative of anatomy or motion imaged.

binary number   group of bits.

bit   binary digit; smallest amount of computer memory.

byte   group of eight bits of computer memory.

cathode ray tube (CRT)   imaging display where the strength of the electron beam determines the brightness.

channel   an independent signal path consisting of a transducer element, delay, and other electronic components.

cine loop   storage of the last several real-time frames.

code excitation   a series of pulses and gaps allowing multiple focal zones and harmonic frequencies.

comet tail   a series of closely spaced reverberation echoes behind a strong reflector.

dynamic range   the ratio of the largest to the smallest amplitude the ultrasound system can handle.

edge shadowing   loss in intensity from bending of the sound beam at a curved surface.

enhancement   the increase in reflection amplitude from structures that lie behind a weakly attenuating structure.

field of view   displayed image of the returning echoes.

frame   a complete scan of the ultrasound beam; individual image composed of multiple scan lines.

frame rate   the number of complete scans (images) displayed per second.

freeze frame   holding and displaying one frame of the real-time sequence.

gain   ratio of amplifier output to input of electric power.

grating lobes   secondary sound beams produced by a multi-element transducer.

line density   number of scan lines per frame; scan line density.

matrix   denotes the rows and columns of pixels in a digital image.

memory   storage of echo information.

mirror image   an artifactual gray-scale, color-flow, or Doppler signal appearing on the opposite side of a strong reflector.

multipath   the path toward and away from a reflector are different.

noise   disturbance that reduces the clarity of the signal.

Nyquist limit   the minimum number of samples required to avoid aliasing; Doppler shift frequency above which aliasing occurs.

panoramic image   an expanded image display beyond the normal limits of the transducer.

pixel   picture element; smallest portion of a digital image.

pixel density   number of picture elements per inch.

pixel interpolation   assigning a brightness value to a missing pixel.

pulse inversion   a harmonic imaging technique using two pulses per scan line where the second pulse is an inverse of the first pulse.

pulse repetition frequency   the number of voltage pulses sent to the transducer each second.

pulse repetition period   time from the beginning of one voltage pulse to the start of the next voltage pulse.

random-access memory (RAM)   allows access of stored data in an unsystematic order.

range ambiguity   produced when echoes are placed too superficially because a second pulse was emitted before all reflections have returned from the first pulse.

read-only memory (ROM)   stored data cannot be modified.

real-time imaging   two-dimensional imaging of the motion of moving structures.

reflection   portion of the sound reflected from the boundary of a medium.

refraction   change of sound direction on passing from one medium to another.

reverberation   multiple reflections between a structure and the transducer or within a structure.

scattering   redirection of sound in several directions on encountering a rough surface.

shadowing   reduction of reflective amplitude from reflectors that lie behind a strongly reflecting or attenuating structure.

signal-to-noise ratio   comparison of meaningful information in an image (signal) to the amount of signal disturbance (noise).

spatial compounding   averaging of frames that view anatomy from different angles.

specular   large, flat, smooth surface.

voxel   the smallest distinguishable part of a three-dimensional image; short for volume pixel.

DISPLAY MODES

A-MODE

- Amplitude mode.
- One-dimensional (1-D) quantitative image using a single sound beam.
- Displays the amplitude of the returning echo vertically (*y*-axis) and distance along the horizontal axis (*x*-axis).

B-MODE

- Brightness mode.
- Creates a 2-D qualitative, cross-sectional image using multiple sound beams.
- Displays the strength of the returning echoes as pixels in various shades of gray.
- The vertical or the *y*-axis represents increasing depth and the horizontal or the *x*-axis represents the medial and lateral or right and left aspects of the body (side to side).
- The stronger the reflection, the brighter the pixel.

M-MODE

- Motion mode
- 1-D quantitative series of B-mode pixels.
- The vertical or the *y*-axis represents the motion of the reflecting echoes and the horizontal or the *x*-axis represents time.

THREE-DIMENSIONAL MODE

- 3-D mode.
- 2-D display of a 3-D volume of echo information.
- Slower acquisition of information.

REAL-TIME IMAGING

- Multiple frames per second make up multiple scan lines per frame.
- Imaging depth determines when the next pulse is transmitted.
- Echo brightness increases with echo amplitude.
- Echo position is determined by the round-trip time of the reflector.

ADVANTAGES

- Rapid location of anatomy.
- Movement can be observed.
- Structures or vessels can be followed.

LIMITATIONS

- Penetration depth is limited by the propagation speed of the medium.
- Exact imaging plane cannot be systematically reproduced.
- Measurement of structures larger than the field of view are estimated.

Real-Time Imaging Parameters

PARAMETER	DESCRIPTION	UNITS	RELATIONSHIP
Contrast resolution	• Ability to distinguish between echoes of slightly different amplitudes • Amount of gray shades prevalent in the image	• None	• High contrast demonstrates fewer shades of gray • Low contrast demonstrates more shades of gray • Dependent on the number of bits per pixel • Related to the frame rate
Detail resolution	• Ability to distinguish detail in the image • Includes axial and lateral resolution	• mm	• Directly related to the number of scan lines • Inversely related to frame rate
Field of view	• Size of the displayed image	• N/A	• Directly related to the pulse repetition frequency (PRF) • Inversely related to frame rate and temporal resolution • Operator-adjustable using depth and region-of-interest settings
Frame rate	• Number of images per second • Typically 30-60 frames/sec are used in real-time imaging • Human eye detects less than 15-20 frames/sec	• Hz • Frames/sec	• Determines temporal resolution • Determined by the propagation speed of the medium and imaging depth • Proportional to the PRF • Inversely proportional to the number of focal zones used, imaging depth, and lines per frame • Operator adjustable using depth and PRF settings
Line density	• Concentration of scan lines within the field of view	• Lines/cm • Lines/degrees	• Directly related to PRF and spatial resolution • Inversely related to the frame rate and temporal resolution
Maximum imaging depth	• Maximum penetration depth for the overall parameters used	• cm	• Dependent on the frame rate, number of lines per frame, and the number of focal zones used • Inversely related to the PRF
Pulse repetition frequency	• Determines the number of scan lines per frame • Equal to the voltage PRF • Typically 2.0-15.0 kHz is used in real-time imaging	• Hz • kHz	• Inversely related to the operating frequency and imaging depth • Indirectly adjusted by the operator using imaging depth setting
Temporal resolution	• Ability to precisely position moving structures • Relates to time and motion	• seconds	• Directly related to the frame rate • Inversely related to the number of focal zones used and imaging depth

Real-Time Imaging Techniques

TYPE	DESCRIPTION
Harmonic frequencies (MHz)	• Even and odd multiples of the fundamental frequency • Generated at a deeper imaging depth reducing reverberation artifact • Generated in the highest intensity and narrowest portion of the beam • Returning harmonic signals are processed separate from the operating signals • Improves lateral resolution • Reduces grating lobes
Multifocal imaging	• Ability to use multiple focal zones during real-time imaging • Directly related to lateral resolution and pulse repetition frequency • Inversely related to the frame rate and temporal resolution
Panoramic imaging	• Expansion of the image display beyond the normal limits of the transducer diameter • Retains previous echo information while adding new echo information parallel to the scanning plane
Pixel interpolation	• Assigns a brightness value to missed pixels • Based on the average brightness of adjacent pixels • Commonly used in sector scanning
Pulse inversion	• A technique in harmonic imaging using two pulses per scan, where the second pulse is the inversion of the first pulse • Allows for a broader bandwidth and shorter pulses • Improves axial resolution • Reduces temporal resolution
Spatial compounding	• Scan lines are directed in multiple directions • Improves visualization of structures beneath a highly attenuating structure • Smoothes specular surfaces • Reduces speckle and noise • Uses phasing to interrogate the structures more than once
Three-dimensional imaging	• Acquired by assembling many parallel 2-D scans into a 3-D volume of echo information • Acquired at rates of up to 30 volumes per second • Obtained by: 1. Manual scanning with transducer position sensors 2. Automated mechanical scanned transducers 3. Electronic scanning with a 2-D element array transducer

PULSE-ECHO INSTRUMENTATION

FUNCTIONS

1. Prepare and transmit electronic signals to the transducer to produce a sound wave.
2. Receive electronic signals from reflections.
3. Process the reflected information for display.

POWER

• Output control.
• Controls the amplitude of transmitted sound beam and the amplitude of the received echoes.
• Ranges from 0 to 500 volts.
• Directly related to the signal-to-noise ratio.
• Directly related to the intensity of acoustic exposure to the patient.
• Acoustic exposure is measured by mechanical index (MI) and thermal index (TI).

TRANSDUCER

- Produces ultrasound pulses for each electrical pulse applied.
- Receives returning echo reflections, producing an electrical voltage.
- Delivers electrical voltages to the memory.
- Generates a small voltage signal (radio frequency) proportional to the amplitude of the returning echo.
- Radio frequency signals are processed by the system.
- Preamplification can occur.

CHANNELS

- Individual signal paths for transmission and reception of the sound beam.
- Number of channels equals the number of transducer elements.
- In ultrasound, typically 64, 128, or 196 channels are used.
- Controlling the characteristics of the sound beam is directly related to the number of channels employed.
- Independent pulse delay and element combination constitutes a transmission channel.
- Each independent element, amplifier, analog-to-digital converter, and delay path constitutes a reception channel.

MASTER SYNCHRONIZER

- Clock that instructs the pulser to send an electrical signal to the transducer.
- Coordinates all the components of the ultrasound system.
- Brain or manager of the ultrasound system.

PULSER (TRANSMITTER)

- Range, 10 to 500 volts.
- Generates the electric pulses to the crystal producing pulsed ultrasound waves.
- Determines the pulse repetition frequency, pulse repetition period, and pulse amplitude.
- Drives the transducer through the pulse delays with one voltage pulse per scan line.
- Adjusts the PRF appropriately for imaging depth.
- Communicates with the receiver the moment the crystal is excited to help determine the distance to the reflector.

DIGITAL BEAM FORMER

- Considered part of the pulser.
- Computer chip is the most common form.
- Determines the firing delay for array systems.
- During reception, establishes time delays used in dynamic focusing.
- Advantages: software programming and extremely stable with a wide range of frequencies.

PULSE DELAYS

- Part of the beam former used to control the beam steering and focusing in phased array scanning.
- Controls the size of the element and apodization in phased array operation.

TRANSMIT AND RECEIVER SWITCH (T/R SWITCH)

- Part of the beam former.
- Directs the driving voltages from the pulser and pulse delays to the transducer during transmission.

- Directs the returning echo voltages from the transducer to the receiver during reception.
- Protects the receiver components from the large driving voltages of the pulse.

SIGNAL PROCESSING

- Determines time of flight (location) and amplitude of the echo reflections.
- Transforms the returning echo reflections into signals suitable for display.

RECEIVER

- Receives, amplifies, and modifies echo information returning from the transducer.
- Five functions of the receiver:
  1. Amplification.
  2. Compensation.
  3. Compression.
  4. Demodulation.
  5. Rejection.

AMPLIFICATION

- Units—dB.
- Increases small electric voltages received from the transducer to a level suitable for processing.
- Operator adjustable using overall gain setting.
- Allows identical amplification no matter the depth.
- Does NOT improve the signal-to-noise ratio.
- Typically 60 to 100 dB of gain is available.

COMPENSATION (Fig. 4-1)

- Units—dB.
- Mechanism that compensates for the loss of echo strength caused by the depth of the reflector.
- Operator adjustable using time-gain compensation or depth-gain compensation settings.
- Provides equal amplitude for all similar structures regardless of depth.
- Compensates for attenuation by boosting amplitudes of deep reflections and suppressing superficial reflections.

FIG. 4-1
Gain compensation curve.

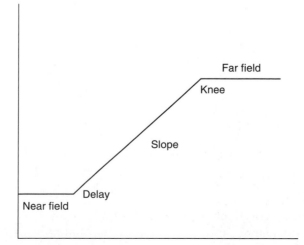

- Near field—area of minimum amplification.
- Delay—depth at which variable compensation begins.
- Slope—available region for depth compensation.
- Knee—deepest region attenuation compensation can occur.
- Far field—area of maximum amplification.

COMPRESSION

- Units—dB.
- Internal process in which larger echoes are equalized with smaller echoes.
- Operator adjustable using the dynamic range or compression settings.
- Changes the gray-scale characteristics of an image without losing the relationship between the largest and smallest amplitudes.
- Ultrasound systems use a compression range of 20 to 40 dB.
- Imaging monitors display a compression range of 10 to 20 dB.

DEMODULATION

- Not operator controlled.
- Process of converting voltages delivered to the receiver to a more useful form for processing.
- Changes the shape of the returning signal to a form the system components can process.
- No visible changes in the image.
- Consists of two components:
  - Rectification.
    - Eliminates the negative half of the signals by turning them into positive voltages.
  - Smoothing.
    - Levels out the rough edges of the signal (envelops).

REJECTION (THRESHOLD, SUPPRESSION)

- Suppression or elimination of smaller-amplitude voltages produced by weak reflections.
- One type is built into the system and another type is operator adjustable.
- Decreases acoustic noise.
- Does not affect intense echoes.

IMAGE STORAGE

SCAN CONVERTER

- Makes gray-scale imaging possible.
- Transfers incoming echo data into a suitable format for display.
- Properly locates each series of echoes in individual scan lines for storage.

Analog Scan Converter

- Found in older ultrasound systems.
- Charges vary the brightness of the display.

Digital Scan Converter

- Stores echo reflection amplitudes as a series of binary numbers.
- Provides stability, uniformity, and accuracy compared to an analog converter.
- Consists of:

Analog-to-Digital Converter

- Changes the voltage of received signals into numeric values.

Digital Memory

- Stores image as binary numbers.

Digital-to-Analog Converter

- Converts binary numbers from memory into analog voltages for CRT display.
- Determines the brightness of the displayed echoes.

MEMORY

- Computer memory stores the echo amplitude and location in a binary (digital) format.
- Memory divides the image into numerous pixels (squares).

Functions

1. Accepts signals from the receiver.
2. Stores information in memory.
3. Assigns the returning signals a shade of gray.
4. Sends the returning signal to display.

Random-Access Memory (RAM)

- Stores echo amplitude and location.
- Information stored will be lost if the power is switched off.

Read-Only Memory (ROM)

- Data cannot be modified.

Bit

- Binary digit.
- Smallest amount of computer memory.
- Two levels of storage: 0 = Off; 1 = On.
- Determines the number of gray shades.
  - Number of memory bits = 2^n shades of gray.
  - 3-bit memory = 2^3 = $2 \times 2 \times 2$ = 8 shades of gray.
  - 5-bit memory = 2^5 (to the 5th power) = $2 \times 2 \times 2 \times 2 \times 2$ = 32 shades of gray.
- Multiple-bit memories allow for numerous shades of gray.
- Ultrasound systems typically employ 6- to 8-bit memories.

BINARY NUMBERS

- Binary numbers in digital systems determine the number of gray shades
- Off = 0; On = 1

Shades of Gray Using Binary Numbers

BINARY NUMBER	64	32	16	8	4	2	1	DECIMAL NUMBER
0100101 =	0	1	0	0	1	0	1	= 32 + 4 + 1 = 37
1010010 =	1	0	1	0	0	1	0	= 64 + 16 + 2 = 82

PREPROCESSING

- Part of the scan converter.
- Processes a signal or image prior to storing in memory.
- Operator adjustable.
- Accentuates boundaries.
- Examples of preprocessing include time gain compensation, dynamic range, write zoom, region of interest/expansion, persistence, pixel interpolation, spatial compounding, panoramic imaging, and 3-D acquisition.

Persistence

- Frame averaging.
- Reduces noise and smoothes the image.

Region of Interest/Expansion

- Condenses the scan lines into a smaller image area.
- Increases detail resolution.

Write Zoom

- Rescans only in the area of interest.
- Acquires new data.
- Increases the number of pixels or scan lines.
- Improves spatial resolution.

POSTPROCESSING (CONTRAST VARIATION)

- Assignments of display brightness before or after data are stored in memory.
- Examples of postprocessing include Read zoom, measurement calipers, B-color, and 3-D presentation.

B-Color

- Presentation of different echo intensities in various colors.
- Improves contrast resolution.

3-D Presentation

- Surface rendering—popular in obstetrical imaging.
- 2-D slices through a 3-D volume—image plane orientation can be presented.
- Transparent views—allow a see-through image of anatomy similar to an x-ray film.

Read Zoom

- Displays only the original data.
- Number of pixels or scan lines are the same as in the original image.

IMAGE DISPLAY

- Receives electrical impulses and translates them into a picture display.
- Each image is divided into multiple small squares similar to a checkerboard-termed matrix.
- Each square of the matrix is assigned either a number 0 = Off or 1 = On.

MATRIX

- The greater the number of rows and columns, the better the spatial resolution.
- Cathode ray tubes typically use a 512×512 matrix, or 262,144 pixels.

PIXEL

- Smallest visible picture element of a display.
- Each pixel stores one shade of gray.

PIXEL DENSITY

- Number of picture elements per inch.
- Directly related to spatial and detail resolution.
- Inversely related to pixel size.

CATHODE RAY TUBE (CRT)

- Provides color and gray-scale capabilities.
- Consists of a vacuum glass envelope containing an electron gun and phosphor fluorescent screen.

- When electrons strike the fluorescent screen, light is emitted.
- Images are produced by modulating the intensity of the electron beam with a received video signal.
- Presents an image by scanning a spot of light in horizontal lines from upper left to lower right, top to bottom.
- The strength of the electron beam determines the brightness of the display.
- Presents images at a rate of 30 frames/sec or 60 fields/sec.
- Flickering occurs below 20 frames/sec.
- Employs 525 horizontal lines interlaced as odd and even line fields.

COMPUTER MONITOR

- A CRT that presents data retrieved from memory in a 2-D pixel matrix.
- Refreshes the display approximately 60 times per second.
- Presents image information in the form of horizontal lines.
- Uses magnetic instead of electrostatic deflection.

LIQUID-CRYSTAL DISPLAY (LCD)

- Thin, flat display device made up of any number of color or monochrome pixels arranged in front of a light source or reflector.
- By controlling the voltage applied across the liquid-crystal layer in each pixel, light may pass through in varying amounts, forming different levels of gray.
- Generally displayed in a 1024×768 rectangular matrix.

RECORDING TECHNIQUES

HARD COPY IMAGING

X-ray Film

- Single emulsion x-ray film.
- Cellulose acetate sheet coated with a gelatin emulsion that contains silver bromide crystals.
- After exposure to light from the monitor, the film is chemically developed.

Thermal Processors

- Use a paper medium to record the image.
- Small heat elements create the image.
- Decreased resolution and gray scale.
- Less stable than an x-ray film.
- Color thermal printers contain a ribbon of color inks.
- Colors include cyan, magenta, yellow, and black.

Laser Imaging

- Automated film handling and developing.
- 15 or more images per sheet of film.
- Higher resolution, better gray scale with less distortion.

Digital Recording Device

- Stores images on computer disks or memory.
- Allows viewing on monitors and film transfer.

Videotape Player

- Used to record motion or real-time imaging.

ARCHIVE STORAGE

MAGNETIC—OPTICAL DISK

- Safely stores information on an optical disk.
- Disk can be rewritten and erased.

PICTURE ARCHIVING AND COMMUNICATION SYSTEM (PACS)

- Also known as digital imaging network (DIN), information management archiving and communication stations (IMACS).
- Electronically communicates images and associated information to workstations external from the ultrasound system.
- Acquisition, display, hard copy, and computer components are interconnected using a local area network (LAN).
- Allows virtual access to archived studies of multiple imaging modalities.
- Ultrasound data are digitized and transferred to the network.
- Data do not deteriorate over time.

STANDARDS FOR ARCHIVING MEDICAL FILES

AMERICAN COLLEGE OF RADIOLOGY (ACR)

- Develops standards for encoding patient file information and interpretation.

DIGITAL IMAGING AND COMMUNICATIONS IN MEDICINE (DICOM)

- Standardizes protocols for communicating image systems.

NATIONAL ELECTRICAL MANUFACTURERS ASSOCIATION (NEMA)

- Develops standards for encoding patient file information and interpretation.

ARTIFACTS OF ULTRASOUND

- Reflection not properly indicative of the structure imaged.
- An apparent echo for which distance, direction, or amplitude do not correspond to a real target.
- Include reflections that are not real, missing, improperly positioned, or of improper brightness, shape, or size.
- When corrective measures are taken, artifacts typically disappear.

CAUSED BY

1. Ultrasound system assumptions.
2. Operator error.
3. Physics of ultrasound.
4. Equipment malfunction.
5. Improper use of equipment.

ASSUMPTIONS IN THE DESIGN OF ULTRASOUND SYSTEMS

1. Image plane is thin.
2. Sound only travels in a straight line.
3. Echoes originate only from objects on the central axis.
4. Distance to a reflector is proportional to the time it takes for an echo to return.
5. Intensity of an echo corresponds to the strength of a reflector.
6. Sound travels directly to and from a reflector.
7. Sound travels in soft tissue at exactly $1.54 \, mm/\mu s$.

Imaging Artifacts

ARTIFACT	DEFINITION	CAUSE	MANIFESTATION
Acoustic speckle	• Low-intensity sound waves interfering with each other • Constructive interference—echoes reinforce each other • Destructive interference—echoes completely or partially cancel each other out	• Interference of echoes from the distribution of scatterers in tissue	• Added objects • Grainy image • Interferes with the ability to detect low-contrast objects
Comet tail	• Dense, tapering trail of echoes just distal to a strong reflector • Located parallel to the sound beam	• Reverberation • Caused by two closely spaced strong reflectors in soft tissue • Foreign body, calcium, or air	• Added objects • Appears as multiple small echogenic bands
Duplication	• Redirection of the sound beam, passing through the medial edges of the abdominus rectus muscle	• Refraction • Unique to the abdominus rectus muscle	• Added objects • Incorrect object size
Edge shadowing	• Redirection of the sound beam at the edge of round or oval structures • Beam hits the edge of a structure larger than the beam width	• Refraction	• Incorrect object brightness • Missed objects
Enhancement	• Increased brightness behind a weakly attenuating structure • Sound beam passes through an area of low attenuation	• Attenuation	• Incorrect object brightness
Focal banding	• Product of horizontal enhancement or banding at focal zone(s)	• Increase in the intensity of the sound beam in the focal zone(s)	• Improper brightness
Grating lobes	• Minor secondary sound beams of an array transducer traveling in different directions than the primary beam • Reduced by subdicing and apodization	• Spacing of the active elements	• Incorrect object location • Duplicates structures lateral to the real structures
Mirror image	• Objects on one side of a strong reflector are duplicated on the other side of the reflector • True and false images are equidistant from the strong reflector • False image is placed deeper	• Reflection • Diaphragm, pleura, and bowel	• Added objects
Multipath	• Paths toward and away from the reflector are different • Beam strikes an interface at an angle and is reflected from a second interface back toward the transducer	• Reflection	• Incorrect object location • Improper brightness • Degrades image quality and axial resolution
Propagation speed error	• Reflectors appear in correct number but at improper locations • Slow speeds place reflectors too deep	• Speed error	• Incorrect object location • Displaces structures axially
Range ambiguity	• All echoes are not received before the next pulse is emitted	• Pulse repetition frequency is too high	• Incorrect object location
Refraction	• Change in direction of the sound beam from one medium to the next	• Bending of the transmitted beam • Sound wave strikes a boundary at an oblique angle	• Displaces structures laterally • Incorrect object size • Incorrect object shape • Degrades lateral resolution
Resolution	• Failure to distinguish two separate adjacent objects	• Beam width • Spatial pulse length	• Missing object • Incorrect object size or shape

Continued

Imaging Artifacts—cont'd

ARTIFACT	DEFINITION	CAUSE	MANIFESTATION
Reverberation	• Equally spaced reflections of diminishing amplitude with increased imaging depth • Two or more strong reflectors are encountered in the sound path; multiple reflections will occur • More reflections than actually exist	• Multiple reflections between the transducer and soft tissue • Created when a sound wave bounces back and forth between two strong reflectors	• Added objects • Appears in multiples • Located parallel to the sound beam
Ring down	• Appears as a series of parallel bands or a solid streak behind a reflector	• Reverberation • Resonance phenomenon associated with a gas bubble	• Added objects
Shadowing	• Reduction in reflection brightness from reflectors that lie behind a strongly attenuating structure or from the edges of reflecting structures	• Attenuation • Refraction	• Incorrect object brightness
Side lobes	• Minor secondary sound beams of a single-element transducer traveling in directions different from the primary beam	• Transducer element changing thickness	• Incorrect object location
Slice or section thickness	• Thickness of the scanned tissue volume • Determined by the thickness of the imaging plane • Imaging plane is not thin or uniform in thickness	• Beam width is greater than the reflector's	• Added objects • True reflector lies outside of the assumed imaging plane

Doppler Artifacts

DOPPLER ARTIFACT	DEFINITION	CAUSE	MANIFESTATION
Aliasing	• Doppler shift exceeding the Nyquist limit	• Doppler shift exceeds one half of the pulse repetition frequency (PRF) • Undersampling of the Doppler shift	• Improper representation of the information sampled • Wrap-around of the pulse wave or color Doppler display • Incorrect flow direction
Flash	• Sudden burst of color Doppler	• Tissue motion • Transducer motion	• Extension of color Doppler beyond the region of blood flow
Mirror image	• Duplication of a vessel or Doppler shift on the opposite side of a strong reflector	• Doppler gain is set too high	• Added vessel or Doppler shift

Chapter Formulas

$$\text{Maximum depth (cm)} = \frac{77}{\text{PRF (kHz)}}$$

Maximum depth (cm) × Number of focal zones × Lines per frame × Frame rate ≤ 77,000

Pulse repetition frequency (Hz) = Lines per frame × Frame rate (frames/sec)

PULSE-ECHO INSTRUMENTATION REVIEW

1. The motion of moving structures in a 2-D image display describes:
   a. static imaging
   b. motion mode
   c. amplitude mode
   d. real-time imaging
   e. temporal resolution

2. In a brightness-mode display, the y-axis represents the:
   a. frame rate
   b. penetration depth
   c. compensation slope
   d. amplitude of the reflector
   e. right or left aspect of the body

3. The number of images per second defines the:
   a. frame rate
   b. line density
   c. field of view
   d. pulse repetition period
   e. pulse repetition frequency

4. The frame rate in real-time imaging can be modified by adjusting the:
   a. output power
   b. dynamic range
   c. amplification
   d. imaging depth
   e. postprocessing

5. Which of the following terms defines the number of scan lines in a single image?
   a. frame rate
   b. frequency
   c. line density
   d. channeling
   e. pulse repetition frequency

6. Which of the following display modes demonstrates the strength of the reflections along the vertical axis?
   a. M-mode
   b. B-mode
   c. A-mode
   d. C-mode
   e. E-mode

7. Frame rate is determined by penetration depth and:
   a. temporal resolution
   b. operating frequency
   c. pulse repetition frequency
   d. thickness of the active element
   e. propagation speed of the medium

8. If the line density is increased, which of the following is most likely to occur?
   a. frame rate will decrease
   b. field of view will increase
   c. spatial resolution will decrease
   d. temporal resolution will increase
   e. pulse repetition frequency will decrease

9. Propagation speed of a medium limits which of the following?
   a. penetration depth
   b. temporal resolution
   c. pixel interpolation
   d. harmonic frequencies
   e. spatial compounding

10. A pulse repetition frequency of 10,000 Hz will demonstrate a maximum penetration depth of:
    a. 7-8 cm
    b. 8-10 cm
    c. 10-11 cm
    d. 12-14 cm
    e. 16-18 cm

11. The maximum amount of lines per frame a transducer can employ at a depth of 10 cm when using 30 frames/sec and two focal zones is:
    a. 85
    b. 116
    c. 128
    d. 135
    e. 178

12. Which of the following is directly related to pulse repetition frequency?
    a. line density
    b. imaging depth
    c. spatial resolution
    d. contrast resolution
    e. operating frequency

13. Increasing the amplitude of the sound beam by 3 dB will:
    a. quadruple the acoustic intensity
    b. increase the signal-to-noise ratio
    c. decrease the intensity by one-quarter
    d. increase the pulse repetition frequency
    e. increase the frequency of the transducer

14. Which of the following describes a function of the T/R switch?
    a. controls the width of the sound beam
    b. delivers electric voltage to the memory
    c. generates electric pulses to the crystal
    d. protects the receiver components from the pulse voltage
    e. adjusts the pulse repetition frequency with imaging depth

15. Output of a diagnostic ultrasound system ranges between just above zero to:
    a. 100 V
    b. 200 V
    c. 500 V
    d. 300 W
    e. 600 W

16. All of the following can be controlled by delays in the transmitted pulse EXCEPT:
    a. aperture
    b. suppression
    c. apodization
    d. beam steering
    e. beam focusing

17. Which of the following offsets for attenuation of the sound beam?
    a. amplifier
    b. suppression
    c. compression
    d. demodulation
    e. compensation

18. Which of the following describes a function of the transducer?
    a. stores echo amplitudes and locations
    b. delivers acoustic voltages to the display
    c. delivers electrical voltages to the memory
    d. controls the amplitude of the received signals
    e. adjusts the pulse repetition frequency for imaging depth

19. The knee of a time gain compensation curve represents the:
    a. area of minimum amplification
    b. area of maximum amplification
    c. region of depth compensation availability
    d. depth at which variable compensation begins
    e. deepest region attenuation compensation can occur

20. Which component of the ultrasound system adjusts the pulse repetition frequency with changes in imaging depth?
    a. pulser
    b. channel
    c. T/R switch
    d. beam former
    e. master synchronizer

21. The transmit and receiver switch is part of which of the following instruments?
    a. pulser
    b. receiver
    c. transducer
    d. beam former
    e. digital scan converter

22. Which of the following constitutes a transmission channel?
    a. an electrical voltage and an element
    b. an individual element and amplifier
    c. an electrical voltage and firing delay
    d. a delay path and an individual element
    e. an independent pulse delay and an element

23. Which of the following statements accurately describes demodulation?
    a. Demodulation suppresses low-level echoes.
    b. Demodulation changes the gray-scale characteristics of an image.
    c. Structure boundaries are accentuated when using demodulation
    d. Processing the received signal is made possible by demodulation
    e. Demodulation provides equal amplitude for structures regardless of depth

24. Which of the following receiver functions decreases acoustic noise?
    a. smoothing
    b. threshold
    c. rectification
    d. compression
    e. amplification

25. Which of the following allows for multiple focal zones and harmonic frequencies?
    a. channeling
    b. code excitation
    c. dynamic focusing
    d. constructive interference
    e. multi-frequency transducers

26. Which of the following is a postprocessing feature?
    a. cine loop
    b. persistence
    c. write zoom
    d. dynamic range
    e. 3-D acquisition

27. The binary number 0110010 corresponds to a decimal number of:
    a. 25
    b. 36
    c. 50
    d. 74
    e. 100

28. How many shades of gray are in a 6-bit memory?
    a. 18
    b. 32
    c. 48
    d. 64
    e. 96

29. What is the term used to describe a picture element?
    a. bit
    b. byte
    c. pixel
    d. frame
    e. matrix

30. What is the frame rate of a cathode ray tube display?
    a. 15 images/sec
    b. 20 frames/sec
    c. 30 images/sec
    d. 40 frames/sec
    e. 60 images/sec

31. Which of the following is a disadvantage of a single-emulsion x-ray film?
    a. transfers data to a local area network
    b. allows easy access to archived studies
    c. old data files are purged from the system
    d. stores images and associated information
    e. communicates information to workstations

32. Which of the following is a characteristic of read zoom?
    a. acquires new data
    b. displays only original data
    c. improves spatial resolution
    d. rescans only in the area of interest
    e. increases the number of pixels per inch

33. The number of frames per second necessary for a real-time image to be free of flicker is:
    a. 10
    b. 20
    c. 30
    d. 40
    e. 60

34. Which of the following is most likely related to pixel density?
    a. log compression
    b. spatial resolution
    c. contrast resolution
    d. temporal resolution
    e. number of gray shades

35. Storage of several preceding real-time frames describes:
    a. cine loop
    b. freeze frame
    c. preprocessing
    d. video imaging
    e. frame averaging

36. Which of the following best describes a digital matrix?
    a. storage of picture elements
    b. smallest element in a digital image
    c. smallest amount of computer memory
    d. number of picture elements in a digital image
    e. rows and columns of picture elements in a digital image

37. Which of the following improves contrast resolution?
    a. rejection
    b. B-color
    c. persistence
    d. write zoom
    e. compression

38. Which of the following components increases the number of scan lines?
    a. read zoom
    b. B-color
    c. persistence
    d. write zoom
    e. cine-loop

39. Which of the following artifacts improperly displays a true reflector's location?
    a. comet tail
    b. mirror image
    c. reverberation
    d. focal banding
    e. range ambiguity

40. When the Doppler gain setting is too high, which of the following artifacts is most likely to occur?
    a. aliasing
    b. shadowing
    c. mirror image
    d. range ambiguity
    e. acoustic speckle

41. Which of the following decreases the likelihood of range ambiguity artifact?
    a. perpendicular incidence
    b. decreasing the receiver gain
    c. increasing the overall output
    d. decreasing the operating frequency
    e. decreasing the pulse repetition frequency

42. The design of ultrasound systems assumes:
    a. the thickness of the imaging plane is uniform
    b. sound travels at variable speeds in soft tissue
    c. sound travels directly to and from a reflector
    d. echoes may originate lateral to the central beam
    e. secondary beams travel lateral to the primary beam

43. Weakening of echoes distal to a strongly attenuating structure describes:
    a. refraction
    b. ring-down
    c. shadowing
    d. enhancement
    e. reverberation

44. Errors in propagation speed will display reflectors:
    a. of improper size
    b. at an improper depth
    c. of improper shape
    d. at an improper brightness
    e. with an improper intensity

45. Enhancement of echo reflections occur distal to a:
    a. nonspecular reflector
    b. strongly reflecting structure
    c. weakly attenuating structure
    d. structure of high impedance
    e. strongly attenuating structure

46. A change in direction of the ultrasound beam is more commonly a result of:
    a. the resonance phenomenon
    b. interference from multiple scatterers
    c. striking a boundary at an oblique angle
    d. reflection from a strongly attenuating structure
    e. secondary sound beams emitted from a phased array

47. Spaces between the active elements of a phased array transducer result in:
    a. multipath reflections
    b. the production of side lobes
    c. enhancement in the focal zone
    d. the production of grating lobes
    e. multiple reflections between the transducer and soft tissue

48. The distance to a reflector is determined by the:
    a. type of transducer used
    b. intensity of the returning echo
    c. thickness of the imaging plane
    d. time it takes for an echo to return
    e. propagation speed of the medium

49. A surgical clip will most likely demonstrate which of the following artifacts?
    a. refraction
    b. multipath
    c. comet tail
    d. mirror image
    e. acoustic speckle

50. Shadowing and enhancement are a result of which type of imaging artifacts?
    a. reflection
    b. refraction
    c. attenuation
    d. reverberation
    e. propagation speed error

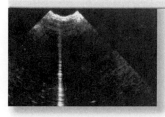

CHAPTER 5

Doppler Instrumentation and Hemodynamics

KEY TERMS

aliasing a misrepresentation of the Doppler shift in a negative direction occurring when the pulse repetition frequency is set too low.

arterioles smallest arteries in the circulatory system controlling the needs of organs and tissues.

Bernoulli effect pressure reduction in a region of high flow speed.

bruit auscultatory sound within an artery produced by turbulent blood flow.

capillaries are the smallest of the body's blood vessels connecting the arterioles and venules and allowing the interchange of oxygen or carbon dioxide and nutrients to the tissue cells.

clutter noise in the Doppler signal caused by high-amplitude Doppler shifts.

Doppler effect observed frequency change of the reflected sound resulting from movement relative to the sound source or observer.

Doppler shift the frequency shift created between the transmitted frequency and received frequency by an interface moving with velocity at an angle to the sound.

energy gradient energy difference between two points.

flow to move in a stream continually changing position and direction.

gate electronic device controlling the transmission or reception of a Doppler signal; Size of the gate is determined by the beam diameter, receiver gate length, and the length of the ultrasound pulse.

helical flow twisting type of blood flow.

hemodynamics science or physical principles concerned with the study of blood circulation.

hue color map the perceived color; any one or a combination of primary colors.

hydrostatic pressure the pressure created in a fluid system, such as the circulatory system.

inertia the resistance to acceleration.

microcirculation consists of the arterioles, capillaries, and venules.

Nyquist limit The highest frequency in a sampled signal represented unambiguously; equal to one-half the pulse repetition frequency.

packet positioning of multiple pulsed Doppler gates over the area of interest.

peak velocity maximum velocity at any given time.

plug flow speed is constant across the vessel.

Poiseuille's equation predicts volume flow in a cylindrical vessel.

pressure gradient difference in pressure required for flow to occur.

pulsatility index a parameter used to convey the pulsatility of a time-varying waveform.

Reynolds number predicts the onset of turbulent flow.

resistant index the difference between the maximum and minimum Doppler frequency shifts divided by the maximum Doppler frequency shift; also known as Pourcelot index.

sample volume electronic device that controls the region of Doppler flow detection.

saturation color map degree to which the original color is diluted with white; the paler the color (or the less saturated it is), the faster the flow velocity; the purer the color, the slower the flow velocity.

spectral broadening increase in the range of Doppler shift frequencies displayed resulting in a loss of the spectral window; usually seen with stenosis.

variance mode the average velocity is calculated, with the colors placed side-to-side.

velocity the rate of motion with respect to time.

velocity mode all measured velocities for each gate are averaged, then the colors are arranged up and down.

venules the smallest veins that receive blood from the capillaries and drain into larger-caliber veins.

volume flow rate the quantity of blood moving through the vessel per unit of time.

HEMODYNAMICS

- A difference in pressure (pressure gradient) is required for flow to occur.
- Pressure difference can be generated by the heart or gravity.
- Blood flows from the higher pressure to the lower pressure.
- Equal pressure at both ends will result in no flow.
- The greater the pressure difference, the greater the volume of blood flow.

CARDIAC CIRCULATION

- Deoxygenated blood flows from the superior and inferior vena cava into the right atrium.
- From the right atrium, blood courses through the tricuspid valve to the right ventricle.
- Blood flows into the lungs through the pulmonary arteries from the right ventricle.
- Oxygenated blood flows into the left atrium through the pulmonary veins.
- Blood continues to flow through the mitral valve into the left ventricle.
- From the left ventricle, blood is pumped into the aorta and systemic circulation.
- Valves are present in the heart to permit forward flow and prevent reverse flow.
- Malfunctioning valves can restrict forward flow (stenosis) or allow reverse flow by not closing completely (insufficiency or regurgitation).

Blood Flow Variables

CONTRIBUTING FACTORS	DESCRIPTION
Density	• Mass per unit volume
Fluid	• Substances that flow and conform to the shape of their containers
	• Gases and liquids
Kinetic energy	• Proportional to its density and velocity squared
Mass	• Measure of an object's resistance to acceleration
	• Directly related to the inertia and force to accelerate
Pressure	• Force per unit area
	• Driving force behind blood flow
	• Directly related to the blood flow volume
	• With each cardiac contraction, the blood is pressure-waved into the arteriole system and microcirculation
	• Equally distributed throughout a static fluid and is forced in all directions
Pressure gradient	• Pressure difference required for flow to occur
	• Proportional to the flow rate
Resistance	• The resistance of the arterioles accounts for about one-half of the total resistance in the systemic system
	• The muscular walls of the arterioles can constrict or relax, producing dramatic changes in flow resistance
	• Directly related to the length of the vessel and fluid viscosity
	• Inversely related to the vessel radius
Velocity	• Speed at which red blood cells (RBCs) travel in a vessel
	• Not constant or uniform across a vessel
	• Dependent on the left-ventricular output, resistance of the arterioles, cross-sectional area, and course of the vessel
Viscosity	• A fluid's ability to resist a change in shape or flow
	• Resistance to flow offered by a fluid in motion
	• Directly related to the number of RBCs
	• Blood is 4 times more viscous than water
	• Units—Poise or kg/m × s

VOLUMETRIC FLOW RATE

- Volume of blood passing a point per unit time.
- Adult cardiac flows at a rate of 5000 mL/min.

- Determined by the pressure difference and the resistance to flow.
- Depends on the pressure difference, length and diameter of the tube, and viscosity of the fluid.

CONTINUITY RULE

- Volumetric flow rate must be constant because blood is neither created nor destroyed as it flows through a vessel.
- The average flow speed in a stenosis must be greater than that proximal and distal to it so that the volumetric flow rate is constant throughout the vessel.
- Concerns a short portion of a vessel.

Poiseuille's Equation

$$\text{Volume flow rate} = \frac{\text{Change in pressure} \times \pi \times \text{Vessel radius}^4}{8 \times \text{Viscosity of blood} \times \text{Length of the vessel}}$$

DEFINITION	RELATIONSHIP
• Predicts flow volume in a long, straight cylindrical vessel	• **Directly related** to the pressure difference and the size or radius of the vessel • **Inversely related** to the vessel length, resistance, and fluid viscosity • Relates to a steady flow in a long **unobstructed tube**

Bernoulli Effect

DEFINITION	RELATIONSHIP
• Region of decreased pressure in an area of high flow speed • Pressure decreases before a stenosis to allow the fluid to accelerate into the stenosis and decelerate out of it	• If flow speed increases, pressure energy decreases • Relates to short **obstructed vessel**

TYPES OF BLOOD FLOW

- Blood flow is typically nonuniform through a specific vessel or throughout the body.
- The muscular walls of the arterioles can constrict or relax, controlling blood flow to specific tissues and organs according to their needs.

Types of Arterial Blood Flow

TYPE	DESCRIPTION
Laminar	• Flow where layers of fluid slide over each other • Maximum flow velocity located in the center of the artery • Minimum flow velocity located near the arterial wall • Found in smaller arteries
Parabolic flow	• Type of laminar flow • Average flow velocity is equal to one-half the maximum flow speed at the center
Plug	• Constant velocity across the vessel • Found in large arteries (i.e., aorta)
Pulsatile	• Steady flow with acceleration and deceleration over the cardiac cycle • Includes added forward flow and/or flow reversal over the cardiac cycle in some locations in the circulatory system • Arterial diastolic flow reveals the state of downstream arterioles
Disturbed	• Altered or interrupted forward flow • Found at bifurcations and mild obstructions • Form of laminar flow
Turbulent	• Random and chaotic flow pattern • Characterized by eddies and multiple flow velocities • Maintains a net forward flow • Onset predicted by a Reynolds number greater than 2000 • Caused by a curve in a vessel's course or a decrease in vessel diameter

VENOUS HEMODYNAMICS

- Veins offer little resistance to flow.
- Venous system demonstrates low-pressure, nonpulsatile flow.
- Pressure is lowest when the patient is lying flat.
- Greatest portion of the circulating blood is located in the venous system.
- Veins accommodate larger changes in blood volume with little change in pressure.

Venous Flow Characteristics

CHARACTERISTIC	DESCRIPTION
Augmentation	• Increased flow velocity after one or more distal compression maneuvers

Phasic	• Flow variation during respiration
	• Inspiration
	  • Increases abdominal pressure, decreasing venous flow from the lower extremities
	  • Decreases thoracic pressure, increasing venous flow from the upper extremities
	• Expiration
	  • Increases the thoracic pressure, decreasing venous flow from the upper extremities
	  • Decreases the abdominal pressure, increasing venous flow from the lower extremities

Proximal pressure	• Manual pressure or Valsalva maneuver impedes venous return • Evaluates valvular competency
Spontaneous	• Unprompted venous flow
Unidirectional	• Flow in only one direction • Exceptions include the hepatic veins and the proximal inferior vena cava

DOPPLER SHIFT

- The **change** in frequency caused by motion.
- Difference between the emitted frequency and the echo frequency returning from moving scatterers.
- Doppler shift is **proportional** to the flow speed and source frequency.
- Doppler shift is dependent on the Doppler angle.
- Cosine values are inversely related to the Doppler angle.

DOPPLER EQUATION

- Relates the Doppler shift to the flow speed and operating frequency.

$$\text{Doppler shift} = \frac{2 \times \text{Transducer freq (MHz)} \times \text{Blood velocity (m/sec)} \times \text{cosine Doppler angle}}{\text{Propagation speed of the medium}}$$

- "2" in the equation is a result of a Doppler shift as a moving receiver and a Doppler shift as the moving emitter.

DOPPLER EFFECT

- Units—Hz.
- Result of the motion of blood.
- Observed frequency or wavelength change of the reflected sound due to reflector movement relative to the source or observer.
- Used to determine the flow velocity and direction of moving reflectors.

DETECTION OF DOPPLER SHIFT

- RBCs are smaller than the wavelength of the sound beam, resulting in Rayleigh scattering.
- Doppler shift occurs in the audible range.
- If the received and transmitted frequencies are the same, there is no Doppler shift.
- A positive Doppler shift occurs when the received frequency is greater than the transmitted frequency.
- A negative Doppler shift occurs when the received frequency is lower than the transmitted frequency.

FACTORS INFLUENCING THE DOPPLER SHIFT

- The angle between the source and reflector is **inversely related** to the Doppler shift.
- Concentration of RBCs may **directly** affect the intensity of the Doppler shift.
- Operating frequency is **directly related** to the Doppler shift.
- A lower-frequency transducer may be necessary to achieve Doppler shifts at deeper depths.

Doppler Instrumentation

DOPPLER TYPE	INSTRUMENTATION	ADVANTAGES/DISADVANTAGES
Continuous wave Doppler	• Uses two crystals—one to transmit and another to receive Doppler information • Displays only a waveform • Large sample volume in the region where the transmitting and receiving sound beams converge • Sound is transmitted 100% of the time	**Advantages** • Ability to measure high velocities (no aliasing) • Ability to use high frequencies • Highly sensitive to low flow velocities • Small probe size • Simplest form of Doppler **Disadvantages** • Lack of imaging ability • Interrogates all vessels in the sampling area (range ambiguity)
Pulse wave Doppler	• Uses a single crystal to transmit and receive Doppler information • Displays a sonographic image of the vessel and Doppler information • Sample volume or gate is placed within a specific vessel • Minimum of 5 cycles per pulse and up to 30 cycles per pulse	**Advantages** • Operator-adjusted placement of the sample volume (range resolution) • Allows a smaller sample volume • Duplex imaging capabilities **Disadvantages** • Maximum detectable Doppler shift is determined by aliasing
Duplex imaging	• Combination of 2-D gray-scale imaging and Doppler information • Electronic scanning permits switching between imaging and Doppler functions several times per second, giving the impression of simultaneous imaging • Imaging frame rates are decreased to allow for interlaced acquisition of Doppler information	**Advantages** • Ability to place sample volume in a specific vessel **Disadvantages** • Decrease in gray-scale imaging frame rate
Spectral analysis	• Allows visualization of the Doppler signal • Provides quantitative data used for evaluating the Doppler shift • High and low impedance conditions downstream give rise to different spectral displays • Vertical axis represents frequency shift (velocity) • Horizontal axis represents time • Uses a fast Fourier transform (FFT) to convert Doppler shift information into a visual spectral analysis • FFT breaks down the complex signals of the Doppler shift into individual frequencies	**Advantages** • Allows measurement of peak, mean, and minimum flow velocities, flow direction, and characteristics of the blood flow • Presents Doppler shift frequencies in frequency order **Disadvantages** • Cannot accurately measure high velocities without aliasing

Continued

Doppler Instrumentation—cont'd

DOPPLER TYPE	INSTRUMENTATION	ADVANTAGES/DISADVANTAGES
Color flow Doppler	• Presents 2-D color-coded information of motion imposed over a gray-scale image • Displays color-coded flow velocity and direction • Color is mapped in velocity or variance mode • Faster velocities will display lighter colors or hues • Color information is obtained in packets (positioning of multiple sample gates over the area of interest) • 3-32 pulses are used to obtain one scan line of color information • Approximately 100-400 Doppler samples per scan line • 4-60 frames per second are used depending on the size of the color box • Increases in length of the color box decreases frame rate • Changing the Doppler angle in an image produces various colors in different locations • Autocorrelation is necessary for rapid obtainment of Doppler shift frequencies	**Advantages** • Ability to detect blood flow quickly • Aids in distinguishing low flow velocities • Determines blood flow direction • Demonstrates nonvascular motion (ureteral jets) • Increasing packet size will increase sensitivity and accuracy **Disadvantages** • Overgaining of the gray-scale image decreases color sensitivity • Displays mean velocities • Less accurate than spectral analysis • Increasing packet size will decrease frame rate and temporal resolution
Power Doppler	• A real-time image of the amplitude of the signal (z-axis) • Displays a 2-D color image representing blood flow imposed over a gray-scale image	**Advantages** • Increased sensitivity to Doppler shifts • Insensitive to Doppler angle effects and aliasing • Better wall definition **Disadvantages** • Does not demonstrate flow direction, speed, or character information

Doppler Artifacts

ARTIFACT	DEFINITION	METHODS OF OVERCOMING ARTIFACT
Aliasing	• Misrepresenting the pulse wave Doppler shift in a negative direction • Exceeding the Nyquist limit	• Increase the pulse repetition frequency (PRF) (scale) • Increase Doppler angle • Adjust baseline to zero • Decrease operating frequency • Decrease depth of the sample volume • Change to continuous wave
Flash	• Sudden burst of color Doppler extending beyond the region of blood flow caused by tissue or transducer motion	• Increase the PRF • Decrease the color gain • Increase filtering of low flow velocities
Mirror imaging	• Duplication of a vessel or Doppler shift on the opposite side of a strong reflector	• Decrease color gain • Use a different acoustic window
Range ambiguity	• Doppler shifts received are not all from the same vessel	• Readjust placement of sample volume

SPECTRAL RATIOS

• Indexes are used to obtain information involving blood flow and vascular impedance that cannot be obtained by absolute velocity information alone.
• Indexes **depend on ratios** involving peak systole, end diastole, and mean velocity throughout the cardiac cycle so **angle correction is not necessary**.

PULSATILITY INDEX

- Most sensitive ratio.
- A parameter used to convey the pulsatility of a time-varying waveform.
- Equal to peak systole minus end diastole divided by the mean velocity.
- Used in abdominal and obstetrical imaging.

RESISTANT INDEX (POURCELOT INDEX)

- Index of pulsatility and opposition to flow.
- Low-resistance waveforms demonstrate broad systolic peaks and forward flow through diastole.
- High-resistance waveforms demonstrate tall, narrow, sharp systolic peaks and reversed or absent diastolic flow.

HEMODYNAMICS AND DOPPLER REVIEW

1. A major cellular component of blood is the:
   a. plasma
   b. platelet
   c. leukocyte
   d. lymphocyte
   e. erythrocyte

2. Which of the following is an auscultatory consequence of turbulent flow?
   a. bruit
   b. stenosis
   c. disturbed flow
   d. high resistance
   e. velocity increase

3. Which of the following is the most accurate definition of hemodynamics?
   a. The pressure created in a fluid system
   b. Predicts flow volume in a cylindrical vessel
   c. A fluid's ability to resist change in shape or flow
   d. The pressure difference required for blood to flow
   e. The physical principles concerned with the study of blood circulation

4. What type of arterial blood flow exhibits a constant velocity across the vessel?
   a. plug
   b. laminar
   c. pulsatile
   d. turbulent
   e. parabolic

5. The microcirculation consists of the:
   a. arteries and veins
   b. arterioles and venules
   c. arterioles, capillaries, and venules
   d. arteries, veins, venules, and capillaries
   e. arteries, arterioles, capillaries, venules, and veins

6. Which portion of the circulatory system exchanges vital nutrients with tissue cells?
   a. aorta
   b. venules
   c. arterioles
   d. capillaries
   e. inferior vena cava

7. Which of the following will most likely resolve aliasing?
   a. decreasing the Doppler gain
   b. decreasing the Doppler angle
   c. increasing the operating frequency
   d. increasing the pulse repetition period
   e. decreasing the depth of the sample volume

8. A positive Doppler shift occurs when the:
   a. spectral information is displayed below the baseline
   b. received frequency is less than the transmitted frequency
   c. received frequency is greater than the transmitted frequency
   d. transmitted frequency is greater than the received frequency
   e. spectral information is displayed on both sides of the baseline

9. Which of the following will most likely increase the system's sensitivity of the Doppler shifts?
   a. increasing the Doppler angle
   b. repositioning the sample volume
   c. increasing the operating frequency
   d. decreasing the size of the sample gate
   e. increasing the pulse repetition frequency

10. If the received and transmitted frequencies are identical, which of the following will occur?
    a. no Doppler shift
    b. positive Doppler shift
    c. negative Doppler shift
    d. ambiguous Doppler shift
    e. proportional Doppler shift

11. A major advantage of continuous wave Doppler is the:
    a. ease of use
    b. small probe size
    c. placement of the sample volume
    d. ability to measure high velocities
    e. interrogation of multiple vessels simultaneously

12. The Doppler equation determines the:
    a. volume flow rate
    b. Reynolds number
    c. cosine of the Doppler angle
    d. viscosity of the red blood cells
    e. change in the transmitted and received frequencies

13. Which of the following is the most consistent predictor of turbulent flow?
    a. Doppler shift
    b. cardiac output
    c. resistive index
    d. pressure gradient
    e. Reynolds number

14. Which of the following is required for blood flow to occur?
    a. Doppler shift
    b. kinetic energy
    c. pressure gradient
    d. high cardiac output
    e. hydrostatic pressure

15. The speed at which blood travels through a vessel is more likely dependent on which of the following?
    a. volume flow rate
    b. size of the capillaries
    c. left-ventricular output
    d. resistance of the venules
    e. type of arterial blood flow

16. In which of the following positions is venous pressure the lowest?
    a. erect
    b. supine
    c. oblique
    d. decubitus
    e. semierect

17. The greatest portion of circulating blood is located in the:
    a. brain
    b. heart
    c. venous system
    d. arterial system
    e. lower extremities

18. What type of blood flow occurs if the average flow velocity is equal to one-half the maximum flow speed in the center?
    a. plug flow
    b. laminar flow
    c. pulsatile flow
    d. disturbed flow
    e. parabolic flow

19. Normal respiratory variations in venous blood flow is termed:
    a. phasic
    b. laminar
    c. pulsatile
    d. spontaneous
    e. bidirectional

20. Which of the following is a disadvantage of duplex imaging?
    a. decrease in imaging frame rate
    b. inability to position sample gate
    c. combines imaging and Doppler information
    d. allows measurement only of mean velocities
    e. inability to use high operating frequencies

21. Noise within the Doppler signal is known as:
    a. flash
    b. clutter
    c. aliasing
    d. acoustic speckle
    e. range ambiguity

22. Which of the following is the driving force of blood flow?
    a. density
    b. velocity
    c. pressure
    d. resistance
    e. volume flow rate

23. Observed frequency changes in moving structures most accurately defines:
    a. aliasing
    b. Doppler shift
    c. Nyquist limit
    d. Doppler effect
    e. pressure gradient

24. The Nyquist limit is equal to:
    a. the operating frequency
    b. the peak systolic velocity
    c. the pulse repetition frequency
    d. the length of the ultrasound pulse
    e. one-half of the pulse repetition frequency

25. What type of color Doppler mapping displays a combination of primary colors?
    a. hue
    b. mosaic
    c. aliasing
    d. variance
    e. saturation

26. Thickening of the spectral trace is most likely a result of:
    a. the reverberation artifact
    b. low-amplitude Doppler shifts
    c. a decrease in vascular resistance
    d. an increase in the range of Doppler shift frequencies
    e. the quantity of blood moving through the sample volume

27. This spectral thickening is termed:
    a. clutter
    b. aliasing
    c. saturation
    d. spectral broadening
    e. low-resistance blood flow

28. The size of the sample volume is determined by the beam diameter, length of the ultrasound pulse, and:
    a. Doppler shift
    b. Doppler angle
    c. operating frequency
    d. receiver gate length
    e. left-ventricular output

29. Which of the following converts Doppler shift information into a visual spectral display?
    a. beam former
    b. scan converter
    c. autocorrelation
    d. fast Fourier transform
    e. digital–analog converter

30. In color-flow Doppler, multiple sample gates positioned in the area of interest are termed:
    a. bytes
    b. pixels
    c. matrix
    d. packets
    e. color volumes

31. Which of the following color modes calculates the mean velocities with the colors placed side-to-side?
    a. hue mode
    b. velocity mode
    c. primary mode
    d. variance mode
    e. saturation mode

32. Which of the following correctly describes the hemodynamics of blood flow?
    a. Blood only flows when pressures are equal
    b. Blood flows from low pressure to high pressure
    c. Blood flows from low resistance to high resistance
    d. Blood flows from higher pressure to lower pressure
    e. Blood flows from higher velocity to lower velocity

33. Increasing the operating frequency will:
    a. overcome aliasing
    b. increase the packet size
    c. increase the Nyquist limit
    d. increase temporal resolution
    e. increase sensitivity to low Doppler shifts

34. Which of the following is an advantage of spectral ratios?
    a. angle correction is unnecessary
    b. only uses peak systolic velocity
    c. increased sensitivity to the Doppler shifts
    d. ability to obtain information involving blood flow
    e. can accurately display high velocities without aliasing

35. The greater the pressure gradient, the greater the:
    a. flow velocity
    b. flow resistance
    c. chance of aliasing
    d. Reynolds number
    e. blood flow volume

36. Resistance to blood flow is proportional to the
    a. Nyquist limit
    b. flow velocity
    c. Reynolds number
    d. blood flow volume
    e. length of the vessel

37. Which of the following occurs during inspiration?
    a. abdominal and thoracic pressure decrease
    b. abdominal and thoracic pressure increase
    c. abdominal pressure decreases and thoracic pressure increases
    d. abdominal pressure increases and thoracic pressure decreases
    e. abdominal pressure decreases and thoracic pressure remains unchanged

38. Which of the following is the simplest form of Doppler?
    a. color
    b. power
    c. amplitude
    d. pulse wave
    e. continuous wave

39. The vertical axis of a spectral analysis represents:
    a. time
    b. motion
    c. intensity
    d. amplitude
    e. frequency

40. Rate of motion with respect to time defines:
    a. energy
    b. inertia
    c. velocity
    d. pressure
    e. acceleration

41. Poiseuille's equation predicts:
    a. the onset of aliasing
    b. the onset of turbulence
    c. the mean flow velocity
    d. resistance to acceleration
    e. flow volume in a cylindrical vessel

42. Pulse wave Doppler uses a maximum of:
    a. 5 cycles per pulse
    b. 10 cycles per pulse
    c. 15 cycles per pulse
    d. 20 cycles per pulse
    e. 30 cycles per pulse

43. Color Doppler frequency shifts are obtained using:
    a. pulser
    b. beam profiler
    c. scan converter
    d. autocorrelation
    e. fast Fourier transfer

44. Which of the following Doppler techniques is sound transmission incessant?
    a. color Doppler
    b. power Doppler
    c. duplex imaging
    d. pulse wave Doppler
    e. continuous wave Doppler

45. Demonstrating nonvascular motion is generally accomplished using:
    a. color Doppler
    b. duplex imaging
    c. spectral analysis
    d. pulse wave Doppler
    e. continuous wave Doppler

46. Power Doppler imaging displays the signal's:
    a. energy
    b. velocity
    c. resistance
    d. amplitude
    e. frequency shift

47. A disadvantage to power Doppler imaging is:
    a. decreased sensitivity
    b. decreased Doppler shifts
    c. decreased range resolution
    d. low pulse repetition frequency
    e. inability to demonstrate flow direction

48. Increasing the Doppler angle is a method of overcoming:
    a. flash
    b. clutter
    c. aliasing
    d. mirror imaging
    e. range ambiguity

49. Smaller arteries commonly demonstrate:
    a. plug flow
    b. laminar flow
    c. parabolic flow
    d. disturbed flow
    e. turbulent flow

50. Increasing the packet size of color Doppler will decrease the:
    a. accuracy
    b. frame rate
    c. sensitivity
    d. Doppler shift
    e. axial resolution

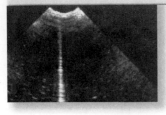

CHAPTER 6

Quality Assurance, Quality Control of Equipment

KEY TERMS

accuracy the quality of being near to the true value; the number of correct test results divided by the total number of tests.

beam profiler a device that plots the reflection amplitudes received by the transducer.

dead zone distance closest to the transducer in which imaging cannot be performed.

hydrophone testing device that measures acoustic output.

quality assurance (QA) the routine, periodic evaluation of data collected on the performance of the ultrasound system and transducers.

quality control (QC) testing used to collect data on the operation and acoustic output of the ultrasound system.

negative predictive value the ability of a test to predict normal findings; the number of correct negative test results divided by the total number of tests.

phantom tissue-equivalent testing device with characteristics that are representative of tissues.

positive predictive value the ability of a test to predict abnormal findings; the number of correct positive test results divided by the total number of tests.

preventive maintenance (PM) service periodic internal cleaning and overall evaluation of the ultrasound system function; generally performed by the system manufacturer.

registration accuracy ability to place echoes in proper position when imaging from different orientations.

sensitivity the ability of a diagnostic technique to identify the presence of disease when disease is actually present; the number of correct positive test results divided by the total number of positive tests.

specificity the ability of a diagnostic technique to identify the absence of disease (normalcy) when no disease is actually present; the number of correct negative test results divided by the total number of negative tests.

system sensitivity measure of how weak a reflection the system can display.

test objects devices without tissue-like properties designed to measure some characteristics of the imaging system.

QUALITY ASSURANCE (QA)

- Routine monthly assessment of the ultrasound system.
- Ensures diagnostic image quality and consistency.
- Prevents poor image quality and system breakdowns.
- Testing devices are available for determining whether sonographic or Doppler instruments are operating correctly and consistently.

METHODS OF EVALUATION

OPERATION TESTING

- Takes into account the entire ultrasound instrument.
- Evaluates the ultrasound system as a diagnostic tool.

ACOUSTIC OUTPUT TESTING

- Considers only the pulser and transducer.
- Evaluates the safety and biological effects of ultrasound and Doppler imaging.
- Requires specialized equipment and is generally performed by the manufacturer.

Methods for Evaluating Operation

TESTING DEVICE	DESCRIPTION	PARAMETERS EVALUATED
AIUM 100 test object	• A device without tissue properties designed to measure some system characteristics • Provides measurement of system performance • Uses 0.75-mm stainless steel rods placed in a mixture with a propagation speed of 1540 m/s	• Dead zone • Compensation • Axial resolution • Lateral resolution • Vertical and horizontal calibration • Registration accuracy • System sensitivity Cannot evaluate • Gray scale • Penetration • Compression
Beam profiler	• A device that plots 3-D reflection amplitudes received by the transducer	• Reflected amplitudes received by the transducer
Tissue-mimicking phantom	• A device with properties representative of different tissue types • Tissue properties include soft tissue, cystic, and solid structures • Small fibers are used to evaluate axial and lateral resolution	• Dead zone • Penetration • Compression • Compensation • Axial resolution • Lateral resolution • Contrast resolution • Slice thickness resolution • Vertical and horizontal calibration • System sensitivity • Registration accuracy
Doppler phantom	• A device using a blood-mimicking fluid • Simulates clinical conditions • Velocity, pulse rates, and durations are known • Some may contain a stenosis OR • Moving string scatters the sound beam • Easy to calibrate • Can produce pulsatile and retrograde motion	• Penetration of the Doppler beam • Flow direction • Accuracy of gate location • Accuracy of measured flow velocity • Image congruency

AIUM, American Institute of Ultrasound in Medicine.

Methods for Evaluating Acoustic Output

TESTING DEVICE	DESCRIPTION	PARAMETERS EVALUATED
Force-balance system	• A device that measures the force (pressure) of the sound beam	• Measures the intensity or power of the sound beam
Hydrophone	• A small transducer element mounted on the end of a hollow needle OR • A large piezoelectric membrane with small metallic electrodes centered on each side • Membrane is made of polyvinylidene fluoride (PVDF)	• Relationship between the amount of acoustic pressure and the voltage produced • Measures acoustic output • Measures pressure and intensities across the sound beam • Measures period, pulse repetition period, and pulse duration

SYSTEM MAINTENANCE

- Transducers and keyboard are cleaned after each patient examination.
- Transducer cables and connections, display monitor, and fan filters are cleaned and evaluated on a weekly or biweekly basis.
- Preventive maintenance service is generally completed two to three times per year.

RECORD KEEPING

- Helps detect gradual or sporadic system changes.
- Documents the need for replacement of existing equipment.
- Necessary for hospital and outpatient clinic accreditation.
- Files for each ultrasound unit should contain:
  - Original purchase order and warranty.
  - Equipment specifications.
  - Results of prior QA tests.
  - Documentation of problems.
  - Service and preventive maintenance reports or invoices.

QUALITY ASSURANCE REVIEW

1. The number of correct test results divided by the total number of tests defines:
   a. accuracy
   b. sensitivity
   c. specificity
   d. registration accuracy
   e. positive predictive value

2. Specificity is defined as the number of correct:
   a. test results divided by the total number of tests
   b. positive test results divided by the total number of tests
   c. negative test results divided by the total number of negative tests
   d. positive test results divided by the total number of positive tests
   e. negative test results divided by the total number of tests

3. Which testing device measures acoustic output?
   a. test object
   b. hydrophone
   c. beam profiler
   d. tissue phantom
   e. string phantom

4. Which of the following most accurately describes quality assurance?
   a. routine evaluation of the ultrasound system
   b. periodic evaluation of the ultrasound transducers
   c. periodic internal cleaning of the ultrasound system
   d. routine evaluation of the transducers and ultrasound system
   e. ability to place reflections in the proper location using different acoustic windows

5. The beam profiler is a testing device that measures:
   a. acoustic output
   b. depth accuracy
   c. flow characteristics
   d. temperature changes
   e. transducer characteristics

6. Preventive maintenance service is generally completed:
   a. annually
   b. once a day
   c. biannually
   d. once a week
   e. once a month

7. The ability to place reflections in proper positions no matter the imaging orientation describes:
   a. accuracy
   b. system sensitivity
   c. quality assurance
   d. system specificity
   e. registration accuracy

8. Routine periodic evaluation of the ultrasound system illustrates:
   a. system sensitivity
   b. an examination protocol
   c. the as low as reasonably achievable (ALARA) principle
   d. a quality assurance program
   e. preventive maintenance service

9. A testing device with characteristics of specific soft tissue is termed a:
   a. phantom
   b. test object
   c. hydrophone
   d. tissue profiler
   e. silhouette object

10. Cleaning of transducers should be performed:
    a. daily
    b. hourly
    c. weekly
    d. monthly
    e. after each patient

11. The American Institute of Ultrasound in Medicine (AIUM) 100 test object **cannot** evaluate:
    a. dead zone
    b. compression
    c. axial resolution
    d. vertical calibration
    e. system performance

12. Record keeping of each ultrasound unit is necessary for:
    a. service requests
    b. scheduling cleaning of the air filters
    c. hospital and outpatient clinic accreditation
    d. detection of gradual or sporadic system changes
    e. scheduling the next preventive maintenance service

13. What is the test accuracy if 10 of 100 examinations are misdiagnosed?
    a. 1%
    b. 9%
    c. 10%
    d. 50%
    e. 90%

14. The positive predictive value is determined by the number of correct:
    a. test results divided by the total number of tests
    b. diagnoses divided by the number of positive test results
    c. positive test results divided by the total number of tests
    d. positive test results divided by the total number of positive tests
    e. positive test results divided by the total number of negative tests

15. The AIUM 100 test object evaluates which of the following?
    a. contrast resolution
    b. system sensitivity
    c. direction of blood flow
    d. sample volume location
    e. gray-scale characteristics

16. Which testing device employs a small transducer element?
    a. hydrophone
    b. beam profiler
    c. AIUM test object
    d. force–balance system
    e. tissue-equivalent phantom

17. Quality assurance programs provide assessment of:
    a. image quality
    b. sonographer accuracy
    c. examination protocols
    d. department productivity
    e. preventive maintenance service

18. Which testing device will a quality assurance program most likely use?
    a. hydrophone
    b. beam profiler
    c. Doppler phantom
    d. AIUM 100 test object
    e. tissue-equivalent phantom

19. A force–balance system measures:
    a. image congruency
    b. horizontal calibration
    c. the power of the sound beam
    d. the pulse repetition frequency
    e. accuracy of measured flow speed

20. The hydrophone measures:
    a. temporal resolution
    b. registration accuracy
    c. blood flow direction
    d. pulse repetition period
    e. transducer characteristics

21. The number of correct positive test results divided by the total number of positive tests yields the:
    a. specificity
    b. accuracy
    c. sensitivity
    d. registration accuracy
    e. positive predictive value

22. Which testing device plots reflection amplitudes received by the transducer?
    a. hydrophone
    b. beam profiler
    c. moving string
    d. force–balance system
    e. tissue-equivalent phantom

23. Which of the following evaluates the operation of the ultrasound system?
    a. beam former
    b. hydrophone
    c. force–balance system
    d. tissue-equivalent phantom
    e. preventive maintenance service

24. Which of the following evaluates the safety and biological effects of ultrasound imaging?
    a. operation testing
    b. transducer testing
    c. acoustic output testing
    d. quality assurance program
    e. system maintenance program

25. Negative predictive value is the ability of a diagnostic test to:
    a. predict normal findings
    b. predict abnormal findings
    c. predict the presence of actual disease
    d. identify the absence of actual disease
    e. identify the presence of actual disease

26. The output of the hydrophone indicates the:
    a. likelihood of cavitation
    b. pressure of the sound beam
    c. long-term effects on humans
    d. likelihood of biological effects
    e. acoustic exposure to the patient

27. Periodic internal cleaning and overall evaluation of the ultrasound system describes:
    a. operation testing
    b. acoustic output testing
    c. registration and accuracy
    d. quality assurance program
    e. preventive maintenance service

28. Which of the following testing devices measures the pulse repetition period?
a. hydrophone
b. beam profiler
c. tissue phantom
d. force–balance system
e. AIUM 100 test object

29. Each sonographer should routinely evaluate the:
a. system sensitivity
b. equipment specifications
c. previous quality assurance reports
d. amount of aqueous gel in the warmer
e. integrity of the transducers and connections

30. Tissue-mimicking phantoms are unable to evaluate:
a. penetration
b. compression
c. direction of flow
d. lateral resolution
e. system sensitivity

31. Acoustic output testing considers only the:
a. pulser
b. receiver and pulser
c. pulser and transducer
d. transducer and receiver
e. fast Fourier transform and autocorrelation

32. The width of the sound beam determines the:
a. dead zone
b. axial resolution
c. lateral resolution
d. penetration depth
e. contrast resolution

33. Development of a quality assurance program ensures:
a. lab accreditation
b. image consistency
c. increase in productivity
d. teamwork among the staff
e. continuing education credits

Using the research below, answer questions 34-37.

One hundred abdominal aorta examinations performed over a 6-month period correctly diagnosed 20 of 25 positive examinations and all negative examinations.

34. The positive predictive value of this study is:
a. 20%
b. 50%
c. 75%
d. 80%
e. 100%

35. The sensitivity of this study is:
a. 50%
b. 75%
c. 80%
d. 95%
e. 100%

36. The overall accuracy of this study is:
a. 50%
b. 75%
c. 80%
d. 95%
e. 100%

37. The negative predictive value of this study is:
a. 50%
b. 75%
c. 80%
d. 95%
e. 100%

38. Fan filters on the ultrasound system should be cleaned:
a. daily
b. weekly
c. annually
d. biannually
e. only by the manufacturer

39. The dead zone is located:
a. near the transducer face
b. adjacent to the focal zone
c. superior to the focal zone
d. lateral to the transducer face
e. farthest from the transducer face

40. The ability of a diagnostic technique to identify the presence of genuine disease is termed:
a. specificity
b. sensitivity
c. precision
d. positive predictive value
e. negative predictive value

41. Use of a piezoelectric membrane is found in a:
a. hydrophone
b. beam profiler
c. tissue phantom
d. force–balance system
e. moving-string phantom

42. Which of the following testing devices simulates clinical conditions?
a. hydrophone
b. beam profiler
c. Doppler phantom
d. AIUM 100 test objects
e. force–balance system

43. The ability to identify correctly the absence of disease is termed:
    a. sensitivity
    b. specificity
    c. registration accuracy
    d. positive predictive value
    e. negative predictive value

44. Preventive maintenance service is usually performed by a:
    a. physicist
    b. sonographer
    c. lead sonographer
    d. department manager
    e. biomedical engineer

45. Accuracy of a diagnostic test is most accurately defined as the:
    a. percentage of error
    b. identification of disease
    c. prediction of documenting disease
    d. quality of being near to the true value
    e. average amount of exceptional results

46. Tissue-mimicking phantoms **cannot** evaluate:
    a. dead zone
    b. gray scale
    c. blood flow
    d. compression
    e. axial resolution

47. A device that plots three-dimensional reflection amplitudes received by the transducer evaluates:
    a. acoustic output
    b. transducer characteristics
    c. intensity of the sound beam
    d. accuracy of the sample gate
    e. penetration of the Doppler beam

48. Which of the following testing devices can simulate pulsatile or retrograde flow?
    a. hydrophone
    b. beam profiler
    c. AIUM 100 test object
    d. moving string phantom
    e. tissue-mimicking phantom

49. The relationship between the amount of acoustic pressure and the voltage produced is evaluated by the:
    a. hydrophone
    b. beam profiler
    c. force–balance system
    d. AIUM 100 test object
    e. moving string phantom

50. What is the accuracy of a diagnostic test if 2 examinations of 20 are misdiagnosed?
    a. 50%
    b. 65%
    c. 75%
    d. 90%
    e. 95%

SONOGRAPHY PRINCIPLES AND INSTRUMENTATION MOCK EXAM

1. Reducing the likelihood of bioeffects from acoustic energy is the mission of the:
   a. Nyquist limit
   b. Reynolds number
   c. Huygens principle
   d. ALARA principle
   e. Poiseuille principle

2. The number of cycles in a pulse directly relates to the:
   a. duty factor
   b. spatial pulse length
   c. operating frequency
   d. pulse repetition frequency
   e. propagation speed of the medium

3. The Doppler shift frequency is proportional to the:
   a. cosine values
   b. Doppler angle
   c. operating frequency
   d. velocity of the reflector
   e. propagation speed of the medium

4. In the Fraunhofer zone the beam:
   a. width diverges
   b. is conical in shape
   c. intensity is greatest
   d. intensity is inconsistent
   e. widens toward the focal zone

5. Artifacts consisting of parallel equally spaced lines are characteristic of:
   a. multipath
   b. grating lobes
   c. reverberation
   d. range ambiguity
   e. acoustic shadowing

6. An increase in reflection amplitudes from reflectors behind a weakly attenuating structure is termed:
   a. comet-tail artifact
   b. acoustic shadowing
   c. slice thickness artifact
   d. acoustic enhancement
   e. propagation speed error

7. The ratio of the largest power to the smallest power the ultrasound system can handle describes:
   a. amplitude
   b. bandwidth
   c. compensation
   d. dynamic range
   e. contrast resolution

8. Axial resolution directly relates to the:
   a. penetration depth
   b. spatial pulse length
   c. temporal resolution
   d. transducer diameter
   e. operating frequency

9. When voltage is applied to the piezoelectric crystal, the crystal will:
   a. vibrate
   b. increase in size
   c. decrease in size
   d. remain unchanged
   e. increase or decrease according to the polarity

10. The resistance of the arterioles accounts for about what percentage of the total systemic resistance
    a. 10%
    b. 25%
    c. 33%
    d. 50%
    e. 75%

11. Rayleigh scattering is mostly likely to occur when encountering the:
    a. liver
    b. pleura
    c. diaphragm
    d. red blood cells
    e. urinary bladder

12. Which color always represents the baseline in color Doppler imaging?
    a. red
    b. blue
    c. white
    d. black
    e. yellow

13. Which of the following correctly defines acoustic frequency?
    a. length of one cycle
    b. number of pulses in a cycle
    c. number of cycles in a second
    d. strength of the compression wave
    e. amount of time to complete one cycle

14. What component is not present in A-mode but is necessary for B-mode imaging?
    a. clock
    b. display
    c. amplifier
    d. transducer
    e. scan converter

15. Grating lobes are caused by:
    a. high frame rates
    b. dynamic focusing
    c. reverberation artifact
    d. interference phenomenon
    e. spacing of the array elements

16. Clutter can be reduced using which of the following controls?
    a. wall filter
    b. smoothing
    c. baseline shift
    d. dynamic range
    e. pulse repetition frequency

17. Regions of high density in an acoustic wave are termed:
    a. cycles
    b. reflections
    c. rarefactions
    d. transmissions
    e. compressions

18. Decibel is the unit of measurement for:
    a. intensity
    b. pressure
    c. amplitude
    d. duty factor
    e. compression

19. Transmission of the sound wave from one medium to the next is determined by the media:
    a. density
    b. stiffness
    c. amplitude
    d. impedance
    e. propagation speed

20. Focusing of the sound beam:
    a. decreases beam intensity
    b. improves lateral resolution
    c. increases specular reflections
    d. widens the sound beam in the near zone
    e. creates a spacious sound beam over a specified area

21. As the transducer diameter increases, the:
    a. near zone length decreases
    b. thickness of the element decreases
    c. intensity in the focal zone increases
    d. divergence in the far field decreases
    e. propagation speed of the element decreases

22. Holding a single image of sonographic information for display is termed a:
    a. byte
    b. pixel
    c. scan line
    d. cine loop
    e. freeze frame

23. Convert the binary number 0010011 to a decimal equivalent.
    a. 10
    b. 19
    c. 21
    d. 35
    e. 41

24. The thickness of the matching layer is equal to:
    a. the wavelength
    b. twice the wavelength
    c. one-half of the frequency
    d. one-half of the wavelength
    e. one-quarter of the wavelength

25. Which of the following is most likely to improve axial resolution?
    a. increasing the frame rate
    b. decreasing the beam width
    c. increasing the penetration depth
    d. decreasing the angle of incidence
    e. increasing the transducer frequency

26. What pulse wave transducer displays a trapezoidal image?
    a. vector
    b. linear
    c. sector
    d. convex
    e. endocavity

27. Heat sterilization of ultrasound transducers is not recommended because:
    a. it will void the warranty
    b. the transducer's stability decreases
    c. heat will damage the electric cables
    d. the piezoelectric properties will be lost
    e. the transducer assembly cannot withstand the temperature

28. The formation of a beam from an aperture is explained by:
    a. Snell's law
    b. ALARA principle
    c. piezoelectric effect
    d. Huygens principle
    e. Poiseuille equation

29. The Fresnel zone is another name for the:
    a. far zone
    b. dead zone
    c. near zone
    d. focal zone
    e. focal length

30. Which of the following must remain constant proximal to, at, and distal to a stenosis?
    a. velocity
    b. pressure
    c. resistance
    d. fluid viscosity
    e. volumetric flow rate

31. The greater the impedance difference between two structures, the greater the:
    a. refraction
    b. reflection
    c. attenuation
    d. transmission
    e. reverberation

32. Which Doppler angle yields the greatest Doppler shift?
    a. 0°
    b. 10°
    c. 35°
    d. 45°
    e. 60°

33. Increasing the transducer frequency will:
    a. decrease image quality
    b. decrease contrast resolution
    c. increase the penetration depth
    d. increase the amount of attenuation
    e. decrease sensitivity to Doppler shifts

34. Image quality is improved by:
    a. decreasing the output
    b. decreasing the frame rate
    c. increasing the beam width
    d. shortening the pulse length
    e. decreasing the operating frequency

35. What is the purpose of the damping material in the transducer assembly?
    a. increase sensitivity
    b. reduce pulse duration
    c. eliminate grating lobes
    d. improve sound transmission into the body
    e. diminish reflections at the transducer surface

36. Which of the following instruments generates the pulse of sound?
    a. pulser
    b. amplifier
    c. transducer
    d. beam former
    e. master synchronizer

37. Firing delays found in array systems are determined by the:
    a. receiver
    b. transducer
    c. beam former
    d. master synchronizer
    e. transmitter/receiver switch

38. The speed at which a wave travels through a medium is determined by the:
    a. frequency of the sound source
    b. distance from the sound source
    c. stiffness and density of the medium
    d. resistance and impedance of the medium
    e. amplitude and intensity of the sound beam

39. Which of the following is a method for overcoming aliasing?
    a. shift the baseline
    b. increase imaging depth
    c. decrease the Doppler angle
    d. increase the operating frequency
    e. decrease the pulse repetition frequency

40. Brightening of echoes in the focal zone is a result of:
    a. acoustic speckle
    b. mirror image artifact
    c. slice thickness artifact
    d. horizontal enhancement
    e. propagation speed error

41. A disadvantage of duplex imaging is a(n):
    a. decrease in imaging frame rate
    b. inability to display peak velocities
    c. inability to demonstrate flow direction
    d. decrease in maximum penetration depth
    e. inability to accurately place the sample gate

42. Which of the following transducers will produce a longer focal length if the crystal diameter remains constant?
    a. 5-MHz focused transducer
    b. 10-MHz focused transducer
    c. 5-MHz unfocused transducer
    d. 10-MHz unfocused transducer
    e. 2.5-MHz phased array transducer

43. The duty factor in pulse ultrasound is proportional to the:
    a. pulse duration
    b. penetration depth
    c. operating frequency
    d. pulse repetition period
    e. propagation speed of the medium

44. Depth gain compensation is necessary to:
    a. counteract attenuation
    b. increase axial resolution
    c. decrease contrast resolution
    d. store echo amplitudes and locations
    e. adjust the pulse repetition frequency

45. The Reynolds number predicts the onset of:
    a. aliasing
    b. turbulent flow
    c. parabolic flow
    d. a Doppler shift
    e. biological effects

46. Which of the following types of resolution does the wavelength have the greatest effect on?
    a. axial
    b. lateral
    c. contrast
    d. temporal
    e. enhancement

47. The objective of the matching layer in the assembly of an ultrasound transducer is to reduce the:
    a. pulse duration
    b. spatial pulse length
    c. number of cycles in each pulse
    d. electrical energy applied to the crystal
    e. impedance difference between the element and skin

48. What is the minimum number of memory bits necessary to display 128 shades of gray?
    a. 2
    b. 5
    c. 7
    d. 10
    e. 32

49. Which of the following is a function of read zoom?
    a. frame averaging
    b. improve temporal resolution
    c. magnify and display stored data
    d. acquire and magnify new information
    e. increase the number of pixels per inch

50. Averaging the frame rate is operator adjustable using which of the following functions?
    a. read zoom
    b. persistence
    c. dynamic range
    d. contrast variation
    e. time gain compensation

51. At a stenosis, pressure will:
    a. double
    b. increase
    c. decrease
    d. remain unchanged
    e. vary with cardiac cycle

52. Reducing a 30-dB compensation gain by one-half would display a new gain setting of:
    a. 10 dB
    b. 15 dB
    c. 24 dB
    d. 27 dB
    e. 33 dB

53. Reduction in the intensity of the sound wave is a result of:
    a. heat, reflection, and, transmission
    b. absorption, scattering, and reflection
    c. scattering, refraction, and absorption
    d. reflection, transmission, and refraction
    e. absorption, scattering, and transmission

54. Divergence of the sound beam is demonstrated in the:
    a. focal zone
    b. dead zone
    c. Fresnel zone
    d. Fraunhofer zone
    e. near zone length

55. The ability of a sonogram to identify the true absence of disease is a test's:
    a. accuracy
    b. specificity
    c. sensitivity
    d. positive predictive value
    e. negative predictive value

56. No confirmed significant biological effect in mammalian tissue for exposures:
    a. below 100 W/cm^2 with unfocused and 1 W/cm^2 with focused transducers
    b. above 100 W/cm^2 with unfocused and 1 W/cm^2 with focused transducers
    c. above 1 mW/cm^2 with unfocused and 100 W/cm^2 with focused transducers
    d. below 1 mW/cm^2 with unfocused and 1 mW/cm^2 with focused transducers
    e. below 100 mW/cm^2 with unfocused and 1 W/cm^2 with focused transducers

57. List the intensity ranges from smallest to highest:
    a. SPTP, SATP, SPTA, SATA
    b. SATA, SATP, SPTA, SPTP
    c. SPTP, SPTA, SATP, SATA
    d. SATA, SPTA, SATP, SPTP
    e. SATA, SATP, SPTP, SPTA

58. Diagnostic ultrasound transducers operate on which of the following theories?
    a. Snell's law
    b. Doppler effect
    c. ALARA principle
    d. Piezoelectric effect
    e. Huygens principle

59. Uniform intensity of the sound beam is located in the:
    a. far field
    b. near field
    c. focal point
    d. near zone length
    e. center of the beam

60. The amplitude of the transmitted and received signals is the responsibility of the:
    a. pulser
    b. amplifier
    c. transducer
    d. system output
    e. master synchronizer

61. Which receiver function eliminates the weaker reflections?
    a. threshold
    b. compression
    c. amplification
    d. compensation
    e. demodulation

62. Line density is directly related to the:
    a. duty factor
    b. imaging depth
    c. temporal resolution
    d. pulse repetition period
    e. pulse repetition frequency

63. Which of the following are even harmonic frequencies of a 2-MHz transducer?
    a. 2, 4, 6
    b. 3, 5, 7
    c. 4, 6, 8
    d. 5, 7, 9
    e. 4, 8, 12

64. Which of the following will most likely occur if the pulse repetition frequency is set too high?
    a. flash
    b. aliasing
    c. acoustic speckle
    d. range ambiguity
    e. propagation speed error

65. The mechanical index predicts the likelihood of:
    a. aliasing
    b. cavitation
    c. turbulence
    d. a Doppler shift
    e. thermal damage

66. Mirror imaging artifact is a result of a(n):
    a. weak reflector
    b. strong reflector
    c. impedance difference
    d. weak attenuating structure
    e. strong attenuating structure

67. Approximately what percentage of the sound beam will reflect from a media boundary with perpendicular incidence, if the impedances are different?
    a. 1
    b. 10
    c. 33
    d. 50
    e. 99

68. Placement of an echo is determined by the reflector's round-trip time and:
    a. density
    b. stiffness
    c. amplitude
    d. impedance
    e. propagation speed

69. An early gate time means the sample volume is placed:
    a. deep
    b. shallow
    c. to the left
    d. to the right
    e. at the focal zone

70. Which of the following determines the number of scan lines per frame?
    a. contrast resolution
    b. operating frequency
    c. temporal resolution
    d. pulse repetition frequency
    e. propagation speed of the medium

71. When coursing from a medium of lower propagation speed to a medium of higher propagation speed, the frequency of the sound wave will:
    a. double
    b. increase
    c. decrease
    d. quadruple
    e. remain constant

72. Flow reversal in diastole indicates:
    a. a stenosis
    b. an aneurysm
    c. an obstruction
    d. high resistance distally
    e. high resistance proximally

73. Additional focusing of the sound beam is available in the:
    a. far field
    b. near field
    c. focal zone
    d. focal region
    e. near and far fields

74. How wide are the elements of a linear phased-array transducer?
    a. one wavelength
    b. two wavelengths
    c. one half wavelength
    d. one tenth wavelength
    e. one quarter wavelength

75. In a time-gain compensation curve, the delay represents:
    a. area of minimum amplification
    b. area of maximum amplification
    c. available region for depth compensation
    d. depth at which variable compensation begins
    e. deepest region attenuation compensation can occur

76. Which instrument properly locates each series of reflectors in individual scan lines for storage?
    a. cine loop
    b. scan converter
    c. autocorrelation
    d. fast Fourier transfer
    e. random access memory

77. Specular reflections occur when the sound wave:
    a. strikes a rough surface
    b. encounters a weak reflector
    c. encounters a strong reflector
    d. encounters a smaller reflector
    e. strikes a smooth, large reflector

78. The sonographer can improve lateral resolution by:
    a. increasing the frame rate
    b. increasing the imaging depth
    c. decreasing the resonant frequency
    d. decreasing the spatial pulse length
    e. increasing the number of focal zones

79. Contrast resolution is the ability to distinguish:
    a. different points in time
    b. between echoes analogous to the sound path
    c. between echoes of slightly different amplitudes
    d. two separate structures parallel to the sound path
    e. two separate structures perpendicular to the sound path

80. Operating frequency is determined by the:
    a. frequency of the active element
    b. thickness and diameter of the crystal
    c. diameter and propagation speed of the crystal
    d. propagation speed and thickness of the element
    e. frequency of the sound pulse and diameter of the element

81. The portion of time the transducer is transmitting a pulse is termed:
    a. period
    b. duty factor
    c. a longitudinal wave
    d. pulse repetition period
    e. pulse repetition frequency

82. If the duration of the pulse is shortened, the:
    a. duty factor will increase
    b. pulse repetition period will increase
    c. pulse repetition frequency will decrease
    d. number of cycles in a pulse will increase
    e. number of pulses per second will decrease

83. A large packet size in color-flow imaging will:
    a. increase the frame rate
    b. increase the flow velocity
    c. decrease Doppler sensitivity
    d. increase the volume flow rate
    e. decrease the temporal resolution

84. Multiple focal zones result in a reduction in:
    a. frame rate
    b. pulse duration
    c. frame averaging
    d. lateral resolution
    e. distance to the reflector

85. Which of the following controls adjusts the range of displayed signal amplitudes?
    a. rejection
    b. compression
    c. amplification
    d. compensation
    e. demodulation

86. Which adjustable system control affects the frame rate?
    a. image depth
    b. compression
    c. amplification
    d. compensation
    e. transmit power

87. Varying the excitation voltage to each element in the array forming the ultrasound pulse is termed:
    a. subdicing
    b. apodization
    c. dynamic focusing
    d. pixel interpolation
    e. spatial compounding

88. Ratio of acoustic power and the power required to raise tissue temperature is termed the:
    a. thermal index
    b. Nyquist limit
    c. system sensitivity
    d. mechanical index
    e. registration accuracy

89. The mechanical index is inversely proportional to the:
    a. beam width
    b. acoustic output
    c. acoustic pressure
    d. temporal resolution
    e. operating frequency

90. A linear phased array sweeps the ultrasound beam:
    a. mechanically, by rotating the crystal elements in the array
    b. electronically, by delayed activation of crystals in the array
    c. mechanically, by sequential activation of crystals in the array
    d. electronically, by sequential rotation of the crystals in the array
    e. electronically, by sequential activation of the crystals in the array

91. Which of the following is a technique most likely used in harmonic imaging?
    a. apodization
    b. pulse inversion
    c. pixel interpolation
    d. panoramic imaging
    e. spatial compounding

92. Which of the following uses a variable receiving focus?
    a. subdicing
    b. diffraction
    c. apodization
    d. dynamic aperture
    e. dynamic focusing

93. Which of the following denotes the rows and columns of pixels in a digital image?
    a. bit
    b. byte
    c. matrix
    d. channels
    e. pixel density

94. Which of the following is equal to one-half of the pulse repetition frequency?
    a. Nyquist limit
    b. pulsatility index
    c. Reynolds number
    d. attenuation coefficient
    e. transmission coefficient

95. Equal intensity for all similar structures regardless of the depth is a function of:
    a. suppression
    b. rectification
    c. amplification
    d. compensation
    e. dynamic range

96. Which imaging technique is most likely to visualize structures beneath a highly attenuating structure?
    a. pulse inversion
    b. dynamic focusing
    c. pixel interpolation
    d. spatial compounding
    e. harmonic frequencies

97. Contrast agents improve visualization by increasing:
    a. scatter
    b. reflection
    c. refraction
    d. transmission
    e. reverberation

98. Frequency is proportional to:
    a. period
    b. attenuation
    c. wavelength
    d. penetration depth
    e. propagation speed

99. During reception, diagnostic ultrasound transducers convert:
    a. kinetic energy into electrical voltage
    b. acoustic energy into electrical energy
    c. electrical energy into acoustic energy
    d. electrical voltage into kinetic energy
    e. propagation speed into distance to a reflector

100. What type of blood flow demonstrates a constant speed across the vessel?
    a. plug
    b. laminar
    c. pulsatile
    d. turbulent
    e. parabolic

101. If the amplitude of a wave doubles, the intensity will:
    a. double
    b. quadruple
    c. remain constant
    d. decrease by one half
    e. decrease by one tenth

102. Structures that have lower amplitude echoes than adjacent tissues are termed:
    a. anechoic
    b. isoechoic
    c. echogenic
    d. hypoechoic
    e. hyperechoic

103. For refraction to occur, which of the following must take place?
    a. perpendicular incidence and a change of velocity
    b. perpendicular incidence and a change in impedance
    c. oblique incidence and a change of propagation speed
    d. perpendicular incidence and a change in impedance
    e. oblique incidence and a change in the transmission angle

104. Power Doppler imaging displays flow:
    a. rate
    b. velocity
    c. presence
    d. direction
    e. characteristics

105. The concentration of scan lines within the field of view directly relates to the:
    a. frame rate
    b. contrast resolution
    c. temporal resolution
    d. pulse repetition period
    e. pulse repetition frequency

106. A hydrophone is an instrument used to measure:
    a. cavitation
    b. thermal index
    c. acoustic output
    d. mechanical index
    e. transducer characteristics

107. A rise in tissue temperature is significant when it exceeds:
    a. 1°C
    b. 2°C
    c. 5°C
    d. 9°C
    e. 11°C

108. For an unfocused transducer, two near-zone lengths are equal to the:
    a. transducer diameter
    b. distance to the focus
    c. distance to the reflector
    d. active element thickness
    e. propagation speed of the crystal

109. What artifact displays a series of closely spaced echoes distal to a strong reflector?
    a. speckle
    b. multipath
    c. comet tail
    d. shadowing
    e. enhancement

110. Angling the color Doppler box to the right or left changes the:
    a. frame rate
    b. flow velocity
    c. Doppler shift
    d. dynamic range
    e. pulse repetition frequency

111. Propagation speed less than that of soft tissue will place reflectors too:
    a. deep
    b. bright
    c. medial
    d. lateral
    e. superficial

112. To overcome range ambiguity, the:
    a. duty factor should be increased
    b. imaging depth should be increased
    c. Reynolds number should be reduced
    d. pulse repetition period should be reduced
    e. pulse repetition frequency should be reduced

113. Steering of the sound beam is accomplished by:
    a. increasing the number of focal zones
    b. reducing the pulse repetition frequency
    c. altering the frequency with increasing depth
    d. emitting pulses from different starting points
    e. altering the electronic excitation of the elements

114. Which of the following techniques provides quantitative data?
    a. amplitude mode
    b. duplex imaging
    c. spectral analysis
    d. color flow imaging
    e. power flow imaging

115. Which of the following structures demonstrates the highest attenuation coefficient?
    a. fat
    b. air
    c. liver
    d. kidney
    e. muscle

116. The range of frequencies contained in a pulse is termed the:
    a. spectrum
    b. bandwidth
    c. harmonics
    d. resonant frequencies
    e. pulse repetition frequency

117. Which of the following frequencies is in the infrasound range?
    a. 10 Hz
    b. 25 Hz
    c. 10 kHz
    d. 25 kHz
    e. 10 MHz

118. Which of the following techniques use separate transmitter and receiver elements?
    a. duplex imaging
    b. motion mode
    c. amplitude mode
    d. real-time imaging
    e. continuous wave Doppler

119. The majority of imaging artifacts are likely a result of:
    a. operator error
    b. system assumptions
    c. propagation speed errors
    d. weakly attenuating structures
    e. strongly attenuating structures

120. Structures within the focal zone may display an improper:
    a. size
    b. number
    c. location
    d. brightness
    e. resolution

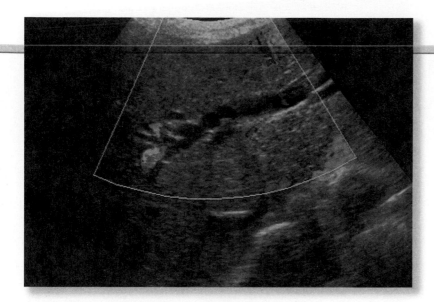

Abdomen

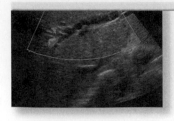

CHAPTER 7

Liver

KEY TERMS

bare area a large triangular area devoid of peritoneal covering located between the two layers of the coronary ligament.

Budd-Chiari syndrome thrombosis of the main hepatic veins.

cavernous hemangioma most common benign neoplasm of the liver consisting of large blood-filled cystic spaces.

cirrhosis a general term used for chronic and severe insult to the liver cells leading to fibrosis and formation of regenerating nodules.

collateral an accessory blood pathway developed through enlargement of secondary vessels.

Couinaud anatomy divides the liver into eight segments in an imaginary *H* pattern.

echinococcal cyst an infectious cystic disease associated with underdeveloped sheep-herding areas of the world.

fatty infiltration excessive deposition of neutral fat within the parenchymal cells.

functional lobar–segmental anatomy divides the liver into the right, left, and caudate lobes.

hepatofugal blood flowing away from the liver.

hepatomegaly enlargement of the liver.

hepatopetal blood flowing into the liver.

liver function tests (LFTs) generic term used for the laboratory values determining liver function (i.e., alt, alkaline phosphatase).

porta hepatis region in the hepatic hilum containing the proper hepatic artery, common duct, and main portal vein.

portal hypertension increased venous pressure in the portal circulation associated with compression or occlusion of the portal or hepatic veins.

Reidel lobe extension of the right lobe inferior and anterior to the lower pole of the right kidney.

shunt a passageway between two natural channels.

stent a tube designed to be inserted in a passageway or vessel to keep it patent.

traditional lobar anatomy divides the liver into the right, left, caudate, and quadrate lobes.

true hepatic cyst congenital cyst formation associated with weakening of the bile duct wall.

varix an enlarged or tortuous vein, artery, or lymph vessel.

PHYSIOLOGY

FUNCTIONS OF THE LIVER

- Breaks down red blood cells, producing bile pigments.
- Secretes bile into the duodenum through the bile ducts.
- Converts excess amino acids into urea and glucose.
- Manufactures glycogen from glucose and store it for future use.
- Releases glycogen as glucose.
- Manufactures heparin.

ANATOMY (Figs. 7-1 and 7-2)

- The liver is the largest solid organ in the body, weighing up to 1600 grams in males and 1400 grams in females.
- It is covered by Glisson capsule.

LIVER DIVISIONS

Left Lobe

- Divided into medial and lateral segments by the left hepatic vein and ligamentum of Teres.

FIG. 7-1
Liver anatomy.

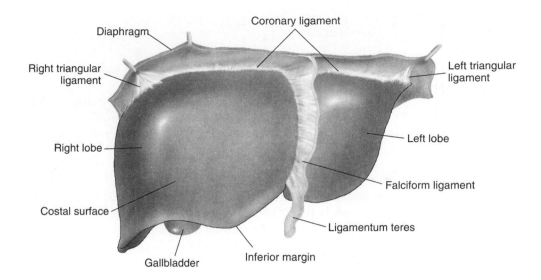

FIG. 7-2
Liver anatomy.

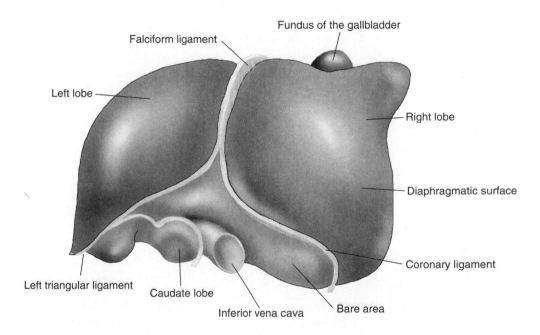

- Separated from the caudate lobe by the ligamentum of venosum.
- Separated from the right lobe by the middle hepatic vein superiorly and the main lobar fissure inferiorly.

Right Lobe

- Divided into the anterior and posterior segments by the right hepatic vein.
- Six times larger than the left lobe.
- Three posterior fossae: gallbladder, porta hepatis, and inferior vena cava.

Caudate Lobe

- Smallest lobe of the liver.
- Separated from the left lobe by the ligamentum of venosum.
- Arterial supply through the portal veins or hepatic arteries.

LIVER LIGAMENTS

- The liver is attached to the diaphragm, anterior abdominal wall, stomach, and retroperitoneum by ligaments.

Coronary

- Consists of an upper and a lower layer.
- The upper layer is formed by the peritoneum from the upper margin of the bare area to the undersurface of the diaphragm.
- The lower layer is reflected from the lower margin of the bare area to the right kidney and is termed the hepatorenal ligament.
- The right and left triangular ligaments are part of the coronary ligament.
- Connects the liver to the body wall.

Falciform

- Attaches the liver to the anterior abdominal wall.
- Extends from the diaphragm to the umbilicus.
- Separates the right and left subphrenic spaces.

Gastrohepatic

- Connects the lesser curvature of the stomach to the liver.

Hepatoduodenal

- Connects the liver to the proximal duodenum.

Teres

- Lies within the falciform ligament.
- Previous fetal umbilical vein.

Triangular

- The most lateral portion of the coronary ligament.
- Connects the liver to the body wall.

Venosum

- Separates the left lobe from the caudate lobe of the liver.
- Obliterated ductus venosum.
- Lesser omentum attaches to the liver in the fissure of the ligamentum venosum.

LIVER SPACES

Morison Pouch (Hepatorenal Pouch)

- Located lateral to the right lobe of the liver and anterior to the right kidney.
- Communicates with the right paracolic space.

Subhepatic Space

- Space located between the inferior edge of the right lobe and anterior to the right kidney.

Subphrenic Space

- Space located between the diaphragm and the superior border of the liver.

VASCULAR ANATOMY

HEPATIC ARTERIES

- Proper hepatic artery enters the liver at the porta hepatis and divides into the right, middle, and left hepatic arteries.
- Thirty percent of the liver's blood supply is through the hepatic artery.
- Lies medial to the common hepatic duct and anterior to the main portal vein.
- Normal diameter of the proper hepatic artery is 2 to 4 mm.

HEPATIC VEINS

- Right, middle, and left hepatic veins converge to empty into the inferior vena cava.
- Transport deoxygenated blood from the liver cells to the inferior vena cava.
- Course between lobes (interlobar) and between segments (intersegmental).
- Have a minimum amount of collagen in the walls.
- Follow a straight longitudinal course increasing in caliber closer to the diaphragm.

PORTAL VEINS

- Main portal vein enters the porta hepatis, dividing into the right and left portal veins.
- Left portal vein subdivides into the left medial and left lateral portal veins.
- Right portal vein subdivides into the right anterior and right posterior portal veins.
- Provide approximately 70% of the liver's blood supply.
- Transport nutrient-rich blood from the digestive tract to the liver cells for metabolic processing and storage.
- Are located within the lobes (intralobar) or within the segments (intrasegmental) of the liver.
- Walls contain fibrin.
- Normal diameter of the main portal vein should not exceed 13 mm.

LOCATION

- Liver is an intraperitoneal organ.

LEFT LOBE

- Lies anterior to the porta hepatis and middle hepatic vein.
- Located inferior to the diaphragm.

RIGHT LOBE

- Lies anterior to the right kidney.
- Located posterior to the middle hepatic vein.

CAUDATE LOBE

- Lies anterior and medial to the inferior vena cava.
- Located posterior to the ligamentum of venosum and porta hepatis.
- Located lateral to the lesser sac.

Congenital Anomalies

ANOMALY	DESCRIPTION	SONOGRAPHIC FINDINGS	DIFFERENTIAL CONSIDERATIONS
Left lobe variants	• Extension into the left upper quadrant • Small left lobe	• Extension of the left lobe into the subphrenic space or across midline • Echogenicity equal to the liver parenchyma	• Splenomegaly • Hepatomegaly • Splenic neoplasm
Reidel lobe	• Extension of the right lobe • Female prevalence	• Extension of the right lobe inferior and anterior to the lower pole of the kidney • Echogenicity equal to the liver parenchyma • Left lobe rarely extends across the midline	• Hepatomegaly • Renal neoplasm

Size

SIZE	ETIOLOGY	CLINICAL FINDINGS	SONOGRAPHIC FINDINGS	DIFFERENTIAL CONSIDERATIONS
Normal adult			• 15-17 cm in length • 10-12.5 cm in height • 20-22.5 cm in width	
Hepatomegaly	• Congestive heart failure • Inflammatory processes • Polycystic disease • Fatty infiltration • Biliary obstruction • Neoplasm • Budd-Chiari syndrome	• Asymptomatic • Right upper quadrant (RUQ) pain • Palpable RUQ mass	• Length exceeding 18 cm • AP diameter exceeding 15 cm	• Reidel lobe • Left lobe variant • Technical error

SONOGRAPHIC APPEARANCE

LIVER

- Homogeneous, moderately echogenic parenchyma.
- Anechoic tubular structures within the parenchyma representing blood vessels and biliary ducts.

BILE DUCTS

- Anechoic tubular structures coursing through the liver parenchyma.
- Smooth hyperechoic wall margins.

HEPATIC VEIN

- Anechoic tubular structures coursing toward the inferior vena cava.
- Caliber increases closer to the inferior vena cava.
- Smooth wall margins.
- Multiphasic hepatofugal blood flow pattern.

PORTAL VEIN

- Anechoic tubular structures coursing from the hepatic hilum through the liver parenchyma.
- Caliber increases closer to the hepatic hilum.
- Prominent smooth hyperechoic wall margins.
- Phasic hepatopetal blood flow pattern.

HEPATIC ARTERY

- Anechoic tubular structure coursing through the liver parenchyma.
- Smooth wall margins.
- Low-resistance hepatopetal blood flow pattern, demonstrating continuous flow throughout diastole.
- Not typically visualized within the liver parenchyma.

TECHNIQUE

PREPARATION

- Nothing by mouth (NPO) 6 to 8 hours prior to examination.
- Emergency examinations may be performed without preparation.

EXAMINATION TECHNIQUE

- Use the highest-frequency abdominal transducer possible to obtain optimal resolution for penetration depth.
- Proper focal zone and depth placement.
- Systematic approach to evaluate and document the entire liver in both the longitudinal and transverse planes.
- Longitudinal and anteroposterior diameter measurements of the liver should be included.
- Anteroposterior diameter measurement of the common hepatic or common bile duct should be included.
- Color Doppler imaging to evaluate vascular structures within the liver parenchyma.
- Evaluation and documentation of intrahepatic and extrahepatic bile ducts.
- Documentation and measurement of any abnormality should also be included in two imaging planes.

INDICATIONS FOR EXAMINATION

- Abnormal liver function tests (LFTs).
- Hepatocellular disease.
- Biliary disease.
- Abdominal pain.
- Postprandial pain.
- Palpable liver or spleen.
- Pancreatitis.

LABORATORY VALUES

ALKALINE PHOSPHATASE

- Normal adult range 35 to 150 U/L.
- An enzyme produced primarily by the liver, bone, and placenta and excreted through the bile ducts.
- Marked elevation is associated with obstructive jaundice.

ALPHA-FETOPROTEIN

- A protein normally synthesized by the liver, yolk sac, and GI tract of the fetus.
- A nonspecific marker for malignancy.

ALANINE AMINOTRANSFERASE

- Normal range 1 to 45 U/L.
- An enzyme found in high concentration in the liver and lower concentrations in the heart, muscle, and kidneys.
- Remains elevated longer than aspartate aminotransferase (AST).
- Elevation associated with cirrhosis, hepatitis, and biliary obstruction.
- Mild elevation associated with liver metastasis.

ASPARTATE AMINOTRANSFERASE

- Normal range 1 to 36 U/L.
- An enzyme present in many kinds of tissue and is released when cells are injured or damaged; levels will be proportional to the amount of damage and the time between cell injury and testing.
- Elevation associated with cirrhosis, hepatitis, and mononucleosis.

BILIRUBIN

- Normal total bilirubin 0.3 to 1.1 mg/dL.
- Normal direct bilirubin 0.1 to 0.4 mg/dL.

- A product from the breakdown of hemoglobin in old red blood cells; a disruption in the process may cause abnormal levels; leakage into tissues gives the skin a yellow appearance.
- Reflects the balance between production and excretion of bile.
- Elevation of direct or conjugated bilirubin is associated with obstruction, hepatitis, cirrhosis, and liver metastasis.
- Elevation of indirect or nonconjugated bilirubin is associated with nonobstructive conditions.

PROTHROMBIN TIME

- Normal clotting time is 10 to 15 seconds.
- Enzyme produced by the liver.
- Production depends on amount of vitamin K.
- Elevation associated with cirrhosis, malignancy, malabsorption of vitamin K, and clotting failure.

SERUM ALBUMIN

- Normal 3.3 to 5.2 g/dL.
- Decrease suggests a decrease in protein synthesis.

Hepatic Cysts

CYSTS	ETIOLOGY	CLINICAL FINDINGS	SONOGRAPHIC FINDINGS	DIFFERENTIAL CONSIDERATIONS
Cyst	• Acquired secondary to parasitic infection, inflammation, or trauma • True cyst is caused by a weakening of a bile ductile	• Asymptomatic • Dull right upper quadrant (RUQ) pain	• Anechoic round- or oval-shaped mass • Well-defined, smooth wall margins • Posterior acoustic enhancement • May contain septations or low-level internal echoes	• Resolving hematoma • Abscess • Polycystic disease • Cystadenoma • Echinococcal cyst
Cystadenoma	• Benign neoplasm containing cystic structures within the lesion • Rare • Middle-aged women	• Hepatomegaly • Palpable RUQ mass	• Multiloculated cystic mass • Well-defined margins • Thin septations demonstrating thin wall margins • Thick septations or mural nodules are suspicious for malignancy	• Resolving hematoma • Hemorrhagic cyst • Echinococcal cyst • Abscess • Adenoma
Polycystic disease	• An inherited disorder • Occurs in 1:500 • Female prevalence • Middle age	• Asymptomatic • Hepatomegaly • Palpable RUQ mass • RUQ pain	• Multiple cystic structures within the liver tissue • Difficult to distinguish normal liver parenchyma • Posterior acoustic enhancement • Multiple cysts may also be found in the kidneys, pancreas, and spleen	• Multiple simple cysts • Cystic metastasis • Cystadenoma

Hepatic Inflammation and Infection

INFLAMMATION/ INFECTION	ETIOLOGY	CLINICAL FINDINGS	SONOGRAPHIC FINDINGS	DIFFERENTIAL CONSIDERATIONS
Abscess, includes: **Amebic** **Fungal** **Pyogenic**	• Ascending cholangitis is most common • Recent travel abroad • Biliary infection • Appendicitis • Diverticulitis	• Abdominal pain • Fever and chills • Leukocytosis • Elevated alkaline phosphatase • Jaundice • Hepatomegaly	• Complex mass • Right lobe is the most common location (80%) • Oval or round in shape • Irregular wall margins • Usually solitary • Posterior acoustic enhancement	• Resolving hematoma • Complicated cyst • Cavernous hemangioma • Metastases
Candidiasis	• Fungal infection	• Immune-suppressed patients • Abdominal pain • Fever and chills • Palpable liver	• Uniformly hypoechoic lesions within the liver parenchyma • Thick wall margins • Hepatomegaly • May demonstrate a target or "wheel within a wheel" appearance • Hyperechoic lesions with posterior acoustic shadowing	• Metastases • Resolving hematoma
Echinococcal cyst	• Parasite *Echinococcus granulosum* • Recent travel to underdeveloped countries	• Right upper quadrant (RUQ) pain • Leukocytosis • Fever • Hepatomegaly	• Septated cystic mass (honeycomb) • Mobile internal echoes (snowflakes) • Cyst containing smaller cysts (daughter cysts) • Collapsed cyst within a cyst (water lily sign) • Round or oval in shape • Smooth wall margins	• Septated liver cyst • Resolving abscess • Resolving hematoma • Cystadenoma • Complicated cyst
Hepatitis	Type A • Viral infection • Incubation of 30-40 days Type B • Viral infection, transmitted by inoculation of infected blood or body fluids • Increases risk of developing a hepatoma Type C • Blood transfusion or "dirty" needle • Increases risk of developing cirrhosis or hepatic neoplasm	• Fatigue • Loss of appetite • Fever and chills • Nausea • Nonobstructive jaundice • Marked elevation in aspartate aminotransferase, alanine aminotransferase, and bilirubin	• Normal-appearing liver parenchyma • Hypoechoic liver parenchyma • Prominence of the portal veins (star effect) • Hepatomegaly • Associated splenomegaly • Increased parenchymal echogenicity in chronic cases	• Normal liver • Biliary obstruction
Peliosis hepatitis	• Occurs in chronically ill patients • Rare disorder	• Hepatomegaly	• Focal or diffuse cystic liver masses • Development of necrotic, blood-filled liver spaces communicating with the hepatic veins	• Cystic metastases • Abscess • Cystadenoma

Continued

Hepatic Inflammation and Infection—cont'd

INFLAMMATION/ INFECTION	ETIOLOGY	CLINICAL FINDINGS	SONOGRAPHIC FINDINGS	DIFFERENTIAL CONSIDERATIONS
Schistosomiasis	• Parasite entering the skin or mucosa and traveling to the lung and then liver • Symptoms may take 4-6 weeks to appear • May even take several years to develop	• Rash • Fever • Diarrhea • Lymphadenopathy	• Increase in echogenicity of the portal walls • Thick portal wall margins • Atrophy of the right lobe • Hypertrophy of the left lobe • Thickening of the gallbladder wall • Portosystemic collaterals	• Hepatitis • Cirrhosis • Fatty infiltration

Benign Hepatic Conditions

CONDITION	ETIOLOGY	CLINICAL FINDINGS	SONOGRAPHIC FINDINGS	DIFFERENTIAL CONSIDERATIONS
Adenoma	• Long history of usage of oral contraceptives • Associated with Type 1 glycogen storage disease	• Asymptomatic • Normal labs • Right upper quadrant (RUQ) pain	• Solid slightly hypoechoic mass • Hypoechoic halo • Complex mass is demonstrated with hemorrhage or necrosis	• Cavernous hemangioma • Focal nodular hyperplasia • Hematoma • Abscess
Cavernous hemangioma	• Benign congenital neoplasm consisting of large blood-filled cystic spaces • Female prevalence • Most common benign liver mass	• Asymptomatic • RUQ pain	• Homogeneous hyperechoic mass • Well-defined wall margins • Round in shape • May increase in size • Complex echo pattern from hemorrhage or necrosis	• Metastases • Focal nodular hyperplasia • Adenoma • Abscess
Cirrhosis	• Alcoholism is most common • Biliary obstruction • Viral hepatitis • Budd-Chiari syndrome • Nutritional deficiencies • Cardiac disease	• Weakness and fatigue • Weight loss • Abdominal pain • Ascites • Elevated aspartate aminotransferase, alanine aminotransferase, and bilirubin • Skin changes and hair loss • Nonobstructive jaundice	• Diffuse increase in parenchymal echogenicity • Irregular nodular contour • Inability to distinguish portal vein wall margins • Increase in sound attenuation • Enlargement of the caudate lobe • Splenomegaly • Ascites	• Fatty infiltration • Diffuse metastases
Fatty infiltration	• Obesity • Diabetes • Cirrhosis • Hepatitis • Alcohol abuse • Hyperlipidemia • Metabolic disorder • Ulcerative colitis	• Asymptomatic • Elevated liver function tests • Hepatomegaly	• Diffuse increase in parenchymal echogenicity • Normal vessel wall margins • Normal liver parenchyma appears as a hypoechoic mass adjacent to the IVC or anterior to the porta hepatis	• Cirrhosis • Glycogen storage disease
Focal nodular hyperplasia	• Hormone influence • Congenital vascular malformation • Second most common benign liver mass	• Asymptomatic	• Hyperechoic or isoechoic liver mass • Well-defined wall margins • Subcapsular in location • Frequently found in the right lobe	• Adenoma • Cavernous hemangioma • Metastases

Benign Hepatic Conditions—cont'd

CONDITION	ETIOLOGY	CLINICAL FINDINGS	SONOGRAPHIC FINDINGS	DIFFERENTIAL CONSIDERATIONS
Glycogen storage disease	• Autosomal recessive disorder • Excessive deposition of glycogen in the liver, kidneys, and GI tract • Type 1—Von Gierke disease is the most common	• Hepatomegaly • Stunted growth • Kidney failure • Hypoglycemia • Bruising	• Marked diffuse increase in echogenicity of the liver parenchyma • Increase in acoustic attenuation • Hepatomegaly • Solid liver masses • Associated with nephromegaly, liver adenoma, and focal nodular hyperplasia	• Fatty infiltration • Cirrhosis
Hemochromatosis	• Rare disease characterized by excess iron deposits throughout the body • May cause cirrhosis	• Fatigue • Shortness of breath • Heart palpitations • Chronic abdominal pain	• Hepatomegaly • Uniform increase in parenchymal echogenicity	• Fatty infiltration • Cirrhosis

Malignant Hepatic Neoplasm

MALIGNANCY	ETIOLOGY	CLINICAL FINDINGS	SONOGRAPHIC FINDINGS	DIFFERENTIAL CONSIDERATIONS
Hepatoblastoma	• Germ cell tumor	• Abdominal distention • Nausea/vomiting • Weight loss • Precocious puberty	• Heterogeneous, hyperechoic mass • Cystic mass with internal septations	• Metastasis
Hepatocellular carcinoma (hepatoma)	• Cirrhosis • Chronic hepatitis B • Exposure to carcinogens in food or environment	• Palpable mass • Abdominal pain • Weight loss • Unexplained fever • Elevated alanine aminotransferase (ALT), aspartate aminotransferase (AST), and alkaline phosphatase • Positive alpha-fetoprotein • Jaundice	• Solid mass with variable echogenicity • May demonstrate a hypoechoic halo • Multiple nodules or diffuse infiltrative masses may also be demonstrated • Hepatomegaly • Ascites	• Metastases • Abscess • Cavernous hemangioma • Adenoma • Cirrhosis
Metastases	• Majority from colon • Pancreas • Breast • Lung	• Hepatomegaly • Right upper quadrant (RUQ) pain • Weight loss • Loss of appetite • Jaundice • Increase in AST, ALT, and bilirubin • Mild increase in alkaline phosphatase	Five Patterns • Bull's-eye or target lesion • Hyperechoic masses • Cystic masses • Complex masses • Diffuse pattern	• Multiple abscesses • Nodular cirrhosis • Fatty infiltration • Multiple cavernous hemangiomas

Hepatic Vascular Abnormalities

VASCULAR CONDITION	ETIOLOGY	CLINICAL FINDINGS	SONOGRAPHIC FINDINGS	DIFFERENTIAL CONSIDERATIONS
Budd-Chiari syndrome	• Hepatoma • Tumor extension	• Abdominal pain • Hepatomegaly • Lower-extremity edema • Mild increase in alkaline phosphatase	• Hypoechoic intraluminal echoes in the hepatic veins (thrombus) • Dilated hepatic veins • Vein wall thickening • Absence of or altered hepatic venous flow • Hepatomegaly • Enlarged caudate lobe • Ascites • Hyperechoic liver parenchyma • Thrombosis in the portal veins	• Cirrhosis • Portal vein thrombosis • Technical error

Portal hypertension	• Cirrhosis
	• Hepatitis
	• Fatty infiltration
	• Portal vein obstruction
		• Splenomegaly
		• Hepatomegaly
		• Increase in liver function tests
		• Hematemesis
		• Jaundice
			• Intrinsic liver disease
			• Main portal vein diameter exceeding 13 mm
			• Splenic and superior mesenteric vein exceeding 10 mm
			• Changes in portal venous flow
			  a. hepatofugal
			  b. pulsatile
			  c. decrease in velocity
			• Portosystemic collaterals
			• Resistive index exceeding 0.8 in the hepatic artery implies portal hypertension
				• Cirrhosis
				• Budd–Chiari syndrome
				• Portal vein thrombosis

Portal vein thrombosis	• Hepatoma or liver metastasis • Sepsis • Blood coagulation disorders • Cirrhosis • Idiopathic	• Severe abdominal pain • Loss of appetite	• Hypoechoic intraluminal echoes in the portal vein(s) • Increase in portal vein diameter • Prominence of the intrahepatic arteries • Absence or altered portal venous blood flow	• Budd-Chiari syndrome • Cirrhosis • Technical error
Transjugular intrahepatic portosystemic shunt (TIPS)	• A shunt is placed between a portal vein and a hepatic vein • Commonly placed between the right portal vein and the right hepatic vein	• Asymptomatic • Symptoms may vary with underlying liver disease	*Normal Gray Scale* • Brightly echogenic, nonshadowing tubular structure • Connects a portal vein to the right hepatic vein • Stent should measure 8 to 12 mm in diameter throughout *Abnormal Gray Scale* • Diameter less than 8 mm • New onset of ascites *Normal Doppler* • Hepatopetal flow in main portal vein at 20 to 60 cm/sec • Hepatofugal flow in right and left portal veins • Flow velocity within stent ranges from 65 to 225 cm/sec *Abnormal Doppler* • Elevated velocity within the stent • Velocity within the stent less than 60 cm/sec • Decrease in main portal vein velocity • Retrograde flow within the stent	• Technical error

Portal Hypertension Collaterals and Portal Caval Shunts

COLLATERAL	DESCRIPTION
Coronary vein	• Located in the mid epigastric area superior to the portosplenic junction
Gastroesophageal	• Located posterior to the left lobe of the liver near the gastroesophageal junction • Tend to rupture and cause internal bleeding
Mesoenterocaval	• Detection of retrograde flow in the superior mesenteric vein implies mesoenterocaval shunting • Collaterals in the pelvis
Paraumbilical vein	• Courses within the falciform ligament from the left portal vein to the umbilicus • Hepatofugal flow
Splenorenal	• Shunts blood from the splenic vein to the left renal vein • Associated with enlargement of the left renal vein
PORTAL CAVAL SHUNTS	
Mesocaval	• Surgical attachment of the mid to distal portion of the superior mesenteric vein to the inferior vena cava
Portacaval	• Surgical attachment of the main portal vein at the portosplenic confluence to the anterior aspect of the inferior vena cava
Splenorenal	• Surgical removal of the spleen with anastomosis of the splenic vein to the left renal vein

HEPATIC TRANSPLANT

- Hepatic artery provides the ONLY blood supply to the biliary tree.

PREOPERATIVE PROTOCOL

- Measure the diameter of the portal vein and hepatic artery.
- Document patency of the portal and hepatic veins, superior mesenteric vein, hepatic artery, and the inferior vena cava.
- Evaluate for portosystemic collaterals.
- Measure the length of the spleen.
- Evaluate liver and biliary tree for pathology.
- Evaluate abdominal cavity for ascites.

POSTOPERATIVE COMPLICATIONS

- Vascular thrombosis.
- Hepatic artery stenosis.
- Infection or fluid collections.
- Rejection.

LIVER REVIEW

1. The adult liver is considered enlarged once the anteroposterior diameter exceeds:
   a. 10 cm
   b. 12 cm
   c. 15 cm
   d. 20 cm
   e. 22 cm

2. Sonographic findings commonly associated with portal hypertension include all of the following EXCEPT:
   a. hepatomegaly
   b. splenomegaly
   c. dilated main portal vein
   d. hypoechoic liver parenchyma
   e. formation of venous collaterals

3. Organs most commonly associated with the development of polycystic disease include all of the following EXCEPT:
   a. liver
   b. kidney
   c. spleen
   d. pancreas
   e. adrenal gland

4. A cavernous hemangioma most commonly appears on ultrasound as a(n):
   a. irregular complex mass
   b. smooth hyperechoic mass
   c. large complex mass
   d. smooth hypoechoic mass
   e. irregular hypoechoic mass

5. Which of the following ligaments separates the left lobe from the caudate lobe of the liver?
   a. coronary
   b. falciform
   c. venosum
   d. gastrohepatic
   e. hepatoduodenal

6. The most common cause of cirrhosis is:
   a. viral hepatitis
   b. anorexia nervosa
   c. alcohol abuse
   d. biliary obstruction
   e. congestive heart failure

7. All of the following symptoms are associated with hepatocellular carcinoma EXCEPT:
   a. weight loss
   b. hepatomegaly
   c. abdominal pain
   d. unexplained fever
   e. elevated serum albumin

8. In the United States, a hepatic abscess is most likely to develop in which of the following conditions?
   a. acute pancreatitis
   b. biliary obstruction
   c. ascending cholangitis
   d. portal vein thrombosis
   e. Budd-Chiari syndrome

9. The left lobe of the liver is separated from the right lobe by which of the following structures?
   a. right hepatic vein and right intersegmental fissure
   b. middle hepatic vein and ligamentum of venosum
   c. left hepatic vein and main lobar fissure
   d. left hepatic vein and right intersegmental fissure
   e. middle hepatic vein and main lobar fissure

10. The right lobe of the liver is divided into anterior and posterior segments by the:
    a. right hepatic artery
    b. main portal vein
    c. right portal vein
    d. right hepatic vein
    e. middle hepatic vein

11. A patient presents with a history of right upper quadrant pain, fever, and leukocytosis. Upon further questioning, the patient admits to recently traveling abroad. A complex mass is identified in the right lobe of the liver. This most likely represents a(n):
    a. hepatoma
    b. abscess
    c. adenoma
    d. cystadenoma
    e. echinococcal cyst

12. Patients with a history of hepatitis B have a predisposing risk factor for developing:
    a. an adenoma
    b. an abscess
    c. a hepatoma
    d. focal nodular hyperplasia
    e. a cavernous hemangioma

13. "Daughter cysts" are associated with which of the following pathologies?
    a. adenoma
    b. hepatoma
    c. fungal abscess
    d. cystadenoma
    e. echinococcal cyst

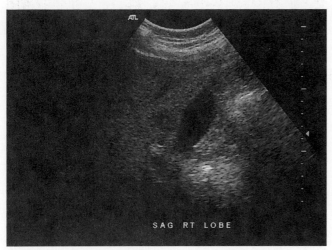

FIG. 7-3 Sagittal sonogram of the right upper quadrant.

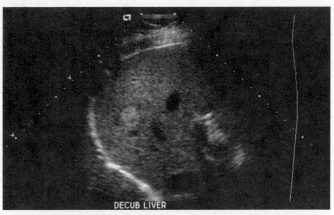

FIG. 7-4 Longitudinal sonogram of the liver.

14. Which of the following hepatic structures is interlobar in location?
    a. hepatic artery
    b. portal vein
    c. hepatic vein
    d. biliary duct
    e. inferior vena cava

15. The normal blood flow pattern in the main portal vein is described as:
    a. phasic
    b. hepatofugal
    c. pulsatile
    d. continuous
    e. retrograde

Using Fig. 7-3, answer questions 16 and 17.

16. An asymptomatic obese patient presents with elevated aspartate aminotransferase (AST) and alanine aminotransferase (ALT) levels discovered during a life insurance physical. The patient admits to drinking alcoholic beverages on social occasions. The hypoechoic area documented in the sonogram most likely represents
    a. nodular fibrosis
    b. a malignant lesion
    c. a hepatic abscess
    d. normal liver tissue
    e. a lymph node

17. The hepatic pathology demonstrated in this sonogram most likely represents:
    a. lymphoma
    b. candidiasis
    c. fatty infiltration
    d. liver metastasis
    e. cirrhosis

Using Fig. 7-4, answer question 18.

18. A postmenopausal patient presents with a history of right upper quadrant pain and normal liver function tests. She denies hormone replacement therapy or previous abdominal surgery. A solitary mass is identified in the right lobe of the liver. This mass most likely represents a(n):
    a. adenoma
    b. hematoma
    c. abscess
    d. cavernous hemangioma
    e. focal nodular hyperplasia

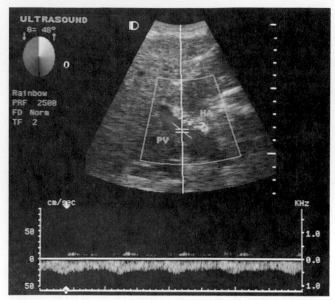

FIG. 7-5   Duplex sonogram of the main portal vein.

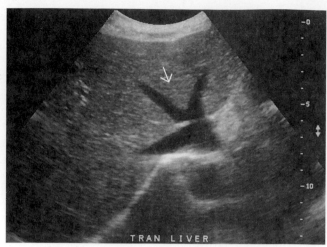

FIG. 7-6   Transverse image of the liver.

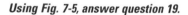

Using Fig. 7-5, answer question 19.

19. A patient presents with a history of hepatitis C and abdominal distention. The finding in this duplex image of the porta hepatis is most commonly associated with which of the following conditions?
   a. hepatitis
   b. fatty infiltration
   c. liver metastasis
   d. portal hypertension
   e. Budd-Chiari syndrome

Using Fig. 7-6, answer question 20.

20. Which of the following hepatic lobes is identified by the arrow?
   a. caudate lobe
   b. lateral left lobe
   c. medial left lobe
   d. anterior right lobe
   e. posterior right lobe

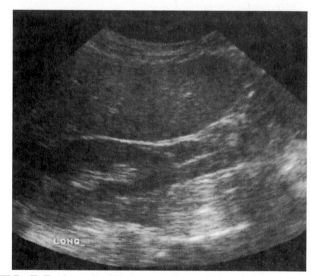

FIG. 7-7   Longitudinal sonogram of the right upper quadrant.

Using Fig. 7-7, answer question 21.

21. A female patient presents with a history of postprandial pain. The left lobe of the liver does not extend across the midline. This image of the right lobe is most likely demonstrating which of the following conditions?
   a. hepatitis
   b. cirrhosis
   c. hepatomegaly
   d. Reidel lobe
   e. fatty infiltration

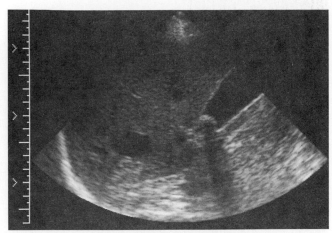

FIG. 7-8 Right upper quadrant.

Using Fig. 7-8, answer questions 22 and 23.

22. An asymptomatic patient presents to the ultrasound department for evaluation of a solitary hepatic mass documented on a recent computed tomography (CT) examination. A nonvascular anechoic structure is identified in the area in question. Based on this clinical history and sonogram, the mass identified is most consistent with a(n):
    a. simple cyst
    b. echinococcal cyst
    c. resolving hematoma
    d. hepatic varix
    e. polycystic disease

23. Which of the following pathologies is also demonstrated in the sonogram?
    a. cholecystitis
    b. choledocholithiasis
    c. cholelithiasis
    d. fatty infiltration
    e. cavernous hemangioma

24. Which of the following liver pathologies is associated with immune-suppressed patients?
    a. adenoma
    b. candidiasis
    c. cavernous hemangioma
    d. polycystic disease
    e. echinococcal cyst

25. Metastatic lesions involving the liver most commonly originate from a primary malignancy of the:
    a. pancreas
    b. kidney
    c. colon
    d. stomach
    e. gallbladder

26. Which of the following ligaments serves as a barrier between the subphrenic space and Morison pouch?
    a. falciform
    b. venosum
    c. coronary
    d. gastrohepatic
    e. hepatoduodenal

27. An abnormally enlarged or dilated vein is most commonly termed a(n):
    a. shunt
    b. varix
    c. stent
    d. aneurysm
    e. perforator

28. Traditional lobar anatomy divides the liver into:
    a. three lobes
    b. four lobes
    c. six lobes
    d. eight lobes
    e. ten lobes

29. Severe insult to the liver cells leading to subsequent necrosis describes:
    a. cirrhosis
    b. portal hypertension
    c. fatty infiltration
    d. Budd-Chiari syndrome
    e. focal nodular hyperplasia

30. Von Gierke disease is most commonly associated with:
    a. cirrhosis
    b. polycystic disease
    c. schistosomiasis
    d. focal nodular hyperplasia
    e. glycogen storage disease

31. Prominence of the portal veins is most commonly associated with which of the following pathologies?
    a. cirrhosis
    b. hepatitis
    c. polycystic disease
    d. fatty infiltration
    e. glycogen storage disease

32. A transjugular intrahepatic portosystemic shunt (TIPS) is commonly placed between the:
    a. right hepatic vein and the right portal vein
    b. middle hepatic vein and the inferior venal cava
    c. right portal vein and the inferior vena cava
    d. left portal vein and the inferior vena cava
    e. left hepatic vein and right portal vein

33. The paraumbilical vein courses from the umbilicus to the:
    a. left hepatic vein
    b. superior mesenteric vein
    c. middle hepatic vein
    d. left portal vein
    e. coronary vein

34. Which of the following conditions describes a congenital extension of the liver anterior and inferior to the right kidney?
    a. sinus inversus
    b. hepatomegaly
    c. Reidel lobe
    d. left lobe variant
    e. hyperplastic caudate lobe

35. Which of the following spaces is located superior to the liver and inferior to the diaphragm?
    a. lesser sac
    b. pleura
    c. subhepatic space
    d. subphrenic space
    e. Morison pouch

36. Enlargement of the caudate lobe is most commonly associated with which of the following pathologies?
    a. cirrhosis
    b. candidiasis
    c. fatty infiltration
    d. liver metastasis
    e. polycystic disease

37. On spectral Doppler, the hepatic veins are characterized by which of the following flow types?
    a. monophasic
    b. parabolic
    c. multiphasic
    d. laminar
    e. turbulent

38. Which of the following ligaments attaches the liver to the anterior abdominal wall?
    a. venosum
    b. falciform
    c. triangular
    d. hepatorenal
    e. right coronary ligament

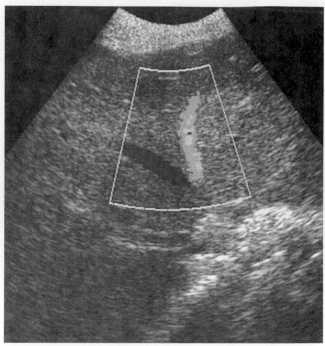

FIG. 7-9   Sagittal image of the liver (see color plate 1).

Using Fig. 7-9 (and color plate 1), answer question 39.

39. A transverse duplex image of the liver displays:
    a. a portosystemic shunt
    b. normal portal venous flow
    c. normal hepatic venous flow
    d. normal and abnormal portal venous flow
    e. normal and abnormal hepatic venous flow

40. Which of the following most accurately describes the location of the caudate lobe?
    a. posterior to the inferior vena cava
    b. medial to the lesser sac
    c. posterior to the porta hepatis
    d. lateral to the inferior vena cava
    e. anterior to the ligamentum venosum

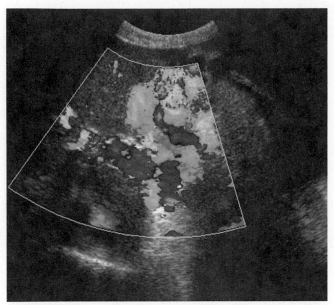

FIG. 7-10 Doppler image of the left upper quadrant (see color plate 2).

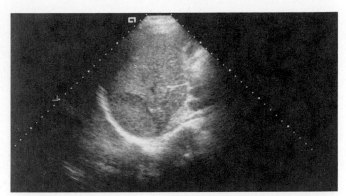

FIG. 7-11 Transverse sonogram of the liver.

44. The diameter of a transjugular portosystemic shunt (TIPS) should measure a minimum of:
a. 2 mm
b. 4 mm
c. 6 mm
d. 8 mm
e. 10 mm

Using Fig. 7-10 (and color plate 2), answer question 41.

41. A patient presents with a history of cirrhosis. Based on this clinical history, the duplex image of the left upper quadrant is most suspicious for:
a. flash artifact
b. gastric varices
c. bowel peristalsis
d. Budd-Chiari syndrome
e. abdominal aortic aneurysm

42. Hepatomegaly is commonly associated with all of the following EXCEPT:
a. hepatitis
b. fatty infiltration
c. acute pancreatitis
d. congestive heart failure
e. polycystic liver disease

43. The most common symptom associated with acute thrombosis of the portal veins is:
a. jaundice
b. tachycardia
c. weight loss
d. severe abdominal pain
e. lower-extremity edema

Using Fig. 7-11, answer question 45.

45. A 30-year-old female patient presents to the ultrasound department with postprandial pain. Gallstones are identified along with a mass in the right lobe of the liver. The patient has been taking oral contraceptives for 10 years. Based on this clinical history and sonogram, the mass is most suspicious for:
a. an adenoma
b. fatty infiltration
c. a hepatoma
d. a cavernous hemangioma
e. focal nodular hyperplasia

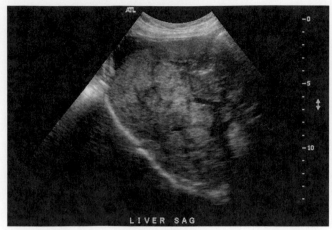

FIG. 7-12 Sagittal sonogram of the liver.

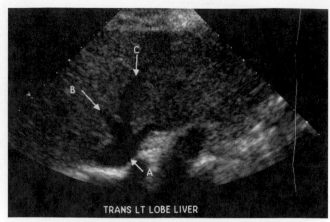

FIG. 7-13 Transverse sonogram of the liver.

Using Fig. 7-12, answer questions 46 and 47.

46. A 70-year-old patient presents with elevated alkaline phosphatase, right upper quadrant pain, and rectal bleeding. A sagittal sonogram of the right upper quadrant is documented. Based on this clinical history the sonographic findings are most consistent with which of the following pathologies?
   a. cirrhosis
   b. fatty infiltration
   c. portal hypertension
   d. liver metastasis
   e. candidiasis

47. The fluid collection identified in this image is located in which of the following spaces?
   a. right pleura
   b. lesser sac
   c. subhepatic space
   d. right paracolic gutter
   e. right subphrenic space

Using Fig. 7-13, answer questions 48-50.

48. Which of the following vascular structures is identified by arrow **A**?
   a. left hepatic vein
   b. left portal vein
   c. middle hepatic vein
   d. right hepatic vein
   e. inferior vena cava

49. Which of the following vascular structures is identified by arrow **B**?
   a. left hepatic vein
   b. left portal vein
   c. middle hepatic vein
   d. right hepatic vein
   e. inferior vena cava

50. Which of the following vascular structures is identified by arrow **C**?
   a. left hepatic vein
   b. left portal vein
   c. middle hepatic vein
   d. right hepatic vein
   e. main portal vein

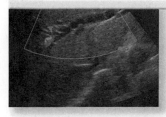

CHAPTER 8

Biliary System

KEY TERMS

acute cholecystitis   acute inflammation of the gallbladder.

adenoma   a benign epithelial tumor; histologically similar to a bowel wall polyp; most common benign neoplasm.

adenomyomatosis   hyperplasia of epithelial and muscle layers in the gallbladder wall; a small polypoid mass of the gallbladder wall; diverticulosis of the gallbladder.

ampulla of Vater   opening in the duodenum for the entrance of the common bile duct.

ascariasis   roundworm that inhibits the intestine.

bile   a fluid secreted by the liver, concentrated in the gallbladder, and poured into the small intestine via the bile ducts; plays a role in emulsification, absorption, and digestion of fats.

bilirubin   yellow pigment in bile formed by the breakdown of red blood cells.

biliary atresia   partial or complete absence of the biliary system.

biliary colic   visceral pain associated with passing of stone(s) through the bile ducts; also called cholecystalgia.

biliary dilatation   dilated bile duct(s).

biloma   an extrahepatic collection of extravasated bile from trauma, surgery, or gallbladder disease.

Bouveret syndrome   paroxysmal tachycardia.

Caroli disease   a segmental, saccular, or beaded appearance to the intrahepatic biliary ducts.

cholangitis   inflammation of a bile duct.

cholangiocarcinoma   carcinoma of a bile duct.

cholecystitis   inflammation of the gallbladder.

cholecystokinin   a hormone secreted in the small intestine that stimulates gallbladder contraction and secretion of pancreatic enzymes; stimulation occurs once food reaches the duodenum.

choledochal cyst   cystic dilatation of the common bile duct.

choledocholithiasis   calculus in the common duct; stones contain bile pigments, bile calcium salts, and cholesterol.

cholelithiasis   the presence or formation of gallstones; stones contain cholesterol, calcium bilirubinate, and calcium carbonate.

cholesterolosis   a form of hyperplastic cholecystosis caused by the accumulation of triglycerides and esterified sterols in the macrophage of the gallbladder wall.

cholesterosis   type of cholesterolosis associated with a strawberry appearance to the gallbladder.

chronic cholecystitis   recurrent attacks of acute cholecystitis.

clonorchiasis   parasite that typically resides in the intrahepatic ducts; the gallbladder and pancreas may also be affected.

common bile duct   portion of the extrahepatic biliary system formed at the junction of the common hepatic and cystic ducts; empties into the second portion of the duodenum.

common duct   term used to include the extrahepatic common hepatic duct and common bile duct.

common hepatic duct   the right and left hepatic ducts join to form the common hepatic duct in the porta hepatis (hepatic hilum).

Courvoisier sign   painless jaundice associated with an enlarged gallbladder caused by the obstruction of the distal common bile duct by an external mass (typically adenocarcinoma of the pancreatic head).

cystic duct   small duct that drains the gallbladder.

emphysematous cholecystitis   gas in the gallbladder wall or lumen.

gallbladder   reservoir for bile.

Hartmann pouch   small posterior pouch near the gallbladder neck.

jaundice   yellowish discoloration of the skin or sclera related to an increased level of bilirubin in the blood.

junctional fold   fold or septation of the gallbladder at the junction of the neck and body.

Klatskin tumor   carcinoma located at the junction of the right and left hepatic ducts.

main lobar fissure   a hyperechoic line extending from the portal vein to the gallbladder fossa; a boundary between the left and right lobes of the liver.

Mirizzi syndrome   impacted stone in the cystic duct causing compression on the common hepatic duct resulting in jaundice.

parallel channeling   condition in biliary obstruction representing imaging of the dilated hepatic duct and adjacent portal vein.

phrygian cap   fold in the gallbladder fundus.

pneumobilia   air in the biliary tree.

polyp   a soft tissue mass protruding from the gallbladder wall.

porcelain gallbladder   calcification of the gallbladder wall.

sludge echogenic bile; viscous bile; contains calcium bilirubinate.

sludgeball mobile, echogenic, nonshadowing mass in the dependent portion of the gallbladder.

tumefactive sludge echogenic bile that does not layer evenly; resembles a polypoid mass.

WES sign wall-echo-shadow sign; "double arc" sign; seen with a stone-filled gallbladder.

BILIARY SYSTEM

FUNCTIONS OF THE BILIARY SYSTEM

- Transport bile to the gallbladder through the bile ducts.
- Store and concentrate bile in the gallbladder.
- Transport bile through the bile ducts to the duodenum.

BILIARY ANATOMY (Fig. 8-1)

BILE DUCTS

- The biliary system originates in the liver as a series of ductules coursing between the liver cells.
- Biliary ducts are subdivided into intrahepatic and extrahepatic ducts.
- Intrahepatic ducts follow the course of the portal veins and hepatic arterial branches.
- Extrahepatic ducts include the cystic and common ducts.
- Bile flows if intraductal pressure is lower than the hepatic secretory pressure. Pressure differences are affected by the activity of the sphincter of Oddi, filling and resorption of the bile in the gallbladder, and the bile flow from the liver.

Common Hepatic Duct

- The right and left hepatic ducts join near the level of the porta hepatis, forming the common hepatic duct (CHD).

Cystic Duct

- Drains the gallbladder.
- 2 to 6 cm in length.
- Contains the spiral valves of Heister.
- Courses posterior and inferiorly merging with the CHD to form the common bile duct (CBD).
- Not routinely visualized on ultrasound.

FIG. 8-1
Biliary anatomy.

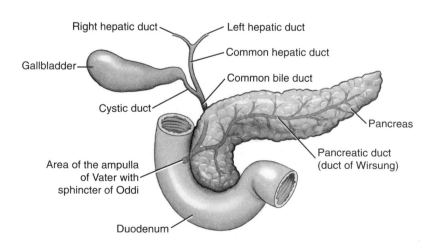

Right hepatic duct — Left hepatic duct
— Common hepatic duct
Gallbladder —
— Common bile duct
Cystic duct —
— Pancreas
— Pancreatic duct (duct of Wirsung)
Area of the ampulla of Vater with sphincter of Oddi
Duodenum

Common Bile Duct

- The common hepatic duct is joined by the cystic duct to form the CBD.
- Courses inferiorly, joining the main pancreatic duct at the ampulla of Vater to enter the descending portion of the duodenum.
- Lies anterior to the main portal vein and lateral to the proper hepatic artery.

Size of the Normal Bile Duct

- Average intraluminal diameter of the CHD is 4 mm and should not exceed 6 mm.
- Starting at age 60, the CBD may increase in diameter by 1 mm per decade.
- Postcholecystectomy patients may demonstrate a slight increase in diameter.
- The CBD will decrease in size or remain unchanged after a fatty meal.

SONOGRAPHIC APPEARANCE

NORMAL INTRAHEPATIC BILE DUCTS

- Anechoic nonvascular tubular structures coursing within the hepatic parenchyma.
- Smooth hyperechoic walls.
- Intraluminal diameter measuring 4 mm. The right and left hepatic bile ducts generally lie anterior to the corresponding portal vein.
- Intrahepatic bile ducts are not routinely visualized on ultrasound.

NORMAL EXTRAHEPATIC BILE DUCTS

Longitudinal Plane

- Anechoic nonvascular tubular structure anterior to the main portal vein and proper hepatic artery.
- Smooth hyperechoic walls.
- Intraluminal diameter 6 mm or less.

Transverse Plane

- Anechoic nonvascular tubular structure anterior to the main portal vein and lateral to the proper hepatic artery.
- Smooth hyperechoic walls.

ABNORMAL INTRAHEPATIC AND EXTRAHEPATIC DUCTS

- Intraluminal diameter exceeding 6 mm.
- Thick, irregular, or nonparallel walls.

GALLBLADDER PHYSIOLOGY AND ANATOMY

FUNCTIONS OF THE GALLBLADDER

- Concentrates bile through the gallbladder epithelium.
- Stores concentrated bile.
- Contracts to release bile when the hormone cholecystokinin is released into the bloodstream.

GALLBLADDER DIVISIONS

- **Fundus:** most inferior and anterior portion; blind end.
- **Body:** mid portion between the neck and fundus.
- **Neck:** narrow, tapering tube-like structure; most superior portion; smallest transverse diameter; fixed anatomic relationship to the main lobar fissure and right portal vein.

LAYERS OF THE GALLBLADDER WALL

1. Outer serosal layer.
2. Subserous layer.
3. Muscular layer.
4. Inner epithelial layer.

GALLBLADDER LOCATION

- An intraperitoneal organ.
- Located in the gallbladder fossa on the posterior surface of the liver.
- Lies lateral to the inferior vena cava and anterior and medial to the right kidney.
- Lies posterior and inferior to the main lobar fissure.
- Gallbladder neck lies most superior.

GALLBLADDER ANATOMICAL VARIANTS

- **Hartmann pouch:** small posterior pouch near the gallbladder neck.
- **Junctional fold:** fold or septation of the gallbladder at the junction of the neck and body.
- **Phrygian cap:** fold in the gallbladder fundus.

CONGENITAL ANOMALIES

- Agenesis.
- Duplication.
- Hourglass shape.
- Intrahepatic or ectopic location.
- Multiseptated.

GALLBLADDER SIZE

- The normal fasting adult gallbladder measures approximately 8 to 10 cm in length and 3 to 5 cm in diameter.

SONOGRAPHIC APPEARANCE

NORMAL FASTING GALLBLADDER

- An ellipsoid anechoic structure located in the gallbladder fossa demonstrating posterior acoustic enhancement.
- Demonstrates smooth hyperechoic walls measuring 3 mm or less in thickness.
- Located in the inferior medial aspect of the liver.

ABNORMAL FASTING GALLBLADDER

- Transverse diameter exceeding 5 cm.
- Thick or edematous wall exceeding 3 mm in thickness.
- Irregular wall contour.
- Intraluminal focus or echoes.
- Acoustic shadowing posterior to the gallbladder fossa.

REASONS FOR NONVISUALIZATION OF THE GALLBLADDER

- Nonfasting patient.
- Surgically absent.
- Obliteration of the gallbladder lumen by intestinal air or gallstones.
- Patient body habitus.

- Ectopic location.
- Agenesis.

NONINFLAMMATORY CAUSES OF GALLBLADDER WALL THICKENING

- Nonfasting patient.
- Ascites.
- Cirrhosis.
- Congestive heart failure.
- Hypoalbuminemia.
- Acute hepatitis.

TECHNIQUE

PREPARATION

- Patient should have nothing by mouth (NPO) for 6 to 8 hours prior to examination.
- Appointments are typically made at the beginning of the patient's day.
  1. decreases the amount of intestinal air.
  2. patient is fasting.
- Emergency examinations may be performed without preparation.

EXAMINATION TECHNIQUE

- Use the highest-frequency abdominal transducer possible to obtain optimal resolution for penetration depth.
- Proper focal zone and depth placement.
- Begin with the patient in the supine position.
- Intrahepatic ducts, extrahepatic ducts, gallbladder, and pancreas should always be evaluated.
- After the supine evaluation, the patient is positioned in the oblique, decubitus, or erect views to demonstrate mobility of gallstones or avoid obscuring bowel gas patterns.
- Transverse and longitudinal images of the intrahepatic ducts, gallbladder, and pancreas must be documented.
- Intraluminal measurement and images of the common hepatic and common bile ducts must be documented. (Only the inner diameter is measured.)
- In the jaundice patient, careful evaluation of the intrahepatic ducts is warranted.

INDICATIONS FOR ULTRASOUND EXAMINATION

- RUQ pain—may radiate to the upper back and chest.
- Increase in liver function tests.
- Nausea/vomiting.
- Intolerance to fatty foods.
- Postprandial pain.
- Positive Murphy sign.
- Jaundice.

LABORATORY VALUES

ALKALINE PHOSPHATASE

- Normal adult range 35 to 150 U/L.
- An enzyme produced primarily by the liver, bone, and placenta and excreted through the bile ducts.
- Marked increase is seen typically with obstructive jaundice.

ALANINE AMINOTRANSFERASE

- Normal range 1 to 45 U/L.
- An enzyme found in high concentration in the liver and in lower concentrations in the heart, muscle, and kidneys.
- Remains elevated longer than aspartate aminotransferase (AST).
- Elevation associated with cirrhosis, hepatitis, and biliary obstruction.
- Mild elevation associated with liver metastasis.

ASPARTATE AMINOTRANSFERASE

- Normal range 1 to 36 U/L.
- An enzyme present in many types of tissue that is released when cells are injured or damaged; levels will be proportional to amount of damage and the time between cell injury and testing.
- Elevation associated with cirrhosis, hepatitis, and mononucleosis.

BILIRUBIN

- Normal total bilirubin 0.3 to 1.1 mg/dL.
- Normal direct bilirubin 0.1 to 0.4 mg/dL.
- A product from the breakdown of hemoglobin in old red blood cells; a disruption in the process may cause abnormal levels; leakage into tissues gives the skin a yellow appearance.
- Reflects the balance between production and excretion of bile.
- Elevation of direct or conjugated bilirubin is associated with obstruction, hepatitis, cirrhosis, and liver metastasis.
- Elevation of indirect or nonconjugated bilirubin is demonstrated in nonobstructive conditions.

Intrahepatic Pathology

PATHOLOGY	ETIOLOGY	CLINICAL FINDINGS	SONOGRAPHIC FINDINGS	DIFFERENTIAL CONSIDERATIONS
Biliary Dilatation	• Biliary obstruction	• Asymptomatic • Right upper quadrant (RUQ) pain • Jaundice • Elevated bilirubin and alkaline phosphatase	• Dilated intra hepatic and/or extrahepatic bile ducts • Parallel channeling • Portal vein may appear flattened with progressive dilatation	• Normal biliary tree • Portal hypertension
Biliary Atresia	• Congenital anomaly • Viral infection	• Persistent jaundice	• Absent hepatic biliary radicles • Small or absent gallbladder • Absent common hepatic duct (CHD) • Hepatomegaly	• Normal biliary tree • Hepatitis
Pneumobilia	• Surgical procedure • Trauma • Infection	• Asymptomatic • RUQ pain	• Hyperechoic focus(i) in the intrahepatic bile ducts • Comet tail reverberation artifact • Often centrally located	• Foreign body • Biliary calculus • Arterial calcification
Caroli disease		• Abdominal pain • Abdominal cramping • Fever • Intermittent jaundice	• Segmental, saccular, or beaded appearance to the intrahepatic bile ducts • Multiple cystic structures in the liver that communicate with the biliary tree	• Polycystic liver disease • Biliary obstruction

Intrahepatic Pathology—cont'd

PATHOLOGY	ETIOLOGY	CLINICAL FINDINGS	SONOGRAPHIC FINDINGS	DIFFERENTIAL CONSIDERATIONS
Clonorchiasis	• Ingestion of raw freshwater fish	• RUQ pain • Fever • Leukocytosis	• Dilatation of the intrahepatic bile ducts • Diffuse thickening of the bile duct walls • Echogenic focus within the bile duct	• Cholangitis • Cholangiocarcinoma
Klatskin tumor		• Jaundice • Acute onset of abdominal pain • Biliary colic • Weight loss • Elevated bilirubin and alkaline phosphatase levels • Mild increase in aspartate aminotransferase and alanine aminotransferase levels	• Small echogenic mass near the hepatic hilum • Dilatation of the intrahepatic bile ducts • Normal extrahepatic bile ducts	• Artifact • Portal vein thrombosis • Hepatic tumor • Lymphadenopathy

Extrahepatic Pathology

PATHOLOGY	ETIOLOGY	CLINICAL FINDINGS	SONOGRAPHIC FINDINGS	DIFFERENTIAL CONSIDERATIONS
Biloma	• Surgery • Trauma • Gallbladder disease	• Right upper quadrant (RUQ) pain	• Anechoic fluid collection near the porta hepatis • Fluid may demonstrate mobility with patient position changes • Check pelvis and paracolic gutters for free fluid	• Seroma • Fluid in the stomach or intestines • Ascites
Cholangitis	• Congenital or acquired stricture • Infection • Parasitic infestation • Biliary stasis • Ulcerative colitis • Autoimmune deficiency syndrome (AIDS)	• Abdominal pain • Fever • Leukocytosis • Jaundice • Mild elevation in aspartate aminotransferase (AST) and alanine aminotransferase (ALT) levels • Marked elevation in bilirubin and alkaline phosphatase levels	• Biliary dilatation • Thickening of the bile duct walls • Pneumobilia • Gallbladder hydrops	• Biliary obstruction • Caroli disease
Cholangio-carcinoma	Risk Factors • Ulcerative colitis • Cholangitis • Choledochal cyst • Male prevalence	• Jaundice • Acute onset of abdominal pain • Biliary colic • Weight loss • Fatigue • Elevated bilirubin and alkaline phosphatase levels • Mild increase in AST and ALT	• Echogenic mass within a bile duct • Dilatation of the intrahepatic and extrahepatic bile ducts • Gallbladder hydrops • Hepatomegaly • Gallstones (30% of cases) • Ascites	• Artifact • Portal vein thrombosis • Lymphadenopathy • Choledocholithiasis • Pancreatic mass

Continued

Extrahepatic Pathology—cont'd

PATHOLOGY	ETIOLOGY	CLINICAL FINDINGS	SONOGRAPHIC FINDINGS	DIFFERENTIAL CONSIDERATIONS
Choledocholithiasis Complications: • **Biliary obstruction** • **Cholangitis** • **Pancreatitis**	• Stone within the common duct • Majority have migrated from the gallbladder	• RUQ colicky pain • Elevated bilirubin and alkaline phosphatase • Mild increase in AST and ALT levels	• Echogenic focus(i) within the common duct • Posterior acoustic shadowing (60-80% of cases) • Biliary dilatation	• Surgical clip • Tortuous bile duct • Cystic duct remnant • Intestinal air • Intraductal tumor
Choledochal cyst	• Congenital weakness of the ductile wall • Reflux of pancreatic juices into the bile duct	• Asymptomatic • Jaundice • RUQ mass • RUQ pain	• Nonvascular cystic mass medial to the gallbladder and lateral to the head of the pancreas • Dilated CHD, CBD, or cystic duct entering the cystic mass • Dilated intrahepatic bile ducts	• Hepatic cyst • Pancreas cyst • Normal junction of the common hepatic and cystic ducts • Gallbladder duplication
Ascariasis	• Ingestion of contaminated water or food	• RUQ pain • Fever • Leukocytosis	• Spaghetti-like echogenic structure within a bile duct • Nonshadowing • Posterior acoustic enhancement	• Stent • Cholangitis • Cholangiocarcinoma • Choledocholithiasis

Gallbladder Pathology

PATHOLOGY	ETIOLOGY	CLINICAL FINDINGS	SONOGRAPHIC FINDINGS	DIFFERENTIAL CONSIDERATIONS
Adenoma (polyp)	• Benign epithelial tumor	• Asymptomatic • Dull right upper quadrant (RUQ) pain • Intolerance to fatty foods	• Echogenic intraluminal focus(i) • Immobile • Nonshadowing • Thickening of the gallbladder wall	• Cholelithiasis • Fold in the gallbladder • Carcinoma
Adenomyomatosis	• Hyperplasia of the epithelial and muscle layers of the gallbladder wall	• Asymptomatic • Dull RUQ pain • Intolerance to fatty foods	• Echogenic intraluminal focus • Diffuse comet tail reverberation artifact • Immobile	• Cholelithiasis • Fold in the gallbladder • Carcinoma
Cholesterolosis	• Local disturbance in cholesterol metabolism • Not associated with serum cholesterol levels • Two types— cholesterosis and cholesterol polyps	• Asymptomatic • Abdominal pain	• Echogenic intraluminal foci • Nonshadowing • Normal gallbladder in the majority of cases • Strawberry appearance with cholesterosis	• Cholelithiasis • Carcinoma • Fold in the gallbladder

Gallbladder Pathology—cont'd

PATHOLOGY	ETIOLOGY	CLINICAL FINDINGS	SONOGRAPHIC FINDINGS	DIFFERENTIAL CONSIDERATIONS
Cholelithiasis	• Abnormal bile composition • Bile stasis • Infection Risk Factors • Family history • Obesity • Pregnancy • Diabetes • Female prevalence (4:1)	• Asymptomatic • RUQ pain • Epigastric pain • Chest or shoulder pain • Elevated liver function tests • Nausea/vomiting • Postprandial pain • Fatty food intolerance	• Hyperechoic intraluminal focus(i) • Posterior acoustic shadowing • Mobile • Wall-echo-shadow (WES)	• Intestinal air • Adenomyomatosis • Polyp • Fold in the gallbladder • Surgical clip
Porcelain gallbladder	• Decrease in vascular supply to the gallbladder • Cystic duct obstruction causing bile stasis • Chronic low-grade infection Risk Factors • Female prevalence	• Asymptomatic • Vague RUQ pain	• Gallstones (95%) • Hyperechoic wall • Marked posterior acoustic shadowing • Diffuse or localized	• Contracted gallbladder with stones (WES) • Intestinal air • Adenomyomatosis
Mirizzi syndrome	• Impacted stone in the cystic duct or gallbladder neck • Obstruction of the CHD • Jaundice • Dilated CHD superior to the obstruction	• RUQ pain • Jaundice • Elevated bilirubin and alkaline phosphatase • Increase in aspartate aminotransferase (AST) and alanine aminotransferase (ALT) levels	• Immobile calculus in the cystic duct or neck of the gallbladder • Dilatation of the intrahepatic and common hepatic ducts • Normal common bile duct	• Choledocholithiasis
Sludge	• Prolonged fasting • Biliary stasis • Biliary obstruction • Cholecystitis • Sickle cell anemia	• Asymptomatic • RUQ pain • Nausea/vomiting	• Nonshadowing low-amplitude echoes layering in the dependent portion of the gallbladder • Echoes move slowly with position change • May fill entire gallbladder	• Technical factors • Intestinal air • Carcinoma
Gallbladder carcinoma Fifth most common malignancy	• Adenocarcinoma in 80% of cases Risk Factors • Cholelithiasis • Porcelain gallbladder • Cholecystitis • Female prevalence (4:1) • 60-70 years of age	• Asymptomatic • RUQ pain • Palpable mass • Jaundice • Anorexia • Nausea/ vomiting • Elevated alkaline phosphatase • Mild increase in AST and ALT levels	• Thick, irregular gallbladder wall • Irregular intraluminal mass • Immobile mass • Cholelithiasis (90% cases) • Lymphadenopathy	• Adenoma • Sludge • Cholecystitis • Adenomyomatosis • Metastases
Metastatic gallbladder disease	Direct Extension: • Pancreas • Stomach • Bile duct Indirect Extension: • Melanoma • Lung • Kidney • Esophagus	• Asymptomatic • RUQ pain • Jaundice • Nausea/vomiting • Elevated alkaline phosphatase	• Focal gallbladder wall thickening • Intraluminal mass • Nonshadowing • Absence of gallstones	• Cholecystitis • Adenoma • Primary carcinoma

Gallbladder Inflammation

INFLAMMATION	ETIOLOGY	CLINICAL FINDINGS	SONOGRAPHIC FINDINGS	DIFFERENTIAL CONSIDERATIONS
Acute cholecystitis **Complications** • **Ascending cholangitis** • **Empyema** • **Perforation** • **Pericholecystic or liver abscess** • **Septicemia**	• Obstruction of the cystic duct • Infection • Idiopathic	• Severe epigastric or RUQ pain • Biliary colic • Positive Murphy sign • Nausea/vomiting • Jaundice • Elevated aspartate aminotransferase (AST), bilirubin, and alkaline phosphatase • Leukocytosis	• Thick, edematous gallbladder wall; "halo sign" • Impacted stone in the cystic duct or gallbladder neck • Cholelithiasis (90% cases) • Pericholecystic fluid • Positive Murphy sign • Sludge	• Liver abscess • Ascites • Nonfasting patient
Emphysematous cholecystitis	• Cholelithiasis • Idiopathic	• RUQ pain • Nausea/vomiting • Fever • Leukocytosis	• Echogenic focus(i) within the gallbladder wall or lumen • Ill-defined posterior acoustic shadowing • Cholelithiasis • Pericholecystic fluid	• Acute cholecystitis • Porcelain gallbladder • Large gallstone • Intestinal air
Gangrenous cholecystitis	Risk Factors • Diabetes • Elderly • Male prevalence	• RUQ pain radiating to the back • Positive Murphy sign • Fever • Leukocytosis • Elevated AST, bilirubin, and alkaline phosphatase	• Diffuse echogenic focus within the lumen • Immobile • Nonshadowing • Nonlayering	• Acute cholecystitis • Emphysematous cholecystitis • Adenoma • Carcinoma
Gallbladder perforation	Risk Factors • Diabetes • Elderly • Infection • Cholelithiasis • Trauma	• RUQ mass • Severe RUQ or epigastric pain • Positive Murphy sign • Nausea/vomiting • Leukocytosis	• Edematous, thick gallbladder wall • Pericholecystic fluid • Cholelithiasis	• Ascites • Hepatic abscess • Perforated peptic ulcer
Chronic cholecystitis	• Recurrent inflammation secondary to infection, obstruction, or metabolic disorders	• Asymptomatic • Vague RUQ pain • Heartburn • Fatty food intolerance • Intermittent nausea/vomiting • Mild increase in aspartate aminotransferase and alanine aminotransferase levels • Possible increase in alkaline phosphatase and bilirubin	• Small or contracted gallbladder • Thick, hyperechoic walls • Cholelithiasis (90% of cases) • Posterior acoustic shadowing • Sludge	• Nonfasting patient • Cholelithiasis • Porcelain gallbladder • Carcinoma
Hydrops	• Obstruction of the cystic duct • Prolong biliary stasis • Surgery • Hepatitis • Gastroenteritis • Diabetes	• Asymptomatic • RUQ or epigastric pain • Nausea/vomiting • Palpable mass	• Enlargement • Gallbladder diameter exceeding 5 cm • Thin, hyperechoic walls	• Normal gallbladder • Hepatic cyst • Phrygian cap
Gallbladder varices	• Portal hypertension • Portal vein thrombosis • Cholecystitis	• Dependent on etiology	• Multiple tortuous tubular structures in the gallbladder periphery • Vascular flow	• Intestinal fluid • Normal vessels

BILIARY REVIEW TEST

1. Cholangiocarcinoma located at the junction of the right and left hepatic ducts is termed a(n):
   a. biloma
   b. phrygian cap
   c. phlegmon
   d. hepatoma
   e. Klatskin tumor

2. Which of the following patient positions may aid in visualization of the cystic duct?
   a. supine
   b. prone
   c. Trendelenburg
   d. left posterior oblique
   e. left lateral decubitus

3. A small septation located between the neck and body of the gallbladder BEST describes:
   a. a junctional fold
   b. a phrygian cap
   c. Hartmann pouch
   d. adenomyomatosis
   e. diverticulosis of the gallbladder

4. A 73-year-old patient complains of vague right upper quadrant pain. A hyperechoic focus with marked posterior acoustic shadowing is demonstrated in the anterior wall of the gallbladder. This history is most consistent with which of the following pathologies?
   a. emphysematous cholecystitis
   b. porcelain gallbladder
   c. cholelithiasis
   d. Mirizzi syndrome
   e. adenomyomatosis

5. Nonshadowing, low-amplitude echoes located in the dependent portion of the gallbladder BEST describes:
   a. polypoid masses
   b. cholelithiasis
   c. cholecystitis
   d. biliary sludge
   e. adenomyomatosis

6. All of the following are associated with cholesterolosis EXCEPT:
   a. cholesterosis
   b. cholesterol polyp
   c. serum cholesterol levels
   d. local disturbance in cholesterol metabolism
   e. accumulation of triglycerides and esterified sterols in the gallbladder wall

7. The spiral valves of Heister are located in which of the following structures?
   a. common bile duct
   b. duct of Santorini
   c. common hepatic duct
   d. cystic duct
   e. duct of Wirsung

8. A patient presents with a sudden onset of abdominal pain and extreme tenderness over the gallbladder fossa. Localized gallbladder wall thickening is visualized on ultrasound. This most likely represents:
   a. acute cholecystitis
   b. a porcelain gallbladder
   c. a hydropic gallbladder
   d. adenomyomatosis
   e. a nonfasting gallbladder

Using Fig. 8-2, answer questions 9 and 10.

9. A 43-year-old female presents to the emergency department complaining of right upper quadrant pain and a sudden onset of jaundice. Which of the following findings is identified in this sonogram?
   a. cholangitis
   b. choledocholithiasis
   c. cholangiocarcinoma
   d. cholecystitis
   e. pancreas neoplasm

10. Complications with this abnormality would most likely include:
    a. biliary obstruction
    b. cholecystitis
    c. cholelithiasis
    d. lymphadenopathy
    e. portal hypertension

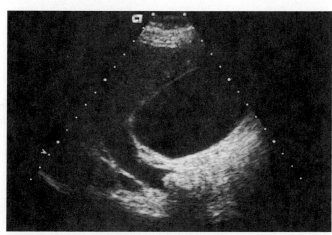

FIG. 8-2 Longitudinal sonogram of the right upper quadrant.

Using Fig. 8-3, answer question 11.

11. A patient presents with a two-day history of acute right upper quadrant tenderness and elevated liver function tests. A sonogram of the gallbladder demonstrates cholelithiasis and:
    a. emphysematous cholecystitis
    b. acute cholecystitis
    c. tumefactive sludge
    d. adenomyomatosis
    e. metastatic gallbladder disease

Using Fig. 8-4, answer questions 12 and 13.

12. The arrows are identifying which of the following structures?
    a. phrygian cap
    b. gallbladder duplication
    c. junctional fold
    d. adenomyomatosis
    e. gallbladder diverticulum

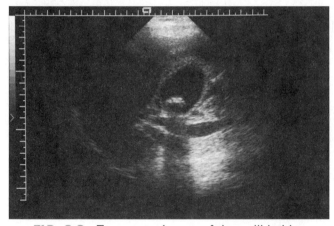

FIG. 8-3   Transverse image of the gallbladder.

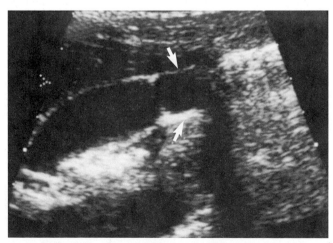

FIG. 8-4   Sagittal image of the gallbladder.

13. Which type of sonographic artifact is demonstrated adjacent to this structure?
    a. grating lobe
    b. refraction
    c. reverberation
    d. mirror image
    e. slice thickness

14. The biliary system has three main functions. Which of the following describes one of these functions?
    a. produces bile
    b. produces cholesterol
    c. stores enzymes
    d. stores fats
    e. stores bile

15. Which of the following conditions is most likely to occur with an episode of prolonged fasting?
    a. cholelithiasis
    b. biliary sludge
    c. cholangitis
    d. gallbladder carcinoma
    e. polypoid mass

16. All of the following are considered layers of the gallbladder wall EXCEPT:
    a. epithelial
    b. serosal
    c. muscular
    d. endothelial
    e. subserosal

17. The distal portion of the common bile duct terminates in which of the following structures?
    a. gallbladder
    b. pylorus
    c. hepatic hilum
    d. duodenum
    e. pancreas

18. In the portal hepatis, the common hepatic duct is located:
    a. posterior to the main portal vein
    b. lateral to the proper hepatic artery
    c. medial to the proper hepatic artery
    d. anterior to the common hepatic artery
    e. medial to the main portal vein

19. Indications for a biliary sonogram include all of the following EXCEPT:
    a. abdominal pain
    b. postprandial pain
    c. positive McBurney sign
    d. elevation of liver function tests
    e. intolerance to fatty foods

20. Which of the following hormones stimulates gallbladder contraction and the secretion of pancreatic enzymes?
    a. amylase
    b. lipase
    c. gastrin
    d. cholecystokinin
    e. bilirubin

21. The diameter of a normal fasting adult gallbladder should **not** exceed:
    a. 3 cm
    b. 5 cm
    c. 7 cm
    d. 10 cm
    e. 15 cm

Using Fig. 8-5, answer question 22.

22. An afebrile patient presents with a 2-week history of moderate right upper quadrant pain and a lack of appetite. The findings demonstrated in this sonogram most likely represent:
    a. an abscess
    b. empyema
    c. a large adenoma
    d. carcinoma
    e. biliary sludge

Using Fig. 8-6, answer questions 23 and 24.

23. The hyperechoic linear structure identified by the arrow is the:
    a. ligamentum venosum
    b. ligamentum teres
    c. main lobar fissure
    d. falciform ligament
    e. intrasegmental fissure

24. This hyperechoic structure is routinely used as a sonographic landmark to locate which of the following structures?
    a. caudate lobe
    b. head of the pancreas
    c. gallbladder
    d. left lobe of the liver
    e. common hepatic duct

Using Fig. 8-7, answer questions 25 and 26.

25. A patient presents with a history of moderate right upper quadrant pain over the last few months. A sonogram of the gallbladder reveals which of the following pathologies?
    a. cholelithiasis
    b. adenomyomatosis
    c. acute cholecystitis
    d. porcelain gallbladder
    e. tumefactive sludge

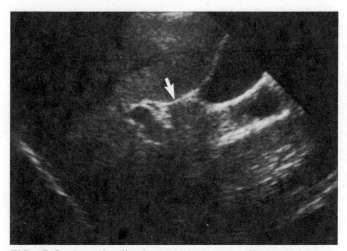

FIG. 8-6 Longitudinal sonogram near the porta hepatic.

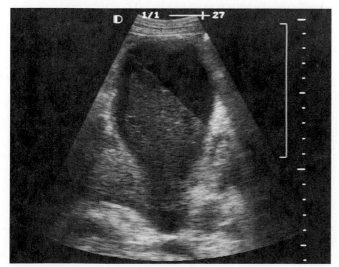

FIG. 8-5 Supine transverse sonogram of the gallbladder.

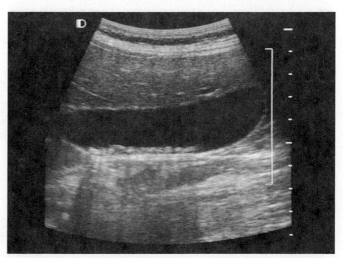

FIG. 8-7 Longitudinal image of the gallbladder.

26. Which of the following technical factors would aid in the diagnosis of this pathology?
    a. fatty meal
    b. drinking 12 oz of water
    c. an intercostal approach
    d. deep inspiration
    e. patient position change

27. Complications in biliary atresia include all of the following EXCEPT:
    a. death
    b. cirrhosis
    c. cholangitis
    d. portal hypertension
    e. hydropic gallbladder

28. Which of the following enzymes is produced primarily by the liver, bone, and placenta?
    a. alanine aminotransferase (ALT)
    b. alkaline phosphatase
    c. aspartate aminotransferase (AST)
    d. bilirubin
    e. prothrombin

29. A decrease in diameter of the common bile duct after ingestion of a fatty meal is associated with:
    a. normal findings
    b. cholecystitis
    c. distal pathology
    d. obstructive jaundice
    e. proximal pathology

30. Thickness of the gallbladder wall in a normal fasting patient should NOT exceed:
    a. 2 mm
    b. 3 mm
    c. 6 mm
    d. 8 mm
    e. 10 mm

31. Dilatation of the intrahepatic ducts with normal extrahepatic ducts is characteristic of:
    a. cholangitis
    b. a choledochal cyst
    c. a Klatskin tumor
    d. choledocholithiasis
    e. a pancreatic neoplasm

32. All of the following are possible complications of acute cholecystitis EXCEPT:
    a. septicemia
    b. cholelithiasis
    c. liver abscess
    d. empyema
    e. perforation of the gallbladder

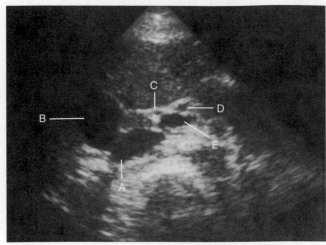

FIG. 8-8 Transverse image of the hepatic hilum.

33. As dilatation of the intrahepatic biliary tree progresses, the portal system becomes:
    a. rounded
    b. fusiform
    c. saccular
    d. flattened
    e. beaded

Using Fig. 8-8, answer questions 34-36.

34. Which of the following letters corresponds to the hepatic artery?
    a. A
    b. B
    c. C
    d. D
    e. E

35. Which of the following letters corresponds to the inferior vena cava?
    a. A
    b. B
    c. C
    d. D
    e. E

36. Which of the following letters corresponds to the main portal vein?
    a. A
    b. B
    c. C
    d. D
    e. E

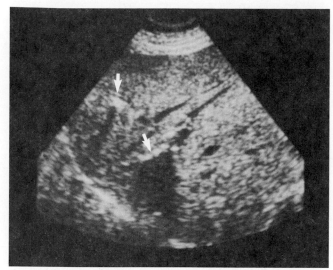

FIG. 8-9 Longitudinal sonogram of the liver.

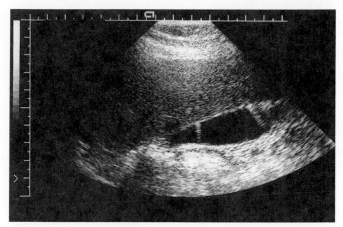

FIG. 8-10 Longitudinal sonogram of the right upper quadrant.

Using Fig. 8-9, answer question 37.

37. An asymptomatic patient with a history of choledochojejunostomy 3 years prior presents for an abdominal ultrasound. Hyperechoic foci are documented in the liver and identified by the arrows. Based on the clinical history, these foci most likely represent:
    a. ascariasis
    b. pneumobilia
    c. arterial calcifications
    d. choledocholithiasis
    e. abscess formation

Using Fig. 8-10, answer questions 38 and 39.

38. A 30-year-old asymptomatic patient presents with a history of hepatitis B. A sonogram is ordered to rule out pathology. The gallbladder demonstrates multiple echogenic foci. Based on this clinical history, the sonographic findings are most consistent with:
    a. cholelithiasis
    b. acute cholecystitis
    c. chronic cholecystitis
    d. adenomyomatosis
    e. malignant neoplasm

39. Which of the following acoustic artifacts is associated with this finding?
    a. comet tail artifact
    b. edge artifact
    c. mirror image
    d. posterior acoustic enhancement
    e. posterior acoustic shadowing

40. A small protrusion near the neck of the gallbladder describes:
    a. fetal lobulation
    b. a junctional fold
    c. Hartmann pouch
    d. a choledochal cyst
    e. Morison's pouch

41. In biliary obstruction, identifying multiple anechoic tubular structures in the left lobe of the liver is termed:
    a. parallel channeling
    b. star effect
    c. Murphy sign
    d. varices
    e. mouse sign

42. Which of the following liver function tests is produced from the breakdown of hemoglobin?
    a. aspartate aminotransferase
    b. alkaline phosphatase
    c. bilirubin
    d. alpha fetoprotein
    e. alanine aminotransferase

43. Predisposing factors linked to the development of cholelithiasis include all of the following EXCEPT:
    a. pregnancy
    b. obesity
    c. diabetes mellitus
    d. hepatitis
    e. female gender

44. Which of the following technical factors would most likely aid in demonstrating shadowing posterior to small-caliber gallstones?
    a. increased transducer frequency
    b. decreased overall gain
    c. increased dynamic range
    d. decreased image depth
    e. fewer number of focal zones

45. Intraductal pressure differences are affected by all of the following EXCEPT:
  a. resorption of bile in the gallbladder
  b. bile flow from the liver
  c. activity of the sphincter of Oddi
  d. filling of the bile in the gallbladder
  e. location of the bile duct

46. All of the following are potential differential considerations in cases of pneumobilia **except:**
  a. stent
  b. cavernous hemangioma
  c. biliary calculus
  d. arterial calcification
  e. surgical clip

Using Fig. 8-11, answer questions 47 and 48.

47. An inpatient presents with a history of abdominal pain and weight loss. Echogenic foci are identified in the gallbladder. Differential considerations for these findings may include all of the following EXCEPT:
  a. polypoid masses
  b. gallbladder carcinoma
  c. metastatic gallbladder disease
  d. tumefactive sludge
  e. adenomas

48. Additional clinical history of pancreatic carcinoma is documented in the patient's chart. Multiple target-shaped lesions are demonstrated within the liver. Given this additional information, the echogenic foci are most suspicious for:
  a. polypoid masses
  b. gallbladder carcinoma
  c. metastatic gallbladder disease
  d. tumefactive sludge
  e. adenomas

Using Fig. 8-12, answer question 49.

49. Which of the following congenital gallbladder anomalies is MOST LIKELY demonstrated in this sonogram of the gallbladder?
  a. strawberry gallbladder
  b. hourglass shape
  c. gallbladder duplication
  d. multiseptated gallbladder
  e. intrahepatic location

Using Fig. 8-13 (and color plate 3), answer question 50.

50. A patient presents with a positive Murphy sign and elevated bilirubin level. Based on this clinical history, the sonogram is most suspicious for:
  a. Wall-echo-shadow (WES)
  b. biliary sludge
  c. acute cholecystitis
  d. cholangiocarcinoma
  e. chronic cholecystitis

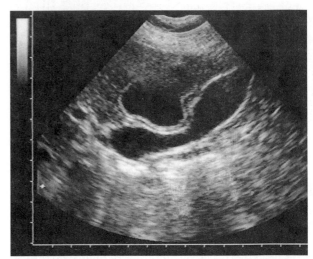

FIG. 8-12   Longitudinal image of the gallbladder fossa.

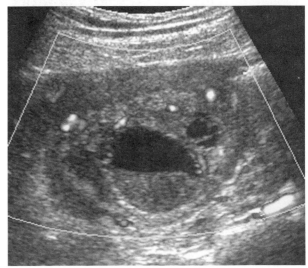

FIG. 8-13   Transverse power Doppler image (see color plate 3).

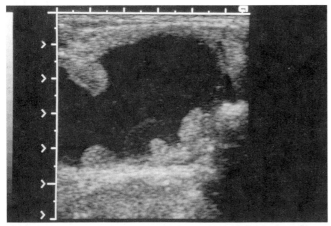

FIG. 8-11   Left lateral decubitus image of the gallbladder.

CHAPTER 9

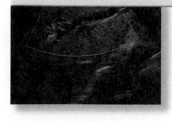

Pancreas

KEY TERMS

acute pancreatitis   acute inflammation causing escape of pancreatic enzymes from the acinar cells into the surrounding tissue. Most commonly caused by biliary disease followed by alcohol abuse.

amylase   digestive enzyme produced in the pancreas that aids in converting starches to sugars; also produced in the salivary glands, liver, and fallopian tubes.

ampulla of Vater   opening in the duodenum for the entrance of the common bile duct.

annular pancreas   anomaly caused by the failure of a normal regression of the left ventral bud.

chronic pancreatitis   multiple, persistent, or prolonged episodes of pancreatitis.

cystic fibrosis   autosomal recessive exocrine gland disorder where organs become clogged with mucus secreted by the exocrine glands.

endocrine   pertaining to a process in which a group of cells secrete into the blood or lymph circulation a substance (i.e., hormone) that has a specific effect on tissues in another part of the body (*Mosby's Dictionary 2006*).

exocrine   the process of secreting outwardly through a duct to the surface of an organ.

duct of Santorini   secondary secretory duct of the pancreas.

duct of Wirsung   primary secretory duct of the pancreas.

lipase   enzyme produced primarily by the pancreas that changes fats to fatty acids and glycerol; increases after damage has occurred to the pancreas.

pancreaticoduodenal   pertaining to the pancreas and duodenum.

pancreatoduodenectomy   also known as Whipple procedure; a surgical resection of the pancreatic head or periampullary area; relieves obstruction of the biliary tree often due to a malignant tumor. The remaining normal pancreatic tissue is attached to the duodenum.

phlegmon   an extension of pancreatic inflammation into the peripancreatic tissues.

portosplenic confluence   the joining of the portal, splenic, and superior mesenteric veins.

pseudocyst   a space or cavity without a lining membrane, containing gas or liquid; caused by a leakage of pancreatic enzymes into surrounding tissues.

sphincter of Oddi   a sheath of muscle fibers surrounding the distal common bile and pancreatic ducts as they cross the wall of the duodenum.

Whipple procedure   see pancreatoduodenectomy.

PANCREAS PHYSIOLOGY

FUNCTIONS OF THE PANCREAS

Exocrine

- Highly digestive enzymes are secreted by the acinar cells and drain into the duodenum through the pancreatic ducts.
  a. amylase—breaks down carbohydrates.
  b. lipase—breaks down fats.
  c. trypsin—breaks down proteins into amino acids.
- Releases hormones once food enters the duodenum.
  a. cholecystokinin—stimulates secretion of pancreatic enzymes and contraction of the gallbladder.
  b. gastrin—stimulates secretion of gastric acids.
  c. secretin—stimulates secretion of bicarbonate.

Endocrine

- Islet cells of Langerhans secrete hormones directly into the bloodstream.
  a. alpha cells secrete glucagon (increases blood glucose).
  b. beta cells secrete insulin (decreases blood glucose).
  c. delta cells secrete somatostatin (autoregulator).

PANCREAS ANATOMY (Fig. 9-1)

- An elongated organ lying transverse and obliquely in the epigastric and hypochondriac regions of the body.
- Retroperitoneal organ located posterior to the lesser sac.

PANCREAS DIVISIONS AND LOCATION

Tail

- Most superior portion of the pancreas lying anterior and parallel with the splenic vein.
- Lies anterior to the upper pole of the left kidney, posterior to the stomach, and lateral to the spine.
- Generally extends toward the splenic hilum (occasionally left renal hilum).

Body

- Largest and most anterior aspect of the pancreas.
- Lies anterior to the aorta, superior mesenteric artery, superior mesenteric vein, splenic vein, left renal vein, and spine.
- Lies posterior to the antrum of the stomach.

Neck

- Lies directly anterior to the superior mesenteric vein and portosplenic confluence.
- Lies posterior to the pylorus of the stomach.

Head

- Lies in the descending portion of the duodenum, lateral to the superior mesenteric vein and anterior to the inferior vena cava.
- Main portal vein and hepatic artery lie inferior to the pancreatic head.
- Gastroduodenal artery lies in the anterolateral portion of the pancreatic head.
- Common bile duct is situated in the posterolateral and inferior portion of the pancreatic head.

Uncinate Process

- Portion of the pancreatic head directly posterior to the superior mesenteric vein and anterior to the aorta and inferior vena cava.
- Variable in size.

FIG. 9-1
Pancreas anatomy.

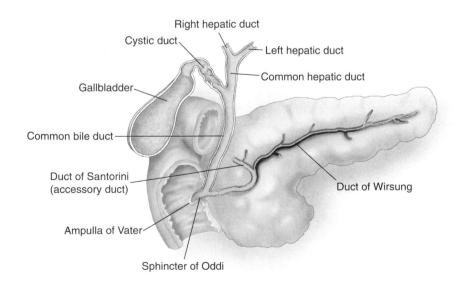

DUCTS OF THE PANCREAS

- Contain smooth muscles that aid in transportation of the pancreatic enzymes.

Duct of Wirsung

- Primary secretory duct extending the entire length of the pancreas.
- Joins the distal common bile duct entering the descending portion of the duodenum through the ampulla of Vater.
- Frequently visualized in the body of the pancreas.

Duct of Santorini

- Secondary secretory duct draining the upper anterior portion of the pancreas.
- Enters the duodenum at the minor papilla approximately 2 cm proximal to the ampulla of Vater.

CONGENITAL ANOMALIES

PANCREATIC DIVISUM

- Failure of the normal fusion of the ducts of Wirsung and Santorini.
- Duct of Wirsung is small and only drains the inferior portion of the pancreatic head.
- Duct of Santorini drains the majority of the pancreas.
- Associated with a higher incidence of pancreatitis.

ANNULAR PANCREAS

- Rare anomaly caused by the failure of a normal regression of the left ventral bud.
- The head of the pancreas surrounds the duodenum, resulting in obstruction of the biliary tree or duodenum.
- Male prevalence.

ECTOPIC PANCREATIC TISSUE

- Ectopic tissue located in the stomach, duodenum, and small or large intestines.
- Small, polypoid-appearing mass.

CYSTIC FIBROSIS

- Autosomal recessive exocrine gland disorder in which organs become clogged with mucus secreted by the exocrine glands.
- Pancreas becomes hyperechoic as a result of fibrosis or fatty replacement.
- Small cysts may be present.

Pancreas Size			
	HEAD	**NECK**	**BODY**	**TAIL**
Adult	2.0-3.0 cm	1.0-2.0 cm	1.0-3.0 cm	2.0-3.0 cm

SONOGRAPHIC APPEARANCE

NORMAL PANCREAS

- Smooth or coarse homogeneous parenchyma.
- Adult pancreas is either isoechoic or hyperechoic when compared to the normal liver.
- May appear hypoechoic in young children and hyperechoic in older adults.

ABNORMAL PANCREAS

- Irregular or heterogeneous parenchyma.
- Calcifications.

NORMAL PANCREATIC DUCT

- Anechoic nonvascular tubular structure.
- Smooth parallel hyperechoic walls measuring ≤3 mm in the head/neck and ≤2 mm in the body.
- Most commonly visualized in the body of the pancreas.

ABNORMAL PANCREATIC DUCT

- Anechoic nonvascular tubular structure.
- Irregular or nonparallel hyperechoic walls.
- Measurement exceeding 3 mm in the head/neck or 2 mm in the body.

TECHNIQUE

PREPARATION

- Patients should have nothing by mouth 6 to 8 hours prior to examination.
- Emergency examinations may be performed without preparation.

EXAMINATION TECHNIQUE

- Use the highest-frequency abdominal transducer possible to obtain optimal resolution for penetration depth.
- Proper focal zone and depth placement.
- The pancreas lies obliquely in the abdomen and may be difficult to visualize. Use the liver as an acoustical window.
- The entire pancreas and surrounding vascular landmarks must be examined and documented in two scanning planes from the level of the celiac axis to below the renal veins.
- Varying patient position and imaging windows should aid in visualization.
- Suspended inspiration, expiration, or Valsalva maneuver may optimize visualization.
- Distending the stomach with water may aid in outlining the pancreas.

INDICATIONS FOR ULTRASOUND EXAMINATION

- Severe epigastric pain.
- Elevated pancreatic enzymes.
- Biliary disease.
- Abdominal distension with hypoactive bowel sounds.
- Pancreatitis.
- Weight loss.
- Anorexia.
- Pancreas neoplasm.
- Evaluate mass from previous imaging study (i.e., CT).

LABORATORY VALUES

SERUM AMYLASE

- Normal range 25 to 125 U/L.
- Increases with pancreatitis and peptic ulcer disease.
- Decreases with hepatitis and cirrhosis.
- Remains elevated for approximately 24 hours in episodes of acute pancreatitis.

URINE AMYLASE

- Remains increased longer than serum amylase in episodes of acute pancreatitis.

SERUM LIPASE

- Normal range 10 to 140 U/L.
- Remains elevated for a longer period of time (up to 14 days).
- Increases with pancreatitis, obstruction of the pancreatic duct, pancreatic carcinoma, acute cholecystitis, cirrhosis, and severe renal disease.

Pancreas Inflammation

PANCREAS INFLAMMATION	ETIOLOGY	CLINICAL FINDINGS	SONOGRAPHIC FINDINGS	DIFFERENTIAL CONSIDERATIONS
Acute pancreatitis	• Biliary disease • Alcohol abuse • Trauma • Peptic ulcer disease • Idiopathic	• Abrupt onset of epigastric pain • Nausea/vomiting • Elevated lipase and amylase	• Normal findings • Decrease in parenchymal echogenicity • Smooth borders • Enlargement	• Normal pancreas • Neoplasm
Chronic pancreatitis	• Repeated, prolonged, or persistent attacks of pancreatitis • Hypocalcemia • Hyperlipidemia	• Chronic right upper quadrant (RUQ) or epigastric pain • Nausea/vomiting • Weight loss • Abnormal glucose tolerance test • Normal amylase and lipase values	• Increase in parenchymal echogenicity • Irregular borders • Calcifications • Pseudocyst formation • Atrophy • Prominent pancreatic duct	• Fatty replacement • Neoplasm
Cystic fibrosis	• Exocrine gland disorder	• Variable	• Increase in parenchymal echogenicity • Small cysts • Nonvisualization of the gallbladder • Biliary sludge • Thick, irregular folds in the GI tract ("donut sign")	• Chronic pancreatitis • Fatty replacement • Polycystic disease

Complications of Pancreatitis

COMPLICATIONS	DESCRIPTION	CLINICAL FINDINGS	SONOGRAPHIC FINDINGS
Abscess	• Develops due to infection of the necrotic pancreas	• Abdominal pain • Leukocytosis • Nausea/vomiting • Fever	• Ranges from anechoic to echogenic • Irregular or smooth borders • Fluid-debris levels
Duodenal obstruction	• High protein concentration in the pancreas enzymes can irritate the duodenum	• Abdominal pain • Abdominal distention • Nausea/vomiting • Constipation	• Limited bowel peristalsis
Hemorrhage	• Rapid development of inflammation causing necrosis and hemorrhage	• Severe abdominal pain • Nausea/vomiting • Elevated amylase • Decrease in hematocrit level	• Well defined homogeneous mass • Cystic mass with debris • Fluid-debris levels

Continued

Complications of Pancreatitis—cont'd

COMPLICATIONS	DESCRIPTION	CLINICAL FINDINGS	SONOGRAPHIC FINDINGS
Phlegmon	• Extension of pancreatic inflammation into the peripancreatic tissues	• Severe abdominal pain • Nausea/vomiting • Elevated amylase	• Hypoechoic solid mass • Posterior acoustic enhancement • Irregular borders • Usually involves the lesser sac and anterior pararenal space
Pseudocyst	• Focal collection of inflammatory necrotic tissue, blood, and pancreas secretions • Most often located in the lesser sac followed by the anterior pararenal space	• Abdominal pain • Palpable mass • Elevated amylase	• Anechoic or complex mass • Thick, irregular borders • Variable shape

Cysts of the Pancreas

PATHOLOGY	ETIOLOGY	CLINICAL FINDINGS	SONOGRAPHIC FINDINGS	DIFFERENTIAL CONSIDERATIONS
Cyst	• Congenital anomalous development of the pancreatic duct Acquired: • Retention cyst • Parasitic cyst • Neoplastic cyst	• Asymptomatic • Dyspepsia • Jaundice	• Anechoic mass • Smooth borders • Posterior acoustic enhancement	• Fluid-filled stomach • Pseudocyst • Polycystic disease
Cystadenoma	Microcystic: • Accounts for 50% of cystic neoplasms involving the pancreas Macrocystic: • Arise from the ducts • Malignant potential	• Asymptomatic • Abdominal pain • Palpable mass • Female prevalence	• Majority are located in the body and tail Microcystic: • Echogenic or complex mass Macrocystic: • Multiloculated cystic mass • Irregular margins • Solid nodules • Displacement of the common bile duct, pancreatic duct, and splenic vein may occur	• Pseudocyst • Polycystic disease • Abscess • Fluid-filled stomach
Polycystic disease	• Associated with polycystic liver or kidney disease	• Asymptomatic • Abdominal pain	• Multiple cysts • Associated with multiples cysts in the liver, kidney, or spleen	• True cyst • Fluid-filled loops of bowel • Cystadenoma
Pseudocyst	• Inflammation of the pancreas	• Abdominal pain • Palpable mass • Elevated amylase	• Anechoic or complex mass • Thick, irregular borders • Variable in size and shape	• Fluid-filled stomach • Neoplasm • Dilated pancreatic duct • Left renal vein • Omental cyst • Cystadenoma

Pancreas Neoplasms

NEOPLASM	ETIOLOGY	CLINICAL FINDINGS	SONOGRAPHIC FINDINGS	DIFFERENTIAL CONSIDERATIONS
Carcinoma	• Adenocarcinoma in 90% of cases • 75% involve the head of the pancreas • 20% involve the body	• Abdominal pain • Severe back pain • Weight loss • Painless jaundice • Anorexia • New onset of diabetes	• Hypoechoic mass in the pancreas • Irregular borders • Dilated biliary tree • Hydropic gallbladder • Liver metastasis • Ascites	• Focal pancreatitis • Adenoma • Caudate lobe of the liver
Islet cell tumor	Functional: • Insulinoma • Gastrinoma Nonfunctional: • 90% are malignant • Comprise one-third of all islet cell tumors	Insulinoma: • Increase in insulin levels Gastrinoma: • Gastric hyperstimulation associated with peptic ulcer disease	• Small, well-defined hypoechoic mass • Large tumors are more echogenic • Typically located in the body or tail • Calcifications • Necrotic cystic areas are more likely malignant	• Adenoma • Carcinoma • Complex cyst

FIG. 9-2
Pancreatoduodenectomy.

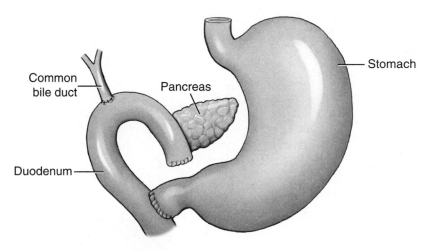

PANCREATODUODENECTOMY (WHIPPLE PROCEDURE)
(Fig. 9-2)

PREOPERATIVE CRITERIA

- Absence of extrapancreatic metastasis.
- Portal, splenic, and superior mesenteric veins are evaluated for patency and absence of tumor or thrombus.
- Celiac axis and superior mesenteric arteries are evaluated for patency.

BASIC PROCEDURE

- Gallbladder is removed.
- Common duct is ligated superior to the cystic duct and anastomosed to the duodenum distal to the pancreas.
- Remaining pancreas tissue is attached to the duodenum.
- Stomach is anastomosed distal to the bile duct.

PANCREAS REVIEW QUESTIONS

1. Demonstration of the pancreatic head surrounding the duodenum is consistent with:
   a. pancreas divisum
   b. ectopic pancreas tissue
   c. a phlegmon
   d. an annular pancreas
   e. the uncinate process

2. Indications for a sonogram of the pancreas include all of the following EXCEPT:
   a. flank pain
   b. biliary disease
   c. weight loss
   d. severe epigastric pain
   e. elevated serum amylase

3. Which of the following enzymes is responsible for the breakdown of proteins into amino acids?
   a. amylase
   b. gastrin
   c. lipase
   d. trypsin
   e. cholecystokinin

4. The location of the uncinate process is described as:
   a. superior to the aorta
   b. anterior to the main portal vein
   c. posterior to the superior mesenteric vein
   d. lateral to the gastroduodenal artery
   e. posterior to the inferior vena cava

5. The most common complication associated with acute pancreatitis is a(n):
   a. abscess
   b. phlegmon
   c. insulinoma
   d. pseudocyst
   e. bowel obstruction

6. Islet cells of Langerhans secrete hormones directly into the:
   a. duodenum
   b. common bile duct
   c. bloodstream
   d. lymphatic circulation
   e. main pancreatic duct

7. In a Whipple procedure, normal pancreatic tissue is attached to the:
   a. liver
   b. stomach
   c. duodenum
   d. spleen
   e. common bile duct

8. Extension of pancreatic inflammation into the peripancreatic tissues is called a(n):
   a. annular pancreas
   b. pseudocyst
   c. phlegmon
   d. abscess
   e. pancreatic divisum

9. The **most common** cause of acute pancreatitis is:
   a. trauma
   b. hyperlipidemia
   c. alcohol abuse
   d. peptic ulcer disease
   e. biliary disease

Using Fig. 9-3, answer question 10.

10. A 59-year-old male inpatient presents with a history of acute pancreatitis. His clinical symptoms include abdominal pain, palpable left upper quadrant mass, and extreme elevation in pancreatic enzymes. Based on this clinical history, the calipers in this sonogram are MOST LIKELY measuring a(n):
    a. biloma
    b. phlegmon
    c. pseudocyst
    d. islet cell tumor
    e. duodenal obstruction

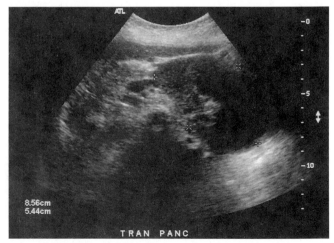

FIG. 9-3 Transverse image of the pancreas.

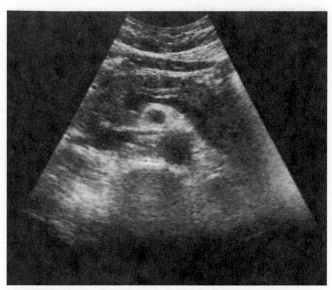

FIG. 9-4 Transverse image of the pancreas.

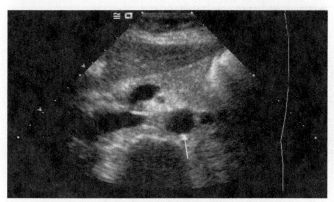

FIG. 9-5 Transverse image of the pancreas.

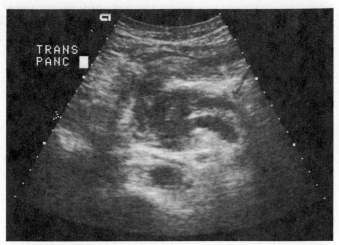

FIG. 9-6 Transverse image of the pancreas.

Using Fig. 9-6, answer questions 13 and 14.

13. A 91-year-old woman presents to the ultrasound department complaining of severe back pain, weight loss, and jaundice. Based on this clinical history, the findings in this sonogram are most suspicious for a(n):
    a. islet cell tumor
    b. abscess
    c. malignant neoplasm
    d. pseudocyst
    e. cystadenoma

14. The anechoic tubular structure demonstrated anterior to the splenic vein is most likely a(n):
    a. abscess
    b. gastric varix
    c. dilated pancreatic duct
    d. tortuous splenic artery
    e. enlarged superior mesenteric vein

15. Pseudocyst formation is most commonly located in which of the following abdominal recesses?
    a. lesser sac
    b. perirenal space
    c. anterior pararenal space
    d. subhepatic space
    e. subphrenic space

16. Which of the following enzymes changes fats into fatty acids and glycerol?
    a. amylase
    b. gastrin
    c. lipase
    d. secretin
    e. trypsin

17. Which region of the pancreas is located most superiorly?
    a. head
    b. body
    c. neck
    d. tail
    e. uncinate process

Using Fig. 9-4, answer question 11.

11. Which of the following structures is demonstrated directly anterior to the splenic vein?
    a. splenic artery
    b. superior mesenteric vein
    c. common bile duct
    d. gastroduodenal artery
    e. pancreatic duct

Using Fig. 9-5, answer question 12.

12. Which of the following vascular structures is identified by the arrow?
    a. aorta
    b. splenic vein
    c. splenic artery
    d. left renal vein
    e. superior mesenteric artery

18. Ectopic pancreatic tissue is most commonly located in which of the following organs?
    a. liver
    b. spleen
    c. stomach
    d. lung
    e. kidney

19. The pancreas and surrounding vascular landmarks should be examined from the level of the:
    a. celiac axis to below the renal veins
    b. superior mesenteric artery to below the renal arteries
    c. main portal vein to below the renal veins
    d. splenic artery to below the superior mesenteric vein
    e. superior mesenteric artery to below the superior mesenteric vein

20. Which of the following pathologies accounts for half of the cystic neoplasms involving the pancreas?
    a. retention cyst
    b. cystic fibrosis
    c. parasitic cyst
    d. polycystic disease
    e. microcystic cystadenoma

21. In acute pancreatitis, which of the following laboratory tests remains elevated longest?
    a. lipase
    b. amylase
    c. bilirubin
    d. glucose
    e. alkaline phosphatase

22. The main pancreatic duct is most commonly visualized in which section of the pancreas?
    a. head
    b. body
    c. neck
    d. tail
    e. uncinate process

23. The majority of nonfunctioning islet cell tumors are:
    a. malignant
    b. hyperechoic in echo texture
    c. located in the head of the pancreas
    d. dependent on insulin levels
    e. associated with peptic ulcer disease

24. All of the following sonographic characteristics are associated with chronic pancreatitis EXCEPT:
    a. increase in parenchymal echogenicity
    b. calcifications
    c. irregular borders
    d. pseudocyst formation
    e. enlargement

25. Clinical findings commonly associated with pancreatic carcinoma may include:
    a. chest pain
    b. weight gain
    c. abdominal bloating
    d. new onset of diabetes
    e. lower-extremity edema

Using Fig. 9-7, answer questions 26.

26. A patient presents with a history of elevating insulin levels. An abdominal ultrasound is ordered to rule out pancreatic disease. Based on this history, the sonographic finding is most suspicious for a(n):
    a. adenoma
    b. focal pancreatitis
    c. cystadenoma
    d. islet cell tumor
    e. adenocarcinoma

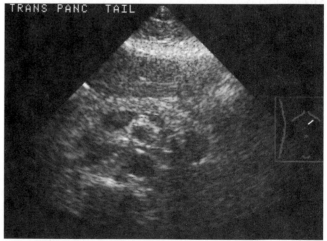

FIG. 9-7 Transverse image of the pancreas.

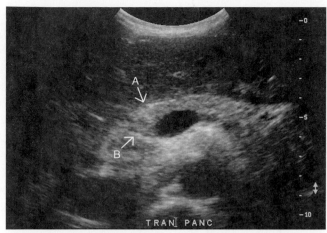

FIG. 9-8   Transverse image of the pancreas.

Using Fig. 9-8, answer questions 27 and 28.

27. Which of the following structures is most likely identified by arrow **A**?
    a. common bile duct
    b. proper hepatic artery
    c. gastroduodenal artery
    d. pancreatic cyst
    e. cystic artery

28. Which of the following structures is most likely identified by arrow **B**?
    a. common bile duct
    b. proper hepatic artery
    c. gastroduodenal artery
    d. cystic artery
    e. duodenum

29. An endocrine function of the pancreas includes secretion of:
    a. gastrin
    b. lipase
    c. insulin
    d. trypsin
    e. cholecystokinin

30. Which of the following vascular landmarks is located superior to the pancreas?
    a. splenic vein
    b. celiac axis
    c. superior mesenteric artery
    d. main portal vein
    e. superior mesenteric vein

31. The tail of the pancreas generally extends toward the:
    a. left renal hilum
    b. stomach
    c. splenic hilum
    d. pararenal space
    e. left adrenal gland

32. Which of the following vascular structures is used as a sonographic landmark in locating the tail of the pancreas?
    a. splenic artery
    b. left renal vein
    c. superior mesenteric vein
    d. splenic vein
    e. portosplenic confluence

33. The diameter of the pancreatic duct in the head/neck region should not exceed:
    a. 2 mm
    b. 3 mm
    c. 6 mm
    d. 10 mm
    e. 15 mm

34. Which of the following structures is responsible for the secretion of pancreatic enzymes?
    a. beta cells
    b. acinar cells
    c. alpha cells
    d. red blood cells
    e. islet cells of Langerhans

35. Which of the following best describes the location of the pancreatic neck?
    a. posterior to the superior mesenteric vein
    b. superior to the celiac axis
    c. anterior to the portosplenic confluence
    d. posterior to the superior mesenteric artery
    e. inferior to the renal veins

36. The majority of pancreatic malignancies involve which portion of the pancreas?
    a. head
    b. neck
    c. body
    d. tail
    e. uncinate process

37. In which section of the pancreas are islet cell tumors most commonly located?
    a. body and tail
    b. head and body
    c. neck and body
    d. head and tail
    e. tail and neck

38. The secondary secretory duct of the pancreas is termed the duct of:
    a. Whipple
    b. Langerhans
    c. Santorini
    d. Wirsung
    e. Vater

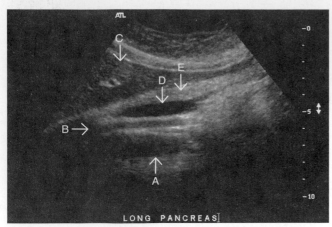

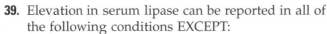

FIG. 9-9 Sagittal image of the pancreas.

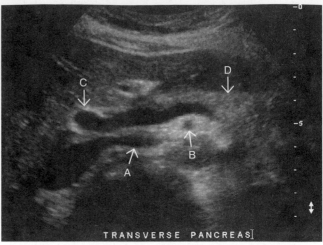

FIG. 9-10 Transverse image of the pancreas.

39. Elevation in serum lipase can be reported in all of the following conditions EXCEPT:
a. cirrhosis
b. acute pancreatitis
c. mononucleosis
d. acute cholecystitis
e. severe renal disease

Using Fig. 9-9, answer questions 40-42.

40. The superior mesenteric vein corresponds to which of the following letters?
a. A
b. B
c. C
d. D
e. E

41. The body of the pancreas corresponds to which of the following letters?
a. A
b. B
c. C
d. D
e. E

42. The left lobe of the liver corresponds to which of the following letters?
a. A
b. B
c. C
d. D
e. E

Using Fig. 9-10, answer questions 43 and 44.

43. Letter **B** corresponds to which of the following vascular structures?
a. splenic artery
b. celiac axis
c. left renal vein
d. right renal artery
e. superior mesenteric artery

44. Letter **C** corresponds to which of the following vascular structures?
a. splenic vein
b. coronary vein
c. portal vein
d. hepatic vein
e. superior mesenteric vein

45. The majority of cystadenomas involving the pancreas are located in the:
a. body and tail
b. head and neck
c. head and body
d. uncinate process
e. body and neck

46. The largest and most anterior section of the pancreas is the:
a. head
b. neck
c. body
d. tail
e. uncinate process

47. Preoperative criteria in a pancreatoduodenectomy include all of the following EXCEPT:
   a. absence of extrapancreatic metastasis
   b. patent portal vein
   c. patent celiac axis
   d. absence of cholelithiasis
   e. patent superior mesenteric vein

48. Rapid progression of pancreatic inflammation is a complication associated with:
   a. acute cholecystitis
   b. polycystic disease
   c. cystic fibrosis
   d. acute pancreatitis
   e. biliary obstruction

49. A sheath of muscle fibers surrounding the distal common bile duct describes the:
   a. ampulla of Vater
   b. minor papilla
   c. sphincter of Oddi
   d. major papilla
   e. duct of Wirsung

50. The leakage of pancreatic enzymes into the surrounding peritoneal space describes a(n):
   a. abscess
   b. seroma
   c. pseudocyst
   d. phlegmon
   e. biloma

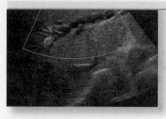

CHAPTER 10

Urinary System

KEY TERMS

acute tubular necrosis (ATN)   ischemic necrosis of tubular cells; most common cause of renal failure.

angiomyolipoma   benign tumor composed of blood vessels, smooth muscle, and fat.

angiotensin   polypoid in the blood that causes vasoconstriction, increase in blood pressure, and the release of aldosterone.

dromedary hump   cortical bulge on the lateral aspect of the kidney.

fascia   fibrous connective membrane of the body that may be separate from other structures.

fetal lobulation   immaturity of renal development resulting in a lobulated renal contour.

Gerota's fascia   protective covering of tissue surrounding each kidney.

glomerulonephritis   inflammation of the glomerulus of the kidney.

glomerulus   structure composed of blood vessels or nerve fibers.

hypertrophied column of Bertin   enlargement of a column of Bertin that extends into the renal pyramid.

junctional parenchymal defect   embryonic remnant of the fusion site between the upper and lower poles of the kidney.

medullary pyramid   renal pyramid.

papilla   blunt apex of the renal pyramid.

parapelvic cyst   cyst beside the renal pelvis; may obstruct the kidney.

peripelvic cyst   cyst around the renal pelvis; does not obstruct the kidney.

renal colic   sharp, severe flank pain radiating to the groin.

renal failure   the inability of the kidneys to excrete waste, concentrate urine, and conserve electrolytes.

renal insufficiency   partial kidney function failure characterized by less than normal urine output.

renal parenchyma   the functional tissue of the kidney consisting of the nephrons.

renal sinus lipomatosis   excessive accumulation of fat in the renal sinus.

renin   renal enzyme that affects blood pressure.

urachus   epithelial tube connecting the apex of the urinary bladder to the umbilicus.

ureterocele   prolapse of the distal ureter into the urinary bladder.

PHYSIOLOGY

- The nephron is the basic functional unit of the kidney.
- Each kidney contains over one million nephrons.

FUNCTIONS OF THE URINARY SYSTEM

- Produces urine and erythroprotein.
- Influences blood pressure, blood volume, and intake or excretion of salt and water through the renin–angiotensin system.
- Regulates serum electrolytes.
- Regulates acid–base balance.

Renal Anatomy (Fig. 10-1)

ANATOMY	DESCRIPTION
Renal capsule	• Fibrous capsule (true capsule) surrounding the cortex
Renal cortex	• Outer portion of the kidney • Bound by the renal capsule and arcuate vessels • Contains glomerular capsules and convoluted tubules
Medulla	• Inner portion of the renal parenchyma • Within the medulla lie the renal pyramids • Renal pyramids contain tubules and the loops of Henle
Column of Bertin	• Inward extension of the renal cortex between the renal pyramids
Renal sinus	• Central portion of the kidney • Contains the major and minor calyces, peripelvic fat, fibrous tissues, arteries, veins, lymphatics, and part of the renal pelvis
Renal hilum	• Contains the renal artery, renal vein, and ureter

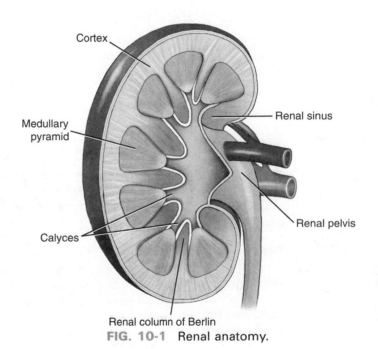

FIG. 10-1   Renal anatomy.

Labels: Cortex; Medullary pyramid; Calyces; Renal column of Berlin; Renal sinus; Renal pelvis

Renal Vasculature

RENAL VESSEL	DESCRIPTION
RENAL ARTERY	• Arises from the lateral aspects of the aorta • May have multiple ipsilateral arteries • A single ipsilateral artery may divide into multiple renal arteries at the hilum • Courses posterior to the renal vein • Main renal artery arises 1.0-1.5 cm inferior to the origin of the superior mesenteric artery • Demonstrates low-resistance blood flow • Supplies the kidney, ureter, and adrenal gland
• Segmental artery	• After entering the renal hilum the artery divides into 4-5 segmental arteries • Demonstrates low-resistance blood flow
• Interlobar artery	• Branch of the segmental artery • Course alongside the renal pyramids • Demonstrates low-resistance blood flow

Continued

Renal Vasculature—cont'd

RENAL VESSEL	DESCRIPTION
• **Arcuate artery**	• Boundary between the cortex and medulla • Branch of the interlobar artery located at the base of the medulla • Arcuate arteries give rise to the interlobular arteries • Demonstrates low-resistance blood flow
• **Interlobular artery** **RENAL VEIN**	• Branch of the arcuate arteries entering the renal glomeruli • Formed from the junction of tributaries in the renal hilum • Courses anterior to the renal artery • Left renal vein receives the left suprarenal and left gonadal vein • Dilatation of the left renal vein due to mesenteric compression may be demonstrated

Arterial Supply to the Ureter

- Renal artery.
- Testicular or ovarian artery.
- Superior vesical artery.

Support Structure of the Kidneys

Psoas muscle	• Major groin muscle • Primary flexor of the hip joint • Lies posterior to the inferior pole of each kidney
Quadratus lumborum muscle	• Muscle of the posterior abdominal wall • Lies posterior and medial to each kidney
Transversus abdominus muscle	• Deepest layer of flat muscles of the anterolateral wall • Lies lateral to each kidney
Gerota's fascia	• Fibrous covering of tissue surrounding each kidney • Also known as Gerota's capsule; renal fascia
Perinephric fat	• Fatty tissue surrounding each kidney
Renal capsule	• Protective connective tissue capsule surrounding each kidney

ANATOMY

LOCATION

- Paired bean-shaped structures lying in a sagittal oblique plane in the retroperitoneal cavity.
- Located between the first and third lumbar vertebrae.
- Superior poles lie more posterior and medial.
- Inferior poles lie more anterior and lateral.
- Left kidney lies superior to the right kidney.

Each Kidney Is Located

- Anterior to the psoas and quadratus lumborum muscles.
- Medial to the transverse abdominus muscle and liver or spleen.
- Lateral to the quadratus lumborum muscle.

Renal Anatomical Variants

VARIANT	DESCRIPTIONS	CLINICAL FINDINGS	SONOGRAPHIC FINDINGS	DIFFERENTIAL CONSIDERATIONS
Dromedary hump	• Cortical bulge on the lateral aspect of the kidney • Demonstrated most often on the left	• Asymptomatic	• Lateral outward cortical bulge • Echogenicity equal to the cortex	• Carcinoma • Hematoma • Renal cyst • Hypertrophied column of Bertin
Extrarenal pelvis	• Renal pelvis extrudes from the renal hilum	• Asymptomatic	• Anechoic oval-shaped structure medial to the renal hilum • No vascular flow	• Hydroureter • Renal cyst • Renal vein
Fetal lobulation	• Immature renal development	• Asymptomatic	• Lobulations in the renal contour	• Junctional parenchymal defect • Dromedary hump
Hypertrophied column of Bertin	• Enlarged column of Bertin	• Asymptomatic	• Mass extending from the cortex into the renal pyramids • Echogenicity similar to cortex	• Carcinoma • Renal duplication • Abscess
Junctional parenchymal defect	• Embryonic remnant of the fusion site between the upper and lower portions of the kidney	• Asymptomatic	• Triangular echogenic area in the anterior aspect of the kidney	• Technical factors • Calcified artery • Angiomyolipoma • Fetal lobulation

Congenital Anomalies

ANOMALY	DESCRIPTION	CLINICAL FINDINGS	SONOGRAPHIC FINDINGS	DIFFERENTIAL CONSIDERATIONS
Agenesis	• Absence of the kidney(s) • Unilateral or bilateral	• Asymptomatic when unilateral • Fatal when bilateral • Associated with genital anomalies	• Empty renal fossa(e) • Large, contralateral kidney	• Pelvic kidney • Surgical removal • Crossed fused ectopia
Cake kidney	• Variant of a horseshoe kidney • Found in the pelvis	• Asymptomatic • Pelvic mass	• Fusion of entire medial aspect of both kidneys • Anterior rotation of the renal pelvis	• Crossed fused ectopia • Renal mass
Crossed fused ectopia	• Both kidneys are fused in the same quadrant • Two separate collecting systems • Two normally located adrenal glands	• Asymptomatic • Abdominal mass	• One single, large kidney • Irregular contour • Inferior pole is directed medially	• Renal mass • Cake kidney • Sigmoid kidney
Duplication	• Two distinct collecting systems • May involve kidney, ureter and/or renal pelvis • May be partial or complete	• Asymptomatic • Flank pain	• Increase in renal length • Two distinct collecting systems • The superior system is most likely to obstruct	• Hypertrophied column of Bertin • Renal mass

Continued

Congenital Anomalies—cont'd

ANOMALY	DESCRIPTION	CLINICAL FINDINGS	SONOGRAPHIC FINDINGS	DIFFERENTIAL CONSIDERATIONS
Horseshoe Kidney	• Fusion of the kidneys usually at the inferior poles • Connected by an isthmus of functioning parenchyma or nonfunctioning fibrotic tissue • Anterior rotation of the renal pelves and ureters • Separate collecting systems • Most common form of renal fusion	• Asymptomatic • Pulsatile abdominal mass	• Bilateral low-lying medially placed kidneys with partial or complete fusion of the inferior poles • "Dipping effect" of both inferior poles • Isthmus of tissue demonstrated anterior to the abdominal aorta • Isthmus echo texture is similar to the renal cortex	• Renal mass • Lymphadenopathy • Bowel • Retroperitoneal tumor
Pelvic kidney	• Failure to ascend with development • Associated with a short ureter • Renal artery and vein are located more inferior • Renal vein drains directly into the inferior vena cava	• Asymptomatic • Pelvic pain	• Elongated core of echogenic tissue surrounded by less echogenic parenchyma • Located in the lower abdomen or pelvis • Empty ipsilateral renal fossa • Lies in an oblique plane	• Bowel • Pelvic mass
Renal Ptosis	• Unusual mobile kidney that descends from the normal position toward the pelvis • Poor support structures	• Asymptomatic	• Abnormal mobility of a kidney	• Pelvic kidney • Horseshoe kidney
Sigmoid kidney	• Variant of the horseshoe kidney	• Asymptomatic • Abdominal mass	• Superior pole of one kidney is fused with the inferior pole of the contralateral kidney • S-shaped	• Bowel • Abdominal mass
Thoracic kidney	• Kidney migrates into the chest through a herniation in the diaphragm • Rare finding	• Chest mass	• Elongated core of echogenic tissue surrounded by less echogenic parenchyma • Located in the chest • Not easily demonstrated on ultrasound	• Chest mass

SIZE

ADULT

• 9.0 to 12.0 cm in length.
• 4.0 to 5.0 cm in width.
• 2.5 to 3.0 cm in height.
• Minimum of 1 cm in cortical thickness.

CHILD

• 7.0 to 8.0 cm in length.
• Formula: (© *SDMS Abdominal National Certification Examination Review; Third Edition*).
  Renal length (cm) = 6.79 + [0.22 × age (years)].

INFANT

- 5.0 to 6.0 cm in length.
- Formula: (© *SDMS Abdominal National Certification Examination Review; Third Edition*).
  Renal length (cm) = 4.98 + [0.155 × age (months)].

Normal Sonographic Appearance—Adult Kidney

DIVISION	SONOGRAPHIC APPEARANCE
Renal capsule	• Well-defined echogenic line surrounding the kidney
Renal cortex	• Fine, moderate, to low-level echogenicity
	• Less echogenic compared to the normal liver parenchyma
Medulla	• Hypoechoic; may appear anechoic
Columns of Bertin	• Moderate to low-level echogenicity
Renal sinus	• Hyperechoic; most echogenic
Arcuate vessels	• Small echogenic foci at the corticomedullary junction
Cortical thickness	• Minimum 1 cm

Normal Sonographic Appearance—Pediatric Kidney

DIVISION	SONOGRAPHIC APPEARANCE
Renal capsule	• Sparse amount of perinephric fat makes it difficult to distinguish the capsule
Renal cortex	• Moderate to highly echogenic
Medulla	• Commonly anechoic
	• Do not mistake for hydronephrosis
Renal sinus	• Barely visible in infants

TECHNIQUE

PREPARATION

- Kidneys—patient should be hydrated.
- Renal vessels—nothing by mouth for 6 to 8 hours before the examination.
- Bladder—drink 8 to 16 ounces of water before the examination.

EXAMINATION TECHNIQUE

- Use the highest-frequency abdominal transducer possible to obtain optimal resolution for penetration depth.
- Proper focal zone and depth placement.
- Evaluation and documentation of the superior, inferior, medial, and lateral aspects of each kidney in the coronal or sagittal plane.
- Evaluation and documentation of the superior pole, renal hilum, and inferior pole of each kidney in the transverse plane.
- Measurements of maximum length, thickness, and width of each kidney.
- Measurement of the cortical thickness of each kidney.
- Evaluation and documentation of the bladder wall.
- Prevoid and postvoid bladder volumes may be included.
- Kidneys are best evaluated with an empty urinary bladder.
- Documentation and measurements of any abnormality should be included.

Patient Positions	
PATIENT POSITION	**DEMONSTRATES/BENEFITS**
Supine	• Right superior pole with intercostal approach • Right inferior pole with subcostal approach
Left posterior oblique (LPO)	• Allows bowel to move away from right kidney • Subcostal or intercostal approach
Left lateral decubitus	• Liver and kidney "fall" from the rib cage • Aids in obese or gassy patients
Right posterior oblique (RPO)	• Left superior pole with intercostal approach • Posterior subcostal approach for left inferior pole
Right lateral decubitus	• Left posterior approach with deep inspiration
Prone	• Demonstrates mid and inferior poles of both kidneys • Great for infants and small children • Superior poles may be visualized • Used in renal biopsies

INDICATIONS FOR EXAMINATION

- Increase in creatinine or BUN levels.
- Urinary tract infection.
- Flank pain.
- Hematuria.
- Hypertension.
- Decrease in urine output.
- Trauma.
- Evaluate mass from previous medical imaging study (i.e., CT).

LABORATORY VALUES

CREATININE

- Normal 0.6 to 1.2 mg/dL.
- A waste product produced from meat protein and normal wear and tear on the muscles in the body.
- More specific in determining renal dysfunction than BUN levels.
- Elevated in renal failure, chronic nephritis or urinary obstruction.

BLOOD UREA NITROGEN

- Normal 11 to 23 mg/dL.
- Produced from the breakdown of food proteins.
- Elevated in urinary obstruction, renal dysfunction, or dehydration.
- Decreased levels associated with overhydration, pregnancy, liver failure, decrease in protein intake, and smoking.

HEMATURIA

- Visible or microscopic red blood cells in the urine.
- Associated with early renal disease.

PROTEINURIA

- Abnormal amount of proteins in the urine.
- Associated with nephritis, nephrolithiasis, carcinoma, polycystic disease, hypertension, and diabetes mellitus.
- Increases risk of developing progressive renal dysfunction.

CONCENTRATION–DILUTION URINALYSIS

- Used to detect chronic renal disease.

Cystic Pathology of the Kidneys

PATHOLOGY	ETIOLOGY	CLINICAL FINDINGS	SONOGRAPHIC FINDINGS	DIFFERENTIAL CONSIDERATIONS
Simple cyst	• Acquired condition • Found in 50% of patients over the age of 55	• Asymptomatic	• Anechoic mass • Hyperechoic thin walls • Smooth margins • Posterior acoustic enhancement	• Liver cyst • Adrenal cyst
Parapelvic cyst	• Acquired condition originating from the renal parenchyma	• Asymptomatic • Hypertension • Hematuria	• Anechoic mass located in the renal hilum • Does not communicate with the collecting system • Hyperechoic thin walls • Smooth margins • Posterior acoustic enhancement	• Hydronephrosis • Renal vein • Extrarenal pelvis • Renal artery aneurysm
Peripelvic cyst	• Acquired condition which may develop from the lymphatic system or an obstruction	• Asymptomatic	• Anechoic mass located near or around the renal pelvis • Hyperechoic thin walls • Smooth margins • Posterior acoustic enhancement	• Prominent renal pyramid • Localized hydronephrosis
Adult polycystic kidney disease	• Inherited disorder • Normal renal parenchyma is replaced with cysts	• Palpable abdominal mass • Hypertension • Hematuria • Colicky pain • Elevated BUN and creatinine	• Bilateral disease • Multiple cysts • Irregular margins • Normal renal parenchyma may not be visualized	• Multiple simple cysts • Hydronephrosis
Childhood polycystic kidney disease	• Inherited disorder • Normal renal parenchyma is replaced with cysts	• Palpable abdominal mass • Hypertension • Hematuria • Colicky pain	• Bilateral disease • Hyperechoic enlarged kidneys	• Chronic renal failure • Renal sinus lipomatosis
Multicystic dysplasia	• Noninherited disorder • Urinary obstruction in early embryology	• Palpable abdominal mass • Flank pain • Hypertension	• Unilateral disease • Numerous cysts of variable shape and size • Associated with ureteropelvic junction obstruction and malrotation • Normal renal parenchyma may not be visualized	• Multiple simple cysts • Hydronephrosis

Inflammatory Conditions

INFLAMMATORY CONDITION	ETIOLOGY	CLINICAL FINDINGS	SONOGRAPHIC FINDINGS	DIFFERENTIAL CONSIDERATIONS
Renal abscess	• Infection	• Flank pain • Fever or chills • Leukocytosis	• Hypoechoic or complex mass • Thick irregular wall margins • Shadowing associated with gas formation	• Neoplasm • Focal pyelonephritis • Complicated cyst • Resolving hematoma
Acute tubular necrosis (ATN)	• Toxic drug exposure • Hypotension • Trauma • Surgery of the heart or aorta • Jaundice • Sepsis	• Asymptomatic • Renal failure	• Bilateral enlarged kidneys • Hyperechoic renal pyramids	• Renal sinus lipomatosis • Chronic pyelonephritis • Renal failure
Chronic renal failure	• Glomerulonephritis • Hypertension • Vascular disease • Diabetes mellitus • Chronic hydronephrosis	• Elevated BUN and creatinine • Proteinuria • Polyuria • Headaches • Fatigue • Weakness • Anemia	• Renal atrophy • Hyperechoic parenchyma • Thin renal cortex • Difficult to distinguish the kidney from surrounding structures	• Renal sinus lipomatosis • Hypoplastic kidney
Glomerulonephritis	• Immune diseases • Infection • Strep throat • Lupus • Chronic hepatitis C • Vasculitis	• Asymptomatic • Proteinuria • Decrease in urine output • Hypertension • Hematuria • Fatigue • Edema	• Hyperechoic renal cortex • Enlarged kidney(s)	• Renal sinus lipomatosis
Pyelonephritis	• Bacteria ascends from the bladder	• Flank pain • Fever or chills • Dysuria • Pyuria • Leukocytosis	• Generalized or focal swelling of the kidney(s) • Well-defined renal pyramids	• Renal abscess • Neoplasm

Obstruction and Calculus of the Kidney

OBSTRUCTION	ETIOLOGY	CLINICAL FINDINGS	SONOGRAPHIC FINDINGS	DIFFERENTIAL CONSIDERATIONS
Hydronephrosis	• Obstruction of the urinary tract	• Flank pain • Hematuria • Fever • Leukocytosis	Grade I (mild) • Slight dilatation of the calyces Grade II (moderate) • Extensive dilatation of the calyces • Thinning of the renal pelvis • Splaying of calyces similar to a bear claw Grade III (severe) • Massive dilatation of the calyces • Loss of renal parenchyma • Resistive index (RI) > 0.7	• Extrarenal pelvis • Parapelvic cyst • Polycystic disease • Reflux
Medullary sponge kidney	• Benign congenital condition	• Asymptomatic	• Hyperechoic foci in the region of the renal papillae • Widening of the distal collecting system	• Nephrolithiasis • Angiomyolipoma
Nephrolithiasis	• Urinary stasis	• Asymptomatic • Renal colic • Flank pain • Hematuria	• Hyperechoic focus within the kidney • Occurs in the corticomedullary junction • Posterior acoustic shadowing	• Calcified vessel • Angiomyolipoma

Benign Pathology of the Kidney

BENIGN PATHOLOGY	ETIOLOGY	CLINICAL FINDINGS	SONOGRAPHIC FINDINGS	DIFFERENTIAL CONSIDERATIONS
Adenoma	• Glandular epithelium • Most common cortical tumor	• Asymptomatic • Hematuria	• Well-defined hypoechoic mass • Generally small	• Abscess • Complicated cyst
Angiomyolipoma	• Composed of fat, blood vessels, and muscle • Tends to hemorrhage	• Asymptomatic • Flank pain • Gross hematuria	• Well-defined hyperechoic mass • May distort renal architecture	• Carcinoma • Junctional parenchymal defect • Lipoma
Lipoma	• Composed of fat	• Asymptomatic	• Well-defined hyperechoic mass	• Angiomyolipoma • Junctional parenchymal defect
Renal sinus lipomatosis	• Obesity • Previous urinary obstruction • Chronic renal infection • Steroid therapy	• Asymptomatic • Elevated creatinine	• Increase in echogenicity of the renal sinus • Thinning of the renal cortex • Normal renal contour	• Chronic renal failure

Malignant Pathology of the Kidney

MALIGNANT PATHOLOGY	ETIOLOGY	CLINICAL FINDINGS	SONOGRAPHIC FINDINGS	DIFFERENTIAL CONSIDERATIONS
Renal carcinoma Stages: 1. Confined to the kidney 2. Spread to perinephric fat 3. Extension to the renal vein, inferior vena cava, or lymph nodes 4. Extension to near or distant structures	• Adenocarcinoma in 85% of cases (renal cell) • Transitional cell carcinoma	• Painless hematuria • Uncontrolled hypertension	• Irregular mass with echogenicity ranging from hypoechoic to hyperechoic • Indistinct borders • Hypervascular mass • Metastasis to the lung, liver, and long bones • Extension into the renal vein and inferior vena cava	• Adrenal tumor • Abscess • Focal pyelonephritis • Adenoma • Angiomyolipoma

Continued

Malignant Pathology of the Kidney—cont'd

MALIGNANT PATHOLOGY	ETIOLOGY	CLINICAL FINDINGS	SONOGRAPHIC FINDINGS	DIFFERENTIAL CONSIDERATIONS
Wilms tumor (nephroblastoma)	Risk Factors: • Beckwith-Wiedemann syndrome • Hemihypertrophy • Sporadic aniridia • Male prevalence • Omphalocele • 5 years of age or less	• Palpable mass • Abdominal pain • Nausea/vomiting • Gross hematuria • Hypertension	• Predominately solid, well-defined renal mass • Variable echo pattern • Echogenic rim • Calcification	• Neuroblastoma • Renal carcinoma

Vascular Disorders of the Kidneys

VASCULAR DISORDER	ETIOLOGY	CLINICAL FINDINGS	SONOGRAPHIC AND DOPPLER FINDINGS	DIFFERENTIAL CONSIDERATIONS
Renal artery stenosis	• Atherosclerosis • Fibromuscular hyperplasia (mid to distal)	• Hypertension • Renal insufficiency	• Peak systolic velocity greater than 180 cm/sec • Spectral broadening • Absence of diastolic flow • Delayed acceleration time • Renal artery ratio greater than 3.5 • Visual narrowing of the renal artery by atherosclerosis or thickening of the arterial wall • Kidney atrophy • Kidney infarct	• Tortuous artery • Poor Doppler angle
Renal artery aneurysm Risk factor • Pregnancy	• Fibromuscular dysplasia • Blunt trauma • Kawasaki disease • Intraluminal catheter–induced injury • Atherosclerosis	• Asymptomatic • Hypertension • Flank pain • Hematuria	• Doubling of the normal artery • Artery diameter of 1.5 cm or greater • Risk of rupture when the diameter exceeds 2 cm	• Tortuous renal artery • Bifurcation of the renal artery • Renal vein
Arteriovenous fistula	• Congenital malformation • Trauma • Renal biopsy complication	• Asymptomatic	• High peak systolic velocity associated with high diastolic velocity • Extremely turbulent flow	• Renal artery stenosis
Renal vein thrombosis Risk factors • Malignancy • Primary renal disease • Lupus • Diabetes • Sickle cell anemia • Amyloidosis • Pancreatitis	• Renal disease • Surgery • Trauma • Dehydration	• Flank pain • Hematuria	• Increase in vein diameter • Hypoechoic or complex echoes within the renal vein • Continuous, minimal, or absent intraluminal venous flow • Enlarged kidney	• Renal vein tumor extension • Improper gain or focal zone settings • Improper Doppler settings or angle
Renal vein tumor extension	• Renal carcinoma • Renal lymphoma • Nephroblastoma	• Depends on the underlying cause	• Increase in vein diameter • Echogenic mass within the renal vein • Vascular flow within the mass • Continuous, minimal, or absent intraluminal venous flow	• Renal vein thrombosis • Improper gain or focal zone settings • Improper Doppler settings or angle

RENAL DIALYSIS

- Renal dialysis is a process of diffusing blood across a membrane to remove substances a normal kidney would eliminate.
- Renal dialysis may restore electrolytes and acid–base balance.
- Renal dialysis patients have an increased incidence of developing a renal:
  a. cyst.
  b. adenoma.
  c. carcinoma.

RENAL TRANSPLANT

- Transplanted kidney is usually placed in the anterior right iliac fossa.
- Renal artery is anastomosed to the ipsilateral internal iliac artery.
- Renal vein is anastomosed to the ipsilateral external iliac vein.
- Ureter is implanted into the superior portion of the urinary bladder.
- Fat from around the bladder is placed over the ureter to act as a valve.

Renal Transplant Complications

TRANSPLANT COMPLICATION	DESCRIPTION
Renal artery stenosis	• Occurs months to years posttransplant
Renal artery thrombosis	• Occurs in the first few days
Primary renal vein thrombosis	• Originates in the renal vein
Secondary renal vein thrombosis	• Extends into the iliac vein
	• Can result from iliac compression
Hematoma	• Hypoechoic when acute
	• Complex when subacute
	• Anechoic when chronic
Urinoma	• Develops in the first few weeks
	• Rapid increase in size on serial examinations
	• Anechoic fluid collection
Lymphocele	• Usually found medial to the transplant
	• Anechoic fluid collection frequently containing septations
Abscess	• Usually develops in the first few weeks
	• Variable sonographic appearance

NORMAL SONOGRAPHIC APPEARANCE OF THE RENAL TRANSPLANT

- Renal sinus appears hyperechoic.
- Renal cortex appears hypoechoic.
- Prominent renal pyramids.
- Arcuate vessels may be demonstrated.

ABNORMAL SONOGRAPHIC APPEARANCE OF THE RENAL TRANSPLANT

- Increase in renal size (circular in appearance).
- Increase in size of the renal pyramids.
- Increase in echogenicity of the renal cortex.
- Decrease in echogenicity of the renal sinus.
- Loss of corticomedullary definition.
- Hypoechoic areas within the renal parenchyma.

NORMAL DOPPLER APPEARANCE OF THE RENAL TRANSPLANT

- Low-resistance vascular flow in the renal, segmental, and arcuate arteries.
- Resistive index (RI) of 0.7 or less.

ABNORMAL DOPPLER APPEARANCE OF THE RENAL TRANSPLANT

- Monophasic or absence of vascular flow.
- RI of 0.9 suggests rejection.

URINARY BLADDER ANATOMY

- Normal bladder wall thickness is 3 mm when distended.
- Normal bladder wall thickness is 5 mm when empty.
- Normal bladder wall is thicker in infants than adults.
- Ureters enter the bladder wall at an oblique angle approximately 5 cm above the bladder outlet.
- Postvoid residual normally should not exceed 20 mL.

APEX

- Superior portion of the bladder.

NECK

- Inferior portion of the bladder continuous with the urethra.

TRIGONE

- Region between the apex and neck of the bladder.

NORMAL SONOGRAPHIC APPEARANCE

- Anechoic fluid-filled structure located in the pelvic midline.
- Ureteric orifices appear as small echogenic protuberances on the posterior aspect of the bladder.
- Bladder wall thickness is dependent on distention of urinary bladder but should not exceed 5 mm.

Congenital Abnormalities of the Urinary Bladder

CONGENITAL ABNORMALITY	ETIOLOGY	CLINICAL FINDINGS	SONOGRAPHIC FINDINGS	DIFFERENTIAL CONSIDERATIONS
Bladder exstrophy	• Failure of the mesoderm to form over the lower abdomen	• Typically discovered in utero	• Lower anterior abdominal wall defect • Mass protruding from this defect • Normal bladder not identified	• Omphalocele • Inguinal hernia • Umbilical hernia
Bladder diverticulum	• Bladder wall muscle weakness	• Asymptomatic • Urinary tract infection • Pelvic pain	• Anechoic pedunculation of the urinary bladder • Neck of diverticulum is small • May enlarge when bladder contracts	• Ovarian cyst • Fluid-filled bowel • Ascites

Congenital Abnormalities of the Urinary Bladder—cont'd

CONGENITAL ABNORMALITY	ETIOLOGY	CLINICAL FINDINGS	SONOGRAPHIC FINDINGS	DIFFERENTIAL CONSIDERATIONS
Bladder ureterocele	• Congenital obstruction of the ureteric orifice	• Asymptomatic • Urinary tract infection	• Hyperechoic septation seen within the bladder at the ureteric orifice • Demonstrated when urine enters the bladder	• Artifact • Bladder tumor • Catheter balloon
Urachal sinus	• Epithelial tube connecting the apex of the bladder with the umbilicus	• Asymptomatic • Fluid draining from the umbilicus	• Linear tubular structure extending from the apex of the urinary bladder to the umbilicus	• Rectus abdominus hematoma • Subcutaneous fat

Pathology of the Urinary Bladder

BLADDER PATHOLOGY	ETIOLOGY	CLINICAL FINDINGS	SONOGRAPHIC FINDINGS	DIFFERENTIAL CONSIDERATIONS
Bladder calculus	• Develops in the bladder • Migrates from the kidney(s)	• Asymptomatic • Hematuria	• Hyperechoic focus within the urinary bladder • Posterior acoustic shadowing • Mobile with patient position change	• Intestinal air • Calcified vessel
Cystitis	• Infection	• Dysuria • Urinary frequency • Leukocytosis	• Increase in bladder wall thickness • Mobile internal echoes	• Bladder sludge • Hematuria
Bladder sludge	• Debris in the bladder	• Asymptomatic	• Homogeneous low-level echoes • Mobile with patient position change	• Cystitis • Hematuria
Bladder malignancy	• Transitional cell carcinoma	• Painless hematuria • Frequent urination • Dysuria	• Echogenic mass • Irregular margins • Immobile with patient position change • Internal vascular blood flow	• Benign tumor • Bladder sludge • Ureterocele
Bladder polyp	• Papilloma	• Asymptomatic • Frequent urination	• Echogenic intraluminal mass • Smooth margins • Immobile with patient position change • Internal vascular flow	• Malignant tumor • Bladder sludge • Ureterocele

URINARY SYSTEM REVIEW

1. Which of the following terms describes the typical sonographic appearance of the medullary pyramids in the neonate?
   a. anechoic
   b. hypoechoic
   c. hyperechoic
   d. echogenic
   e. barely visible

2. Which of the following conditions is associated with a decrease in blood urea nitrogen (BUN)?
   a. dehydration
   b. hydronephrosis
   c. liver failure
   d. polycystic renal disease
   e. renal failure

3. The renal arteries arise from which aspect of the abdominal aorta?
   a. medial
   b. lateral
   c. anterior
   d. inferior
   e. superior

4. Which of the following structures is considered the basic functional unit of the kidney?
   a. glomerulus
   b. nephron
   c. loop of Henle
   d. renal pyramid
   e. collecting tubule

5. The quadratus lumborum is a muscle located in the:
   a. groin
   b. medial abdominal wall
   c. lateral abdominal wall
   d. anterior abdominal wall
   e. posterior abdominal wall

6. Fusion of the entire medial aspect of both kidneys is a congenital anomaly termed:
   a. cross fused ectopia
   b. cake kidney
   c. renal duplication
   d. sigmoid kidney
   e. junctional parenchymal defect

7. Which of the following conditions is most likely to mimic a duplicated urinary system?
   a. junctional parenchymal defect
   b. fetal lobulation
   c. dromedary hump
   d. renal ptosis
   e. hypertrophied column of Bertin

8. Functions of the kidneys include all of the following EXCEPT:
   a. regulation of acid–base balance
   b. urine production
   c. regulation of electrolyte balance
   d. synthesis of amino acids
   e. production of erythroprotein

9. The most common renal neoplasm identified in patients over the age of 55 years is a(n):
   a. simple cyst
   b. renal calculus
   c. angiomyolipoma
   d. multicystic dysplastic kidney
   e. renal cell carcinoma

10. Rejection of a renal transplant is suggested once the resistive index reaches:
    a. 0.3
    b. 0.7
    c. 0.9
    d. 1.5
    e. 2.0

Using Fig. 10-2, answer question 11.

11. A catheterized paraplegic patient is scheduled for a retroperitoneum ultrasound. An anechoic structure is identified in the region of the urinary bladder. This structure most likely represents a(n):
    a. ureterocele
    b. urachal sinus
    c. bladder diverticulum
    d. a catheter balloon
    e. small amount of residual urine

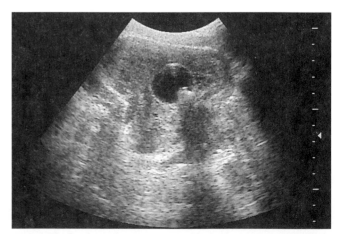

FIG. 10-2   Longitudinal image of the urinary bladder.

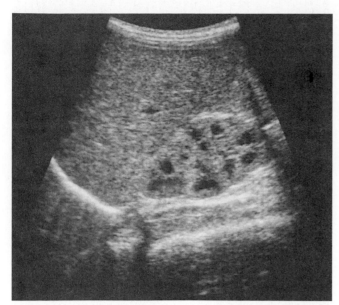

FIG. 10-3 Longitudinal image of the kidney.

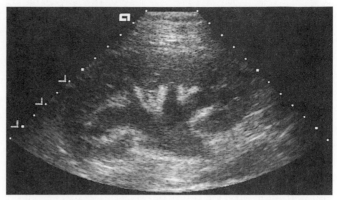

FIG. 10-4 Longitudinal image of the kidney.

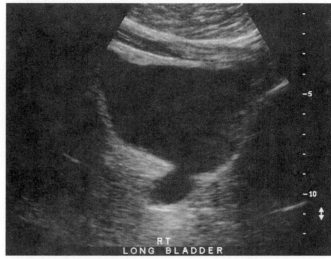

FIG. 10-5 Longitudinal image of the right side of the urinary bladder.

Using Fig. 10-3, answer question 12.

12. A 5-week-old infant presents to the ultrasound department with a history of a single urinary tract infection. The sonogram of the kidney most likely demonstrates:
    a. hydronephrosis
    b. infantile polycystic disease
    c. normal medullary pyramids
    d. acute renal failure
    e. dilated arcuate vessels

Using Fig. 10-4, answer questions 13 and 14.

13. A 25-year-old woman presents to the emergency department complaining of severe left flank pain. A sonogram of the kidney is most likely demonstrating which of the following conditions?
    a. nephrolithiasis
    b. polycystic kidney disease
    c. pyelonephritis
    d. medullary sponge kidney
    e. hydronephrosis

14. The most common etiology for this pathology is:
    a. bladder infection
    b. congenital anomaly
    c. urinary tract obstruction
    d. urinary stasis
    e. steroid therapy

Using Fig. 10-5, answer question 15.

15. A 45-year-old female patient arrives for a pelvic ultrasound complaining of urinary frequency. An anechoic structure is identified contiguous with the urinary bladder. The pathology identified is most suspicious for a(n):
    a. ureterocele
    b. ovarian cyst
    c. dilated urethra
    d. bladder diverticulum
    e. dilated ureter

16. Which of the following renal structures is composed of blood vessels or nerve fibers?
    a. nephron
    b. loop of Henle
    c. renal pyramid
    d. renal tubule
    e. glomerulus

17. A patient complaining of sharp, severe flank pain radiating to the groin is describing:
    a. renal colic
    b. dysuria
    c. mittelsmirtz
    d. dyspareunia
    e. positive McBurney sign

18. Which of the following structures are contained in the renal sinus?
    a. renal artery, renal vein, ureter
    b. lymphatics, perinephric fat, minor calyces
    c. major calyces, renal pelvis, ureter
    d. lymphatics, peripelvic fat, major calyces
    e. renal artery, renal vein, renal pelvis

19. Which of the following muscles is located lateral to each kidney?
    a. psoas
    b. quadratus lumborum
    c. rectus abdominus
    d. internal oblique
    e. transversus abdominus

20. A hyperechoic focus located in the anterior renal cortex in an asymptomatic patient most likely represents:
    a. adenoma
    b. ischemic necrosis
    c. renal carcinoma
    d. a junctional parenchymal defect
    e. renal calculus

21. Normal postvoid residual urine volume should not exceed:
    a. 5 mL
    b. 20 mL
    c. 50 mL
    d. 100 mL
    e. 125 mL

22. A 43-year-old female patient presents to the ultrasound department complaining of right flank pain and dysuria. A generalized swelling of the kidney is demonstrated. The medullary pyramids appear well defined. This is most suspicious for:
    a. acute tubular necrosis
    b. renal carcinoma
    c. hydronephrosis
    d. pyelonephritis
    e. polycystic renal disease

23. Which of the following patient positions is typically used for renal biopsy procedures?
    a. supine
    b. prone
    c. right lateral decubitus
    d. left posterior oblique
    e. reverse Trendelenburg

24. Small echogenic protuberances identified on the posterior wall of the urinary bladder most likely represents:
    a. arcuate vessels
    b. ureteric orifices
    c. bladder diverticulums
    d. bladder calculi
    e. hydroureters

25. Clinical findings associated with acute glomerulonephritis may include all of the following EXCEPT:
    a. polyuria
    b. proteinuria
    c. fatigue
    d. edema
    e. hematuria

Using Fig. 10-6, answer question 26.

26. A 54-year-old female presents to the ultrasound department complaining of right upper quadrant pain. Which of the following anatomical variants is most likely identified in this sonogram?
    a. dromedary hump
    b. fetal lobulation
    c. crossed fused ectopia
    d. junctional parenchymal defect
    e. hypertrophied column of Bertin

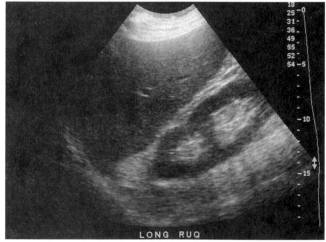

FIG. 10-6 Sagittal image of the right upper quadrant.

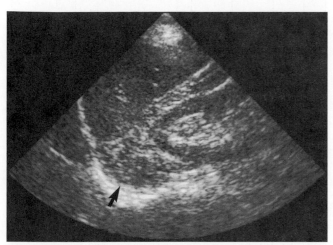

FIG. 10-7   Sagittal image of the right upper quadrant.

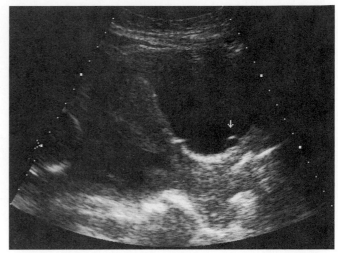

FIG. 10-9   Sagittal image of the urinary bladder.

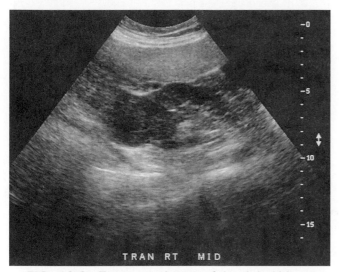

FIG. 10-8   Transverse image of the right kidney.

Using Fig. 10-8, answer question 28.

28. A 70-year-old patient presents with a history of painless hematuria, uncontrolled hypertension, and vague right upper quadrant pain. A mass is identified that demonstrates internal blood flow. Based on this history, the mass identified in the sonogram is most suspicious for a(n):
    a. hematoma
    b. dromedary hump
    c. angiomyolipoma
    d. renal carcinoma
    e. hemorrhagic cyst

Using Fig. 10-9, answer question 29.

29. During a screening obstetrical examination an intermittent bladder abnormality is identified. This incidental finding is most consistent with a(n):
    a. diverticulum
    b. urachal cyst
    c. catheter balloon
    d. ureterocele
    e. ureteral jet

Using Fig. 10-7, answer question 27.

27. A morbidly obese patient presents to the ultrasound department with a history of elevated liver function tests. He denies abdominal or flank pain. The arrow in this sonogram is **mostly likely** identifying:
    a. sinus lipomatosis
    b. perinephric fat
    c. a cavernous hemangioma
    d. an adrenal adenoma
    e. a complicated renal cyst

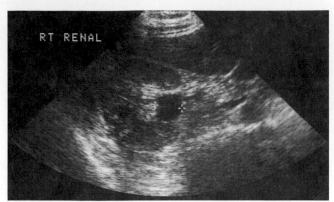

FIG. 10-10   Transverse image of the right kidney.

Using Fig. 10-10, answer question 30.

30. An asymptomatic patient presents to the
ultrasound department with a clinical history of
microscopic hematuria. The anechoic area
demonstrated in the sonogram is MOST
consistent with a(n):
   a. extrarenal pelvis
   b. peripelvic cyst
   c. urinary tract obstruction
   d. parapelvic cyst
   e. hydroureter

31. Predisposing factors for developing a Wilms
tumor include all of the following EXCEPT:
   a. hemihypertrophy
   b. sporadic aniridia
   c. age less than 5 years
   d. diaphragmatic hernia
   e. Beckwith-Wiedemann syndrome

32. A benign tumor composed of fat, blood vessels,
and muscle describes a(n):
   a. adenoma
   b. lipoma
   c. hematoma
   d. fibroma
   e. angiomyolipoma

33. Fibromuscular hyperplasia is most commonly
associated with stenosis in which of the following
renal arteries?
   a. main renal artery
   b. arcuate artery
   c. interlobar artery
   d. segmental artery
   e. abdominal aorta

34. Renal artery stenosis is suggested once the peak
systolic velocity exceeds:
   a. 90 cm/sec
   b. 135 cm/sec
   c. 180 cm/sec
   d. 230 cm/sec
   e. 250 cm/sec

35. Which of the following conditions is most likely
associated with painless hematuria?
   a. hydronephrosis
   b. pyelonephritis
   c. angiomyolipoma
   d. renal cell carcinoma
   e. polycystic renal disease

36. Which of the following conditions is frequently
associated with urinary stasis?
   a. parapelvic cyst
   b. nephrolithiasis
   c. renal carcinoma
   d. chronic renal failure
   e. medullary sponge kidney

37. Fusion of the superior pole of one kidney to
inferior pole of the contralateral kidney is most
consistent with which of the following congenital
anomalies?
   a. cake kidney
   b. cross fused ectopia
   c. pelvic kidney
   d. sigmoid kidney
   e. duplicated kidney

38. Aneurysms involving the renal artery are at an
increased risk of rupturing once the diameter
exceeds:
   a. 0.5 cm
   b. 1.0 cm
   c. 1.5 cm
   d. 2.0 cm
   e. 3.0 cm

39. The complete inability of the kidneys to excrete
waste, concentrate urine, and converse
electrolytes is termed renal:
   a. colic
   b. ptosis
   c. failure
   d. obstruction
   e. insufficiency

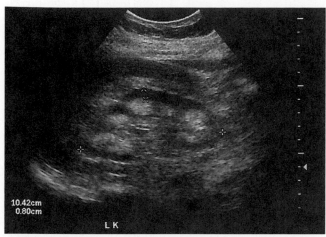

FIG. 10-11 Sagittal sonogram of the left kidney.

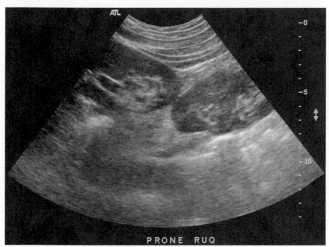

FIG. 10-12 Prone image of the right flank.

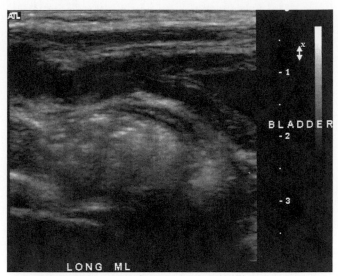

FIG. 10-13 Sagittal sonogram of the pelvis.

Using Fig. 10-12, answer question 41.

41. A middle-aged patient presents with a history of elevated creatinine levels. The left kidney is not identified in the left flank. A sonogram of the right flank is documented. Which of the following congenital anomalies is most likely demonstrated in this sonogram?
a. lump kidney
b. cake kidney
c. renal duplication
d. sigmoid kidney
e. dromedary hump

Using Fig. 10-13, answer question 42.

42. A patient presents with a history of intermittent umbilical discharge. The patient denies a history of abdominal trauma, pain, or fever. A sonogram of the pelvic midline reveals a tubular mass between the urinary bladder and umbilicus. Based on the clinical history, the sonogram is most likely demonstrating which of the following conditions?
a. rectus abdominus hematoma
b. umbilical abscess
c. Meckel's diverticulum
d. urachal sinus
e. umbilical hernia

Using Fig. 10-11, answer question 40.

40. A 51-year-old man complaining of right upper quadrant pain presents to the ultrasound department with a history of gallstones. This sonogram is most likely identifying which of the following conditions?
a. angiomyolipomas
b. medullary sponge kidney
c. glomerulonephritis
d. chronic renal failure
e. renal metastases

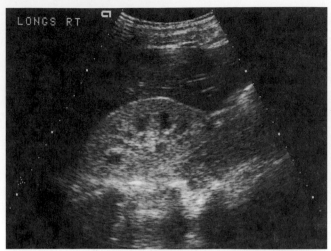

FIG. 10-14   Longitudinal image of the kidney.

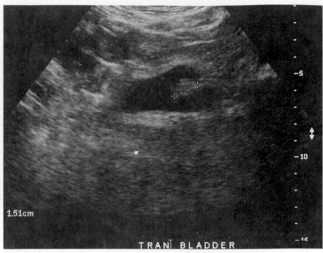

FIG. 10-16   Sonogram of the urinary bladder.

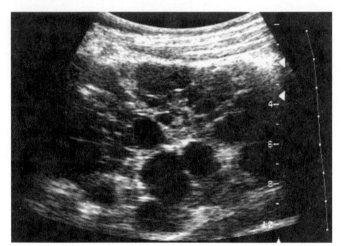

FIG. 10-15   Sagittal image of the right kidney.

Using Fig. 10-14, answer question 43.

43. A patient hospitalized with malaria presents with a history of proteinuria. An enlarged hyperechoic kidney is demonstrated on ultrasound. Based on this clinical history, the sonogram is most suspicious for which of the following conditions?
   a. pyelonephritis
   b. chronic renal failure
   c. glomerulonephritis
   d. renal sinus lipomatosis
   e. medullary sponge disease

Using Fig. 10-15, answer question 44.

44. A 40-year-old patient presents with a history of elevated creatinine levels. A sagittal image of the right kidney demonstrates multiple masses. Based on the clinical and sonographic findings, the masses are most suspicious for:
   a. a nephroblastoma
   b. hydronephrosis
   c. renal sinus lipomatosis
   d. polycystic kidney disease
   e. a medullary sponge kidney

Using Fig. 10-16, answer questions 45 and 46.

45. A 78-year-old patient presents to the ultrasound department to rule out an abdominal aortic aneurysm. An incidental mass was discovered in the urinary bladder. Blood flow was demonstrated within the mass using color Doppler imaging. This incidental finding is most suspicious for a bladder:
   a. diverticulum
   b. adenoma
   c. carcinoma
   d. sludgeball
   e. ureterocele

46. When encountering this type of pathology, which of the following questions in most important for the sonographer to ask the patient?
   a. Do you have high blood pressure?
   b. How often do your urinate each day?
   c. Have you noticed any blood in your urine?
   d. When was your last physical examination?
   e. How much water do you drink each day?

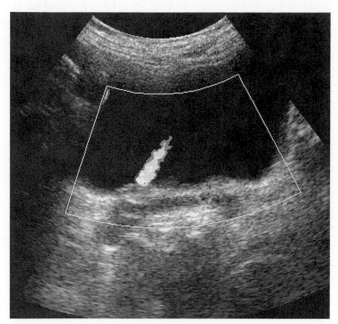

FIG. 10-17 Transverse Doppler sonogram (see color plate 4).

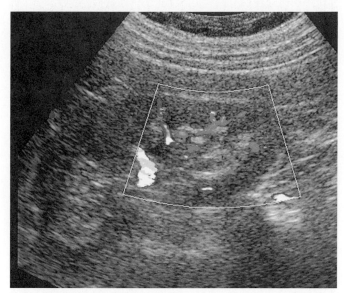

FIG. 10-18 Sagittal Doppler image (see color plate 5).

Using Fig. 10-17 (and color plate 4), answer question 47.

47. This image of the urinary bladder is most likely demonstrating which of the following?
    a. ureterocele
    b. ureteral jet
    c. flash artifact
    d. external iliac artery
    e. internal iliac artery

48. Complications following renal transplant surgery may include all of the following EXCEPT:
    a. abscess
    b. lymphocele
    c. renal artery stenosis
    d. renal vein thrombosis
    e. parapelvic cyst formation

Using Fig. 10-18 (and color plate 5), answer question 49.

49. Duplex imaging of the lower pole of the left kidney most likely demonstrates which of the following?
    a. renal veins
    b. renal arteries
    c. Bertin vessels
    d. arcuate vessels
    e. suprarenal vessels

50. The normal renal cortex measures a minimum of:
    a. 0.5 cm
    b. 0.7 cm
    c. 1.0 cm
    d. 1.5 cm
    e. 2.0 cm

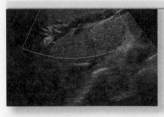

CHAPTER 11

Spleen

KEY TERMS

accessory spleen   a nodule of normal splenic tissue commonly located near the splenic hilum.

anemia   a decrease in hemoglobin levels in the blood.

asplenia syndrome   absence of the spleen associated with two right lungs, a midline liver, and gastrointestinal and urinary anomalies.

hamartoma   a rare benign neoplasm composed of lymphoid tissue. Also known as splenoma.

hematocrit   the percentage of red blood cells in the blood.

hemoglobin   carries oxygen from the lungs to the cells and returns carbon dioxide back to the lungs.

intraparenchymal hematoma   hematoma located within the splenic parenchyma.

leukemia   proliferation of white blood cells.

leukocytosis   white blood cell count above 20,000 mm^3.

leukopenia   white blood cell count below 4,000 mm^3.

lymphoma   malignant disorder involving the lymphoreticular system.

polysplenia   multiple small spleens associated with two left lungs and gastrointestinal, cardiovascular, and biliary anomalies.

splenic artery aneurysm   a localized dilatation of the splenic artery.

splenic infarction   occlusion of the main splenic artery or one of its branches.

subcapsular hematoma   hematoma located between the splenic capsule and parenchyma.

wandering spleen   refers to an abnormal location of the spleen.

PHYSIOLOGY

FUNCTION OF THE SPLEEN

- Removes foreign material from the blood.
- Initiates an immune reaction, resulting in production of antibodies and lymphocytes.
- Major destruction site of old red blood cells; red blood cells are removed and hemoglobin is recycled.
- Reservoir for blood.

ANATOMY (Fig. 11-1)

- Predominant organ in the left upper quadrant.
- Except at the hilum, the spleen is covered by the peritoneum.
- The spleen is divided into the:
  1. Superior and medial portion.
  2. Inferior and lateral portion.
  3. Splenic hilum.

SPLENIC VASCULATURE

- The splenic artery arises from the celiac axis and divides into six branches after entering the splenic hilum.
- The splenic vein joins the superior mesenteric vein, forming the main portal vein.
- In cases of portal hypertension, the splenic vein may shunt blood directly into the left renal vein.

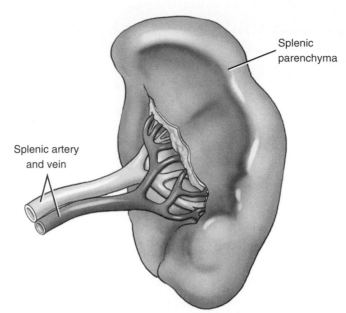

FIG. 11-1 Splenic anatomy.

Splenic
parenchyma

Splenic artery
and vein

LOCATION

- Intraperitoneal organ.
- Located inferior to the diaphragm and anterior to the left kidney.
- Lies posterior and lateral to the stomach.
- Located lateral to the pancreas.

Congenital Anomalies

VARIANT	DESCRIPTION	CLINICAL FINDINGS	SONOGRAPHIC FINDINGS	DIFFERENTIAL CONSIDERATIONS
Accessory spleen	• Improper splenic fusion	• Asymptomatic	• Homogeneous mass typically located medial to the splenic hilum • Echogenicity similar to spleen • Round or oval in shape • Variable size	• Lymphadenopathy • Pancreatic mass • Adrenal mass
Aplasia	• Failure of the spleen to develop	• Asymptomatic	• Absence of the spleen	• Splenectomy • Wandering spleen
Polysplenia	• Multiple small spleens	• Asymptomatic • Varies with associated congenital anomalies	• Multiple small spleens • Located along the greater curvature of the stomach • Associated with gastrointestinal, cardiovascular, and biliary anomalies	• Lymphadenopathy • Retroperitoneal masses
Wandering spleen	• Improper fusion of the dorsal mesentery with the posterior peritoneum	• Asymptomatic	• Abnormal location of the spleen	• Asplenia • Splenic rupture

Splenic Size

SIZE	ETIOLOGY	CLINICAL FINDINGS	SONOGRAPHIC FINDINGS	DIFFERENTIAL CONSIDERATIONS
Normal adult spleen			• Length: 10-12 cm • Width: 7 cm • Height: 3-4 cm	
Splenomegaly	• Congestive heart failure • Cirrhosis • Portal hypertension • Portal vein thrombosis • Infection • Diabetes mellitus • Hypertension • Hepatitis • Trauma • Hemolytic anemia	• Asymptomatic • Dyspepsia • Fatigue • Abdominal pain • Palpable left upper quadrant mass	• Enlargement of the spleen Adults • Length exceeding 13 cm • Hypoechoic parenchyma • Evaluate liver for pathology • Evaluate abdominal cavity for ascites	• Technical error • Splenic rupture

NORMAL SONOGRAPHIC APPEARANCE

- Moderately echogenic homogeneous parenchyma.
- Isoechoic to slightly hypoechoic compared to the normal liver parenchyma.

TECHNIQUE

PREPARATION

- No preparation is necessary for a sonogram of the spleen.
- Nothing by mouth 6 to 8 hours prior to examination is the typical preparation since imaging the spleen is rarely requested alone.

EXAMINATION TECHNIQUE

- Use the highest-frequency abdominal transducer possible to obtain optimal resolution for penetration depth.
- Proper focal and depth placement.
- Patients may lie in the supine, right posterior oblique, or right lateral decubitus position.
- Coronal and transverse scanning planes are used to evaluate the spleen from the left hemidiaphragm to the left kidney.
- Evaluation and documentation of the length, height, and width of the spleen.
- Documentation and measurement of any abnormality should be included.

INDICATIONS FOR EXAMINATION

- Chronic liver disease.
- Infection.
- Leukocytosis.
- Leukopenia.
- Palpable mass.
- Abdominal pain.
- Fatigue.
- Trauma.

LABORATORY VALUES

ERYTHROCYTE

- Red blood cell.
- Normal serum levels:
  Male—4.6-6.2 million/mm^3.
  Female—4.2-5.4 million/mm^3.
- Carries oxygen from the lungs to the tissues in the body.
- Carries carbon dioxide back to the lungs.
- Develops in the bone marrow and has a life span of 120 days.
- Spleen stores red blood cells and destroys old red blood cells.
- Contains hemoglobin.
- Elevation associated with polycythemia vera and severe diarrhea.
- Decreases associated with internal bleeding, hemolytic anemia, Hodgkin disease, and hemangiosarcomas.

LEUKOCYTE

- White blood cell.
- Normal serum levels: 4,500-11,000 mm^3.
- Defends the body from infection.
- Elevation associated with infection, leukemia, hemorrhage, and malignancy.
- Decreases associated with lymphoma, leukemia, viral infection, hypersplenia, and diabetes mellitus.

HEMATOCRIT

- Normal serum levels:
  Male—40-54 mL/dL.
  Female—37-47 mL/dL.
- Percentage of red blood cells in the blood.
- Elevation associated with dehydration, shock, polycythemia vera, and infection.
- Decreases associated with hemorrhage, anemia, and leukemia.

HEMOGLOBIN

- Normal serum levels:
  Male—13-18 g/dL.
  Female—12-16 g/dL.
- Oxygen-carrying pigment of the red blood cell.
- Carries oxygen from the lungs to the cells and carbon dioxide from the cells back to the lungs.
- Developed in the bone marrow inside of the red blood cell.
- Recycled by the spleen into iron.
- Basis of bilirubin.

Splenic Pathology

PATHOLOGY	ETIOLOGY	CLINICAL FINDINGS	SONOGRAPHIC FINDINGS	DIFFERENTIAL CONSIDERATIONS
Abscess	• Infective endocarditis—most common • Infection • Trauma	• Fever • Left upper quadrant (LUQ) pain • Leukocytosis	• Hypoechoic or complex splenic mass • Ill-defined, thick wall margins • May demonstrate posterior acoustic enhancement	• Hematoma • Splenic infarction • Cavernous lymphangioma

Continued

Splenic Pathology—cont'd

PATHOLOGY	ETIOLOGY	CLINICAL FINDINGS	SONOGRAPHIC FINDINGS	DIFFERENTIAL CONSIDERATIONS
Calcifications	• Granulomatosis • Splenic infarction • Calcified cyst • Abscess	• Asymptomatic • Abdominal pain	• Hyperechoic focus(i) disperse within the splenic parenchyma • May demonstrate posterior acoustic shadowing	• Calcified vessel(s)
Cavernous hemangioma	• Consists of large blood-filled cystic spaces • Most common benign neoplasm	• Asymptomatic • LUQ pain	• Well-defined hyperechoic splenic mass • Homogeneous or complex echo texture	• Splenic infarction • Hemangiosarcoma • Metastases
Cavernous lymphangioma	• Malformation of the lymph system	• Asymptomatic	• Hypoechoic solid splenic mass	• Abscess • Hematoma
Cyst	• Rare finding • Congenital • Infective • Neoplastic • Parasitic • Previous trauma	• Asymptomatic	• Well-defined anechoic mass • Smooth wall margins • Posterior acoustic enhancement • May demonstrate septations or debris	• Hematoma • Abscess • Cystic lymphangiomyomatosis
Cystic lymphangiomyomatosis	• Rare neoplasm • Proliferation of the smooth muscle cells in the lymph node	• Asymptomatic • Abdominal mass	• Diffuse or focal multiloculated cystic mass	• Splenic cyst
Hamartoma	• Rare benign neoplasm • Composed of lymphatic tissue	• Asymptomatic	• Hyperechoic parenchymal mass • Well-defined borders • Solitary or multiple in number	• Cavernous hemangioma • Metastases • Hemangiosarcoma
Splenic artery aneurysm Risk factors Atherosclerosis Portal hypertension Infection Trauma Female prevalence	• Localized dilatation of the splenic artery	• Asymptomatic • LUQ pain • Nausea/vomiting • Shoulder pain	• Anechoic dilatation of the splenic artery	• Tortuous artery • Splenic vein
Splenic candidiasis	• Multiple splenic infections • Associated with patients with autoimmune disorders	• Fever • Splenomegaly	• Target lesion or "wheel within a wheel" appearance	• Metastases
Splenic infarction	• Emboli from the heart • Associated with subacute bacterial endocarditis, leukemia, sickle cell anemia, metastasis, and pancreatitis	• Usually asymptomatic • LUQ pain	Acute Stage • Hypoechoic mass • Well-defined margins Chronic Stage • Hyperechoic mass • Well-defined margins • Splenic atrophy	• Hematoma • Cavernous hemangioma
Splenic rupture	• Trauma • Splenomegaly • Infectious disorder	• LUQ pain • Tachycardia • Palpable mass • Abdominal pain • Decrease in hematocrit	• Hypoechoic or complex mass • May demonstrate posterior acoustic enhancement • Subcapsular rupture appears as a crescent-shaped fluid collection • Evaluate abdominal cavity for free fluid	• Recent splenic infarction • Abscess • Cyst

Malignancy of the Spleen

MALIGNANCY	ETIOLOGY	CLINICAL FINDINGS	SONOGRAPHIC FINDINGS	DIFFERENTIAL CONSIDERATIONS
Hemangiosarcoma	• Rare splenic malignancy	• Anemia is most common • Left upper quadrant (LUQ) pain • Leukocytosis • Weight loss	• Hyperechoic or complex mass • Frequently metastasizes to the liver	• Abscess • Hematoma • Cavernous hemangioma
Leukemia	• Proliferation of white blood cells	• Lymphadenopathy • Palpable spleen • Joint pain • Weakness • Fever	• Splenomegaly • Diffuse increase in parenchyma echogenicity • Hypoechoic or hyperechoic nodules	• Lymphoma • Metastases
Lymphoma	• Malignant disorder involving the lymphoreticular system • Divided into Hodgkin and Non-Hodgkin	• Lymphadenopathy • LUQ pain • Fever • Weight loss • Decrease in WBC count	• Hypoechoic splenic masses • Ill-defined margins • May demonstrate splenomegaly	• Metastatic lesion • Hematoma
Metastases	• Melanoma is the most common • Breast • Lung • Pancreas	• Asymptomatic	• Typically hypoechoic or target lesions	• Multiple abscesses • Lymphoma • Splenic candidiasis • Leukemia

SPLEEN REVIEW

1. The most common location of an accessory spleen is near the:
   a. left renal hilum
   b. body of the pancreas
   c. left adrenal gland
   d. splenic hilum
   e. lesser curvature of the stomach

2. All of the following are considered functions of the spleen EXCEPT:
   a. reservoir for blood
   b. filters the blood
   c. recycles hemoglobin
   d. initiates production of antibodies
   e. breaks down old white blood cells

3. Enlargement of the spleen may be associated with all of the following conditions EXCEPT:
   a. cirrhosis
   b. hypotension
   c. diabetes mellitus
   d. portal hypertension
   e. congestive heart failure

4. The most common benign neoplasm of the spleen is a(n):
   a. cyst
   b. accessory spleen
   c. hematoma
   d. cavernous hemangioma
   e. cystadenoma

5. Hematocrit is defined as the percentage of:
   a. platelets in the red blood cell
   b. oxygen in the red blood cell
   c. red blood cells in the blood
   d. platelets in the blood
   e. oxygen in the blood

6. The most common clinical finding associated with a hemangiosarcoma is:
   a. anemia
   b. weight loss
   c. leukopenia
   d. abdominal pain
   e. lymphadenopathy

7. Metastasis to the spleen most commonly originates from which of the following malignancies?
   a. renal cell carcinoma
   b. hepatoma
   c. melanoma
   d. nephroblastoma
   e. adrenocortical carcinoma

8. Multiple splenic infections is a predisposing factor of which of the following conditions?
   a. infarction
   b. candidiasis
   c. arterial calcification
   d. cavernous hemangioma
   e. arterial aneurysm

9. The normal adult spleen measures approximately:
   a. 9 cm in length, 2 cm in width, and 5 cm in height
   b. 13 cm in length, 4 cm in width, and 6 cm in height
   c. 11 cm in length, 7 cm in width, and 4 cm in height
   d. 17 cm in length, 4 cm in width, and 7 cm in height
   e. 15 cm in length, 5 cm in width, and 7 cm in height

10. Hemangiosarcoma involving the spleen frequently metastasizes to which of the following organs?
    a. liver
    b. colon
    c. lung
    d. kidney
    e. pancreas

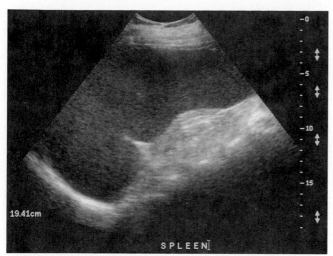

FIG. 11-2 Coronal sonogram of the left upper quadrant.

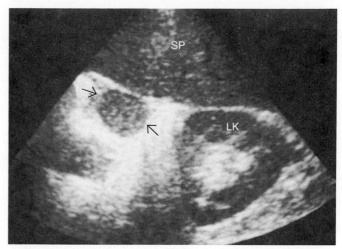

FIG. 11-3 Transverse sonogram of the left upper quadrant.

Using Fig. 11-2, answer questions 11 and 12.

11. A 50-year-old patient with a long history of alcohol abuse presents to the ultrasound department complaining of left upper quadrant pain. This sonogram of the left upper quadrant is most consistent with which of the following conditions?
    a. lymphoma
    b. splenomegaly
    c. lymphangioma
    d. splenic rupture
    e. splenic infarction

12. Based on this history and sonogram, the sonographer should also evaluate for which of the following pathologies?
    a. pancreatitis
    b. portal hypertension
    c. lymphadenopathy
    d. renal obstruction
    e. abdominal aortic aneurysm

Using Fig. 11-3, answer question 13.

13. A patient presents with a history of liver function tests showing elevated levels. The arrows in this sonogram are most likely identifying a(n):
    a. pancreatic mass
    b. enlarged lymph node
    c. wandering spleen
    d. accessory spleen
    e. adrenal hyperplasia

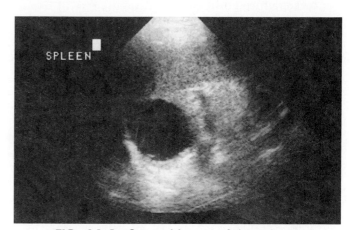

FIG. 11-4 Coronal image of the spleen.

Using Fig. 11-4, answer question 14.

14. An asymptomatic patient presents to the ultrasound department with a history of hepatitis B. An incidental finding is identified in the superior portion of the spleen. This finding is most consistent with a(n):
    a. cyst
    b. hematoma
    c. abscess
    d. cystic lymphangioma
    e. cavernous hemangioma

15. Which of the following splenic abnormalities is most commonly linked to infective endocarditis?
    a. hematoma
    b. abscess
    c. infarction
    d. calcifications
    e. hamartoma

16. The location of the spleen is best described as:
    a. anterior to the stomach
    b. superior to the diaphragm
    c. posterior to the left kidney
    d. lateral to the stomach
    e. medial to the left adrenal gland

17. Predisposing factors for developing an aneurysm of the splenic artery may include all of the following EXCEPT:
    a. trauma
    b. infection
    c. atherosclerosis
    d. male prevalence
    e. portal hypertension

18. A congenital anomaly of the spleen associated with gastrointestinal, cardiovascular, and biliary anomalies is most consistent with:
    a. aplasia
    b. asplenia syndrome
    c. wandering spleen
    d. polysplenia syndrome
    e. accessory spleen

19. The splenic artery is a branch of which of the following vascular structures?
    a. abdominal aorta
    b. celiac axis
    c. gastric artery
    d. thoracic aorta
    e. superior mesenteric artery

20. When compared to the liver, the echogenicity of the normal splenic parenchyma is described as:
    a. hypoechoic
    b. hyperechoic
    c. isoechoic
    d. hypoechoic or isoechoic
    e. hyperechoic or isoechoic

Using Fig. 11-5, answer questions 21 and 22.

21. A retroperitoneal ultrasound is ordered on an elderly patient with a history of elevated creatinine levels. Hyperechoic foci are identified in the splenic parenchyma. These foci are most suspicious for:
    a. candidiasis
    b. pneumobilia
    c. splenic calcifications
    d. multiple small hemangiomas
    e. multiple splenic abscesses

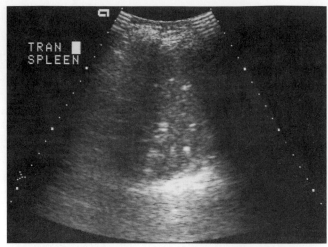

FIG. 11-5   Transverse sonogram of the left upper quadrant.

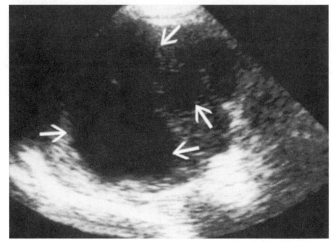

FIG. 11-6   Coronal sonogram of the left upper quadrant.

22. Based on the clinical history, these sonographic findings are most likely considered:
    a. life threatening
    b. incidental findings
    c. postsurgical changes
    d. complications of infection
    e. hypervascular lesions

Using Fig. 11-6, answer question 23.

23. An afebrile 13-year-old female patient presents to the ultrasound department complaining of vague left upper quadrant pain. She admits to "wrestling" with her brother a week ago. She denies blunt force trauma. Laboratory tests are pending. Based on this clinical history, the sonographic findings are most suspicious for which of the following conditions?
    a. lymphoma
    b. hematoma
    c. polycystic disease
    d. loculated abscess
    e. pseudocyst

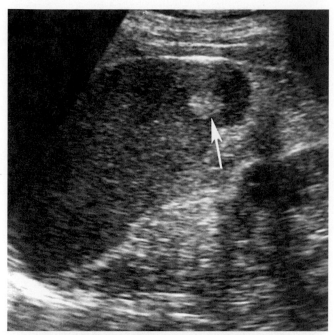

FIG. 11-7 Coronal sonogram of the spleen.

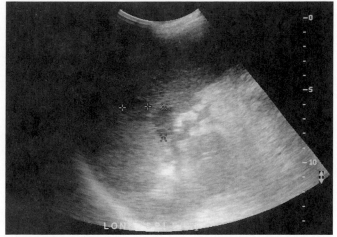

FIG. 11-8 Coronal sonogram of the spleen.

Using Fig. 11-7, answer question 24.

24. An asymptomatic middle-aged patient presents with a history of liver function tests showing elevated levels on an annual physical examination. An abdominal ultrasound is ordered to rule out liver disease. A sonogram of the left upper quadrant demonstrates a hyperechoic mass in the splenic parenchyma. Based on this history, the mass identified most likely represents a(n):
    a. abscess
    b. lipoma
    c. calcified artery
    d. cavernous hemangioma
    e. primary malignant tumor

Using Fig. 11-8, answer question 25.

25. An afebrile patient with a history of leukemia presents to the ultrasound department complaining of left upper quadrant pain. A sonogram of the spleen demonstrates hypoechoic nodules within the splenic parenchyma. These nodules most likely represent:
    a. candidiasis
    b. lymphadenopathy
    c. primary malignant tumors
    d. multiple splenic abscesses
    e. metastatic disease

26. Which of the following structures carries carbon dioxide back to the lungs?
    a. platelet
    b. lymphocyte
    c. hematocrit
    d. hemoglobin
    e. leukocyte

27. Leukemia may be associated with all of the following EXCEPT:
    a. splenomegaly
    b. joint pain
    c. leukopenia
    d. weakness
    e. lymphadenopathy

28. Indications for an ultrasound of the spleen may include all of the following EXCEPT:
    a. fatigue
    b. trauma
    c. abdominal mass
    d. elevated serum amylase
    e. leukocytosis

29. Which of the following splenic pathologies is associated with granulomatosis?
    a. cysts
    b. calcifications
    c. cavernous hemangioma
    d. cystadenoma
    e. cavernous lymphangioma

30. A patient presents with a history of portal hypertension. The spleen is expected to demonstrate:
    a. atrophy
    b. fatty infiltration
    c. enlargement
    d. intraparenchymal calcifications
    e. reversal of flow in the splenic vein

31. Leukocytosis is defined as a white blood cell count:
    a. below 4,000
    b. below 11,000
    c. above 4,000
    d. above 12,000
    e. above 20,000

32. A hematoma located below the splenic capsule most commonly appears on ultrasound as a:
    a. left pleural effusion
    b. lateral anechoic mass
    c. hypoechoic parenchymal mass
    d. crescent-shaped fluid collection inferior to the diaphragm
    e. loculated mass anterior to the left kidney

33. Which of the following pathologies is associated with a "wheel within a wheel" appearance on ultrasound?
    a. candidiasis
    b. infarction
    c. hemangiosarcoma
    d. cavernous hemangioma
    e. cystic lymphangiomatosis

34. Splenic infarction is most commonly associated with an embolism originating from which of the following structures?
    a. heart
    b. liver
    c. spleen
    d. pancreas
    e. lower extremity

35. Which of the following conditions is most likely to demonstrate an elevated hematocrit?
    a. overhydration
    b. infection
    c. leukemia
    d. hemorrhage
    e. splenomegaly

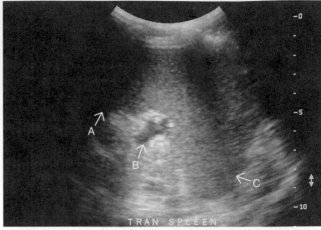
FIG. 11-9   Transverse sonogram of the spleen.

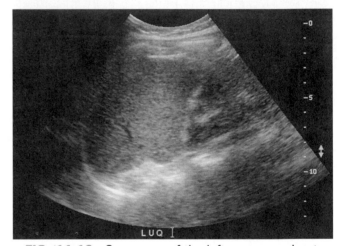
FIG. 11-10   Sonogram of the left upper quadrant.

Using Fig. 11-9, answer questions 36 through 38.

36. Which of the following splenic regions is identified by arrow **A**?
    a. superior portion
    b. inferior portion
    c. splenic hilum
    d. anterior portion
    e. posterior portion

37. Which of the following splenic regions is identified by arrow **B**?
    a. superior portion
    b. inferior portion
    c. splenic hilum
    d. anterior portion
    e. posterior portion

38. Which of the following splenic regions is identified by arrow **C**?
    a. superior portion
    b. inferior portion
    c. splenic hilum
    d. anterior portion
    e. posterior portion

Using Fig. 11-10, answer question 39.

39. Which of the following scanning planes is most likely demonstrated in this sonogram?
    a. anterior
    b. posterior
    c. subcostal
    d. transverse
    e. coronal

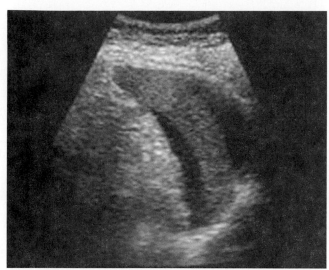

FIG. 11-11 Transverse sonogram of the left upper quadrant.

Using Fig. 11-11, answer question 40.

40. A patient presents with a history of increased abdominal girth and liver function tests showing elevated levels. Which of the following findings is most likely demonstrated in this sonogram of the left upper quadrant?
a. ascites
b. phlegmon
c. pleural effusion
d. hemoperitoneum
e. splenorenal ligament

41. A patient arrives at the emergency department following a motor vehicle accident. An abdominal ultrasound is MOST LIKELY ordered to evaluate for which of the following conditions?
a. pancreatitis
b. biliary obstruction
c. urinary obstruction
d. hemoperitoneum
e. abdominal aortic aneurysm

42. In cases of portal hypertension, the splenic vein is most likely to shunt blood directly into the:
a. gastric vein
b. left renal vein
c. middle hepatic vein
d. inferior vena cava
e. inferior mesenteric vein

43. The splenic vein joins the superior mesenteric vein to form the:
a. coronary vein
b. hepatic vein
c. inferior mesenteric vein
d. portal vein
e. gastric vein

44. Leukopenia is defined as a white blood cell count:
a. below 4,000
b. below 11,000
c. above 4,000
d. above 12,000
e. above 20,000

45. Which of the following structures is recycled into iron by the spleen?
a. erythrocytes
b. platelets
c. leukocytes
d. hemoglobin
e. monocytes

46. Which of the following conditions is most likely associated with a decrease in leukocytes?
a. anemia
b. lymphoma
c. leukemia
d. malignancy
e. cirrhosis

47. Normal hemoglobin levels should not exceed:
a. 5 g/dL
b. 10 g/dL
c. 20 g/dL
d. 50 g/dL
e. 75 g/dL

48. In a 40-year-old patient, splenomegaly is suggested once the length of the spleen exceeds:
a. 7 cm
b. 11 cm
c. 13 cm
d. 18 cm
e. 20 cm

49. A patient with an accessory spleen will most likely present with which of the following symptoms?
a. dyspepsia
b. no symptoms
c. left upper quadrant pain
d. palpable abdominal mass
e. elevated white blood cell count

50. Which of the following benign neoplasms is composed of lymphoid tissue?
a. lipoma
b. adenoma
c. seroma
d. hamartoma
e. cavernous hemangioma

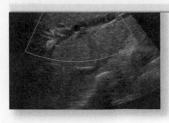

CHAPTER 12

Retroperitoneum

KEY TERMS

Addison disease life-threatening condition caused by partial or complete failure of the adrenocortical function. Also known as adrenocortical insufficiency.

Cushing syndrome a metabolic disorder resulting from chronic and excessive production of cortisol by the adrenal cortex. Results in the inability of the body to regulate secretions of cortisol or adrenocorticotrophic hormone (ACTH). Also known as hyperadrenalism.

diaphragmatic crura fibers that connect the vertebral column and diaphragm. They are identified superior to the celiac axis and lie anterior to the aorta and posterior to the inferior vena cava.

floating aorta enlarged lymph nodes posterior to the aorta giving the impression the aorta is floating above the spine.

hyperaldosteronism excessive production of aldosterone.

lymphadenopathy focal or generalized enlargement of the lymph nodes.

neuroblastoma malignant tumor of the adrenal gland found in young children.

pheochromocytoma a rare vascular tumor of the adrenal medulla.

retroperitoneal pertaining to organs closely attached to the posterior abdominal wall.

retroperitoneal fibrosis dense fibrous tissue proliferation typically confined to the paravertebral and central retroperitoneum areas.

suprarenal glands adrenal glands.

ADRENAL GLANDS (Fig. 12-1)

- A pair of endocrine glands located in the retroperitoneum.

PHYSIOLOGY

FUNCTION OF THE ADRENAL GLANDS

- Produce hormones.

EPINEPHRINE (ADRENALINE)

- Secreted by the medulla.
- Increases in times of excitement or emotional stress.

NOREPINEPHRINE

- Secreted by the medulla.
- Acts to increase blood pressure by vasoconstriction without affecting cardiac output.

GLUCOCORTICOIDS

- Cortisol.
- Normal range:
  serum 4-22 µg/dL (morning)
  3-17 µg/dL (afternoon)
  urine 20-90 µg/dL
- Secreted by the cortex.
- Aids in the body's response to stress.
- Modifies the body's response to infection, surgery, or trauma.
- Aids in controlling the amount of water in the body.

FIG. 12-1
Retroperitoneum
anatomy.

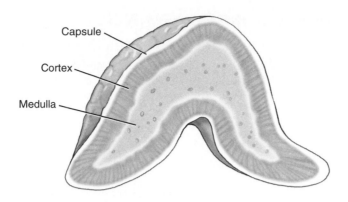

Capsule

Cortex

Medulla

- Controls protein and carbohydrate metabolism.
- Increases with stress and decreases with inflammation.

GONADAL HORMONE

- Androgens, estrogens, and progesterone.
- Secreted by the cortex.

MINERAL CORTICOIDS

- Aldosterone.
- Secreted by the cortex.
- Helps maintain the body's fluid and electrolyte balance by promoting sodium reabsorption and potassium excretion within the kidneys.

ANATOMY

- Consists of two regions.
  - Medulla—inner portion, which comprises 10% of the gland.
  - Cortex—outer portion, which comprises 90% of the gland.

LOCATION

- Retroperitoneal structures located in Gerota fascia within the perinephric space.
- Located anterior, medial, and superior to each kidney.
- Lie lateral to the diaphragmatic crura.
- Right adrenal gland lies posterior and lateral to the inferior vena cava.
- Left adrenal gland lies lateral to the aorta and posterior-medial to the splenic artery and tail of the pancreas.

SIZE

- Adult adrenal gland measures 3 to 5 cm in length, 2 to 3 cm in width, and 1 cm in height.

VASCULAR ANATOMY

- The adrenal glands are supplied by the superior, middle, and inferior suprarenal arteries.
- Superior suprarenal artery arises from the inferior phrenic artery.
- Middle suprarenal artery arises from the lateral aspect of the abdominal aorta.
- Inferior suprarenal artery arises from the renal artery.
- Right suprarenal vein drains directly into the inferior vena cava.
- Left suprarenal vein drains into the left renal vein.

NORMAL SONOGRAPHIC APPEARANCE

- Solid, hypoechoic, crescent-shaped structures surrounded by echogenic fat.
- Prominent in the neonate and children demonstrating a hypoechoic cortex and hyperechoic medulla.
- Difficult to visualize in the adult.

TECHNIQUE

PREPARATION

- No preparation is necessary for a sonogram of the adrenal glands or retroperitoneum.
- Nothing by mouth 6 to 8 hours prior to examination is the typical preparation to decrease intestinal interference.

EXAMINATION TECHNIQUE

- Use the highest-frequency abdominal transducer possible to obtain optimal resolution for penetration depth.
- Proper focal and depth placement.
- Supine, oblique, and/or decubitus positions may be used.
- Sagittal or coronal and transverse planes are used to evaluate and document the adrenal glands and surrounding structures.
- Documentation and measurement of the length, height, and width of each adrenal gland if visualized.
- Evaluation and documentation of the retroperitoneum using a four- or nine-quadrant method.
- Documentation and measurement of any abnormality should be included.

INDICATIONS FOR EXAMINATION

- Hypertension.
- Abdominal distention.
- Severe anxiety.
- Sweating.
- Tachycardia.
- Weight loss.
- Diabetes mellitus.
- Evaluate mass from previous medical imaging study (i.e., CT).

LABORATORY VALUES

ADRENOCORTICOTROPHIC HORMONE (ACTH)

- Normal range: 10-80 pg/mL.
- Regulates cortisol production.
- Produced in the pituitary gland.
- Elevation associated with adrenal tumor, Cushing disease, and lung tumor.

ALDOSTERONE

- Normal range:
  Recumbent 3-10 ng/dL
  Erect 5-30 ng/dL
- Steroid secreted by the cortex.
- Regulates sodium and water levels, which affects blood volume and pressure.
- Elevation associated with hyperaldosteronism.
- Decreases associated with hypoaldosteronism and Addison disease.

POTASSIUM

- Normal range: serum 3.5-5.0 mEq/L.
- Essential to the normal function of every organ system.
- Maintains necessary concentration of nutrients inside and outside of the cell.
- Elevation associated with Addison disease.
- Decreases associated with Cushing disease and hyperaldosteronism.

SODIUM

- Normal range: serum 135-145 mEq/L.
- Major component in determining blood volume.
- Decreases associated with Addison disease.

Benign Adrenal Pathology

PATHOLOGY	ETIOLOGY	CLINICAL FINDINGS	SONOGRAPHIC FINDINGS	DIFFERENTIAL CONSIDERATIONS
Adenoma	• Benign cortical mass • Functioning or nonfunctioning Risk Factors • Diabetes mellitus • Obesity • Hypertension • Elderly population	• Asymptomatic • Elevated adrenal hormones	• Hypoechoic, homogeneous mass • Smooth wall margins • May demonstrate necrosis or hemorrhage	• Adrenal hyperplasia • Adrenocortical carcinoma • Renal or liver mass • Adrenal hemorrhage
Adrenal cyst	• Rare • Unilateral	• Asymptomatic • Hypertension	• Anechoic mass • Well-defined wall margins • Posterior acoustic enhancement • Walls may calcify	• Cyst of the liver, spleen, or kidney • Hydronephrosis
Adrenal hemorrhage	• Adrenal mass • Hypoxia • Traumatic delivery • Septicemia	• Asymptomatic • Palpable abdominal mass • Decrease in hematocrit	• Cystic or complex adrenal mass • Frequently located on the right	• Cyst or neoplasm of the liver, spleen, or kidney • Adenoma • Adrenocortical carcinoma
Adrenal hyperplasia	• Proliferation in adrenal cells • Typically bilateral	• Asymptomatic • Hypertension • Elevated adrenocorticotrophic hormone (ACTH) level	• Enlargement of the adrenal gland(s) • Change in the normal triangular shape	• Adenoma • Adrenocortical carcinoma
Pheochromocytoma	• Rare vascular tumor of the medulla • Small percentage are malignant	• Hypertension • Sweating • Tachycardia • Chest or epigastric pain • Headache • Palpitations • Severe anxiety • Increase in epinephrine and norepinephrine	• Solid mass • Homogeneous texture • May appear complex due to necrosis or hemorrhage • May calcify	• Renal mass • Adrenocortical carcinoma • Adrenal adenoma • Adrenal hemorrhage

Malignant Adrenal Pathology

PATHOLOGY	ETIOLOGY	CLINICAL FINDINGS	SONOGRAPHIC FINDINGS	DIFFERENTIAL CONSIDERATIONS
Adrenocortical carcinoma	• Neoplasm of the adrenal cortex • Functioning or nonfunctioning	• Hypertension • Weakness • Abdominal pain • Weight loss • Weakening of the bones	• Complex or echogenic mass • Irregular wall margins • Tends to invade the IVC • Metastasis to the lungs and bone	• Renal mass • Adrenal hemorrhage • Pheochromocytoma • Metastases
Metastases	• Lung most common • Breast • Stomach	• Hypertension • Abdominal pain	• Variable in appearance	• Renal mass • Adrenal hemorrhage • Pheochromocytoma • Adrenocortical carcinoma
Neuroblastoma	• Neoplasm of the adrenal gland common in young children • Male prevalence	• Palpable mass • Abdominal distention • Sweating • Weight loss • Weakness	• Heterogeneous mass • Poorly defined wall margins • More common on the left • Metastasis to the liver, bone, lung, and lymph nodes	• Nephroblastoma • Lymphoma • Adrenal hemorrhage

Conditions Associated with the Adrenal Glands

CONDITION	DESCRIPTION	ETIOLOGY	CLINICAL FINDINGS
Addison disease	• Life-threatening condition caused by partial or complete failure of adrenocortical function • Destruction of the adrenal cortex • Loss of cortisol and aldosterone secretions • Increased incidence in females • Diagnosis is established if the amount of cortisol in the plasma and steroid in the urine does not increase after stimulation with adrenocorticotrophic hormone (ACTH)	• Auto-immune reaction • Tuberculosis • Adrenal hemorrhage • Chronic infection • Surgical removal of both adrenal glands	• Anorexia • Bronze skin pigmentation • Chronic fatigue • Dehydration • Emotional changes • GI disorders • Hypotension • Weakness • Salt cravings • Elevated serum potassium • Decrease in serum sodium and glucose
Cushing disease	• Rare and serious disorder resulting from excessive production of cortisol • Excessive use of cortical hormones • Results in accumulation of fat on the abdomen, face, upper back, and upper chest	• Pituitary mass is the most common cause • Adrenal mass • Polycystic ovarian disease • Excessive amount of glucocorticoid hormone	• Fatigue • Purplish striae on the skin • Decrease in immunity to infection • Emotional changes • Increase in thirst and urination • Muscle weakness • New onset of diabetes mellitus • Osteoporosis • Elevation in ACTH, white blood cells, and blood glucose levels • Decrease in serum potassium
Hyperaldosteronism	• Excessive production of aldosterone	• Hyperplasia of both adrenal glands • Benign tumor of one adrenal gland (Conn syndrome)	• Hypertension • Elevated aldosterone levels • Decrease in serum potassium level • Normal serum sodium level

RETROPERITONEUM

- Area of the body behind the peritoneum.

BORDERS OF THE RETROPERITONEUM

- Superior border—diaphragm.
- Inferior border—pelvic rim.
- Anterior border—posterior parietal peritoneum.
- Posterior border—posterior abdominal wall muscles.
- Lateral border—transversalis fascia and peritoneal portions of the mesentery.

SPACES IN THE RETROPERITONEUM

Anterior Pararenal

- Fat area between the posterior peritoneum and Gerota fascia.
- Includes: pancreas, descending portion of the duodenum, ascending and descending colon, superior mesenteric vessels and inferior portion of the common bile duct.

Posterior Pararenal

- Space between Gerota fascia and the posterior abdominal wall muscles.
- Includes: iliopsoas and quadratus lumborum muscles and the posterior abdominal wall.

Perirenal

- Space separated from the pararenal space by Gerota fascia.
- Includes: kidneys, adrenal glands, perinephric fat, ureters, renal vessels, aorta, inferior vena cava, and lymph nodes.

LYMPH NODES

FUNCTIONS OF LYMPH NODES

- Filter the lymph of debris and organisms.
- Form lymphocytes and antibodies to fight infection.

DIVISIONS OF LYMPH NODES

Parietal Nodes

- Located in the retroperitoneum and course along the prevertebral vessels.
- Surround the aorta.
- Kidney, adrenal gland, ovarian/testicular nodes drain into the para-aortic nodes.
- Subdivided into:
  Common iliac.
  Epigastric.
  External iliac.
  Iliac circumflex.
  Internal iliac.
  Lumbar.
  Sacral.

Visceral Nodes

- Located in the peritoneum and follow the course along the vessels supplying the major organs.

SONOGRAPHIC APPEARANCE OF THE NORMAL LYMPH NODE

- Hypoechoic solid mass.
- Hyperechoic fatty center.
- Smooth margins.
- Oval shape.
- Internal vascular blood flow.
- Usually measures less than 1 cm.

SONOGRAPHIC APPEARANCE OF THE ABNORMAL LYMPH NODE

- Enlarged hypoechoic mass exceeding 1 cm in size.
- Loss of hyperechoic fatty center.
- Smooth wall margins and oval shape typically caused by infection.
- Irregular margins and round shape suspicious for malignancy.
- Displacement of adjacent structures.

SONOGRAPHIC APPEARANCE OF RETROPERITONEAL MASSES

- Hyperechoic to hypoechoic mass(es).
- Irregular wall margins.
- Anterior displacement of the kidneys, inferior vena cava, aorta, and mesenteric vessels.
- Deformity of the inferior vena cava and urinary bladder.
- Obstruction of the urinary tract or biliary system.
- Loss of organ definition.

Benign Pathology of the Retroperitoneum

PATHOLOGY	DESCRIPTION	SONOGRAPHIC FINDINGS	DIFFERENTIAL CONSIDERATIONS
Lymphadenopathy	• Any disorder characterized by a localized or generalized enlargement of the lymph nodes or lymph vessels	• Hypoechoic mass • May appear complex • Smooth or irregular margins • Exceeds 1 cm in size	• Lipoma • Retroperitoneal fibrosis • Retroperitoneal hemorrhage • Horseshoe kidney
Lymphocele	• A fluid collection containing lymph from an injured lymph vessel	• Anechoic fluid collection • Round or oval in shape • Well-defined borders • Frequently contain septations • Posterior acoustic enhancement	• Hematoma • Urinoma • Ascites • Abscess
Retroperitoneal abscess	• A collection of pus between the peritoneum and the posterior abdominal wall	• Hypoechoic or complex mass • Irregular margins • May demonstrate posterior acoustic shadowing • Mass takes on the shape of the space	• Hemorrhage • Lymphadenopathy • Retroperitoneal fibrosis • Horseshoe kidney
Retroperitoneal fibrosis	• A chronic inflammatory process in which fibrotic tissue surrounds the large blood vessels located in the lumbar area • Usually idiopathic	• Hypoechoic bulky midline mass • Rarely extends above the second lumbar vertebra • May demonstrate associated hydronephrosis	• Lymphadenopathy • Retroperitoneal hemorrhage • Retroperitoneal abscess • Horseshoe kidney

Benign Pathology of the Retroperitoneum—cont'd

PATHOLOGY	DESCRIPTION	SONOGRAPHIC FINDINGS	DIFFERENTIAL CONSIDERATIONS
Retroperitoneal hemorrhage	• Associated with trauma, tumor, aneurysm, cyst, or infarction	• Hypoechoic fluid collections • May demonstrate echogenic clot	• Ascites • Retroperitoneal fibrosis • Lymphadenopathy • Horseshoe kidney
Urinoma	• A cyst filled with urine • Adjacent or within the urinary tract • Typically located in the perinephric space	• Anechoic fluid collection • Smooth, thin walls • Frequently contain septations • Rapid increase in size on serial examinations	• Lymphocele • Hematoma • Cyst • Abscess

Benign Neoplasms of the Retroperitoneum

PATHOLOGY	DESCRIPTION	SONOGRAPHIC FINDINGS	DIFFERENTIAL CONSIDERATIONS
Fibroma	• A neoplasm consisting largely of fibrous connective tissue	• Hyperechoic mass • Well-defined wall margins	• Lipoma • Mesothelioma • Myxoma
Lipoma	• A neoplasm consisting of fatty tissue	• Hyperechoic mass • Well-defined wall margins	• Fibroma • Liposarcoma • Mesothelioma • Myxoma
Mesothelioma	• Abnormal growth of the epithelial cells	• Localized echogenic mass • Irregular wall margins • Similar appearance to the fetal placenta	• Liposarcoma • Lymphadenopathy • Lipoma • Myxoma • Horseshoe kidney
Myxoma	• A neoplasm consisting of connective tissue • Subcutaneous, retroperitoneal, cardiac, and urinary in location • May be extremely large	• Complex or echogenic mass • Lobulated or smooth wall margins	• Fibroma • Lipoma • Mesothelioma • Lymphadenopathy • Horseshoe kidney
Teratoma	• A neoplasm composed of different types of tissues that do not occur together or at the site of the tumor.	• Complex mass	• Leiomyosarcoma • Abscess • Myxoma

Malignant Neoplasms of the Retroperitoneum

PATHOLOGY	DESCRIPTION	SONOGRAPHIC FINDINGS	DIFFERENTIAL CONSIDERATIONS
Fibrosarcoma	• A sarcoma containing fibrous connective tissues	• Hypoechoic or complex mass • May infiltrate surrounding structures	• Lymphadenopathy • Retroperitoneal fibrosis • Retroperitoneal hemorrhage • Horseshoe kidney
Leiomyosarcoma	• A sarcoma containing large spindle cells of smooth muscle	• Echogenic or complex mass • Cystic areas of necrosis may be demonstrated	• Teratoma • Rhabdomyosarcoma • Retroperitoneal abscess
Liposarcoma	• A malignant growth of fat cells • Most common retroperitoneal neoplasm	• Hyperechoic mass • Thick wall margins • May infiltrate surrounding tissues	• Lipoma • Fibroma • Rhabdomyosarcoma • Mesothelioma
Rhabdomyosarcoma	• A highly malignant tumor derived from striated muscle	• Hyperechoic or complex mass	• Teratoma • Liposarcoma • Fibrosarcoma • Leiomyosarcoma

RETROPERITONEUM REVIEW

1. Which of the following hormones modifies the body's response to inflammation?
   a. androgens
   b. aldosterone
   c. norepinephrine
   d. glucocorticoids
   e. epinephrine

2. A malignant neoplasm derived from striated muscle describes a:
   a. myxoma
   b. mesothelioma
   c. leiomyosarcoma
   d. rhabdomyosarcoma
   e. pheochromocytoma

3. All of the following structures are located within the anterior pararenal space EXCEPT:
   a. pancreas
   b. ascending colon
   c. superior mesenteric artery
   d. inferior vena cava
   e. descending colon

4. Bilateral adrenal hyperplasia is associated with:
   a. hyperaldosteronism
   b. Addison disease
   c. Conn syndrome
   d. Bouveret syndrome
   e. Cushing disease

5. Which of the following is considered a function of the lymph node?
   a. modify the body's response to inflammation
   b. aid in controlling the amount of water in the body
   c. maintain the water and sodium balance
   d. form antibodies to fight infection
   e. maintain normal blood circulation

6. Symptoms associated with adrenocortical carcinoma include all of the following EXCEPT:
   a. hypertension
   b. severe anxiety
   c. muscle weakness
   d. weight loss
   e. abdominal pain

7. Indications for a sonogram of the adrenal glands include all of the following EXCEPT:
   a. tachycardia
   b. severe anxiety
   c. hypertension
   d. renal insufficiency
   e. weight loss

8. Which of the following adrenal neoplasms is most likely to infiltrate surrounding structures?
   a. teratoma
   b. liposarcoma
   c. myxoma
   d. mesothelioma
   e. leiomyosarcoma

9. A urinoma is most likely to develop in which of the following regions?
   a. lesser sac
   b. paracolic gutter
   c. perinephric space
   d. subhepatic space
   e. pouch of Douglas

10. The most common neoplasm to develop in the retroperitoneum is a:
    a. liposarcoma
    b. myxoma
    c. fibrosarcoma
    d. mesothelioma
    e. rhabdomyosarcoma

11. Which of the following statements correctly describes the adrenal glands?
    a. The medulla comprises 25% of the gland
    b. The right suprarenal vein drains into the right renal vein
    c. Gonadal hormones are secreted by the medulla
    d. Norepinephrine is secreted by the cortex
    e. The suprarenal arteries arise from the aorta, renal, and inferior phrenic arteries

12. The anterior pararenal space is most accurately defined as the area between the:
    a. perirenal space and the posterior pararenal space
    b. posterior peritoneum and Gerota fascia
    c. anterior abdominal wall and the psoas muscle
    d. posterior retroperitoneum and the perirenal space
    e. anterior peritoneum and Gerota fascia

13. Young children have a predisposing factor for developing which of the following adrenal neoplasms?
    a. nephroblastoma
    b. pheochromocytoma
    c. Wilms tumor
    d. neuroblastoma
    e. liposarcoma

14. Which of the following structures form the anterior border of the retroperitoneum?
    a. diaphragm
    b. pelvic rim
    c. posterior parietal peritoneum
    d. transversalis fascia
    e. posterior abdominal wall muscles

15. All of the following structures are located within the perirenal space EXCEPT:
    a. kidneys
    b. aorta
    c. lymph nodes
    d. psoas muscles
    e. adrenal glands

16. Hemorrhage within the retroperitoneum may be caused by all of the following conditions EXCEPT:
    a. trauma
    b. neoplasm
    c. infarction
    d. ruptured aneurysm
    e. abscess formation

17. Benign adrenal pathology associated with hypertension, tachycardia, and palpitations is most consistent with which of the following pathologies?
    a. hyperplasia
    b. pheochromocytoma
    c. hemorrhage
    d. adenoma
    e. polycystic disease

18. Visceral lymph nodes are located:
    a. around the aorta
    b. in the perineum
    c. along the prevertebral vessels
    d. in the peritoneum
    e. near the adrenal glands

19. The location of the right adrenal gland most accurately correlates to which of the following regions?
    a. lateral to the right kidney
    b. posterior to the inferior vena cava
    c. medial to the diaphragmatic crura
    d. inferior to the right kidney
    e. medial to the inferior vena cava

20. Elevation in which of the following laboratory tests is a clinical finding in Addison disease?
    a. cortisol
    b. aldosterone
    c. serum sodium
    d. serum potassium
    e. adrenocorticotrophic hormone

21. Which of the following conditions is a predisposing factor for development of an adrenal adenoma?
    a. anorexia
    b. hypotension
    c. diabetes mellitus
    d. congestive heart failure
    e. polycythemia vera

22. The "floating aorta" sign is caused by lymphadenopathy in which of the following regions?
    a. lesser sac
    b. perinephric space
    c. anterior to the aorta
    d. surrounding the aorta
    e. posterior to the aorta

23. An adrenal cyst is considered a:
    a. rare finding
    b. bilateral condition
    c. functioning neoplasm
    d. life-threatening neoplasm
    e. proliferation of adrenal cells

24. Which of the following hormones is secreted by the adrenal medulla?
    a. cortisol
    b. epinephrine
    c. estrogen
    d. aldosterone
    e. secretin

25. A condition caused by complete or partial failure of the adrenocortical function describes:
    a. Conn syndrome
    b. Addison disease
    c. Budd-Chiari syndrome
    d. Cushing disease
    e. Graves disease

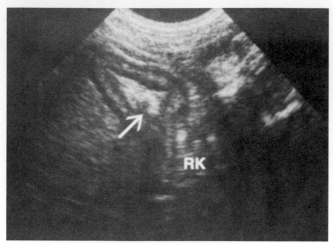

FIG. 12-2   Neonatal adrenal gland.

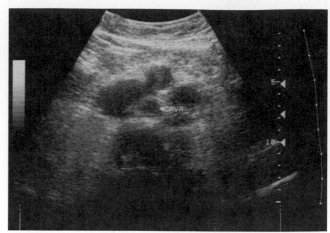

FIG. 12-4   Midline transverse image of the great vessels.

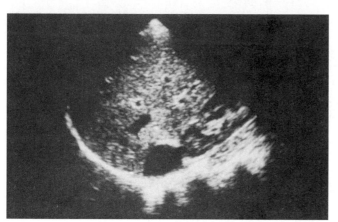

FIG. 12-3   Sagittal image of the right upper quadrant.

Using Fig. 12-2, answer question 26.

26. A 2-day-old neonate presents with a history of decreased urinary output. A sagittal image demonstrates a hyperechoic focus within the right adrenal gland. This finding is most suspicious for a(n):
a. adrenal lipoma
b. normal cortex
c. adrenal hemorrhage
d. normal medulla
e. neuroblastoma

Using Fig. 12-3, answer questions 27 and 28.

27. A 35-year-old male presents with a history of a sudden onset of hypertension. An anechoic area is identified in the right upper quadrant. On the

basis of the clinical history, the anechoic area in this sonogram is most suspicious for a(n):
a. adrenal cyst
b. liver cyst
c. adrenal adenoma
d. pheochromocytoma
e. retroperitoneal hemorrhage

28. The pathology identified in this sonogram is considered a(n):
a. incidental finding
b. result of trauma
c. rare finding
d. malignant lesion
e. rare vascular tumor

Using Fig. 12-4, answer question 29.

29. A 45-year-old female presents with a history of weight loss, severe back pain, and elevated alkaline phosphatase. A sonogram of the great vessels identifies multiple masses anterior to the inferior vena cava and abdominal aorta. These masses are most suspicious for:
a. liposarcoma
b. lymphoceles
c. lymphadenopathy
d. pseudomyxoma peritonei
e. retroperitoneal fibrosis

30. Which of the following abnormalities is the most likely complication of retroperitoneal fibrosis?
a. pancreatitis
b. cholecystitis
c. hydronephrosis
d. portal hypertension
e. abdominal aortic aneurysm

31. An enlarged lymph node demonstrating an oval shape and smooth wall margins is most consistent with an underlying:
    a. malignancy
    b. hemorrhage
    c. infection
    d. infarction
    e. obstruction

32. Which of the following fluid collections is most likely to demonstrate a rapid increase in size following renal transplant surgery?
    a. seroma
    b. abscess
    c. hematoma
    d. urinoma
    e. lymphocele

33. An abnormal growth of epithelial cells is demonstrated in which of the following neoplasms?
    a. myxoma
    b. teratoma
    c. lipoma
    d. leiomyosarcoma
    e. mesothelioma

34. Which of the following malignant neoplasms contains cells of smooth muscle?
    a. fibrosarcoma
    b. liposarcoma
    c. leiomyosarcoma
    d. rhabdomyosarcoma
    e. mesothelioma

35. The sonographic appearance of a liposarcoma is most likely described as a:
    a. hypoechoic mass with thin wall margins
    b. hyperechoic mass with thick wall margins
    c. complex mass with irregular wall margins
    d. hypoechoic mass with irregular wall margins
    e. hyperechoic mass with thin wall margins

Using Fig. 12-5, answer question 36.

36. A neonate presents with a history of decreasing hematocrit levels. A sonogram of the right upper quadrant demonstrates a complex mass in the right adrenal gland. On the basis of the clinical history, the mass is most suspicious for a(n):
    a. abscess
    b. adenoma
    c. complex cyst
    d. hemorrhage
    e. adrenocortical carcinoma

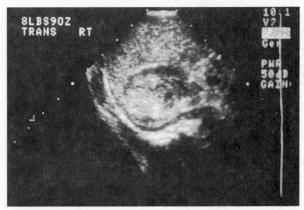

FIG. 12-5 Transverse sonogram of the right upper quadrant.

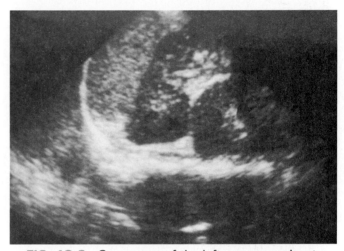

FIG. 12-6 Sonogram of the left upper quadrant.

Using Fig. 12-6, answer question 37.

37. A toddler presents with a history of abdominal distension, weight loss, and fatigue. A complex mass is identified inferior to the spleen and medial to the superior pole of the left kidney. On the basis of the clinical history, the sonogram is most suspicious for which of the following pathologies?
    a. adrenal hemorrhage
    b. nephroblastoma
    c. intussusception
    d. neuroblastoma
    e. splenic rupture

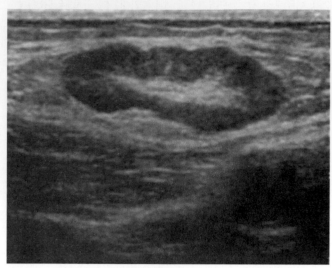

FIG. 12-7   Sonogram of the left groin.

Using Fig. 12-7, answer question 38.

38. A 70-year-old patient presents with a palpable mass in the left groin following a recent invasive procedure. A sonogram of the left groin demonstrates an oval-shaped mass in the superficial tissues of the thigh. This mass is most likely a:
    a. fibroma
    b. lipoma
    c. hematoma
    d. lymph node
    e. pseudoaneurysm

39. The outer portion of the adrenal gland comprises:
    a. 10% of the gland
    b. 25% of the gland
    c. 50% of the gland
    d. 75% of the gland
    e. 90% of the gland

40. The adrenal glands are also known as the:
    a. cortisol glands
    b. adrenaline glands
    c. suprarenal glands
    d. retroperitoneal glands
    e. stress glands

41. The right suprarenal vein empties into which of the following vascular structures?
    a. splenic vein
    b. left renal vein
    c. inferior vena cava
    d. right gonadal vein
    e. superior mesenteric vein

42. Which of the following hormones increases during times of excitement or stress?
    a. renin
    b. cortisol
    c. aldosterone
    d. epinephrine
    e. norepinephrine

43. Which of the following components is a major factor in determining blood volume?
    a. sodium
    b. vitamin K
    c. potassium
    d. calcium
    e. barium sulfate

44. Obesity is most likely a predisposing factor in developing which of the following adrenal neoplasms?
    a. cyst
    b. hemorrhage
    c. adenoma
    d. neuroblastoma
    e. pheochromocytoma

45. Which of the following hormones is produced by the pituitary gland?
    a. trypsin
    b. insulin
    c. epinephrine
    d. aldosterone
    e. adrenocorticotrophic hormone

46. Which of the following is considered a function of the adrenal glands?
    a. produce hormones
    b. release secretin hormones
    c. regulate serum electrolytes
    d. release glycogen as glucose
    e. maintain homeostasis of blood calcium concentrations

47. A rare vascular tumor of the adrenal gland defines a(n):
    a. adenoma
    b. teratoma
    c. neuroblastoma
    d. rhabdomyosarcoma
    e. pheochromocytoma

48. The inner portion of the adrenal gland is termed the:
    a. hilum
    b. cortex
    c. intima
    d. medulla
    e. sinus

49. The location of the left adrenal gland most accurately correlates to which of the following regions?
a. lateral to the kidney
b. medial to the aorta
c. inferior to the kidney
d. posterior to the splenic artery
e. posterior to the inferior vena cava

50. Cushing disease is most commonly caused by which of the following pathologies?
a. adrenal hyperplasia
b. pituitary mass
c. adrenal mass
d. polycystic ovarian disease
e. adrenal insufficiency

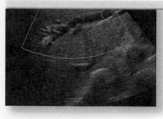

CHAPTER 13

Abdominal Vasculature

KEY TERMS

abdominal aortic aneurysm dilatation of the aorta equal to or exceeding 3 cm in diameter; also known as AAA.

aneurysm a localized widening or dilatation of a blood vessel.

arteriovenous fistula an abnormal connection between an artery and vein; also known as arteriovenous shunting.

berry aneurysm small saccular aneurysms primarily affecting the cerebral arteries.

dissecting aneurysm a result of a tear in the intimal lining of the artery creating a false lumen within the media. This false lumen allows blood to dissect the media and adventitia layers.

ectatic aneurysm dilatation of an artery when compared with a more proximal segment. In the abdominal aorta, the ectatic dilatation does not exceed 3.0 cm.

fusiform aneurysm characterized by a uniform dilatation of the arterial walls; most common type of abdominal aortic aneurysm.

mycotic aneurysm a saccular dilatation of a blood vessel caused by a bacterial infection.

pseudoaneurysm dilatation of an artery as a result of damage to one or more layers of the arterial wall caused by trauma or aneurysm rupture; also known as pulsatile hematoma.

saccular aneurysm dilatation of an artery characterized by a focal out-pouching of one arterial wall; most often caused by trauma or infection.

PHYSIOLOGY AND ANATOMY

FUNCTIONS OF THE VASCULAR SYSTEM

- Arteries and arterioles carry oxygenated blood away from the heart.
- Veins and venules carry blood toward the heart.
- Capillaries connect the arterial and venous systems.
- Extremity veins contain valves.
- Valves extend inward toward the intima.

VESSEL WALL LAYERS

- Venous walls are thinner and less elastic compared with arterial walls.

Tunica Adventitia

- Outer layer.
- Lends greater elasticity to the arteries.

Tunica Media

- Middle muscle layer.
- Helps regulate blood flow by controlling the vessel wall diameter.

Tunica Intima

- Inner layer.
- Composed of a single layer of cells, giving it a smooth surface.

ARTERIAL ANATOMY (Fig. 13-1)

ABDOMINAL AORTA

- Originates at the diaphragm and courses inferiorly until it bifurcates into the right and left common iliac arteries.
- Tapers in size as it courses anterior and inferior in the abdomen.
- Common iliac arteries are the terminal branches of the abdominal aorta.
- Common iliac artery bifurcates into the external and internal (hypogastric) iliac arteries.
- External iliac artery becomes the common femoral artery after passing beneath the inguinal ligament.
- Internal iliac artery bifurcates into anterior and posterior divisions.

MAIN VISCERAL BRANCHES OF THE ABDOMINAL AORTA

Celiac Axis (CA)
- First major branch of the abdominal aorta.
- Arises from the anterior aspect of the aorta.
- Branches into the splenic, left gastric, and common hepatic arteries.
- 1 to 3 cm in length.
- Low-resistance blood flow, with continuous forward flow in diastole.
- Peak systolic velocity remains unchanged after a meal.

FIG. 13-1
Arterial anatomy.

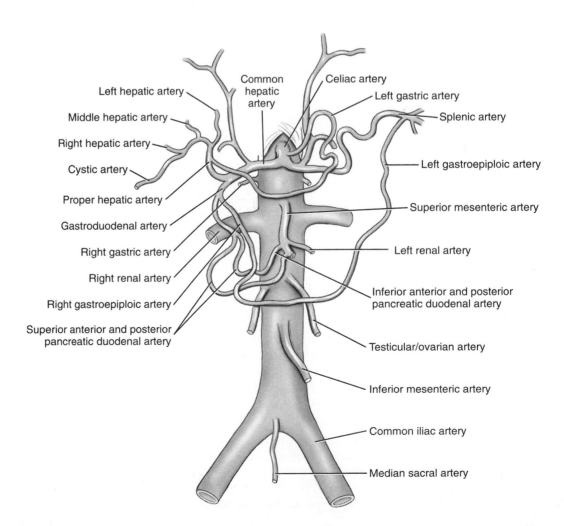

Superior Mesenteric Artery (SMA)

- Second major branch of the abdominal aorta.
- Arises from the anterior surface of the aorta, inferior to the celiac axis.
- Courses inferiorly and parallel to the aorta.
- Branches supply the jejunum, ileum, cecum, ascending colon, portions of the transverse colon, and the head of the pancreas.
- High-resistance multiphasic blood flow when fasting.
- Low-resistance elevated systolic and diastolic velocities, with continuous forward flow in diastole following a meal.
- Distance from the anterior wall of the aorta to the posterior wall of the SMA should not exceed 11 mm.

Middle Suprarenal Arteries

- Arise from the lateral aspect of the abdominal aorta.
- Courses laterally and slightly superior over the crura of the diaphragm to the adrenal glands.

Main Renal Arteries

- Arise from the posterior lateral aspects of the abdominal aorta.
- Located 1.0 to 1.5 cm inferior to the superior mesenteric artery.
- Course posterior to the renal veins.
- Right side arises superior to the left and courses posterior to the inferior vena cava.
- Renal artery bifurcates into segmental arteries at the renal hilum.
- Renal artery gives rise to the inferior suprarenal artery.
- Low-resistance blood flow, with continuous forward flow in diastole.
- Duplicated arteries are found in 10% to 20% of the population.

Gonadal Arteries

- Arise from the anterior aspect of the abdominal aorta inferior to the renal arteries.
- Course parallel to the psoas muscle into the pelvis.
- Low-resistance blood flow, with continuous flow through diastole.
- Not visualized with ultrasound.

Inferior Mesenteric Artery

- Last major branch of the abdominal aorta prior to the aortic bifurcation.
- Arises from the anterior aorta.
- Courses inferior and to the left of midline.
- Supplies the left transverse colon, descending colon, upper rectum, and sigmoid.
- Visualized on ultrasound in an oblique plane, slightly to the left of midline and approximately 1 cm superior to the aortic bifurcation.
- Low-resistance blood flow, with continuous flow through diastole.

MAIN PARIETAL BRANCHES OF THE ABDOMINAL AORTA

Inferior Phrenic Artery

- Arises from the anterior aspect of the abdominal aorta branching into the right and left inferior phrenic arteries just below the diaphragm near the level of the 12th thoracic vertebrae.
- Supplies the inferior portion of the diaphragm.
- Gives rise to the superior suprarenal artery.

Lumbar Arteries

- Four arteries arise on each side of the abdominal aorta.
- Supplies the abdominal wall and spinal cord.
- Located inferior to the gonadal arteries and superior to the inferior mesenteric artery.

Median sacral artery

- Located inferior to the inferior mesenteric artery and superior to the aortic bifurcation.

ADDITIONAL ABDOMINAL ARTERIES

Gastroduodenal Artery (GDA)

- Branch of the common hepatic artery.
- Lies between the superior portion of the duodenum and the anterior surface of the pancreatic head.

Hepatic Artery

- Common hepatic artery is a branch of the celiac axis.
- Gives rise to the gastroduodenal artery and is now termed the proper hepatic artery.
- Courses adjacent to the portal vein.
- The proper hepatic artery bifurcates into the right, middle, and left hepatic arteries at the hepatic hilum.
- Low-resistance blood flow, with continuous flow through diastole.
- Increased flow velocity is associated with jaundice, cirrhosis, lymphoma, and metastases.

Splenic Artery

- Tortuous branch of the celiac axis.
- Gives rise to the left gastroepiploic artery and additional branches to the pancreas and stomach.
- Courses along the superior margin of the pancreatic body and tail.
- Low-resistance blood flow, with continuous flow through diastole.
- May be mistaken for a dilated pancreatic duct.

VENOUS ANATOMY (Fig. 13-2)

INFERIOR VENA CAVA (IVC)

- Formed at the junction of the right and left common iliac veins.
- Carries oxygen-depleted blood from the body superiorly to the right atrium of the heart.
- Major abdominal branches include lumbar veins, right gonadal vein, renal veins, right suprarenal vein, inferior phrenic vein, and hepatic veins.

MAIN VENOUS TRIBUTARIES

Common Iliac Veins

- Drain blood from the lower extremities and pelvis.
- Formed by the junction of the external and internal iliac veins.

FIG. 13-2
Venous anatomy.

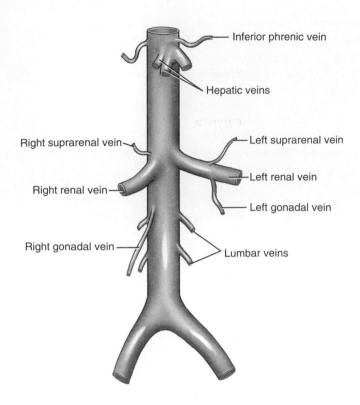

- Inferior phrenic vein
- Hepatic veins
- Right suprarenal vein
- Left suprarenal vein
- Left renal vein
- Right renal vein
- Left gonadal vein
- Right gonadal vein
- Lumbar veins

Renal Veins

- Course anterior to the renal arteries.
- Left renal vein courses posterior to the superior mesenteric artery and anterior to the abdominal aorta.
- Left renal vein receives the left suprarenal and gonadal veins.
- Left renal vein may appear dilated due to compression from the mesentery.
- Right renal vein has a short course to the IVC.
- Demonstrates spontaneous phasic blood flow.

Hepatic Veins

- Lie at the boundaries of the hepatic segments and course toward the IVC.
- Three major branches: left, middle, and right hepatic veins.
- Right hepatic vein courses coronally between the anterior and posterior segments of the right hepatic lobe.
- Middle hepatic vein follows an oblique course between the left and right hepatic lobes.
- Left hepatic vein courses posterior between the medial and lateral segments of the left hepatic lobe.
- Doppler demonstrates spontaneous, multiphasic, and pulsatile blood flow toward the IVC (hepatofugal).
- Increase in blood flow with inspiration and diminished flow with Valsalva maneuver.

ADDITIONAL ABDOMINAL VEINS

Main Portal Vein

- Drains the gastrointestinal tract, pancreas, spleen, and gallbladder.
- Provides approximately 70% of the liver's blood supply.
- Formed by the junction of the splenic and superior mesenteric veins.

- Bifurcates into the right and left portal veins.
- Should not exceed 1.3 cm in diameter.
- Demonstrates phasic low flow velocities toward the liver (hepatopetal).
- Blood flow will decrease with inspiration.
- Diameter will increase after a meal.
- Additional tributaries include:
  a. Coronary vein—enters at the superior border of the portosplenic confluence.
  b. Inferior mesenteric vein—enters at the inferior border of the portosplenic confluence.

Splenic Vein

- Joins the superior mesenteric vein to form the main portal vein.
- Courses posterior to the pancreas and crosses anterior to the superior mesenteric artery.
- Demonstrates spontaneous phasic flow away from the spleen and toward the liver.
- Increase in caliber with inspiration.

Superior Mesenteric Vein

- Courses parallel to the superior mesenteric artery.
- Demonstrates spontaneous phasic flow toward the liver.
- Caliber will increase with inspiration and following a meal.

Gonadal Veins

- Right gonadal vein empties directly into the inferior vena cava.
- Left gonadal vein empties into the left renal vein and occasionally the left suprarenal vein.

Lumbar Veins

- Branches of the common iliac veins.
- Course lateral to the spine and posterior to the psoas muscles.

LOCATION

Abdominal Aorta

- Lies to the left of midline adjacent to the inferior vena cava.
- Courses inferior and anterior in the abdomen to the level of the fourth lumbar vertebra (umbilicus), where it bifurcates into the right and left common iliac arteries.
- Lies anterior to the spine and psoas muscle.
- Separated from the spine by 0.5 to 1.0 cm of soft tissue.

Inferior Vena Cava

- Lies to the right of midline parallel to the abdominal aorta.
- Formed at the level of the fifth lumbar vertebra at the junction of the right and left common iliac veins coursing superiorly in the abdomen to the right atrium of the heart.
- Lies anterior to the spine, psoas muscle, crus of the diaphragm, and right adrenal gland.
- Lies posterior to the head of the pancreas.

SIZE

Abdominal Aorta
- The size of the normal abdominal aorta should not exceed 3 cm in diameter.
- The aorta tapers as it courses inferiorly and measures approximately:
  Suprarenal: 2.5 cm.
  Renal: 2.0 cm.
  Infrarenal: 1.5 cm.
  Common iliac: 1.0 cm.

Inferior Vena Cava
- Usually measures less than 2.5 cm.
- Decrease in caliber is demonstrated in inspiration and an increase in size when respiration is suspended.

SONOGRAPHIC APPEARANCE

- Anechoic tubular structure.
- Thin hyperechoic wall margins.
- Internal vascular flow.
- Aorta demonstrates a high-resistance multiphasic parabolic flow pattern.
- Inferior vena cava demonstrates spontaneous phasic flow and multiphasic pulsatile flow as it nears the diaphragm.

TECHNIQUE

PREPARATION

- Preparation for the abdominal vasculature is typically nothing by mouth 6 to 8 hours prior to the examination.

EXAMINATION TECHNIQUE

- Use the highest-frequency abdominal transducer possible to obtain optimal resolution for penetration depth.
- Proper focal zone and depth placement.
- Decrease in dynamic range.
- Proper Doppler controls (PRF, gain, wall filters).
- Evaluation and documentation of the abdominal aorta, common iliac arteries, and inferior vena cava in the sagittal and transverse planes.
- Evaluation and documentation of the maximum diameter of the abdominal aorta, common iliac arteries, and inferior vena cava.
- Duplex evaluation and documentation of any additional vascular structures requested.
- Duplex evaluation, documentation, and measurement of any abnormality should be included.
- If intraluminal thrombus is present, measurement of the vessel lumen should be included.

INDICATIONS FOR EXAMINATION

- Pulsatile abdominal mass.
- Family history of abdominal aortic aneurysm.
- Hypertension.
- Abdominal pain.
- Lower back pain.
- History of arteriosclerosis.

- Severe postprandial pain.
- Pulmonary embolism.
- Liver disease.
- Evaluate mass from previous medical imaging study (i.e., CT).

Arterial Pathology

ARTERIAL PATHOLOGY	DESCRIPTION
Aneurysm	• Weakening of the arterial wall • All layers of the artery are stretched but intact • Rare in patients under 50 years • Male prevalence 5:1 • Growth rate of 2 mm/year is average and considered normal up to 5 mm/year • Exceeds 3.0 cm in diameter for the abdominal aorta • Exceeds 2.0 cm in diameter for the common iliac artery • Exceeds 1.0 cm in diameter for the popliteal artery • 25% of popliteal aneurysms are associated with an abdominal aortic aneurysm
Arterial stenosis	• Narrowing or constriction of an artery • Caused by atherosclerosis, arteriosclerosis, or fibrointimal hyperplasia
Arteriosclerosis	• Pathologic thickening, hardening, and loss of elasticity of the arterial walls
Atherosclerosis	• Disorder characterized by yellowish plaques of lipids and cellular debris in the inner layers of the arterial walls
Pseudoaneurysm	• Dilatation of an artery caused by damage to one or more layers of the artery as a result of trauma or aneurysm rupture

Aneurysms of the Abdominal Aorta

ANEURYSM	ETIOLOGY	CLINICAL FINDINGS	SONOGRAPHIC FINDINGS	DIFFERENTIAL CONSIDERATIONS
Abdominal aortic aneurysm	• Arteriosclerosis most common • Infection	• Asymptomatic • Pulsatile abdominal mass • Back and/or leg pain • Abdominal pain	• Typically fusiform-shaped dilatation of the aorta • Saccular dilatation of the aorta may be demonstrated • Diameter of 3 cm or greater • Vessel becomes tortuous • Wall calcifications • Intramural thrombus	• Lymphadenopathy • Retroperitoneal tumor • Dissection
Dissecting aneurysm	• Extension of a dissecting thoracic aneurysm • Hypertension • Marfan syndrome • Idiopathic • Pregnancy	• Sharp chest or abdominal pain • Audible bruit	• Thin hyperechoic membrane within the aorta • Membrane flaps with arterial pulsations • Doppler demonstrates opposite flow direction between the membrane during diastole	• Chronic intraluminal thrombus • Postsurgical repair
Ectatic aneurysm	• Weakening of the arterial wall	• Asymptomatic	• Dilatation of the aorta when compared with a more proximal segment • Dilatation measures less than 3 cm in diameter	• Tortuous artery • Technical error
Mycotic aneurysm	• Bacterial infection	• Asymptomatic • Abdominal pain • Pulsatile abdominal mass	• Typically saccular-shaped dilatation of the aorta • Asymmetrical wall thickening	• Lymphadenopathy • Retroperitoneal tumor • Intramural thrombus

Continued

Aneurysms of the Abdominal Aorta—cont'd

ANEURYSM	ETIOLOGY	CLINICAL FINDINGS	SONOGRAPHIC FINDINGS	DIFFERENTIAL CONSIDERATIONS
Pseudoaneurysm	• Trauma to the arterial wall permits the escape of blood into the surrounding tissues • Most common complication of an aortic graft	• Pulsatile mass	• Fluid collection communicating with an artery • Doppler will demonstrate turbulent swirling blood flow within the fluid collection • To and fro blood flow pattern is demonstrated in the neck of the aneurysm	• Hematoma • Lymphadenopathy • Aneurysm • Arteriovenous fistula
Ruptured aneurysm	• Risk of rupture within 5 years 5 cm = 5% 6 cm = 16% 7 cm = 75%	• Severe abdominal pain • Severe groin pain • Hypotension	• Normal aortic size • Aneurysm may still be visualized • Asymmetrical or unilateral para-aortic hypoechoic mass • "Veil appearance" over the aorta and surrounding structures • Free fluid in the peritoneal cavities	• Lymphadenopathy • Chronic intraluminal thrombus
Surgical repair	• Previous history of aneurysm	• Asymptomatic • Abdominal or lower back pain	• Anechoic space between the graft and repaired aorta • Hyperechoic parallel echoes along the arterial walls	• Dissection • Rupture aneurysm • Chronic intraluminal clot • Retroperitoneal pathology

Abdominal Venous Pathology

VENOUS PATHOLOGY	ETIOLOGY	CLINICAL FINDINGS	SONOGRAPHIC FINDINGS	DIFFERENTIAL CONSIDERATIONS
Arteriovenous shunts (AV fistula)	• Trauma • Congenital • Surgery • Inflammation • Neoplasm	• Presence of a bruit or "thrill" • Lower back or abdominal pain • Edema • Hypertension	Doppler demonstrates: • Pulsatile flow within the vein • Increase in arterial flow proximal to site of shunting • Decrease in arterial flow distal to site of shunting • Turbulent waveform with high velocities in both the artery and the vein	• Tortuous vessel • Stenotic vessel
Enlargement	• Congestive heart failure • Thrombosis • Infiltrating neoplasm	• Asymptomatic • Edema	• Inferior vena cava exceeding 3.7 cm in diameter • Main portal vein exceeding 1.3 cm in diameter • Splenic or superior mesenteric vein exceeding 1.0 cm • Intraluminal medium- to low-level echoes seen with neoplasms or thrombus	• Extrinsic compression • Arteriovenous shunting • Portal hypertension • Technical error
Infiltrating neoplasm	• Renal carcinoma	• Asymptomatic • Edema	• Intraluminal medium- to low-level echoes	• Venous thrombosis • Primary caval tumor • Technical error
Primary caval neoplasm	• Leiomyosarcoma is most common	• Asymptomatic • Edema	• Intraluminal medium- to low-level echoes	• Infiltrating tumor • Venous thrombosis • Technical error
Thrombosis	• Extension of thrombus from femoral, iliac, renal, hepatic, or gonadal veins	• Asymptomatic • Edema	• Intraluminal medium- to low-level echoes	• Infiltrating tumor • Primary caval tumor • Technical error

ABDOMINAL VASCULATURE REVIEW

1. A true aortic aneurysm is defined as a dilatation of the abdominal aorta:
   a. when compared with a more proximal segment
   b. measuring 3.0 cm or greater
   c. when compared with a previous imaging study
   d. measuring 2.5 cm or greater
   e. inferior to the renal arteries

2. A fusiform aneurysm is best described as:
   a. a focal out-pouching of one arterial wall
   b. damage to one or more layers of an arterial wall
   c. a uniform dilatation of the arterial walls
   d. asymmetric thrombus formation
   e. an increase in size when compared to a more proximal segment

3. The first visceral branch of the abdominal aorta is the:
   a. gastric artery
   b. celiac axis
   c. inferior phrenic artery
   d. middle suprarenal artery
   e. superior mesenteric artery

4. The left renal vein receives tributaries from which of the following veins?
   a. inferior mesenteric and coronary veins
   b. left suprarenal and inferior mesenteric veins
   c. coronary and splenic veins
   d. coronary and left suprarenal veins
   e. left suprarenal and left gonadal veins

5. The main portal vein bifurcates at the hepatic hilum into the:
   a. anterior and posterior portal veins
   b. right and middle portal veins
   c. medial and lateral portal veins
   d. left and right portal veins
   e. superior and inferior portal veins

6. Which of the following statements most accurately describes the left renal vein?
   a. The left renal vein demonstrates a pulsatile flow pattern.
   b. The left renal artery is located anterior to the left renal vein.
   c. The superior mesenteric artery courses posterior to the left renal vein.
   d. The left renal vein may appear dilated due to compression from the mesentery.
   e. The left renal vein courses posterior to the inferior vena cava.

7. Which of the following structures is located anterior to the inferior vena cava?
   a. spine
   b. psoas muscle
   c. right adrenal gland
   d. diaphragmatic crura
   e. head of the pancreas

8. The abdominal aorta usually bifurcates into the right and left common iliac arteries at the level of the:
   a. 12th thoracic vertebra
   b. 2nd lumbar vertebra
   c. 4th lumbar vertebra
   d. 5th lumbar vertebra
   e. lumbosacral junction

9. The celiac axis branches into which of the following arteries?
   a. proper hepatic, left gastric, and splenic arteries
   b. common hepatic, right gastric, and splenic arteries
   c. common hepatic and splenic arteries
   d. proper hepatic, gastroduodenal, and splenic arteries
   e. common hepatic, left gastric, and splenic arteries

10. The presence of a palpable "thrill" within an artery is suspicious for a(n):
    a. aneurysm
    b. occlusion
    c. stenosis
    d. thrombus
    e. arteriovenous fistula

11. The contour of a mycotic aneurysm is most commonly described as:
    a. berry shaped
    b. saccular shaped
    c. fusiform shaped
    d. heart shaped
    e. teardrop shaped

12. The gonadal arteries arise from the:
    a. renal arteries
    b. abdominal aorta
    c. lumbar arteries
    d. internal iliac arteries
    e. inferior suprarenal arteries

13. Which of the following arteries gives rise to the gastroepiploic artery?
    a. hepatic artery
    b. gastric artery
    c. splenic artery
    d. gastroduodenal artery
    e. superior mesenteric artery

14. Which of the following veins courses in an oblique plane between the right and left lobes of the liver?
    a. right hepatic vein
    b. right portal vein
    c. main portal vein
    d. middle hepatic vein
    e. left hepatic vein

15. The normal diameter of the main portal vein should not exceed:
    a. 0.7 cm
    b. 1.0 cm
    c. 1.3 cm
    d. 1.8 cm
    e. 2.1 cm

Using Fig. 13-3, answer questions 16 through 18.

16. A patient presents with a history of pulmonary embolism. A sagittal image of the inferior vena cava demonstrates an intraluminal mass. On the basis of the clinical history, the mass is most suspicious for a(n):
    a. neoplasm
    b. thrombus
    c. incompetent valve
    d. ulcerative plaque
    e. inflammatory process

17. The arrow is demonstrating which of the following vascular structures?
    a. hepatic artery
    b. portal vein
    c. hepatic vein
    d. right renal artery
    e. superior mesenteric artery

18. The anechoic structure lying anterior to the inferior vena cava and posterior to the liver most likely represents the:
    a. pancreas
    b. gallbladder
    c. right hepatic vein
    d. superior mesenteric vein
    e. caudate lobe of the liver

Using Fig. 13-4, answer questions 19 and 20.

19. Which of the following visceral branches of the abdominal aorta is identified by arrow **A**?
    a. renal artery
    b. celiac axis
    c. gonadal artery
    d. inferior phrenic artery
    e. superior mesenteric artery

20. Which of the following branches of the abdominal aorta is identified by arrow **B**?
    a. celiac axis
    b. renal artery
    c. gonadal artery
    d. superior mesenteric artery
    e. inferior suprarenal artery

21. Which of the following conditions most commonly coexists with a popliteal aneurysm?
    a. carotid stenosis
    b. arteriovenous fistula
    c. venous insufficiency
    d. abdominal aortic aneurysm
    e. dissection of the thoracic aorta

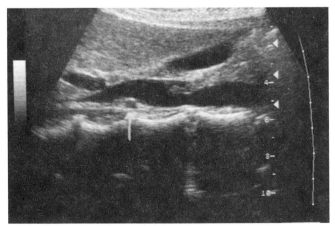

FIG. 13-3 Sagittal sonogram of the right upper quadrant.

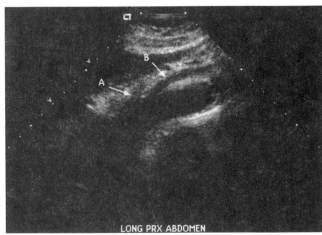

FIG. 13-4 Sonogram of the abdominal aorta.

22. Development of an abdominal aortic aneurysm is most commonly caused by:
    a. trauma
    b. infection
    c. drug addiction
    d. arteriosclerosis
    e. fibrointimal hyperplasia

23. Dissection of the abdominal aorta is linked to all of the following EXCEPT:
    a. trauma
    b. pregnancy
    c. hypotension
    d. Marfan syndrome
    e. dissection of the thoracic aorta

24. The inferior vena cava is considered enlarged once the diameter exceeds:
    a. 1.5 cm
    b. 2.0 cm
    c. 2.5 cm
    d. 3.0 cm
    e. 3.7 cm

25. Development of an arteriovenous fistula may be caused by all of the following conditions EXCEPT:
    a. trauma
    b. surgery
    c. neoplasm
    d. hypertension
    e. inflammation

26. An infiltrating neoplasm within the inferior vena cava most commonly originates from which of the following structures?
    a. liver
    b. spleen
    c. kidney
    d. pancreas
    e. adrenal gland

27. Direct extension of thrombus into the inferior vena cava may originate in all of the following venous structures EXCEPT:
    a. renal vein
    b. femoral vein
    c. hepatic vein
    d. splenic vein
    e. right gonadal vein

28. Berry-shaped aneurysms primarily affect which of the following arteries?
    a. splenic
    b. hepatic
    c. cerebral
    d. extracranial
    e. abdominal aorta

29. Duplication of the main renal arteries is demonstrated in approximately:
    a. 5% to 10% of the population
    b. 10% to 20% of the population
    c. 40% to 50% of the population
    d. 50% to 75% of the population
    e. more than 75% of the population

30. All of the following conditions may demonstrate abnormal blood flow patterns within the hepatic artery EXCEPT:
    a. jaundice
    b. cirrhosis
    c. cholecystitis
    d. lymphoma
    e. metastases

Using Fig. 13-5, answer question 31.

31. A 65-year-old local farmer presents with a history of leukocytosis and an enlarging, pulsatile abdominal mass. The anterior, posterior, and lateral borders of the distal aorta are outlined by the calibers. On the basis of the clinical history, the sonogram is most likely demonstrating which of the following pathologies?
    a. lymphadenopathy
    b. arterial dissection
    c. retroperitoneal fibrosis
    d. mycotic abdominal aortic aneurysm
    e. ectatic abdominal aortic aneurysm

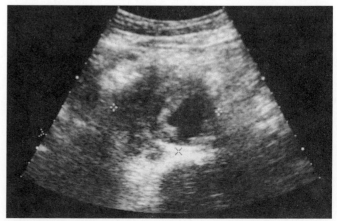

FIG. 13-5 Transverse sonogram of the distal abdominal aorta.

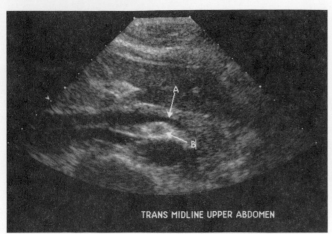

FIG. 13-6 Transverse sonogram of the upper abdomen.

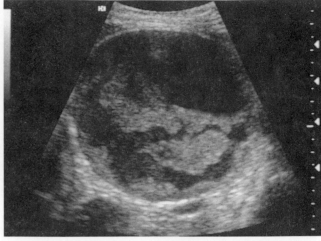

FIG. 13-7 Transverse sonogram of the abdominal aorta.

Using Fig. 13-6, answer questions 32 and 33.

32. Which of the following vascular structures is identified by arrow **A**?
    a. splenic artery
    b. portal vein
    c. splenic vein
    d. left renal vein
    e. superior mesenteric vein

33. Which of the following vascular structures is identified by arrow **B**?
    a. celiac axis
    b. splenic artery
    c. superior mesenteric vein
    d. gastroduodenal artery
    e. superior mesenteric artery

Using Fig. 13-7, answer question 34.

34. An asymptomatic patient presents with a history of an abdominal aortic aneurysm. The findings in this sonogram are most suspicious for which of the following conditions?
    a. pseudoaneurysm
    b. dissecting aneurysm
    c. ruptured aneurysm
    d. aneurysm with chronic thrombus
    e. para-aortic lymphadenopathy

Using Fig. 13-8, answer questions 35 and 36.

35. Arrow **A** is most likely identifying which of the following vascular structures?
    a. hepatic vein
    b. main portal vein
    c. gastroduodenal artery
    d. inferior vena cava
    e. right renal vein

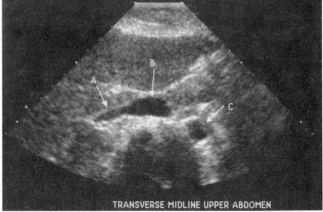

FIG. 13-8 Transverse sonogram of the upper abdomen.

36. The anechoic area identified by arrow **B** is most consistent with which of the following vascular structures?
    a. hepatic vein
    b. splenic vein
    c. inferior vena cava
    d. left renal artery
    e. superior mesenteric artery

37. Dilatation of an artery caused by damage to one or more layers of the arterial wall describes a(n):
    a. berry aneurysm
    b. arteriovenous fistula
    c. dissecting aneurysm
    d. pseudoaneurysm
    e. abdominal aortic aneurysm

38. The common iliac artery is considered enlarged once the diameter exceeds:
    a. 1.0 cm
    b. 1.5 cm
    c. 2.0 cm
    d. 2.5 cm
    e. 3.0 cm

39. Which of the following vascular structures courses posterior to the inferior vena cava?
    a. proper hepatic artery
    b. splenic artery
    c. right renal artery
    d. superior mesenteric artery
    e. inferior mesenteric artery

40. Which of the following vessels lies between the duodenum and the anterior portion of the pancreatic head?
    a. gastric artery
    b. hepatic artery
    c. celiac axis
    d. gastroduodenal artery
    e. superior mesenteric artery

41. The inferior vena cava generally measures less than:
    a. 1.0 cm
    b. 2.5 cm
    c. 3.0 cm
    d. 3.5 cm
    e. 4.0 cm

42. Which of the following arteries supplies the left transverse colon, descending colon, and the sigmoid?
    a. gonadal artery
    b. superior mesenteric artery
    c. gastroepiploic artery
    d. external iliac artery
    e. inferior mesenteric artery

43. Patients with Marfan syndrome have a predisposing risk factor for developing a(n):
    a. pseudoaneurysm
    b. pulmonary embolism
    c. abdominal aortic aneurysm
    d. renal vein thrombosis
    e. stenosis in the common carotid artery

44. The risk of rupture in an abdominal aortic aneurysm measuring 6.0 cm in diameter is approximately:
    a. 5% within 1 year
    b. 15% within 5 years
    c. 25% within 10 years
    d. 50% within 2 years
    e. 75% within 5 years

45. The amount of blood supplied to the liver from the portal venous system is approximately:
    a. 10%
    b. 25%
    c. 35%
    d. 50%
    e. 70%

46. Which of the following vessels course anterior to the abdominal aorta and posterior to the superior mesenteric artery?
    a. portal vein
    b. splenic vein
    c. left renal vein
    d. superior mesenteric vein
    e. common hepatic artery

47. Normal diameter of the splenic vein should not exceed:
    a. 0.5 cm
    b. 1.0 cm
    c. 1.5 cm
    d. 2.0 cm
    e. 2.5 cm

48. Which of the following vascular structures is most commonly mistaken as a dilated pancreatic duct?
    a. splenic vein
    b. celiac axis
    c. splenic artery
    d. superior mesenteric vein
    e. gastroduodenal artery

49. A dilatation of an artery when compared with a more proximal segment describes which of the following abnormalities?
    a. pseudoaneurysm
    b. pulsatile hematoma
    c. arteriovenous fistula
    d. ectatic aneurysm
    e. saccular aneurysm

50. All of the following statements accurately describe the venous system EXCEPT:
    a. Venous walls are thicker than arterial walls.
    b. Lower-extremity veins contain valves.
    c. Venous valves extend inward toward the intima.
    d. Veins carry blood toward the heart.
    e. Perforator veins connect the superficial system with the deep system.

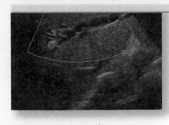

CHAPTER 14

Gastrointestinal Tract

KEY TERMS

alimentary tract digestive tract.

cardiac orifice opening at the upper end of the stomach.

chyme semiliquid mass composed of food and gastric juices.

Crohn disease inflammation of the intestines; occurs most frequently in the ileum.

diverticulum saccular out-pouching of the mucous membrane through a tear in the muscular layer of the gastrointestinal tract.

fecalith a hard compacted mass of feces in the colon.

gastritis inflammation of the stomach.

gastroparesis failure of the stomach to empty; caused by a decrease in gastric mobility.

greater curvature of the stomach longer, convex, left border of the stomach.

haustra a recess or sacculation demonstrated in the walls of the ascending and transverse colon.

ileus obstruction of the small intestines.

intussusception prolapse of one segment of bowel into the lumen of an adjacent segment of bowel.

lesser curvature of the stomach shorter, concave, right border of the stomach.

Meckel diverticulum an anomalous sac protruding from the ileum; caused by an incomplete closure of the yolk stalk.

McBurney point situated midway between the umbilicus and the right iliac crest.

McBurney sign extreme pain or tenderness over McBurney point; associated with an appendicitis.

mucocele distention of the appendix or colon with mucus.

pepsin a protein-digesting enzyme produced by the stomach.

peristalsis rhythmic serial contractions of the smooth muscle of the intestines that forces food through the digestive tract.

pyloric orifice opening at the lower end of the stomach.

pylorospasm spasm of the pyloric sphincter; associated with pyloric stenosis.

rugae ridges or folds in the stomach lining.

target sign a circular structure demonstrating alternate hyper and hypoechoic wall layers. A target sign may or may not signify pathology in the gastrointestinal tract.

GASTROINTESTINAL (GI) TRACT (Fig. 14-1)

- Extends from the mouth to the anus.
- Divisions include the mouth, pharynx, esophagus, stomach, small intestines, and colon.
- Also called digestive tract, alimentary tract or canal, and intestinal tract.
- Lined with a mucous membrane.

PHYSIOLOGY

FUNCTIONS OF THE GI TRACT

- Ingest food.
- Digest food.
- Secrete mucous and digestive enzymes.
- Absorb and break down food.
- Reabsorb fluid in the intestinal walls to prevent dehydration.
- Form solid feces.
- Release fecal waste.

FIG. 14-1
GI anatomy.

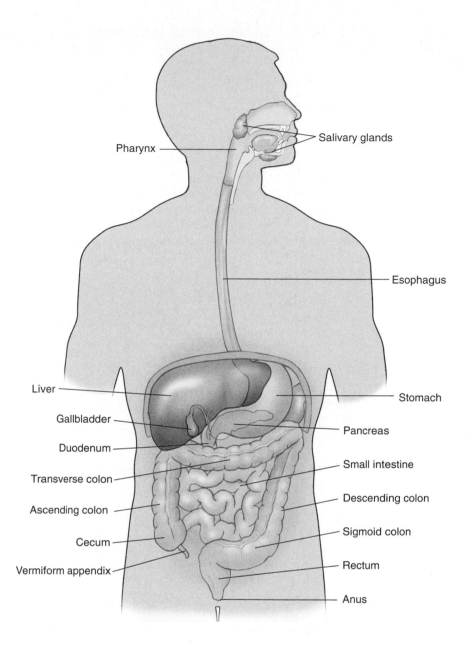

- Pharynx
- Salivary glands
- Esophagus
- Liver
- Stomach
- Gallbladder
- Pancreas
- Duodenum
- Small intestine
- Transverse colon
- Descending colon
- Ascending colon
- Sigmoid colon
- Cecum
- Rectum
- Vermiform appendix
- Anus

ANATOMY

ESOPHAGUS

- Muscular tube extending from the pharynx to the stomach.
- Courses down the chest through the esophageal hiatus of the diaphragm, terminating at the cardiac orifice of the stomach.
- Wall layers from the outer layer to the lumen include:
  - external or fibrous.
  - muscularis.
  - submucosal.
  - mucosal.

STOMACH

- Principal organ of digestion located between the esophagus and small intestines.
- Secretes hydrochloric acid and pepsin.

- Divided into the fundus, body, and pylorus.
- Wall layers from the outer layer to the lumen include:
  - Serosal.
  - Muscularis propria.
  - Submucosal.
  - Muscular.
  - Mucosal or rugae.

SMALL INTESTINES

- Elaborate tube extending from the pyloric opening to the ileocecal valve.
- Secretes mucus and receives digestive enzymes.
- Divided into the duodenum, jejunum, and ileum.
- Majority of food absorption occurs in the small intestines.
- Wall layers from outer layer to lumen include:
  - Serous.
  - Muscular.
  - Submucosal.
  - Mucosal.

DUODENUM

- Divided into the superior, descending, horizontal, and ascending portions.
- Secretes large quantities of mucus, protecting the small intestines from the strongly acidic chyme.
- Enzymes from the duct of Wirsung and bile from the common bile duct empty into the descending portion.

JEJUNUM

- Extends from the duodenum to the ileum.

ILEUM

- Extends from the jejunum to the junction with the cecum (ileocecal junction).

COLON

- Extends from the terminal ileum to the anus.
- Secretes large quantities of mucus.
- Divisions include the cecum, appendix, ascending colon, transverse colon, descending colon, sigmoid, rectum, and anus.
- Bacteria in the colon produce vitamin K and some B complex vitamins.
- Wall layers from the outer layer to the lumen include:
  - Serous.
  - Muscular or haustra.
  - Submucosal.
  - Mucosal.

CECUM

- Blind pouch of the colon located in the right lower quadrant directly posterior to the abdominal wall.

APPENDIX

- Narrow, blind-end, tubular structure communicating with the cecum.
- Nonperistaltic structure generally located in the right lower quadrant.
- Contains lymphoid tissue.

ASCENDING COLON

- Extends superiorly from the cecum.
- Curves to the left, forming the hepatic flexure.

TRANSVERSE COLON

- Courses transversely from the right to the left side of the upper abdomen.
- Curves inferiorly, forming the splenic flexure.

DESCENDING COLON

- Begins inferior to the spleen and terminates at the sigmoid.

SIGMOID

- Narrowest portion of the colon, terminating at the rectum.
- Mobile structure in contact with the psoas muscle.
- Located in the left iliac fossa.

RECTUM

- Terminal portion of the colon located between the sigmoid and anus.

ANAL CANAL

- Lower portion of the rectum.

LOCATION

ESOPHAGUS

- Located to the left of midline, posterior to the left lobe of the liver and anterior to the abdominal aorta.
- Right margin is contiguous with the lesser curvature of the stomach.
- Left margin is contiguous with the greater curvature of the stomach.

STOMACH

- Located in the left upper quadrant extending transversely and slightly to the right of midline.
- Pylorus lies in a transverse plane slightly to the right of midline.

SMALL INTESTINES

- Located in the central and lower portion of the abdominal cavity.
- Surrounded superiorly and laterally by the colon.

DUODENUM

- Located lateral and posterior to the head of the pancreas.

JEJUNUM

- Located in the umbilical and left iliac regions.

ILEUM

- Located in the umbilical and right iliac regions.

COLON

- Forms an upside down U shape extending from the right lower quadrant to the left lower quadrant.

SIZE

- Stomach wall should not exceed 5 mm in thickness when distended.
- Normal bowel wall should not exceed 4 mm in thickness.
- Normal appendix should not exceed 2 mm in wall thickness or 6 mm in diameter.

- Small intestines decrease in size from the pylorus to the ileocecal valve.
- Colon is largest at the cecum and gradually decreases in size toward the rectum.

SONOGRAPHIC APPEARANCE

- Walls of the gastrointestinal tract demonstrate alternating hyperechoic and hypoechoic circular echo patterns (mucosal layer appears hyperechoic).
- Gastroesophageal junction appears as a target structure lying posterior to the liver and slightly to the left of midline.
- Stomach appears as a target structure when empty and an anechoic structure with swirling hyperechoic echoes when distended with fluid.
- Small intestines are usually gas-filled.
- Jejunum and ileum demonstrate small folds in the wall termed the "keyboard sign."
- Ascending and transverse colon are identified by haustral wall markings (3 to 5 cm apart).
- Descending colon is seen as a tubular structure with echogenic wall margins.
- Peristalsis should be observed in the stomach and small and large intestines.
- Rectum is best evaluated with an endorectal transducer.

TECHNIQUE

PREPARATION

- Nothing by mouth 4 to 8 hours prior to a gastrointestinal tract examination.
- Fluid in the stomach is helpful when evaluating for pyloric stenosis.
- Emergency examinations may be performed without preparation.

EXAMINATION TECHNIQUE

- Use the highest-frequency abdominal transducer possible to obtain optimal resolution for penetration depth when surveying the abdomen.
- Use the highest-frequency linear transducer possible to obtain optimal resolution for penetration depth when surveying the appendix.
- Ensure proper focal zone and depth placement.
- Evaluate and document gastrointestinal structures in two imaging planes.
- Evaluate for peristalsis.
- Document compression technique when evaluating the appendix.
- Document length, width, and wall thickness of the pyloric canal when indicated.
- Evaluate and document vascularity of abnormal structures using color and spectral Doppler.

INDICATIONS FOR EXAMINATION

- Abdominal or right lower quadrant pain.
- Leukocytosis.
- Vomiting.
- Weight loss.
- Fever.
- Abdominal mass.
- Diarrhea.
- Absence of bowel sounds.

Pathology of the Stomach

PATHOLOGY	ETIOLOGY	CLINICAL FINDINGS	SONOGRAPHIC FINDINGS	DIFFERENTIAL CONSIDERATIONS
Carcinoma	• Adenocarcinoma in 80% of cases • Male prevalence	• Upper abdominal discomfort • Nausea/vomiting • Decrease in appetite • Fatigue • Weight loss • Abdominal mass	• Target tumor of the stomach • Hypervascular mass • Gastric wall thickening • Left upper quadrant mass	• Polyp • Ulcer • Lymphoma • Metastases
Gastric dilatation	• Gastric obstruction • Gastroparesis • Duodenal ulcer • Inflammation • Pylorospasm • Neurological disease • Neoplasm • Medication	• Abdominal pain • Nausea/vomiting • Bloating	• Fluid-filled mass in the left upper quadrant • Swirling hyperechoic interluminal echoes • Decrease or lack of forward peristalsis of stomach contents • Thin gastric wall margins	• Omental cyst • Renal cyst • Liver cyst • Pancreatic pseudocyst
Gastric ulcer	• Bacterial infection (75%) • Stress • Malignant neoplasm	• Epigastric pain • Postprandial pain • Bloating • Nausea • Heartburn	• Thick gastric wall margins • Hypervascular gastric wall • Most commonly located in the lesser curvature of the stomach	• Gastritis • Neoplasm
Gastritis	• Bacterial infection • Bile reflux • Smoking • Excessive alcohol consumption • Radiation	• Upper abdominal discomfort • Decrease in appetite • Belching • Nausea/vomiting • Fatigue • Fever	• Diffuse or localized thickening in the gastric wall • Enlarged and prominent rugae	• Gastric ulcer • Neoplasm
Hypertrophied pyloric stenosis	• Marked thickening of the circular muscle fibers of the pylorus	• Projectile vomiting • Dehydration • Weight loss • Palpable upper abdominal mass (olive sign)	• Pyloric wall thickness above 3-4 mm • Pyloric diameter exceeding 15 mm • Length of the pyloric canal exceeding 18 mm	• Normal pyloric canal
Leiomyoma	• Benign neoplasm of the smooth muscle	• Asymptomatic	• Intraluminal solid gastric mass • Well-defined wall margins	• Polyp • Leiomyosarcoma • Gastritis
Leiomyosarcoma	• Malignant neoplasm of the smooth muscle	• Asymptomatic • Epigastric pain • Decrease in appetite • Weight loss	• Intraluminal target lesion • May appear hypoechoic	• Leiomyoma • Polyp
Polyp	• Abnormal growth of the mucous membrane tissue • Most common tumor of the stomach	• Asymptomatic	• Hypoechoic lesion protruding from the gastric wall • Smooth wall margins	• Carcinoma • Leiomyoma • Gastritis

Pathology of the Small Intestines

PATHOLOGY	ETIOLOGY	CLINICAL FINDINGS	SONOGRAPHIC FINDINGS	DIFFERENTIAL CONSIDERATIONS
Crohn disease	• Chronic inflammation of the intestines	• Abdominal cramping • Blood in stool • Diarrhea • Fever • Decrease in appetite • Weight loss	• Thick loops of bowel • Matted loops of bowel • Abscess formation • Mesenteric lymphadenopathy	• Ileus • Diverticular abscess
Ileus	• Bowel obstruction • Peritonitis • Renal colic • Acute pancreatitis • Bowel ischemia • Neoplasm	• Abdominal pain • Constipation • Fever • Nausea/vomiting • Absence of bowel sounds	• Distention of the small bowel with air or fluid • Hypoactive or absent bowel sounds	• Intussusception • Crohn disease
Intussusception	• Telescoping of one part of the intestines into the lumen of an adjacent part	• Abdominal pain • Palpable mass • Vomiting • Abnormal stools	• Edematous bowel • Multiple circular rings "Donut sign" • Hypovascular intestinal wall • Hypervascular mesentery	• Ileus • Crohn disease
Lymphoma	• Hodgkin or non-Hodgkin	• Lymphadenopathy • Left upper quadrant pain • Fever • Blood loss • Leukopenia • Weight loss • Anorexia • Abdominal mass	• Irregular complex bowel mass • Mesenteric lymphadenopathy	• Lymphadenopathy • Retroperitoneal pathology
Meckel diverticulum	• Incomplete closure of the yolk stalk	• Asymptomatic • Abdominal or pelvic pain • Rectal bleeding	• Anechoic or complex mass located slightly to the right of the umbilicus • Thick wall margins • Round or oval in shape	• Diverticular abscess • Appendicitis • Ovarian pathology

Pathology of the Colon

PATHOLOGY	ETIOLOGY	CLINICAL FINDINGS	SONOGRAPHIC FINDINGS	DIFFERENTIAL CONSIDERATIONS
Acute appendicitis	• Obstructed appendix	• Periumbilical or right lower quadrant (RLQ) pain • Fever • Nausea/vomiting • Leukocytosis • McBurney sign	• Noncompressible tubular structure generally located in the RLQ • Diameter of the appendix exceeding 6 mm • Wall thickness exceeding 2 mm • Hypervascular structure • Rebound pain at McBurney point • Fecalith or calculus formation	• Bowel obstruction • Diverticulum • Normal cecum • Ovarian pathology • Ectopic pregnancy

Pathology of the Colon—cont'd

PATHOLOGY	ETIOLOGY	CLINICAL FINDINGS	SONOGRAPHIC FINDINGS	DIFFERENTIAL CONSIDERATIONS
Appendiceal abscess	• Infection	• Tender palpable RLQ mass • Spiking fever • Marked leukocytosis • McBurney sign	• Poorly defined hypoechoic mass • Noncompressible	• Diverticular abscess • Tubo-ovarian abscess • Ovarian torsion • Ectopic pregnancy
Carcinoma	• 50% are located in the rectum • 25% are located in the sigmoid	• Asymptomatic • Rectal bleeding • Change in bowel patterns	• Hypoechoic thickening of the bowel wall • Compressed wall layers	• Polyp • Diverticulum • Abscess • Crohn disease
Diverticular abscess	• Infection	• Asymptomatic • Lower abdominal pain • Fever • Leukocytosis • Rectal bleeding	• Hypoechoic circular or oval mass adjacent to the colon • Thickening of the colon wall • Hypervascular periphery	• Neoplasm • Appendicitis • Lymphadenopathy
Mucocele	• Inflammatory scarring—most common • Neoplasm • Fecalith • Polyp	• Palpable abdominal mass • Abdominal pain	• Cystic to hypoechoic intraluminal bowel mass • Posterior acoustic enhancement • Irregular inner wall margin • May demonstrate calcification(s)	• Cystadenoma • Ovarian cyst • Appendiceal abscess • Diverticulum
Polyp	• Abnormal growth of mucous membrane tissue	• Asymptomatic • Rectal bleeding • Abdominal pain • Diarrhea or constipation	• Hypoechoic mass of the bowel wall protruding into the lumen	• Carcinoma • Diverticulum • Fecal material

GASTROINTESTINAL TRACT REVIEW

1. The esophagus begins at the pharynx and terminates at the:
   a. esophageal orifice of the stomach
   b. cardiac orifice of the stomach
   c. pyloric orifice of the stomach
   d. gastric orifice of the stomach
   e. esophageal hiatus of the stomach

2. Male infants have a predisposing factor for developing which of the following gastrointestinal conditions?
   a. ileus
   b. gastritis
   c. intussusception
   d. Meckel diverticulum
   e. hypertrophied pyloric stenosis

3. Clinical symptoms related to an episode of acute appendicitis may include all of the following EXCEPT:
   a. fever
   b. nausea
   c. heartburn
   d. positive McBurney sign
   e. periumbilical pain

4. Which portion of the gastrointestinal tract is most likely to demonstrate rugae?
   a. esophagus
   b. stomach
   c. duodenum
   d. transverse colon
   e. sigmoid colon

5. Which of the following enzymes is produced by the stomach?
   a. gastrin
   b. lipase
   c. secretin
   d. pepsin
   e. amylase

6. Which of the following is considered a function of the duodenum?
   a. secrete pepsin
   b. produce lipase
   c. secrete hydrochloric acid
   d. secrete large quantities of mucus
   e. produce vitamin K and B complex

7. Crohn disease most commonly occurs in which of the following regions?
   a. duodenum
   b. jejunum
   c. ileum
   d. cecum
   e. sigmoid

8. Prolapse of one section of bowel into the lumen of another bowel segment describes which of the following conditions?
   a. ileus
   b. Crohn disease
   c. diverticulitis
   d. intussusception
   e. Meckel diverticulum

9. The walls of the jejunum and ileum demonstrate small folds termed the:
   a. WES sign
   b. olive sign
   c. target sign
   d. keyboard sign
   e. doughnut sign

10. The large intestines include all of the following regions EXCEPT the:
    a. rectum
    b. ileum
    c. cecum
    d. appendix
    e. sigmoid

11. The right margin of the esophagus is contiguous with the:
    a. duodenum
    b. pyloric canal
    c. tail of the pancreas
    d. lesser curvature of the stomach
    e. greater curvature of the stomach

12. Which of the following structures demonstrate haustral wall markings?
    a. cecum
    b. appendix
    c. duodenum
    d. stomach
    e. ascending colon

13. The small intestine is a region of the gastrointestinal tract extending from the:
    a. duodenum to the ileum
    b. pyloric opening to the appendix
    c. duodenum to the cecum
    d. duodenum to the appendix
    e. pyloric opening to the ileocecal valve

14. To be considered within normal limits, the length of the pyloric canal should not exceed:
    a. 10 mm
    b. 12 mm
    c. 15 mm
    d. 18 mm
    e. 21 mm

15. The diameter of the normal adult appendix should not exceed:
    a. 2 mm
    b. 4 mm
    c. 6 mm
    d. 8 mm
    e. 10 mm

16. Extreme pain over McBurney point is most commonly associated with:
    a. cholecystitis
    b. intussusception
    c. an appendicitis
    d. diverticulitis
    e. pancreatitis

17. Malignant neoplasms involving the large intestines are most frequently located in which of the following regions?
    a. ileum
    b. rectum
    c. sigmoid
    d. ascending colon
    e. descending colon

18. The common bile duct enters which of the following sections of the duodenum?
    a. superior
    b. descending
    c. ascending
    d. inferior
    e. horizontal

19. An episode of excessive alcohol consumption is most commonly associated with which of the following conditions?
    a. ileus
    b. colitis
    c. gastritis
    d. appendicitis
    e. diverticulitis

20. Which of the following organs is considered the principal organ of digestion?
    a. mouth
    b. pharynx
    c. esophagus
    d. stomach
    e. small intestines

21. Which of the following gastrointestinal regions is composed of five individual wall layers?
    a. esophagus
    b. stomach
    c. duodenum
    d. cecum
    e. rectum

22. McBurney point is best described as a point between the:
    a. umbilicus and inguinal canal
    b. symphysis pubis and right iliac crest
    c. umbilicus and right iliac crest
    d. xiphoid and right costal margin
    e. right costal margin and right iliac crest

23. Which of the following is **not** a section of the duodenum?
    a. ascending
    b. descending
    c. superior
    d. inferior
    e. horizontal

24. Distention of the small bowel with fluid or air is associated with all of the following conditions EXCEPT:
    a. peritonitis
    b. neoplasm
    c. renal colic
    d. acute pancreatitis
    e. gastroparesis

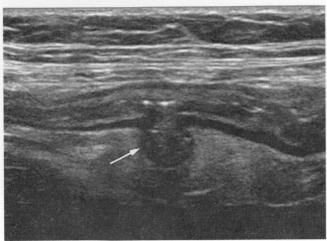

FIG. 14-2   Sonogram of the descending colon.

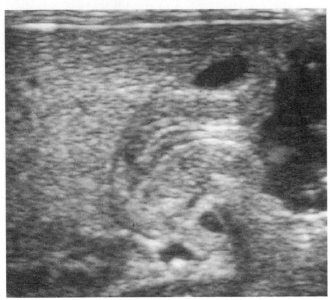

FIG. 14-3   Sonogram of the upper abdomen.

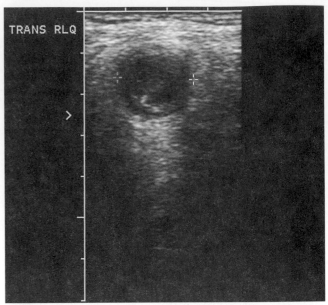

FIG. 14-4   Sonogram of the right lower quadrant.

Using Fig. 14-3, answer question 26.

26. A 4-month-old infant presents with a history of projectile vomiting and a palpable upper abdominal mass. The finding in this sonogram is most suspicious for:
   a. gastritis
   b. pancreatitis
   c. acute cholecystitis
   d. pyloric stenosis
   e. intussusception

Using Fig. 14-4, answer question 27.

27. A 20-year-old woman presents to the emergency department complaining of severe pelvic pain. Laboratory tests reveal a negative pregnancy test and leukocytosis. A pelvic ultrasound is ordered to rule out pelvic pathology. A longitudinal image lateral to the right ovary reveals a noncompressible tender mass. On the basis of the clinical history, this mass is most suspicious for a(n):
   a. hydrosalpinx
   b. appendicitis
   c. paraovarian cyst
   d. external iliac aneurysm
   e. ectopic pregnancy

Using Fig. 14-2, answer question 25.

25. A 50-year-old male patient presents with a history of lower abdominal pain and occasional rectal bleeding. He is afebrile and denies abnormal bowel patterns. On the basis of this clinical history, the sonographic finding is most suspicious for a(n):
   a. polyp
   b. abscess
   c. diverticulum
   d. carcinoma
   e. haustral wall marking

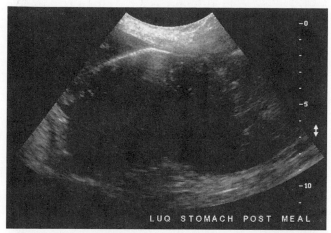

FIG. 14-5 Sonogram of the left upper quadrant.

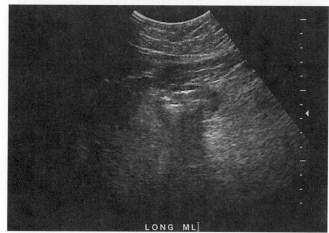

FIG. 14-6 Transverse sonogram of the upper abdomen.

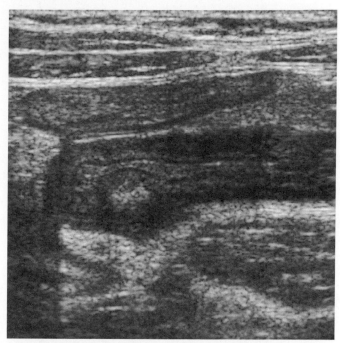

FIG. 14-7 Sonogram of the small intestines.

Using Fig. 14-6, answer question 29.

29. Which of the following normal gastrointestinal structures is demonstrated in this midline sonogram of the upper abdomen?
  a. duodenum
  b. pyloric canal
  c. ascending colon
  d. gastroesophageal junction
  e. greater curvature of the stomach

Using Fig. 14-7, answer question 30.

30. A 30-year-old woman presents with a history of chronic abdominal cramping, weight loss, and diarrhea. On the basis of this clinical history, the findings in this sonogram are most consistent with:
  a. peritoneal ascites
  b. diverticulitis
  c. Crohn disease
  d. acute appendicitis
  e. pelvic inflammatory disease

Using Fig. 14-5, answer question 28.

28. A 90-year-old woman presents with a history of upper abdominal discomfort and weight loss. One hour after ingesting 16 oz of fluid a significant amount of fluid remains in the stomach. This may be associated with all of the following conditions EXCEPT:
  a. gastritis
  b. duodenal ulcer
  c. esophageal reflux
  d. gastroparesis
  e. neurological disease

Using Fig. 14-8, answer question 31.

31. A patient complaining of right lower quadrant pain demonstrates discomfort in the region of the ascending colon. The recesses identified by the arrows are most suspicious for which of the following structures?
  a. polyps
  b. fecaliths
  c. diverticulums
  d. ileocecal valve
  e. haustral wall markings

Using Fig. 14-9, answer question 32.

32. The intestinal wall layer identified by the arrow is most likely the:
  a. fibrous layer
  b. submucosal layer
  c. muscular layer
  d. mucosal layer
  e. serosal layer

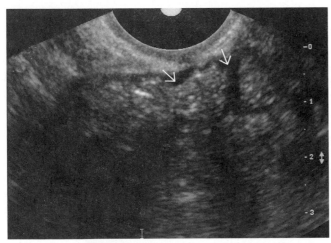

FIG. 14-8   Sonogram of the ascending colon.

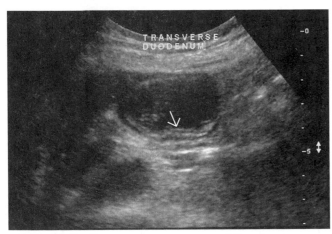

FIG. 14-9   Transverse sonogram of the duodenum.

33. An elderly patient presents with a history of rectal bleeding and a change in normal bowel patterns. An irregular complex mass is identified in the rectum on an endorectal sonogram. On the basis of this history, the finding in this sonogram is most suspicious for:
  a. polyp
  b. fecalith
  c. diverticulum
  d. hemorrhoid
  e. carcinoma

34. To be considered within normal limits, the wall thickness of the pyloric canal should not exceed:
  a. 2 mm
  b. 4 mm
  c. 6 mm
  d. 8 mm
  e. 10 mm

35. Functions of the gastrointestinal tract include all of the following EXCEPT:
  a. digest food
  b. secrete mucus into the intestines
  c. secrete digestive enzymes
  d. release glycogen as glucose
  e. absorb and break down food

36. Ulcers are more commonly located in which of the following regions of the stomach?
  a. body
  b. fundus
  c. pylorus
  d. lesser curvature
  e. greater curvature

37. A patient presents with a history of abdominal distention and pain. A sonogram of the periumbilical area demonstrates distended fluid-filled loops of small bowel. On the basis of the clinical history, the sonographic findings are most suspicious for which of the following conditions?
  a. ileus
  b. intussusception
  c. diverticulitis
  d. Crohn disease
  e. acute appendicitis

38. The wall in an adult appendix is considered abnormal once the thickness exceeds:
  a. 2 mm
  b. 4 mm
  c. 6 mm
  d. 8 mm
  e. 10 mm

39. The duodenum protects the small intestines from chyme by secreting:
    a. bile
    b. pepsin
    c. mucus
    d. sodium bicarbonate
    e. cholecystokinin

40. The ileum is a section of the gastrointestinal tract extending from the:
    a. duodenum to the cecum
    b. jejunum to the appendix
    c. duodenum to the appendix
    d. cecum to the ascending colon
    e. jejunum to the ileocecal junction

41. The majority of food absorption occurs in which portion of the gastrointestinal tract?
    a. stomach
    b. cecum
    c. small intestines
    d. ascending colon
    e. esophagus

42. Which of the following sections of the gastrointestinal tract terminates at the junction with the sigmoid colon?
    a. cecum
    b. rectum
    c. ileum
    d. transverse colon
    e. descending colon

43. Forward movement of intestinal contents caused by rhythmic contractions of the intestines is termed:
    a. rugae
    b. pylorospasm
    c. cramping
    d. peristalsis
    e. haustral contractions

44. A female patient complaining of right lower quadrant pain and vomiting presents to the emergency department. Her last menstrual period was 2 weeks earlier. A pelvic ultrasound might be ordered to rule out all of the following EXCEPT:
    a. appendicitis
    b. pancreatitis
    c. ovarian torsion
    d. hemorrhagic cyst
    e. tubo-ovarian abscess

45. Possible sonographic findings in gastric carcinoma include all of the following EXCEPT:
    a. target lesion
    b. gastric wall thickening
    c. large cystic mass
    d. hypervascular mass
    e. left upper quadrant mass

46. A gastric ulcer is most commonly caused by a(n):
    a. neoplasm
    b. increase in gastrin
    c. bacterial infection
    d. decrease in hydrochloric acid
    e. decrease in sodium bicarbonate

47. Gastritis is most likely described in sonographic terms as a(n):
    a. intraluminal target lesion
    b. absence of rugae in the stomach walls
    c. fluid-filled mass in the left upper quadrant
    d. diffuse thickening of the gastric walls
    e. poorly defined hypoechoic gastric mass

48. Which of the following abnormalities is **not** associated with a mucocele?
    a. polyp
    b. neoplasm
    c. fecalith
    d. gastritis
    e. scarring

49. Which portion of the large intestines demonstrates the narrowest lumen?
    a. cecum
    b. ileum
    c. sigmoid
    d. ascending
    e. descending

50. An asymptomatic patient demonstrates a small, intraluminal hypoechoic mass on ultrasound. The mass appears to protrude from a gastric wall. This is most suspicious for which of the following gastric pathologies?
    a. polyp
    b. ulcer
    c. adenoma
    d. leiomyoma
    e. leiomyosarcoma

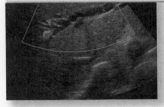

CHAPTER 15

Superficial Structures: Breast, Abdominal Wall, and Musculoskeletal Sonography

KEY TERMS

abdominal hernia protrusion of peritoneal contents through a defect in the abdominal wall.

Achilles tendon attaches the gastrocnemius and soleus muscles.

acini smallest functional unit of the breast.

anisotropy hypoechoic sonographic artifact caused when the ultrasound beam is not perpendicular to the fibrillar structure of a tendon.

Baker cyst a synovial cyst adjacent and posterior to the knee joint.

bursa a fibrous sac found between the tendon and bone; lined with a synovial membrane and secretes synovial fluid.

Cooper ligament strands of connective tissue serving as a support structure of the breast; provides shape and consistency to the breast parenchyma.

fibril a small filamentous fiber that is often a component of a cell.

fibrocystic disease the presence of a single or multiple palpable cysts in the breast.

galactocele a cyst caused by obstruction of a lactating duct.

gynecomastia an abnormal enlargement of a male breast(s).

lactiferous duct one of many channels that carry milk for the lobes of each breast to the nipple.

lactiferous sinus an area of enlargement in a lactiferous duct near the areola.

ligament a flexible band of fibrous tissue binding joints together.

linea alba a midline tendon of the anterior abdominal wall extending from the xiphoid process to the symphysis pubis.

lobe a collection of lobules within the breast parenchyma; approximately 15-20 lobes per breast.

lobule the simplest functional unit of the breast.

mammary zone breast parenchyma lying within the superficial fascia.

muscle tissue composed of fibers and cells that are able to contract, causing movement of the body parts or organs.

musculoskeletal system consists of all the muscles, bones, joints, ligaments, and tendons that function in the movement of the body and organs.

rectus abdominus muscle one of a pair of anterolateral abdominal wall muscles located lateral to the linea alba.

retromammary zone located between the posterior margin of the mammary zone and the pectoralis muscles.

tendon bands of dense fibrous connective tissue that attach muscle to bone.

tendinosis term used to describe degenerative changes in a tendon without signs of tendon inflammation; associated with overuse injuries.

terminal ductal lobular unit (TDLU) small lobular unit formed by the acini and the terminal ducts.

Thompson test a test used to evaluate the integrity of the Achilles tendon where the toes are pointing down while squeezing the calf.

PHYSIOLOGY

FUNCTION OF THE BREAST

- Produces and secretes milk.

FUNCTION OF THE ANTERIOR ABDOMINAL WALL

- Movement of the torso.

FUNCTION OF THE MUSCULOSKELETAL SYSTEM

- Movement of body parts and organs.

THE BREAST

BREAST ANATOMY AND LOCATION (Fig. 15-1)

TERMINAL DUCTAL LOBULAR UNIT

- Formed by the acini and terminal duct.
- Several terminal ductal lobular units join to form a breast lobe.
- Origin of nearly all breast pathology.
- Diameter should not exceed 2 mm.

LOBE

- 15-20 lobes per breast.
- A major duct courses within each lobe toward the nipple.

LACTIFEROUS DUCT

- Contained within each breast lobe.
- Courses toward the nipple.

FIG. 15-1
Breast anatomy

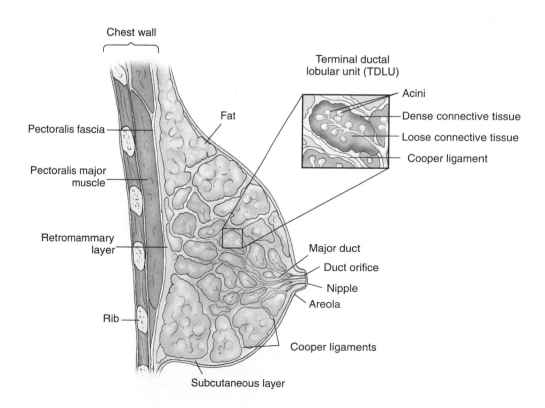

Chest wall

Terminal ductal
lobular unit (TDLU)

Acini

Dense connective tissue

Loose connective tissue

Cooper ligament

Fat

Pectoralis fascia

Pectoralis major
muscle

Retromammary
layer

Major duct

Duct orifice

Nipple

Areola

Rib

Cooper ligaments

Subcutaneous layer

- Enlarge at the areola.
- Lined with epithelial cells.
- Diameter should not exceed 3 mm.

FIBROUS PLANES OF THE BREAST

Skin
- Composed of epidermis and dermis layers.
- Measures 2 to 3 mm in thickness.

Subcutaneous Fat Layer
- Premammary layer.
- Composed of fat and connective tissue.
- Located between the skin and the mammary zone.
- Contain Cooper ligaments.

Cooper ligaments
- Connective breast tissue providing a "skeletal" framework for the breast.
- Located within the subcutaneous layer of the breast.
- Course between the layers of the superficial fascia.

Superficial Fascia
- Lies within the subcutaneous fat anterior to the mammary zone.

Mammary Zone
- Breast parenchyma lying within the superficial fascia.
- Composed of epithelial and stromal tissue.
- Located between the subcutaneous fat and retromammary space.

Retromammary Space
- Houses the deep fascia.
- Composed of small fat lobules.
- Located between the posterior margin of the mammary zone and the pectoral muscles.

Deep Fascia
- Deep layer of the superficial fascia.
- Located within the retromammary space.

Pectoralis Muscles
- Muscular fascia surrounding the chest muscle.

PECTORALIS MAJOR MUSCLE
- Located between the retromammary space and pectoralis minor muscle.

PECTORALIS MINOR MUSCLE
- Located deep to the pectoralis major muscle and anterior to the rib cage.

BREAST VASCULATURE

ARTERIAL SUPPLY
- Lateral thoracic and internal mammary arteries.
- Lateral thoracic artery arises from the axillary artery.
- Internal mammary artery arises from the subclavian artery.

VENOUS SYSTEM

- Superficial veins lie deep to the superficial fascia.
- Superficial veins of the right and left breast communicate.
- Deep veins drain into the internal mammary, axillary, subclavian, and intercostal veins.
- Lymph vessels generally course parallel with the venous system.

CONGENITAL BREAST ANOMALIES

- **Amastia**—complete absence of one or both breasts.
- **Athelia**—complete absence of the nipple.
- **Amazia**—absence of the breast tissue with presence of the nipple.
- **Nipple inversion**—nipple inverts inward.
- **Polymastia**—accessory or supernumerary breast.
- **Polythelia**—accessory nipple; most common breast anomaly.

SONOGRAPHIC APPEARANCE OF THE BREAST

- Skin line appears hyperechoic.
- Superficial and deep fascial planes appear hyperechoic.
- Glandular breast parenchyma appears moderately hyperechoic.
- Fat breast lobules should demonstrate a medium-gray echo pattern.
- Retromammary layer appears hypoechoic.
- Pectoralis muscles appear moderately hyperechoic.
- Cooper ligaments appear as hyperechoic linear structures; may demonstrate posterior acoustic shadowing.
- Lactiferous ducts appear as nonvascular, anechoic tubular structures coursing toward the nipple.

TECHNIQUE

PREPARATION

- No preparation.

BREAST EXAMINATION TECHNIQUE

- 7.5-MHz or higher linear transducer to obtain optimal resolution for penetration depth.
- Multiple focal zones and proper depth placement.
- Gain settings demonstrating breast fat as a medium shade of gray and a simple cyst as an anechoic mass.
- Increase in dynamic range setting.
- Proper Doppler controls for low flow velocity (PRF, gain, wall filters).
- Patient is generally placed in a right or left posterior oblique position.
- Standoff pad should not exceed 1.0 cm in thickness.
- Evaluation and documentation of breast parenchyma in two imaging planes, remaining perpendicular to the chest wall.
- Proper annotation of the image location and scanning plane.
- Images are generally labeled by quadrant and/or the face of a clock.
- Distance from the nipple is described as 1,2,3 ("1" is closest to nipple).
- Depth of the area of interest is described as A,B,C ("C" is closest to the chest wall).
- Documentation and measurement of any abnormality should be included.

INDICATIONS FOR A BREAST EXAMINATION

- Palpable lump.
- Breast inflammation.
- Evaluate mass from a previous medical imaging study (i.e., mammogram).
- Ultrasound-guided interventional procedure.
- Evaluate augmented breast.
- Evaluate male breast parenchyma.
- Serial evaluation of a benign lesion.

Benign Breast Pathology

PATHOLOGY	ETIOLOGY	CLINICAL FINDINGS	SONOGRAPHIC FINDINGS	DIFFERENTIAL CONSIDERATIONS
Cyst	• Obstruction of a duct • Infection • Common around 35-50 years of age	• Asymptomatic • Breast pain or tenderness • Palpable mass	• Anechoic round or oval mass • Smooth, thin wall margins • Posterior acoustic enhancement • No internal vascular flow • Compresses with transducer pressure • Mass does not breach fascial plane(s) • May demonstrate internal echoes	• Lactiferous duct • Fibroadenoma • Carcinoma
Cystosarcoma phyllodes	• Uncommon benign fibroepithelial neoplasm • May undergo malignant transformation	• Sudden onset of a palpable nontender breast mass • Mobile mass	• Oval mass demonstrating a low- to medium-level echo pattern • Unilateral mass • May demonstrate cystic spaces within the mass • Smooth wall margins • Width of mass is larger than the height • Mass does not breach fascial plane(s) • Internal blood flow may be demonstrated	• Complex cyst • Fibroadenoma • Carcinoma • Normal breast fat
Fibroadenoma	• Tumor composed of dense epithelial and fibroblastic tissue • Influenced by estrogen levels	• Asymptomatic • Palpable nontender breast mass • Mobile mass • Firm or rubbery on palpation	• Solid oval-shaped breast mass • Low- to medium-level echo pattern • Posterior acoustic enhancement • Mass does not breach the fascial plane • Width of mass is larger than the height • Can degenerate or calcify • Internal blood flow may be demonstrated	• Complex cyst • Normal breast fat • Carcinoma
Fibrocystic disease	• Presence of palpable breast cyst(s) • Not generally associated with future development of breast carcinoma	• Painful or tender breasts frequently 7-10 days before the start of menses • Increase in pain intensity closer to the start of menses	• Hyperechoic breast parenchyma • Dense breast tissue • Prominent ducts • Numerous breast cysts	• Multiple breast cysts • Mastitis

Benign Breast Pathology—cont'd

PATHOLOGY	ETIOLOGY	CLINICAL FINDINGS	SONOGRAPHIC FINDINGS	DIFFERENTIAL CONSIDERATIONS
Hamartoma	• Proliferation of normal tissues	• Asymptomatic • Palpable mass	• Heterogeneous complex mass • Smooth wall margins • May demonstrate posterior acoustic shadowing • Mass does not breach fascial plane(s) • Mass compresses with moderate transducer pressure	• Complex cyst • Carcinoma • Fibroadenoma
Galactocele	• Obstruction of a lactating duct	• Palpable retroareolar mass	• Round or oval hypoechoic retroareolar mass • Smooth wall margins • Posterior acoustic enhancement	• Fibroadenoma • Complex cyst • Abscess
Gynecomastia	• Abnormal proliferation of ductal, glandular tissue, and stroma • Increased amount of subcutaneous fat • Hormone disorders • Endocrine disorders • Neoplasms	• Abnormal enlargement of the male breast(s) • Painful or tender breast(s)	• Hypoechoic to hyperechoic tissue beneath the areola • Ducts converging toward the areola • Increased amount of breast fat • Unilateral or bilateral	• Neoplasm • Mastitis
Lipoma	• Mature adipose tissue	• Soft, mobile mass	• Homogeneous hyperechoic mass within the subcutaneous fat • Oval in shape • Smooth wall margins • May appear similar to breast fat	• Glandular breast tissue • Fibroadenoma • Complex cyst
Mastitis	• Bacteria infection • Obstructed lactiferous duct • Infected cyst	• Painful or tender breast(s) • Erythema • Fever • Thick nipple discharge • Swelling • Lymphadenopathy • Malaise	• Dilated lactiferous ducts • Hypervascular breast parenchyma	• Fibrocystic disease
Papilloma	• Epithelial neoplasm	• Asymptomatic • Bloody nipple discharge	• Hypoechoic mass commonly found beneath the areola • Single adjacent dilate duct	• Papillary carcinoma • Dilated lactiferous duct • Lactiferous sinus

Malignant Breast Pathology

PATHOLOGY	ETIOLOGY	CLINICAL FINDINGS	SONOGRAPHIC FINDINGS	DIFFERENTIAL CONSIDERATIONS
Invasive ductal carcinoma	• Most common malignancy	• Asymptomatic • Palpable breast mass • Changes in breast or nipple contour	• Hypoechoic breast mass • Heterogeneous mass • Irregular or ill-defined borders • Posterior acoustic shadowing • Adjacent tissue may appear hyperechoic • Mass breaches fascial plane(s) • Cooper ligaments may appear thick and straight in course • Height of mass is larger than the width	• Degenerating fibroadenoma • Hematoma • Breast scarring or fibrosis
Colloid carcinoma	• Malignancy	• Asymptomatic • Soft palpable breast mass • Breast thickening	• Solid hypoechoic breast mass • Round in shape • Smooth wall margins	• Fibroadenoma • Complex cyst • Invasive ductal carcinoma
Medullary carcinoma	• Malignancy	• Asymptomatic • Soft palpable mass • Usually centrally located	• Solid hyperechoic breast mass • Round or oval in shape • Smooth to mildly irregular wall margins	• Fibroadenoma • Fibrotic breast tissue • Fibrosis • Invasive ductal carcinoma
Metastatic breast disease	• Malignant lymphoma • Melanoma • Lung • Ovarian	• Asymptomatic • Superficial breast mass • Multiple masses	• Discrete masses • Heterogeneous low-level internal echoes • Smooth wall margins • Usually found in the subcutaneous tissue	• Lipoma • Enlarged lymph node • Primary carcinoma
Papillary carcinoma	• Uncommon malignancy	• Asymptomatic • Bloody nipple discharge	• Solid mass most commonly located near the areola • Well-defined borders • Small in size • Dilated ducts	• Fibroadenoma • Complex cyst

ANTERIOR ABDOMINAL WALL AND MUSCULOSKELETAL SYSTEM

ANTERIOR ABDOMINAL WALL ANATOMY (Fig. 15-2)

- Consists of several layers of fat, fascia, and muscle.
- Subcutaneous tissue located anterior to the muscle groups.
- Fascial interface located anterior to the peritoneum.

LINEA ALBA

- Midline tendon extending from the xiphoid process to the symphysis pubis.
- Located posterior to the subcutaneous fat.

RECTUS ABDOMINUS MUSCLES

- Located on either side of the linea alba.
- Extend the entire length of the anterior abdominal wall.
- Each rectus muscle is contained within a rectus sheath.

EXTERNAL OBLIQUE MUSCLES

- Composes a portion of the lateral abdominal wall.
- Located anterior to the internal oblique and transverse abdominus muscles.

FIG. 15-2
Anterior abdominal wall anatomy.

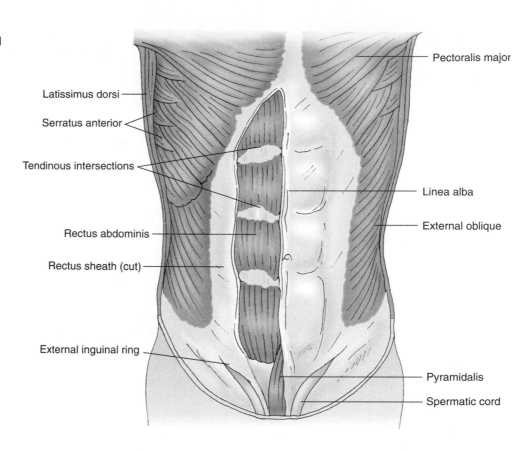

INTERNAL OBLIQUE MUSCLES

- Composes a portion of the lateral abdominal wall.
- Located posterior to the external oblique muscle and anterior to the transverse abdominus muscle.
- Acts with the contralateral external oblique muscle to achieve side bends of the trunk.

TRANSVERSUS ABDOMINUS MUSCLE

- Composes a portion of the lateral abdominal wall.
- Located immediately posterior to the internal and external oblique muscles.

MUSCULOSKELETAL ANATOMY

ACHILLES TENDON

- Tendon of the posterior calf attaching the gastrocnemius and soleus muscles.
- Thickest and strongest tendon in the body.
- Covered by fascia and integument.
- Limited blood supply increases the risk for injury and difficulty in healing.
- Inserts into the posterior surface of the calcaneus.
- Normally 5 to 7 mm in thickness and 12 to 15 mm in diameter.
- Increase in the normal size has been documented in athletes.

HIP JOINT

- A synovial joint between the femur and the acetabulum of the pelvis.

KNEE JOINT

- A complex hinge joint.
- Condyloid joint connecting the femur and the tibia.
- Arthrodial joint connecting the patella and the femur.
- Permits flexion and extension of the leg.

SHOULDER JOINT

- Ball and socket articulation of the humerus with the scapula.
- Joint includes eight bursae and five ligaments.
- Most mobile joint of the body.

SONOGRAPHIC APPEARANCE OF THE ANTERIOR ABDOMINAL WALL

- Superficial fat demonstrates a medium shade of gray echogenicity.
- Muscles demonstrate a low to medium shade of gray echo pattern with hyperechoic striations.
- The peritoneal line appears as a hyperechoic linear structure anterior to the peritoneal cavity in the deepest layer of the abdominal wall.

SONOGRAPHIC APPEARANCE OF THE MUSCULOSKELETAL SYSTEM

- Muscles demonstrate a low to medium shade of gray echo pattern with hyperechoic striations.
- Tendons appear homogeneous with hyperechoic linear bands throughout when viewed in the longitudinal plane.
- Ligaments appear homogeneous with compacted hyperechoic linear bands throughout when viewed in the longitudinal plane.
- Peripheral nerves appear as echogenic structures and tend to be slightly hypoechoic compared with the tendons and ligaments.

TECHNIQUE

PREPARATION

- No preparation.

EXAMINATION TECHNIQUE

- Use the highest-frequency linear transducer possible to obtain optimal resolution for penetration depth.
- Ensure multiple focal zones and proper depth placement.
- Evaluate and document the area of interest in two different scanning planes.
- Measure and document any abnormality in two scanning planes.
- Use Valsalva maneuver when evaluating the abdominal wall.
- Achilles tendon measurements should be made in the transverse plane.

INDICATIONS FOR AN ANTERIOR ABDOMINAL WALL EXAMINATION

- Trauma.
- Hernia.
- Palpable mass.
- Postsurgery.
- Evaluate mass from previous medical imaging study (i.e., CT).

INDICATIONS FOR A MUSCULOSKELETAL EXAMINATION

- Trauma.
- Pain.
- Palpable mass.
- Hernia.
- Decrease in motion.
- Evaluate mass from previous medical imaging study (i.e., CT).

Anterior Abdominal Wall Pathology

PATHOLOGY	ETIOLOGY	CLINICAL FINDINGS	SONOGRAPHIC FINDINGS	DIFFERENTIAL CONSIDERATIONS
Abdominal wall abscess	• Infection	• Palpable abdominal wall mass • Fever • Leukocytosis	• Hypoechoic or anechoic mass anterior to the peritoneal fascial plane • May demonstrate posterior acoustic enhancement or shadowing	• Hematoma • Hernia • Seroma
Rectus sheath hematoma	• Trauma • Pregnancy • Long-term steroid use • Coughing • Sneezing • Heavy exercise • Anticoagulant therapy	• Abdominal pain • Abdominal mass	• Hypoechoic or anechoic mass located in the rectus muscle or between the sheath and muscle	• Abscess • Hernia
Umbilical hernia	• Defect in the abdominal muscles	• Visual or palpable umbilical mass	• Extension of the intestines and/or omentum through a defect in the abdominal wall	• Hematoma • Abscess

Musculoskeletal Pathology

PATHOLOGY	ETIOLOGY	CLINICAL FINDINGS	SONOGRAPHIC FINDINGS	DIFFERENTIAL CONSIDERATIONS
Achilles tendonitis	• Inflammation • Trauma	• Pain or tenderness at the site of insertion • Palpable mass • Decreased range of motion in the foot or ankle joint	• Thickening of the tendon • Tendon thickness exceeding 7 mm • Prominent hypoechoic areas interspersed between the fibrous tissues • Irregular wall margins • Hypervascularity • Calcifications in chronic cases	• Partial tear • Anisotropy artifact • Tendinosis
Achilles tendon tear	• Trauma	• Painful tendon • Positive Thompson test • Focal cleft at tendon insertion	Complete Tear • Irregular tendon contour • Hematoma surrounding the defect • Most commonly located in the distal portion 2-6 cm from the calcaneus Partial Tear • Focal disruption in the tendon • Fluid collection within the tendon • Most commonly located in the distal portion	• Anisotropy artifact • Tendonitis • Tendinosis
Baker cyst	• Knee trauma • Rheumatoid arthritis • Osteoarthritis • Chronic knee dysfunction	• Pain in knee or proximal calf • Knee swelling • Palpable mass	• Anechoic mass in the medial and posterior aspect of the knee • May contain internal echoes • May extend into the calf • Rarely extends into the thigh • Fluid collections dissect inferiorly into the muscular fascial planes when ruptured	• Joint effusion • Abscess • Hematoma
Septic hip	• Infection	• Limping or change in gait • Recent illness	• Asymmetry in the anterior hip recess exceeding 2 mm when compared with the contralateral hip	• Joint effusion

SUPERFICIAL STRUCTURES REVIEW

1. Which of the following is the smallest functional unit in the breast parenchyma?
   a. lobe
   b. acini
   c. lobule
   d. terminal duct
   e. terminal ductal lobular unit

2. Which of the following joints has the largest range of motion?
   a. hip
   b. elbow
   c. wrist
   d. knee
   e. shoulder

3. Which of the following structures is considered the "skeletal" framework in the breast?
   a. acini
   b. deep fascia
   c. superficial fascia
   d. Cooper ligaments
   e. pectoralis major muscle

4. The most common congenital breast anomaly is:
   a. amastia
   b. amazia
   c. athelia
   d. polymastia
   e. polythelia

5. Which of the following most accurately describes the location of the transversus abdominus muscle?
   a. anterior to the internal oblique muscle
   b. medial to the external oblique muscle
   c. posterior to the internal oblique muscle
   d. lateral to the internal oblique muscle
   e. anterior to the external oblique muscle

6. A retroareolar mass developing shortly after childbirth is most suspicious for a(n):
   a. fibroadenoma
   b. galactocele
   c. hamartoma
   d. cystosarcoma phyllodes
   e. invasive ductal carcinoma

7. Which of the following artifacts is likely to occur when the ultrasound beam is not perpendicular with a fibrillar tendon?
   a. duplication
   b. reverberation
   c. refraction
   d. anisotropy
   e. shadowing

8. When imaging the breast parenchyma, the thickness of the standoff pad should not exceed:
   a. 0.5 cm
   b. 1.0 cm
   c. 2.0 cm
   d. 2.5 cm
   e. 3.0 cm

9. Which of the following benign breast neoplasms may undergo malignant transformation?
   a. simple cyst
   b. fibroadenoma
   c. complex cyst
   d. hamartoma
   e. cystosarcoma phyllodes

10. Complete absence of one or both breasts is termed:
    a. amazia
    b. athelia
    c. amaurosis
    d. amastia
    e. amyelia

11. Abnormal enlargement of the male breast parenchyma is most likely a clinical finding in which of the following pathologies?
    a. mastitis
    b. polymastia
    c. hamartoma
    d. galactocele
    e. gynecomastia

12. All of the following correctly describe the venous system of the breast parenchyma EXCEPT:
    a. deep veins may empty into the subclavian vein
    b. superficial veins lie deep to the superficial fascia
    c. deep veins may empty into the axillary vein
    d. lymph vessels generally course parallel with the Cooper ligaments
    e. superficial veins from the left and right breast can communicate

13. The echogenicity of a fatty breast lobule is most commonly described as a(n):
    a. anechoic, oval-shaped mass
    b. smooth, heterogeneous mass
    c. hyperechoic band of tissue
    d. smooth, moderately hypoechoic mass
    e. smooth, hyperechoic mass

14. Breast pathology most commonly originates in which of the following structures?
    a. lymph node
    b. breast lobule
    c. lactiferous duct
    d. connective breast tissue
    e. terminal ductal lobular unit

15. The deep layer of the superficial fascia is located within the:
    a. subcutaneous fat
    b. Cooper ligaments
    c. mammary zone
    d. retromammary space
    e. pectoralis muscles

16. Echogenicity of glandular breast tissue when compared to a fatty breast lobule is best described as:
    a. isoechoic
    b. hyperechoic
    c. heterogeneous
    d. moderately hyperechoic
    e. moderately hypoechoic

17. The diameter of a normal lactiferous duct should not exceed:
    a. 1.0 mm
    b. 1.5 mm
    c. 2.0 mm
    d. 2.5 mm
    e. 3.0 mm

18. Painful breast(s) 1 week prior to the onset of menstruation is a common symptom in which of the following conditions?
    a. mastitis
    b. gynecomastia
    c. fibrocystic disease
    d. metastatic breast disease
    e. inflammatory carcinoma

19. A common malignancy of the breast demonstrating posterior acoustic shadowing describes which of the following neoplasms?
    a. lobular carcinoma
    b. colloid carcinoma
    c. medullary carcinoma
    d. invasive ductal carcinoma
    e. papillary carcinoma

20. A defect in the muscles of the abdominal wall is most likely related to a:
    a. cyst
    b. polyp
    c. hernia
    d. hematoma
    e. diverticulum

21. The Thompson test is used to check the integrity of the:
    a. calf muscles
    b. knee joint
    c. rotator cuff
    d. Achilles tendon
    e. anterior abdominal wall

22. The most common benign breast lesion in women between the ages of 35 and 50 is a:
    a. simple cyst
    b. papilloma
    c. fibroadenoma
    d. cystadenoma
    e. hamartoma

23. Estrogen levels most frequently influence which of the following breast lesions?
    a. mastitis
    b. lipoma
    c. papilloma
    d. fibroadenoma
    e. galactocele

24. Muscle attaches to bone by which of the following structures?
    a. tendon
    b. fibril
    c. bursa
    d. ligament
    e. synovial membrane

25. Which of the following structures provides support to the breast parenchyma?
    a. deep fascia
    b. pectoralis muscles
    c. Cooper ligaments
    d. subcutaneous fat
    e. superficial fascia

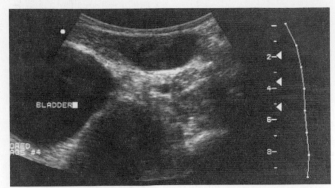

FIG. 15-3   Transverse sonogram of the left anterior abdominal wall.

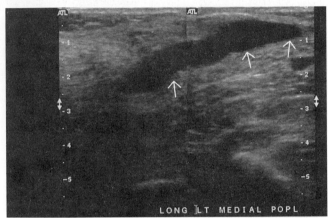

FIG. 15-4   Sonogram of the medial popliteal fossa.

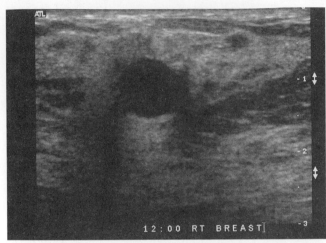

FIG. 15-5   Sonogram of the right breast.

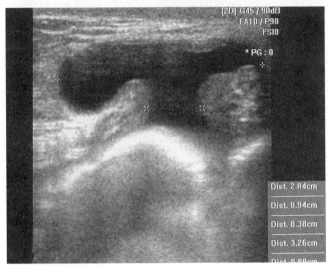

FIG. 15-6   Transverse sonogram of the anterior abdominal wall.

Using Fig. 15-3, answer question 26.

26. An afebrile elderly patient hospitalized with pneumonia presents with a palpable abdominal wall mass. A mass is identified adjacent to the urinary bladder. This finding is most suspicious for a(n):
   a. urachal sinus
   b. umbilical hernia
   c. enlarged lymph node
   d. rectus sheath hematoma
   e. abdominal wall abscess

Using Fig. 15-4, answer question 27.

27. An elderly patient presents with a history of acute ankle swelling. A sonogram is ordered to rule out deep vein thrombosis. A nonvascular anechoic structure is identified in the popliteal fossa. Based on these sonographic findings the anechoic structure is most suspicious for a:
   a. torn ligament
   b. synovial cyst
   c. joint effusion
   d. lymph node
   e. thrombosed superficial vein

Using Fig. 15-5, answer question 28.

28. A 45-year-old female presents with a firm, nontender, palpable breast mass. The finding in this sonogram is most consistent with a:
   a. simple cyst
   b. fibroadenoma
   c. galactocele
   d. cystadenoma
   e. cystosarcoma phyllodes

Using Fig. 15-6, answer question 29.

29. A patient presents to the ultrasound department with a palpable umbilical mass. The finding in this sonogram is most consistent for a(n):
   a. abscess
   b. hematoma
   c. hernia
   d. lipoma
   e. urachal sinus

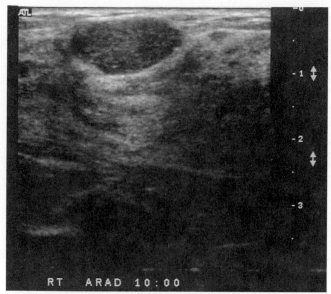

FIG. 15-7 Sonogram of the right breast.

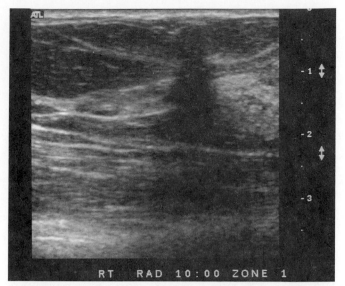

FIG. 15-8 Sonogram of the breast below.

Using Fig. 15-7, answer question 30.

30. A 25-year-old female presents with a firm, nontender, palpable breast mass. An antiradial image of the right breast demonstrates a hypoechoic mass. On the basis of the clinical history, the sonographic finding is most suspicious for a:
a. simple cyst
b. lymph node
c. fibroadenoma
d. galactocele
e. fat lobule

Using Fig. 15-8, answer question 31.

31. A patient is referred for an ultrasound to evaluate a mass identified on a recent mammogram. A radial image of the right breast demonstrates an abnormality most suspicious for:
a. cystosarcoma phyllodes
b. papillary carcinoma
c. fibrocystic disease
d. invasive ductal carcinoma
e. metastatic breast disease

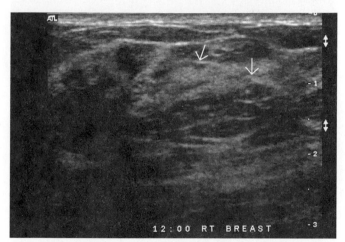

FIG. 15-9 Sonogram of the right breast.

Using Fig. 15-9, answer question 32.

32. The hyperechoic linear structure identified by the arrow is most consistent with:
a. the deep fascia
b. the superficial fascia
c. a Cooper ligament
d. a lactiferous duct
e. microcalcifications

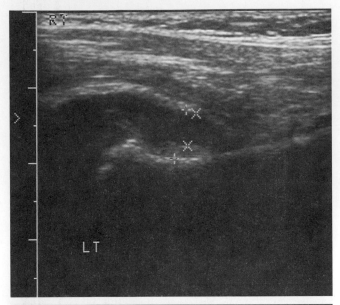

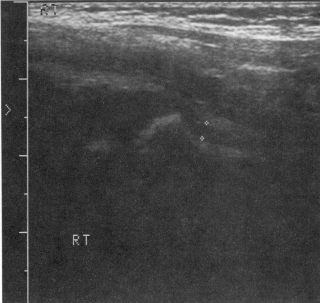

FIG. 15-10   Sonograms of the left and right hip.

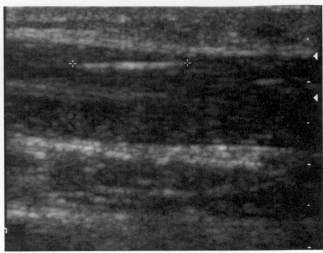

FIG. 15-11   Sonogram of the forearm.

Using Fig. 15-10, answer question 33.

33. A toddler with a recent upper respiratory infection presents with a history of limping. Asymmetric hip joints are identified on ultrasound. On the basis of the clinical history, the sonographic finding is most suspicious for which of the following conditions?
a. septic hip
b. hip dislocation
c. joint effusion
d. deep vein thrombosis
e. synovial cyst formation

Using Fig. 15-11, answer question 34.

34. A patient complains of pain in the forearm following a hiking trip. A soft tissue image over the area of discomfort demonstrates a hyperechoic linear structure outlined by the calibers. This is most suspicious for a:
a. lipoma
b. ligament
c. calcified vessel
d. foreign body
e. fascial plane

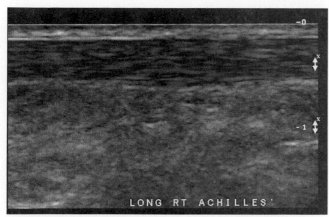

FIG. 15-12 Sagittal sonogram of the Achilles tendon.

Using Fig. 15-12, answer question 35.

35. A patient presents with an aching over the right Achilles tendon. A sagittal image of the tendon reveals which of the following findings?
a. normal tendon
b. tendonitis
c. complete tear
d. hematoma
e. incomplete tear

36. The breast parenchyma is composed of approximately:
a. 1 to 10 lobes
b. 5 to 15 lobes
c. 15 to 20 lobes
d. 20 to 30 lobes
e. 40 to 50 lobes

37. Thickness of a normal Achilles tendon should not exceed:
a. 3 mm
b. 5 mm
c. 7 mm
d. 10 mm
e. 15 mm

38. Possible etiologies of a rectus sheath hematoma may include all of the following conditions EXCEPT:
a. trauma
b. pregnancy
c. severe coughing
d. abdominal wall defect
e. anticoagulant therapy

39. The location of the rectus abdominus muscles is described as lateral to the:
a. iliac crests
b. linea alba
c. external oblique muscles
d. internal oblique muscles
e. psoas muscles

40. The fascial interface of the anterior abdominal wall is located directly anterior to the:
a. linea alba
b. peritoneum
c. retroperitoneum
d. subcutaneous fat
e. rectus abdominus muscles

41. The Valsalva maneuver is a common technique used when evaluating the:
a. pediatric hip
b. rotator cuff
c. Achilles tendon
d. anterior abdominal wall
e. gastrointestinal tract

42. A teenager arrives to the emergency department following a skiing injury. A nonvascular hypoechoic mass is identified in the posterior popliteal fossa. This mass most likely represents a(n):
a. Baker cyst
b. lymph node
c. hematoma
d. aneurysm
e. pseudoaneurysm

43. The sinus of a lactiferous duct is located near the:
a. areola
b. axilla
c. sternum
d. chest wall
e. tail of Spence

44. A mass is identified in the upper outer quadrant of the right breast, near the axilla and chest wall. This mass should be annotated as:
a. 2:00 1A
b. 10:00 3C
c. 2:00 2B
d. 10:00 1C
e. 10:00 3A

45. Sonographic findings associated with invasive ductal carcinoma may include all of the following EXCEPT:
a. hypoechoic mass
b. ill-defined borders
c. posterior acoustic shadowing
d. width of mass is larger than height
e. thick Cooper ligaments

46. Measurement of the Achilles tendon should be made in the:
a. sagittal plane
b. transverse plane
c. coronal plane
d. prone position
e. supine position

47. A complete tear of the Achilles tendon is most commonly located:
  a. at the superior insertion
  b. in the medial portion of the tendon near the medial malleolus
  c. approximately 2 to 6 cm from the superior tendon insertion
  d. in the lateral portion of the tendon near the lateral malleolus
  e. in the distal portion of the tendon near the calcaneus

48. Which of the following muscles extends the entire length of the anterior abdominal wall?
  a. linea alba
  b. psoas
  c. external oblique
  d. rectus abdominus
  e. internal oblique

49. In the breast, the lymph vessels generally course parallel with the:
  a. venous system
  b. lactiferous ducts
  c. Cooper ligaments
  d. retromammary zone
  e. terminal ductal lobular units

50. Clinical symptoms associated with mastitis may include all of the following EXCEPT:
  a. fever
  b. erythema
  c. breast pain
  d. malaise
  e. bloody nipple discharge

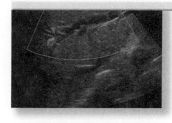

CHAPTER **16**

Scrotum and Prostate

KEY TERMS

appendix testis   a small solid structure located posterior to the epididymal head.

benign prostatic hypertrophy (BPH)   benign enlargement of the prostate gland; noninflammatory condition.

central zone (CZ)   cone-shaped area of the prostate gland located deep in the peripheral zone.

cryptorchidism   undescended testis.

epididymis   long, tightly coiled ducts that carry sperm from the testis to the vas deferens.

epididymitis   inflammation of the epididymis; commonly caused by a urinary tract infection; most common cause of acute scrotal pain.

hydrocele   abnormal accumulation of serous fluid between the two layers of tunica vaginalis.

mediastinum testis   thick portion of the tunica albuginea.

peripheral zone (PZ)   the largest area of the prostate gland located just beneath the capsule.

periurethral glands   glandular tissue lining the proximal prostatic urethra.

polyorchidism   more than two testes.

prostate specific antigen (PSA)   a protein produced by the prostate; elevation is associated with carcinoma of the prostate gland.

orchitis   inflammation of the testis; commonly caused by Chlamydia.

rete testis   network of ducts formed in the mediastinum testis connecting the epididymis with the superior portion of the testis.

seminal vesicles   small paired structures that store sperm.

spermatic cord   supporting structure on the posterior border of the testes that courses through the inguinal canal.

spermatocele   a cyst arising form the rete testis.

surgical capsule   connective tissue dividing the peripheral and central zones.

testicular torsion   twisting of the spermatic cord upon itself, obstructing the blood vessels supplying the epididymis and testis; also known as bell clapper.

transitional zone (TZ)   two small areas of the prostate gland adjacent to the proximal urethral space.

tunica albuginea   fibrous sheath enclosing each testis.

tunica vaginalis   two layers of serous membrane (visceral and parietal) covering the anterior and lateral portions of the testis and epididymis.

TURP   transurethral resection prostatomy.

varicocele   dilatation of the spermatic veins; most common cause of male infertility.

vas deferens   a small tube that transports the sperm from each testis to the prostatic urethra.

verumontanum   divides the urethra into proximal and distal segments.

PHYSIOLOGY

FUNCTION OF THE SCROTUM

- Allows maintenance of a lower body temperature necessary for sperm survival.

FUNCTIONS OF THE EPIDIDYMIS

- Store and transport sperm produced by the testes.
- Mature the sperm.

FUNCTIONS OF THE TESTIS

- Produce testosterone.
- Germinate sperm.

225

FUNCTIONS OF THE PROSTATE GLAND

- Secretes alkaline fluid to transport sperm.
- Secretions contain alkaline phosphatase, citric acid, and prostate specific antigen (PSA).
- Produces 80% to 85% of the ejaculation fluid.
- Produces PSA.

ANATOMY

SCROTUM (Fig. 16-1)

- A two-compartment pouch that contains and supports each testis.
- Divided by a medium raphe or septum.
- Contains a number of tissue layers and vascular structures.

EPIDIDYMIS

- Empties into the ductus deferens (vas deferens).
- Located lateral and posterior to the testis.
- Extends from the superior to the inferior pole of each testis.
- Divided into:
  - Head—located posterior and superior to the testis.
  - Body—located directly posterior to the testis.
  - Tail—located posterior and inferior to the testis.

TESTES

- Paired male reproductive organs located in the scrotum.
- Endocrine and exocrine glands.
- Composed of multiple lobules.

Tunica Albuginea

- Fibrous sheath enclosing each testis.

Tunica Vaginalis

- Two layers of serous membrane (visceral and parietal) covering the anterior and lateral portions of the testis and epididymis.
- Small amount of fluid is normal within these layers to prevent friction.
- Potential space for fluid collections (i.e., hydrocele).

FIG. 16-1
Scrotum anatomy.

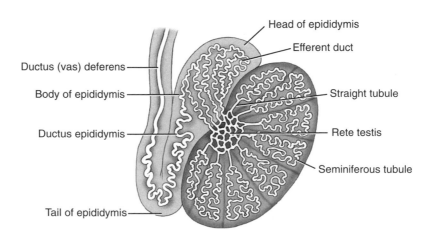

Head of epididymis
Efferent duct
Ductus (vas) deferens
Body of epididymis
Straight tubule
Ductus epididymis
Rete testis
Seminiferous tubule
Tail of epididymis

Mediastinum Testis

- Thick portion of the tunica albuginea.
- Located in the posterior medial border of the testis.

Rete Testis

- Network of ducts formed in the mediastinum testis.
- Transports seminal fluid from the testis to the epididymis.
- Connects the epididymis to the superior testis.

Spermatic Cord

- Support structure located on the posterior border of the testes.
- Courses through the inguinal canal.

Vas Deferens

- A small tube that transports sperm from each testis to the prostatic urethra.
- Also called ductus deferens.

PROSTATE GLAND (Fig. 16-2)

- A cone-shaped retroperitoneal structure.
- Inferior border (apex) provides an exit for the urethra.
- Superior border (base) is in contact with the urinary bladder.
- Consists of five lobes: anterior, middle, posterior, and two lateral lobes.
- Divided into three zones: central, peripheral, and transitional zones.

Central Zone (CZ)

- Comprises approximately 25% of the glandular tissue.
- Resistant to disease.
- Midline wedge at the base of the prostate between the peripheral and transitional zones.

Peripheral Zone (PZ)

- Comprises approximately 70% of the glandular tissue.
- Surrounds the distal urethral segment.
- Separated from the central zone by the surgical capsule.
- Occupies the posterior, lateral, and apical regions of the prostate.
- Site for most prostate cancer.

Transitional Zone (TZ)

- Comprises 5% of the glandular tissue and periurethral glands.
- Two small glandular areas adjacent to the proximal urethral sphincter.

FIG. 16-2
Prostate anatomy.

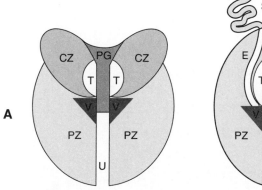
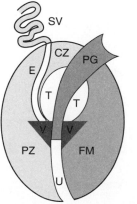

- Bound caudally by the verumontanum.
- Area where benign prostatic hypertrophy (BPH) originates.

Periurethral Glands

- Comprise 1% of glandular tissue.
- Tissue lines the prostatic urethra.

Seminal Vesicles

- Paired structures lying superior to the prostate, posterior to the bladder, and lateral to the vas deferens.
- Ducts of the seminal vesicles enter the central zone.
- Joins the vas deferens to form the ejaculatory ducts.
- Stores sperm.

Surgical Capsule

- Connective tissue separating the peripheral and central zones.
- Surgical boundary line used in transurethral resection procedures.
- Not a true capsule.

Verumontanum

- Divides the urethra into proximal and distal segments.
- Region where the ejaculatory ducts enter the urethra.

VASCULAR ANATOMY

SCROTUM

Testicular Arteries

- Arise from the anterior aspect of the abdominal aorta.
- Branch in the posterior portion of the superior testis.
- Course along the periphery toward the mediastinum testis.
- Low-resistance flow, demonstrating low flow velocity (15 cm/sec).

Centripetal Arteries

- Course away from the mediastinum and branch into multiple rami arteries.
- Low-resistance blood flow, demonstrating low flow velocity.

Cremasteric and Deferential Arteries

- Contained in the spermatic cord.
- Supply the epididymis, scrotal tissue, and testes.

Testicular Veins

- Left testicular vein empties into the left renal vein.
- Right testicular vein empties directly into the inferior vena cava.

Spermatic Vein

- Normal size 1 to 2 mm.
- Dilated when diameter exceeds 4 mm.

PROSTATE

Prostaticovesical Arteries

- Arise from the internal iliac arteries.
- Branches include the prostatic and inferior vesical arteries.

Inferior Vesical Artery

- Supplies the bladder base, seminal vesicles, and the ureter.

Capsular Arteries

- Supplies two thirds of the blood going into the prostate.

Urethral Artery

- Supplies one third of the blood into the prostate.

Congenital Anomalies—Scrotum

ANOMALY	DESCRIPTION	CLINICAL FINDINGS	SONOGRAPHIC FINDINGS	DIFFERENTIAL CONSIDERATIONS
Cryptorchidism	• Undescended testis • 80% are located in the inguinal canal • Associated with a herniated scrotal sac and an increased risk of infertility, torsion, and malignancy • Normal testes will descend by 6 months of age	• Absence of testis in the scrotum • Palpable inguinal mass	• Absence of testis in the scrotum • Oval-shaped hypoechoic mass in the inguinal canal, pelvis, or retroperitoneum • Smaller in size than a normal testis • Generally mobile	• Lymph node • Hematoma • Bowel
Polyorchidism	• Presence of more than two testes • Associated with inguinal hernia, testicular torsion, and malignancy	• Asymptomatic • Enlarged scrotum • Palpable scrotal mass	• Small echogenic extratesticular mass similar to the testis • Usually located in the superior medial aspect of the scrotum	• Epididymal neoplasm • Testicular neoplasm • Epididymitis

SIZE

ADULT

- Testis: 4 cm in length, 2 cm in height, and 3 cm in width.
- Epididymis: 10 mm in the superior portion and 4 mm in the posterior and inferior portions.
- Prostate: 2 cm in length, 3 cm in height, and 4 cm in width.

PREPUBERTY

- Testis: 2.0 to 2.5 cm in length.

INFANT

- Testis: 1.0 to 1.5 cm in length.

SONOGRAPHIC APPEARANCE

SCROTUM

- Thin hyperechoic wall measuring 2 to 8 mm in thickness.
- Small amount of anechoic fluid surrounds each testis.
- Vascular structures are prominent inferiorly.

TESTES

- Homogenous parenchyma demonstrating a medium- to low-level echo pattern.
- Ovoid in shape.
- The mediastinum testis appears as a hyperechoic linear structure located in the medial and posterior aspect of each testis.
- Low-resistance, low-velocity intratesticular blood flow demonstrating continuous flow throughout diastole.
- Hypoechoic parenchyma is demonstrated in infants and children.
- The echogenicity of the testes should be symmetrical.
- Intratesticular Doppler blood flow should be symmetrical.

EPIDIDYMIS

- Homogenous structure demonstrating a medium- to low-level echo pattern.
- Isoechoic to hypoechoic when compared to the normal testis.

PROSTATE

- Homogeneous structure demonstrating a medium-level echo pattern.
- Peripheral zone appears uniform in texture and slightly more echogenic than the central zone.
- Seminal vesicles appear as hypoechoic structures superior to the prostate gland.
- Verumontanum appears hyperechoic compared with the parenchyma.

TECHNIQUE

SCROTUM PREPARATION

- No preparation is necessary to evaluate the male scrotum.

PROSTATE PREPARATION

- Distended urinary bladder with transabdominal imaging of the prostate.
- Empty urinary bladder with transrectal imaging of the prostate.
- Bowel preparations may also be requested.

EXAMINATION TECHNIQUE

Scrotum

- Use the highest-frequency linear transducer possible to obtain optimal resolution for penetration depth.
- Multiple focal zones.
- Proper depth placement, dynamic range, and gain controls.
- Proper Doppler controls for low-velocity flow (PRF, gain, wall filters).
- Patients lie in the supine position with a rolled towel placed underneath the scrotum.
- The penis is placed on the lower abdomen and covered with a towel.
- Sagittal and transverse scanning planes are used to evaluate the scrotum, testes, and epididymis.
- Duplex evaluation and documentation of the scrotum, testes, and epididymis from the superior to inferior walls and medial to lateral walls of the scrotum in both the sagittal and transverse planes.
- Documentation and measurement of the length, height, and width of each testis.
- Duplex evaluation, documentation, and measurement of any abnormality should be included.

Prostate

- Use the highest-frequency transabdominal or endorectal transducer possible to obtain optimal resolution for penetration depth.

- Ensure proper focal zone and depth placement.
- Place patients in the supine position for transabdominal imaging and the left lateral decubitus position for endorectal imaging.
- Evaluate and document from the base of the prostate to the seminal vesicles in the transverse plane.
- Evaluate and document the right and left sides of the prostate gland, the urethra, and the verumontanum in the sagittal plane.

INDICATIONS FOR SCROTAL EXAMINATION

- Scrotal pain.
- Scrotal trauma.
- Enlarged scrotum.
- Palpable scrotal mass.
- Infertility.
- Undescended testis.
- Evaluate mass from previous medical imaging study (i.e., computed tomography).

INDICATIONS FOR PROSTATE EXAMINATION

- Enlarged prostate.
- Decreased urine output.
- Urinary frequency.
- Urinary urgency.
- Dysuria.
- Elevated PSA level.
- Infertility.
- Routine screening starting at age 50.

LABORATORY VALUES

PROSTATE SPECIFIC ANTIGEN

- Normal monoclonal PSA 4.0 ng/mL.
- Protein produced by the prostate.
- Elevation of 20% in 1 year is indicative of carcinoma.
- Increase of 0.75 ng/mL in 1 year is indicative of carcinoma.

Scrotal Pathology

PATHOLOGY	ETIOLOGY	CLINICAL FINDINGS	SONOGRAPHIC FINDINGS	DIFFERENTIAL CONSIDERATIONS
Hernia	• Weak abdominal wall muscles • Inguinal hernia may extend into the scrotum	• Scrotal mass • Abdominal pain	• Complex extratesticular mass • Mass can be traced to the inguinal canal • Peristalsis may be noted	• Testicular torsion • Hematocele
Hydrocele	• Inflammation • Idiopathic • Congenital • Associated with torsion, trauma, or malignancy	• Enlarged scrotum • Asymptomatic • Scrotal mass • Scrotal pain	• Anechoic fluid collection lateral and anterior to the testis • Strong posterior acoustic enhancement • Thin scrotal wall when acute • Diffuse wall thickening when chronic • May demonstrate internal echoes or septations	• Epididymal cyst • Spermatocele • Hematocele • Hernia
Varicocele	• Idiopathic • Incompetent valves in the spermatic vein	• Asymptomatic • Infertility • Tender scrotal mass • Scrotal ache	• Tortuous venous structures exceeding 4 mm in diameter • Most commonly located on the left and in the inferior portion of the scrotum • Veins increase in size with Valsalva maneuver or while patient is standing	• Loculated hydrocele • Epididymal cyst

Epididymal Pathology

PATHOLOGY	ETIOLOGY	CLINICAL FINDINGS	SONOGRAPHIC FINDINGS	DIFFERENTIAL CONSIDERATIONS
Cyst	• Cystic dilatation of epididymal tubules • Vasectomy	• Asymptomatic • Palpable scrotal mass	• Anechoic mass in the epididymis • Compression of the testis	• Spermatocele • Loculated hydrocele • Varicocele
Epididymitis	• Urinary infection • Idiopathic • Trauma	• Acute scrotal pain • Swelling • Leukocytosis • Fever	• Hypoechoic epididymis • Enlarged epididymis • Hyperechoic with calcifications when chronic • Small cysts may be visualized	• Testicular torsion • Varicocele
Spermatocele	• Retention cyst arising from the rete testis • Idiopathic • Infection • Trauma	• Asymptomatic • Palpable scrotal mass	• Anechoic mass lying superior to the testis • Round or oval in shape • Does not compress testis • Generally solitary	• Loculated hydrocele • Epididymal cyst

Testicular Pathology

PATHOLOGY	ETIOLOGY	CLINICAL FINDINGS	SONOGRAPHIC FINDINGS	DIFFERENTIAL CONSIDERATIONS
Cyst	• Incidence increases with age	• Asymptomatic	• Anechoic mass within the testis • Smooth wall margins • Posterior acoustic enhancement	• Resolving hematoma • Vascular structure • Neoplasm
Malignant neoplasm	• Germ cell neoplasm—most common seminoma • Teratoma • Stromal neoplasm • Metastases	• Asymptomatic • Palpable scrotal mass • Scrotal swelling	• Hypoechoic intratesticular mass • May appear complex • Hypervascular mass periphery • Reactive hydrocele	• Abscess • Hematoma • Focal orchitis
Microcalcifications	• Idiopathic • Calcified vessels • Granulomatosis	• Asymptomatic	• Multiple small hyperechoic foci dispersed in the testis parenchyma • Usually bilateral • Associated with a neoplasm in 40% of cases	• Neoplasm • Chronic orchitis • Resolving hematoma
Orchitis	• Chlamydia—most common • Secondary to epididymitis	• Scrotal pain • Scrotal swelling • Fever • Nausea/vomiting	• Enlarged hypoechoic testis parenchyma • Increase in intratesticular vascular flow • Hydrocele • Complex areas of necrosis • Atrophy and intratesticular calcifications are demonstrated in chronic cases	• Testicular torsion • Neoplasm
Tubular ectasia of the rete testis	• Usually associated with epididymal obstruction due to trauma or inflammation	• Asymptomatic	• Cystic lesion demonstrated in the region of the mediastinum testis • Variable in size • Usually bilateral and asymmetrical	• Carcinoma
Testicular rupture	• Trauma	• Scrotal pain • Scrotal swelling • Palpable scrotal mass	• Irregular fibrous testicular capsule • Extrusion of the testis into the scrotal sac • Hematocele	• Neoplasm • Hematoma
Testicular torsion	• Twisting of the spermatic cord upon itself obstructing the blood vessels supplying the epididymis and testis	• Sudden onset of groin or scrotal pain • Lower abdominal pain • Nausea/vomiting • Scrotal swelling	• Hypoechoic parenchyma • May appear enlarged • Markedly absent or decreased intratesticular blood flow • Hydrocele	• Neoplasm • Hematoma • Improper Doppler settings and angle

Prostate Pathology

PATHOLOGY	ETIOLOGY	CLINICAL FINDINGS	SONOGRAPHIC FINDINGS	DIFFERENTIAL CONSIDERATIONS
Benign prostatic hypertrophy	• Noninflammatory enlargement of the prostate gland • Usually occurs in the transitional zone	• Urinary frequency • Dysuria • Decreased urinary output • Urinary tract infection	• Symmetrical prostate enlargement • Hypoechoic parenchyma • May demonstrate nodules, cysts, or calcifications • Associated hydronephrosis	• Carcinoma
Carcinoma	• Idiopathic • Associated with hormone production	• Asymptomatic • Hematuria • Bladder obstruction	• Small hypoechoic nodules • Smooth or irregular wall margins • Elevated PSA • Majority located in the peripheral zone	• Seminal vesicle • Benign prostatic hypertrophy
Prostatitis	• Infection • Acute or chronic inflammation of the prostate gland	• Urinary frequency and urgency • Dysuria	• Diffuse hyperechoic parenchyma • Prostate atrophy in chronic cases	• Calcifications

SCROTUM AND PROSTATE REVIEW

1. A hydrocele is defined as an abnormal fluid collection between the:
   a. tunica albuginea and the tunica vaginalis
   b. spermatic cord and the tunica albuginea
   c. two layers of the tunica vaginalis
   d. spermatic cord and the tunica vaginalis
   e. two layers of the tunica albuginea

2. "Bell clapper" is another term used to describe which of the following abnormalities?
   a. hydrocele
   b. varicocele
   c. microcalcifications
   d. testicular torsion
   e. cryptorchidism

3. Normal testes will descend into the scrotal sac by:
   a. 6 months of age
   b. 12 months of age
   c. 2 years of age
   d. 3 years of age
   e. 5 years of age

4. Carcinoma of the prostate gland most commonly develops in the:
   a. central zone
   b. peripheral zone
   c. seminal vesicles
   d. transitional zone
   e. periurethral gland

5. Which of the following arteries gives rise to the testicular arteries?
   a. gonadal arteries
   b. common iliac arteries
   c. internal iliac arteries
   d. anterior aspect of the abdominal aorta
   e. lateral aspect of the abdominal aorta

6. A fibrous sheath enclosing the testis describes which of the following structures?
   a. rete testis
   b. vas deferens
   c. tunica albuginea
   d. mediastinum testis
   e. tunica vaginalis

7. Which of the following functions is considered a responsibility of the prostate gland?
   a. stores sperm
   b. matures sperm
   c. germinates sperm
   d. produces ejaculation fluid
   e. produces testosterone

8. The thickened portion of the tunica albuginea is termed the:
   a. rete testis
   b. epididymis
   c. vas deferens
   d. seminal vesicles
   e. mediastinum testis

9. Which of the following structures supports the posterior border of the testes?
   a. epididymis
   b. rete testes
   c. spermatic cord
   d. tunica albuginea
   e. mediastinum testis

10. Indications for a scrotal ultrasound may include all of the following EXCEPT:
    a. infertility
    b. groin pain
    c. palpable mass
    d. undescended testis
    e. decreased urine output

11. An anechoic structure arising from the rete testes describes which of the following structures?
    a. epididymal cyst
    b. testicular cyst
    c. hydrocele
    d. spermatocele
    e. prostate cyst

12. Which of the following structures transports sperm from the testes to the prostatic urethra?
    a. rete testis
    b. spermatic cord
    c. vas deferens
    d. seminal vesicles
    e. mediastinum testis

13. A spermatic vein is considered dilated once the diameter exceeds:
    a. 2 mm
    b. 4 mm
    c. 6 mm
    d. 8 mm
    e. 10 mm

14. The scrotum is divided into two separate compartments by the:
    a. medium raphe
    b. tunica vaginalis
    c. rete testes
    d. mediastinum testis
    e. spermatic cord

Using Fig. 16-3, answer question 15.

15. A 35-year-old patient presents with a palpable scrotal mass. He is afebrile and denies any scrotal pain. On the basis of this clinical history, the sonographic finding is most suspicious for which of the following abnormalities?
   a. testicular torsion
   b. acute orchitis
   c. testicular carcinoma
   d. epididymitis
   e. scrotal herniation

Using Fig. 16-4, answer question 16.

16. An 85-year-old patient presents with intermittent scrotal swelling. He states the swelling "comes and goes." On the basis of this clinical history, the sonographic finding is most suspicious for:
   a. testicular rupture
   b. testicular carcinoma
   c. epididymitis
   d. scrotal hernia
   e. testicular torsion

Using Fig. 16-5, answer question 17.

17. Hyperechoic foci are identified in which of the following regions of the prostate gland?
   a. peripheral zone
   b. surgical capsule
   c. central zone
   d. seminal vesicles
   e. periurethral glands

Using Fig. 16-6, answer questions 18 and 19.

18. A 30-year-old patient presents with a tender scrotal mass. The sonographic finding is most suspicious for which of the following abnormalities?
   a. orchitis
   b. a scrotal hernia
   c. a hydrocele
   d. a varicocele
   e. epididymitis

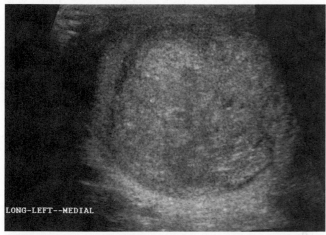

FIG. 16-3   Sagittal sonogram of the left testis.

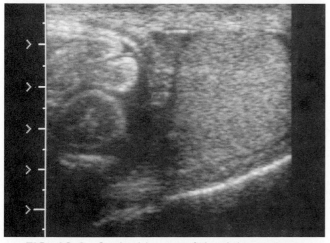

FIG. 16-4   Sagittal image of the right scrotum.

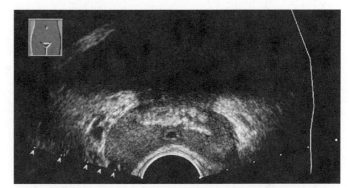

FIG. 16-5   Sonogram of the prostate gland.

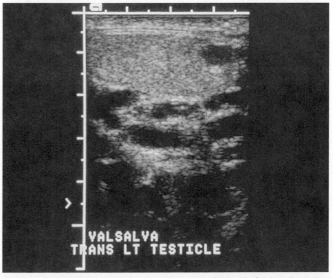

FIG. 16-6   Transverse sonogram of the inferior border of the left scrotum.

19. Which of the following complications is associated with this diagnosis?
    a. infertility
    b. reactive hydrocele
    c. testicular carcinoma
    d. testicular torsion
    e. deep vein thrombosis

Using Fig. 16-7, answer questions 20 and 21.

20. A patient presents with a history of scrotal swelling and tenderness. He denies any scrotal trauma. On the basis of this clinical history, the sonographic findings are most consistent with a:
    a. hydrocele
    b. urinoma
    c. varicocele
    d. spermatocele
    e. hematocele

21. The echogenic structure superior to the testis most likely represents the:
    a. spermatic cord
    b. ductus deferens
    c. medium raphe
    d. mediastinum testis
    e. epididymal head

22. Epididymitis is most commonly caused by which of the following conditions?
    a. hydrocele
    b. varicocele
    c. bladder infection
    d. inguinal hernia
    e. epididymal cyst

23. Which of the following regions in the prostate most commonly develops benign prostatic hypertrophy (BPH)?
    a. central zone
    b. peripheral zone
    c. transitional zone
    d. periurethral glands
    e. verumontanum

24. Twisting of the spermatic cord upon itself is a predisposing factor of which of the following abnormalities?
    a. orchitis
    b. prostatitis
    c. epididymitis
    d. spermatocele
    e. testicular torsion

25. A 30-year-old patient presents with a low-grade fever and acute testicular pain. An enlarged hypoechoic right testis is demonstrated on ultrasound. Hypervascular flow is demonstrated within the testis on color Doppler imaging. On the basis of this clinical history, the sonographic findings are most suspicious for which of the following abnormalities?
    a. orchitis
    b. epididymitis
    c. testicular torsion
    d. tubular ectasia
    e. malignant neoplasm

26. Sudden onset of severe scrotal pain in an adolescent patient is most suspicious for:
    a. orchitis
    b. a hydrocele
    c. epididymitis
    d. testicular rupture
    e. testicular torsion

27. The epididymis connects to the testis by which of the following structures?
    a. medium raphe
    b. vas deferens
    c. rete testis
    d. spermatic cord
    e. tunica vaginalis

28. Which of the following is considered a function of the seminal vesicles?
    a. germinate sperm
    b. transport sperm
    c. store sperm
    d. mature sperm
    e. produce ejaculatory fluid

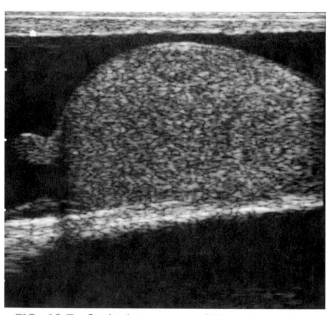

FIG. 16-7   Sagittal sonogram of the right scrotum.

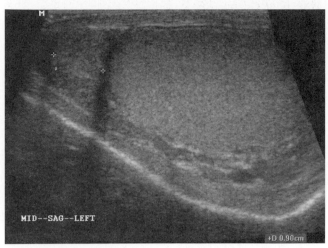

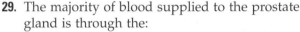

FIG. 16-8   Sonogram of the left scrotum.

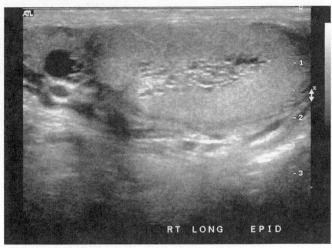

FIG. 16-9   Sagittal sonogram of the right scrotum.

29. The majority of blood supplied to the prostate gland is through the:
  a. urethral artery
  b. capsular artery
  c. cremasteric arteries
  d. inferior vesical artery
  e. prostaticovesical arteries

Using Fig. 16-8, answer questions 30 and 31.

30. A 45-year-old patient presents with acute scrotal pain after a mountain biking trip. On the basis of this clinical history, the sonographic findings are most suspicious for which of the following abnormalities?
  a. hematocele
  b. varicocele
  c. epididymitis
  d. scrotal hernia
  e. testicular torsion

31. An echogenic mass is identified superior to the testis and outlined by the calibers. This most likely represents which of the following structures?
  a. hematoma
  b. spermatocele
  c. seminal vesicle
  d. head of the epididymis
  e. spermatic cord

Using Fig. 16-9, answer questions 32 and 33.

32. A 76-year-old patient presents with a history of a palpable mass in the superior portion of the right scrotal sac. A nonvascular cystic mass is identified in the medial portion of the testis. This mass is most suspicious for which of the following abnormalities?
  a. varicocele
  b. acute orchitis
  c. microcalcifications
  d. malignant neoplasm
  e. tubular ectasia of the rete testis

33. The contralateral testis in this patient will most likely demonstrate a:
  a. spermatocele
  b. cryptorchidism
  c. normal appearance
  d. loculated hydrocele
  e. tubular ectasia of the rete testis

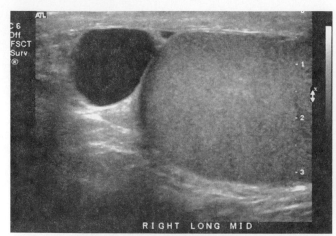

FIG. 16-10   Sagittal image of the right testis.

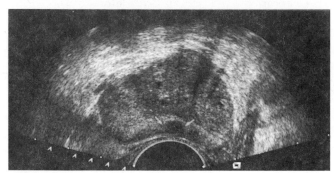

FIG. 16-11   Transrectal image of the prostate gland.

Using Fig. 16-10, answer question 34.

34. An asymptomatic patient presents with a palpable right scrotal mass discovered during a recent physical examination. The sonographic finding is most consistent with which of the following abnormalities?
a. varicocele
b. hydrocele
c. testicular cyst
d. spermatocele
e. cystadenoma

Using Fig. 16-11, answer question 35.

35. A patient presents with a history of hematuria and elevated prostate specific antigen (PSA). The neoplasm identified by the arrows is located in which region of the prostate gland?
a. central zone
b. seminal vesical
c. transitional zone
d. peripheral zone
e. periurethral gland

36. The male urethra is divided into proximal and distal segments by which of the following structures?
a. seminal vesicles
b. surgical capsule
c. vas deferens
d. verumontanum
e. transitional zone

37. The normal monoclonal level of prostate specific antigen (PSA) should not exceed:
a. 2 ng/mL
b. 4 ng/mL
c. 6 ng/mL
d. 8 ng/mL
e. 10 ng/mL

38. Decreased urine output is most commonly linked with an abnormality in which of the following structures?
a. testis
b. scrotum
c. epididymis
d. prostate gland
e. spermatic cord

39. The location of the epididymis is most accurately described as:
a. anterior to the testis
b. posterior to the testis
c. posterior and medial to the testis
d. posterior and lateral to the testis
e. anterior and medial to the testis

40. Blood is supplied directly to the epididymis through which of the following arteries?
a. capsular
b. testicular
c. cremasteric
d. centripetal
e. inferior vesical

41. Which of the following veins receives the left testicular vein?
a. left renal vein
b. inferior vena cava
c. left external iliac vein
d. left suprarenal vein
e. left internal iliac vein

42. Which of the following pathologies is the most common cause of acute scrotal pain?
a. orchitis
b. hydrocele
c. varicocele
d. epididymitis
e. testicular torsion

43. Which of the following most accurately describes the echogenicity and location of the seminal vesicles?
   a. heterogeneous structures located anterior to the urinary bladder
   b. homogeneous structures located inferior to the prostate gland
   c. hyperechoic structures located posterior to the urinary bladder
   d. hypoechoic structures located superior to the prostate gland
   e. homogeneous structures located medial to the vas deferens

44. Which of the following arteries is contained in the spermatic cord?
   a. cremasteric
   b. inferior vesical
   c. centripetal
   d. internal iliac
   e. capsular

45. A 60-year-old patient presents with a history of urinary frequency and a decrease in urinary output. These clinical symptoms are most commonly associated with:
   a. a hydrocele
   b. prostatitis
   c. orchitis
   d. prostate carcinoma
   e. benign prostatic hypertrophy (BPH)

46. Cryptorchism is associated with an increased risk in developing:
   a. orchitis
   b. a varicocele
   c. a spermatocele
   d. testicular torsion
   e. microcalcifications

47. Which region of the prostate gland comprises only 5% of the glandular tissue?
   a. central zone
   b. peripheral zone
   c. transitional zone
   d. verumontanum
   e. periurethral glands

48. The prostatic urethra is lined by which of the following structures?
   a. central zone
   b. vas deferens
   c. verumontanum
   d. periurethral glands
   e. seminal vesicles

49. The lobes of the prostate gland are termed the:
   a. head, body, and tail
   b. anterior, posterior, and two lateral lobes
   c. central, peripheral, and transitional lobes
   d. superior, inferior, anterior, and posterior lobes
   e. anterior, middle, posterior, and two lateral lobes

50. The sonographic appearance of the mediastinum testis is best described as a(n):
   a. hyperechoic linear structure located in the posterior medial aspect of the testis
   b. hypoechoic ovoid-shaped structure located in the posterior lateral aspect of the testis
   c. hypoechoic linear structure located in the anterior medial aspect of the testis
   d. anechoic tubular structure located in the posterior medial aspect of the testis
   e. hyperechoic tortuous structure located in the anterior medial aspect of the testis

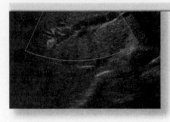

CHAPTER 17

Neck

KEY TERMS

brachial cleft cyst   a congenital diverticulum of the brachial cleft located directly below the angle of the mandible.

exophthalmos   bulging of the eyeballs; associated with hyperthyroidism.

De Quervain syndrome   subacute thyroiditis secondary to a viral infection.

goiter   a pronounced swelling of the neck caused by an enlarged thyroid gland.

Graves disease   a multisystemic autoimmune disorder characterized by pronounced hyperthyroidism; usually associated with an enlarged thyroid and exophthalmos.

Hashimoto disease   a progressive autoimmune inflammatory disorder of the thyroid gland; most common cause of hypothyroidism; associated with an increased risk in developing a thyroid malignancy.

hypercalcemia   an excessive amount of calcium in the blood; associated with hyperparathyroidism.

hyperparathyroidism   excessive function of the parathyroid glands; may lead to osteoporosis and nephrolithiasis.

hyperthyroidism   hyperactivity of the thyroid gland; associated with Graves disease.

hypocalcemia   a deficiency of calcium in the blood; associated with hypoparathyroidism.

hypoparathyroidism   a condition of insufficient secretion of the parathyroid glands; associated with hypocalcemia and primary parathyroid dysfunction.

hypothyroidism   decreased activity of the thyroid gland; associated with Hashimoto disease.

iodide   an anion of iodine.

longus colli muscles   neck muscles located on the anterior surface of the vertebral column, between the atlas and the third thoracic vertebra; commonly associated with whiplash injuries.

myxedema   the most severe form of hypothyroidism; characterized by swelling of the hands, face, and feet; may lead to coma and death.

postpartum thyroiditis   a transient thyroiditis seen following pregnancy.

sternocleidomastoid muscles   lateral and superficial neck muscles that attach to the sternum, clavicle, and the mastoid process of the temporal bone; act to flex and rotate the head.

strap muscles   a group of long and flat muscles located anterior and lateral to each thyroid lobe; includes the sternohyoid, sternothyroid, and omohyoid muscles.

thyroglossal cyst   an embryonic remnant cyst located between the isthmus of the thyroid and the tongue.

PHYSIOLOGY

FUNCTION OF THYROID GLANDS

- Secrete hormones: thyroxine, triiodothyronine, and calcitonin.
- Secretion of thyroid hormones is primarily controlled by the thyroid-stimulating hormone produced by the pituitary gland.

FUNCTION OF THE PARATHYROID GLANDS

- Maintain homeostasis of blood calcium concentrations.

FUNCTION OF THE CAROTID ARTERIES

- Supply blood to the head and neck.

FUNCTION OF THE JUGULAR VEINS

- Drain blood from the head and neck.

ANATOMY (Fig. 17-1)

MUSCLES OF THE NECK

Longus Colli Muscles
- Located on the anterior surface of the vertebral column.
- Lie posterior to the thyroid lobe and common carotid artery.

Platysma Muscles
- Superficial muscles located in the lateral neck.
- Located posterior to the subcutaneous tissues.

Sternocleidomastoid Muscles
- Lateral and superficial neck muscles.
- Located lateral to the thyroid lobes.

Strap Muscles
- A group of long flat neck muscles.
- Located anterior and lateral to the thyroid lobe.

VASCULATURE OF THE NECK

COMMON CAROTID ARTERIES
- Left originates from the aortic arch.
- Right arises from the innominate (brachiocephalic) artery.
- Ascend the anterolateral aspect of the neck.
- Lie medial to the internal jugular vein and lateral to the thyroid lobe.
- Course deep to the sternocleidomastoid muscles.
- Typically no branches.
- Bifurcate into the external and internal carotid arteries.

EXTERNAL CAROTID ARTERIES
- Supplies the neck, scalp, and face with blood.
- Lies anterior and medial to the internal carotid artery.
- Multiple extracranial branches.
- Superior thyroid artery is the first branch of the external carotid arteries.

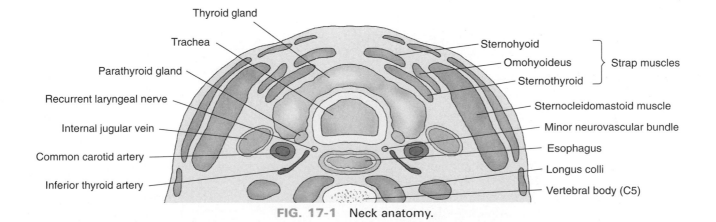

FIG. 17-1   Neck anatomy.

INTERNAL CAROTID ARTERIES

- Main blood supply to the eyes and brain.
- Lie posterior and lateral to the external carotid artery.
- Terminate at the circle of Willis.
- No extracranial branches.
- Ophthalmic artery is the first branch of the internal carotid artery.

VERTEBRAL ARTERIES

- Arise from the first segment of the subclavian artery.
- Provide blood to the posterior brain.
- Lie in the posterior neck, ascending through the transverse processes of the spine.
- Left and right vertebral arteries join to form the basilar artery at the base of the skull.
- Basilar artery terminates in the posterior aspect of the circle of Willis.
- Multiple extracranial branches.

INTERNAL JUGULAR VEINS

- Receive the major portion of blood from the brain, neck, and superficial parts of the face.
- Course lateral to the carotid artery.
- Unite with the subclavian vein, forming the innominate (brachiocephalic) vein.
- Right and left innominate veins join, forming the superior vena cava.

EXTERNAL JUGULAR VEINS

- Receives blood from the exterior cranium and deep parts of the face.
- Located in the superficial fascia of the lateral neck.
- Empties into the subclavian vein.

VERTEBRAL VEINS

- Receive blood from the posterior brain and empties into the brachiocephalic vein.
- Located anterior to the corresponding vertebral artery.

ANATOMY OF THE THYROID GLANDS

- Endocrine glands.
- Divided into the right and left lobes with a connecting isthmus.

VASCULATURE OF THE THYROID GLANDS

- Arterial flow is supplied by the superior and inferior thyroid arteries.
- Superior thyroid artery arises from the external carotid artery.
- Inferior thyroid artery arises from the thyrocervical artery.
- Superior, middle thyroid veins drain into the internal jugular vein; inferior thyroid vein drains into the innominate vein.

ANATOMY OF THE PARATHYROID GLANDS

- Two paired bean-shaped glands located posterior to the thyroid gland.

LOCATION

THYROID LOBES

- Medial and anterior to the corresponding common carotid artery and internal jugular vein.
- Posterior and medial to the sternocleidomastoid and strap muscles.
- Anterior to the longus colli muscle.

THYROID ISTHMUS

- Anterior to the trachea.
- Medial and anterior to the common carotid arteries and internal jugular veins.

PARATHYROID GLANDS

- Posterior to the thyroid glands.
- Anterior to the longus colli muscles.

CONGENITAL ANOMALIES

PYRAMIDAL LOBE

- Third lobe arising from the superior portion of the isthmus.
- Ascends to the level of the hyoid bone.

ABSENT ISTHMUS

- Thyroid consists of two distinct lobes.

ECTOPIC PARATHYROID GLAND LOCATION

- May be found near the carotid bifurcation or posterior to the carotid artery.
- May be located retroesophageal, substernal, or intrathyroid.

SIZE

- **Isthmus**—0.2 to 0.6 cm in height.
- **Thyroid glands**—4.0 cm in length, 2.0 cm in height, and 3 cm in width.
- **Parathyroid glands**—up to 6.0 mm in length, 2 mm in height, and 4 mm in width.

SONOGRAPHIC APPEARANCE

- Thyroid lobes and isthmus appear as homogeneous solid structures demonstrating a medium-gray echo pattern.
- Sternocleidomastoid and strap muscles appear hypoechoic when compared with the normal thyroid gland.
- Longus colli muscles appear hyperechoic when compared with the normal thyroid gland.
- Parathyroid glands are flat bean-shaped hypoechoic structures located posterior and medial to the thyroid lobes.
- Carotid arteries and jugular veins appear as anechoic tubular structures demonstrating internal vascular flow.

TECHNIQUE

PREPARATION

- No preparation.

EXAMINATION TECHNIQUE

- Use the highest-frequency linear transducer possible to obtain optimal resolution for penetration depth.
- Use multiple focal zones and proper depth placement.
- Increase the dynamic range setting when imaging the thyroid glands.
- Use Doppler settings for low- to medium-flow states.
- Place the patient in a supine position with the neck extended.
- A pillow may be placed under the upper back to hyperextend the neck.

- Evaluate and document both thyroid lobes from the superior to inferior borders and the medial to lateral borders in two imaging planes.
- Document length, width, and height of each thyroid lobe.
- Document thickness of isthmus.
- Document length, width, and height of any abnormality.
- With multinodular goiters, include measurements of the largest nodules for serial comparison.

INDICATIONS FOR EXAMINATION

- Palpable neck mass.
- Abnormal thyroid function tests.
- Dysphagia.
- Dyspnea.
- Fatigue.
- Serial evaluation of thyroid nodule(s).
- Evaluate mass from a previous medical imaging study (i.e., CT).

LABORATORY VALUES

THYROID

Thyrotropin (TSH)

- Normal range 3 to 42 ng/mL.
- Thyroid-stimulating hormone (TSH).
- Regulates thyroid hormone secretion and production.
- Secretion controlled by the anterior pituitary gland.
- Prolonged elevation is associated with hyperplasia and thyroid enlargement.
- Decrease in levels is the first indication of thyroid gland failure.

Thyroxine (T_4)

- Normal range 4.5 to 12.0 µg/dL.
- Stimulates consumption of oxygen.
- Secreted by the follicular cells of the thyroid.
- Controlled by thyrotropin (TSH).
- 100 to 200 mg of iodide must be ingested per week for normal thyroxine production.
- Decreases associated with thyroid disease and nonfunctioning pituitary gland.

Triiodothyronine (T_3)

- Normal range 70 to 190 ng/dL.
- Regulates tissue metabolism.
- Decreases associated with Hashimoto thyroiditis.

Calcitonin

- Normal range <100 pg/mL.
- Lowers calcium and phosphorus concentration in the blood.
- Inhibits bone resorption.
- Secreted by the parafollicular cells (C-cells) of the thyroid gland.
- Elevation associated with medullary thyroid carcinoma.
- Decreases are associated with surgical removal or nonfunctioning thyroid glands.

PARATHYROID

Parathormone (PTH)

- Normal range 12 to 68 pg/ml.
- Regulates calcium metabolism in conjunction with calcitonin.

- Released in response to low extracellular concentration of free calcium.
- Elevation associated with hyperparathyroidism.

Calcium

- Normal range 8.5 to 10.5 mg/dL.
- Aids in the transportation of nutrients through the cell membranes.
- Elevation associated with hyperparathyroidism, hyperthyroidism, and malignancy.
- Levels exceeding 14.5 mg/dL can be life threatening.
- Decreases are associated with nonfunctioning or surgical removal of the parathyroid glands.

THYROID PATHOLOGY

HYPERTHYROIDISM

- Hyperactivity of the thyroid gland.
- Symptoms include nervousness, exophthalmos, tremors, constant hunger, weight loss, heat intolerance, palpitations, increased heart rate, and diarrhea.
- If untreated, may lead to cardiac failure.

HYPOTHYROIDISM

- Decreased activity of the thyroid gland.
- Symptoms include weight gain, mental and physical lethargy, skin dryness, feeling cold, muscle cramps, constipation, arthritis, slow metabolic rate, and decreased heart rate.
- If untreated, may lead to myxedema, coma, or death.

THYROID NODULES

- 60% are benign.
- 20% are cysts.
- 20% are malignant.

Benign Thyroid Neoplasms

BENIGN MASS	ETIOLOGY	CLINICAL FINDINGS	SONOGRAPHIC FINDINGS	DIFFERENTIAL CONSIDERATIONS
Adenoma	• Composed of epithelial tissue	• Asymptomatic • Hyperthyroidism	• Homogeneous echogenic mass • Prominent hypoechoic peripheral halo • Peripheral blood flow • May degenerate	• Carcinoma • Cyst • Goiter
Cyst	• Simple cyst	• Asymptomatic • Palpable neck mass	• Anechoic mass • Smooth wall margins • Posterior acoustic enhancement • May demonstrate internal debris	• Cystic degeneration of a solid nodule
Goiter	• Impaired synthesis of thyroid hormones	• Palpable neck mass • Dysphagia • Dyspnea • Hyper- or hypothyroidism	• Enlarged thyroid lobe(s) • Multiple solid nodules	• Thyroiditis
Graves disease	• Autoimmune disorder of the thyroid gland	• Hyperthyroidism • Exophthalmos • Palpable neck mass • Dysphagia • Dyspnea	• Diffuse enlargement of the thyroid glands • Multilocular nodules	• Thyroiditis • Carcinoma

Continued

Benign Thyroid Neoplasms—cont'd

BENIGN MASS	ETIOLOGY	CLINICAL FINDINGS	SONOGRAPHIC FINDINGS	DIFFERENTIAL CONSIDERATIONS
Hashimoto disease	• Chronic lymphatic inflammatory disease	• Often painless • Hypothyroidism • Leukocytosis • Sore throat • Fever	• Enlarged hypoechoic thyroid glands • Hypervascular parenchyma	• Graves disease • Abscess
Thyroiditis	• Hashimoto disease • De Quervain syndrome • Postpartum infection	• Hyperthyroidism followed by hypothyroidism • Fatigue • Fever • Leukocytosis • Neck pain • Dysphagia	• Enlarged hypoechoic gland • Hypervascular parenchyma • Discrete nodules	• Graves disease

Cysts of the Neck

CYST	ETIOLOGY	CLINICAL FINDINGS	SONOGRAPHIC FINDINGS	DIFFERENTIAL CONSIDERATIONS
Brachial cleft cyst	• Congenital diverticulum of the brachial cleft	• Asymptomatic • Lateral neck mass	• Anechoic superficial neck mass • Located directly below the angle of the mandible • Located anterior to the sternocleidomastoid muscle • May demonstrate internal debris	• Thyroglossal cyst • Thyroid cyst
Cystic hygroma	• Inadequate drainage of lymph fluid into the jugular vein • Increased secretion from the epithelial lining	• Asymptomatic • Posterior neck mass	• Thin-walled, multilocular cystic structure	
Thyroglossal cyst	• Embryonic remnant	• Asymptomatic • Superficial anterior neck mass	• Anechoic superficial neck mass • Located between the tongue and the thyroid isthmus • May demonstrate internal debris	• Thyroid cyst • Brachial cleft cyst

Malignant Thyroid Neoplasms

	ETIOLOGY	CLINICAL FINDINGS	SONOGRAPHIC FINDINGS	DIFFERENTIAL CONSIDERATIONS
Carcinoma	• Papillary (65%) • Follicular (25%) • Anaplastic (5%) • Medullary (5%)	• Palpable neck mass • Dysphagia • Dyspnea • Hoarseness • Neck pain • Lymphadenopathy	• Hypoechoic mass • Irregular borders • Thick incomplete peripheral halo • Microcalcification • May degenerate • Increase in size from previous examination • Metastases to cervical lymph nodes, lung, bone, and larynx	• Cystic degeneration of a benign nodule • Nodular goiter • Abscess

PARATHYROID PATHOLOGY

HYPERCALCEMIA

- Elevated calcium in the blood.
- Symptoms include confusion, anorexia, abdominal pain, muscle pain and weakness, stone formation, gout, arthritis, weight loss, and bone demineralization.
- Associated with hyperparathyroidism, metastatic bone tumor, Paget disease, and osteoporosis.
- Extremely high levels may result in coma, shock, kidney failure, or death.

HYPERPARATHYROIDISM

- Excessive function of the parathyroid glands.
- May lead to osteoporosis and nephrolithiasis.

HYPOCALCEMIA

- Deficiency of calcium in the blood.
- Symptoms may include cardiac arrhythmia, hyperparesthesia of the hands, feet, lips, and tongue; muscle cramps; anxiety; and fatigue.
- Associated with hypoparathyroidism, kidney failure, acute pancreatitis, and inadequate amount of magnesium and protein.

HYPOPARATHYROIDISM

- Insufficient function of the parathyroid glands.
- Associated with hypercalcemia and primary parathyroid dysfunction.

Parathyroid Pathology

PATHOLOGY	ETIOLOGY	CLINICAL FINDINGS	SONOGRAPHIC FINDINGS	DIFFERENTIAL CONSIDERATIONS
Adenoma	• Exposure to ionizing radiation	• Hypercalcemia • Decrease in serum phosphorus • Hypertension • Stone formation • Pancreatitis	• Hypoechoic mass located posterior and medial to the thyroid gland • Oval in shape	• Lymph node • Thyroid nodule
Carcinoma	• Epithelial neoplasm • Slow-growing • Tend to infiltrate surrounding tissues	• Hypercalcemia • Elevated parathormone level • Firm palpable neck mass	• Hypoechoic lobulated mass • Round or oval in shape • Attenuation of sound (dense) • Hypervascular	• Parathyroid adenoma • Lymph node • Thyroid neoplasm • Graves disease
Cyst	• Uncommon simple cyst	• Asymptomatic • Female prevalence • 60-70 years of age	• Anechoic mass located posterior and medial to the thyroid gland • Smooth wall margins • Posterior acoustic enhancement	• Thyroid cyst • Thyroglossal cyst
Hyperparathyroidism	• Parathyroid adenoma (80%) • Renal disease • Calcium and vitamin D deficiency	• Elevated parathormone • Hypercalcemia • Abdominal pain • Gout • Painful bones • Nephrolithiasis	• Homogenous hypoechoic nodule • Located posterior and medial to the thyroid gland • Teardrop or oblong in shape	• Complex cyst • Thyroid nodule
Hyperplasia	• Excessive multiplication of normal parathyroid cells • Hyperparathyroidism	• Asymptomatic • Elevated parathormone • Abdominal pain • Gout • Nephrolithiasis • Painful bones	• Multiple hyperechoic homogeneous nodules • Smooth wall margins	• Parathyroid adenoma • Goiter

NECK REVIEW

1. Which of the following veins empties directly into the internal jugular vein?
   a. vertebral
   b. subclavian
   c. brachiocephalic
   d. superior thyroid
   e. external jugular

2. Secretion of thyroid hormones is stimulated by which of the following structures?
   a. cerebellum
   b. thyroid glands
   c. pituitary gland
   d. parathyroid glands
   e. hypothalamus

3. Symptoms of hyperthyroidism may include all of the following EXCEPT:
   a. nervousness
   b. weight loss
   c. exophthalmos
   d. muscle cramps
   e. increased heart rate

4. Which of the following conditions is most commonly associated with hypothyroidism?
   a. Graves disease
   b. Cushing disease
   c. Addison disease
   d. Hashimoto disease
   e. De Quervain syndrome

5. Which of the following is considered a function of the parathyroid gland?
   a. producing hormones
   b. secreting calcitonin
   c. regulating serum electrolytes
   d. initiating an immune reaction
   e. maintaining homeostasis of blood calcium concentrations

6. The vertebral arteries join at the base of the skull to form the:
   a. circle of Willis
   b. basilar artery
   c. carotid sinus
   d. ophthalmic artery
   e. brachiocephalic artery

7. A patient presents with a superficial neck mass located near the angle of the jaw. On ultrasound, the mass demonstrates a few swirling echoes within an anechoic mass. On the basis of this clinical history, the sonographic findings are most suspicious for a:
   a. cystic hygroma
   b. thyroglossal cyst
   c. brachial cleft cyst
   d. carotid body tumor
   e. parathyroid cyst

8. A congenital anomaly associated with an additional thyroid lobe arising from the isthmus is termed a(n):
   a. accessory lobe
   b. pyramidal lobe
   c. ectopic lobe
   d. duplicated isthmus
   e. vertebral lobe

9. Which of the following vascular structures receives blood from the posterior brain and empties into the brachiocephalic vein?
   a. subclavian vein
   b. vertebral vein
   c. innominate vein
   d. external jugular vein
   e. inferior mammary vein

10. The first indication of thyroid gland failure is linked with a decrease in:
    a. thyroxine
    b. calcitonin
    c. thyrotropin
    d. triiodothyronine
    e. progesterone

11. A homogenous mass is identified within the inferior portion of a thyroid lobe. A prominent hypoechoic ring surrounds this mass. These sonographic findings are most consistent with which of the following neoplasms?
    a. lipoma
    b. adenoma
    c. lymph node
    d. complex cyst
    e. papillary carcinoma

12. Tissue metabolism is regulated by which of the following hormones?
    a. thyrotropin
    b. thyroxine
    c. calcitonin
    d. triiodothyronine
    e. parathormone

13. A patient presents with a history of hyperthyroidism followed by hypothyroidism, dysphagia, and leukocytosis. A sonogram demonstrates an enlarged hypervascular thyroid gland. On the basis of this clinical history, the sonographic findings are most suspicious for which of the following conditions?
a. goiter
b. thyroiditis
c. hyperplasia
d. metastatic disease
e. hyperparathyroidism

14. A thyroglossal cyst is located between which of the following structures?
a. hyoid bone and thyroid gland
b. left thyroid lobe and tongue
c. thyroid isthmus and tongue
d. right thyroid lobe and tongue
e. trachea and thyroid gland

15. The majority of blood supplied to the brain is through the:
a. vertebral arteries
b. external carotid arteries
c. circle of Willis
d. internal carotid arteries
e. common carotid arteries

Using Fig. 17-2, answer questions 16-18.

16. The anechoic structures identified by arrow **A** most likely represent which of the following structures?
a. thyroid cyst
b. carotid artery
c. strap muscles
d. parathyroid cyst
e. longus colli muscle

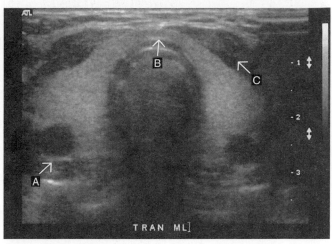

FIG. 17-2 Transverse sonogram of the midline neck.

17. The echogenic structure identified by arrow **B** most likely represents which of the following structures?
a. trachea
b. esophagus
c. strap muscles
d. thyroid isthmus
e. longus colli muscle

18. The hypoechoic structure identified by arrow **C** most likely represents which of the following structures?
a. trachea
b. strap muscles
c. thyroid isthmus
d. longus colli muscle
e. sternocleidomastoid muscle

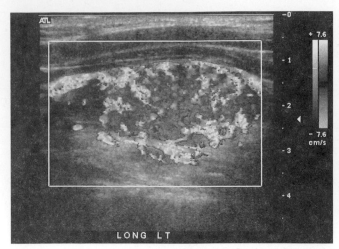 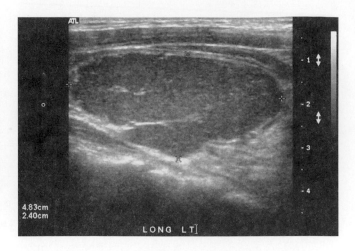

FIG. 17-3   Longitudinal sonograms of the thyroid gland.

Using Fig. 17-3, answer questions 19 and 20.

19. A 32-year-old female presents with a 2-month history of fatigue, sore throat, and dysphagia following an episode of cellulitis. The results of laboratory tests are pending. On the basis of this clinical history, the sonographic findings are most consistent with:
    a. hyperplasia
    b. Graves disease
    c. metastatic disease
    d. Hashimoto disease
    e. carotid body tumor

20. On the basis of the clinical symptoms and sonographic findings, the laboratory results will most likely demonstrate:
    a. hypercalcemia
    b. hypothyroidism
    c. hyperthyroidism
    d. hypoparathyroidism
    e. hyperparathyroidism

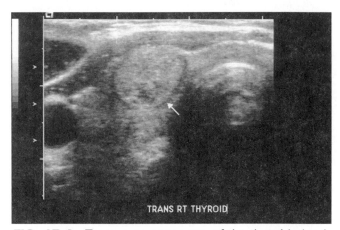

FIG. 17-4   Transverse sonogram of the thyroid gland.

Using Fig. 17-4, answer question 21.

21. A patient presents with a small mass palpated on a recent physical examination and normal laboratory values. A mass is identified in the inferior portion of the right thyroid lobe. On the basis of this clinical history, the sonographic findings are most suspicious for a(n):
    a. goiter
    b. adenoma
    c. carcinoma
    d. complex cyst
    e. hemangioma

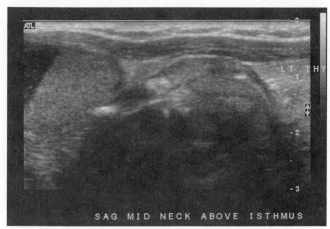

FIG. 17-5 Sagittal sonogram of the midline neck.

Using Fig. 17-5, answer question 22.

22. A patient presents with a palpable anterior neck mass. The patient denies any recent surgery or fever. A nonvascular complex mass is identified extending from the superior portion of the isthmus to the patient's chin. On the basis of this clinical history, the sonographic findings are most suspicious for a:
   a. cystic hygroma
   b. thyroid abscess
   c. thyroglossal cyst
   d. brachial cleft cyst
   e. multinodular goiter

23. How many parathyroid glands are found in the majority of the population?
   a. 2
   b. 3
   c. 4
   d. 5
   e. 6

24. Which of the following arteries arises first from the internal carotid artery?
   a. basilar artery
   b. vertebral artery
   c. ophthalmic artery
   d. superior thyroid artery
   e. middle cerebral artery

25. Which of the following symptoms is most likely related to hypercalcemia?
   a. fatigue
   b. weight gain
   c. palpitations
   d. tingling feet
   e. abdominal pain

26. Pancreatitis, hypertension, and hypercalcemia are clinical findings associated with which of the following neoplasms?
   a. thyroid adenoma
   b. multinodular goiter
   c. parathyroid adenoma
   d. thyroid carcinoma
   e. parathyroid carcinoma

27. Clinical findings associated with Graves disease may include all of the following EXCEPT:
   a. dyspnea
   b. dysphagia
   c. exophthalmos
   d. hypothyroidism
   e. palpable neck mass

28. A cystic hygroma is most likely related to which of the following abnormalities?
   a. thyroglossal cyst
   b. hyperparathyroidism
   c. arteriovenous fistula
   d. inadequate drainage of lymph fluid
   e. impaired synthesis of thyroid hormones

29. Which of the following statements about the carotid artery is TRUE?
   a. The right common carotid artery arises from the aortic arch.
   b. The external carotid artery courses lateral to the internal carotid artery.
   c. The internal carotid artery terminates at the circle of Willis.
   d. The common carotid artery has multiple extracranial branches.
   e. The internal carotid artery lies anterior to the external carotid artery.

30. Inflammation of the thyroid gland secondary to a viral infection is most commonly associated with which of the following conditions?
   a. Graves disease
   b. Caroli disease
   c. Mirizzi syndrome
   d. Addison syndrome
   e. De Quervain syndrome

31. Which of the following muscles is located posterior to the thyroid lobes?
   a. sternohyoid
   b. platysma
   c. omohyoid
   d. longus colli
   e. sternocleidomastoid

32. Indications for a thyroid ultrasound examination may include all of the following EXCEPT:
    a. fatigue
    b. dysphagia
    c. palpitations
    d. audible bruit
    e. palpable neck mass

33. Exposure to ionizing radiation is a predisposing factor for development of which of the following neoplasms?
    a. thyroglossal cyst
    b. cystic hygroma
    c. thyroid adenoma
    d. parathyroid cyst
    e. parathyroid adenoma

34. Primary carcinoma of the thyroid gland is known to extend to all of the following structures EXCEPT:
    a. lung
    b. bone
    c. larynx
    d. liver
    e. lymph nodes

35. Which of the following conditions is considered a predisposing factor for developing a thyroid malignancy?
    a. Graves disease
    b. Hashimoto disease
    c. De Quervain syndrome
    d. Caroli disease
    e. Marfan syndrome

36. The normal length of an adult thyroid lobe is approximately:
    a. 1.0 cm
    b. 2.0 cm
    c. 3.0 cm
    d. 4.0 cm
    e. 6.0 cm

37. Including iodide in your diet is required for the normal production of:
    a. calcium
    b. thyroxine
    c. calcitonin
    d. thyrotropin
    e. triiodothyronine

38. Examination techniques used in thyroid imaging include all of the following EXCEPT:
    a. multiple imaging focal zones
    b. 7.0-MHz or higher linear transducer
    c. decreasing the dynamic range
    d. hyperextension of the patient's neck
    e. low pulse repetition frequency in Doppler imaging

39. Clinical symptoms of hypothyroidism include all of the following EXCEPT:
    a. arthritis
    b. tremors
    c. muscle cramps
    d. weight gain
    e. skin dryness

40. Which of the following arteries is the first branch of the external carotid artery?
    a. lingual artery
    b. fascial artery
    c. superior thyroid artery
    d. ascending pharyngeal artery
    e. superficial temporal artery

41. Serial evaluation of a multinodular goiter should include measurements of the overall length, height, and width of a thyroid lobe along with measurements of the length, height, and width of:
    a. each individual nodule
    b. the largest nodule(s)
    c. the complex nodule(s)
    d. the posterior nodule(s)
    e. the hypervascular nodule(s)

42. The majority of the thyroid nodules identified on ultrasound are:
    a. benign
    b. fluid filled
    c. hypervascular
    d. malignant
    e. multilocular

43. Multilocular nodules are demonstrated on a sonogram of a thyroid gland. This is most consistent with which of the following conditions?
    a. Caroli disease
    b. Graves disease
    c. De Quervain syndrome
    d. Hashimoto disease
    e. Addison syndrome

44. Development of which of the following conditions is linked to hyperthyroidism?
    a. kidney failure
    b. acute pancreatitis
    c. osteoporosis
    d. hepatomegaly
    e. pleural effusion

45. A solitary hypoechoic thyroid nodule demonstrating irregular borders and microcalcifications is most suspicious for:
    a. thyroiditis
    b. carcinoma
    c. an adenoma
    d. diffuse hyperplasia
    e. a hemangioma

46. A parathyroid mass may be suspected when an abnormality is located:
    a. superior to the thyroid isthmus
    b. lateral to a thyroid lobe
    c. posterior to a thyroid lobe
    d. anterior to the thyroid isthmus
    e. posterior to the longus colli muscle

47. Which of the following muscles is located lateral to the thyroid lobes just beneath the subcutaneous tissues in the neck?
    a. longus colli
    b. sternohyoid
    c. platysma
    d. omohyoid
    e. sternocleidomastoid

48. Which of the following muscles is most often affected by a whiplash injury?
    a. scalene
    b. platysma
    c. sternohyoid
    d. longus colli
    e. sternocleidomastoid

49. Pronounced swelling of the neck is most often caused by a(n):
    a. thyroglossal cyst
    b. carotid body tumor
    c. enlarging thyroid gland
    d. thrombosis in the jugular vein
    e. aneurysm of the carotid artery

50. Which of the following is the most common etiology of hyperparathyroidism?
    a. carotid body tumor
    b. cyst of a parathyroid gland
    c. adenoma of a parathyroid gland
    d. hyperplasia of a parathyroid gland
    e. multinodular goiter of a thyroid gland

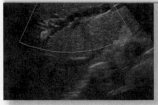

CHAPTER 18

Peritoneum, Noncardiac Chest, and Invasive Procedures

KEY TERMS

ascites   abnormal collection of serous fluid in the peritoneal cavity.

bare area   a large triangular area devoid of peritoneal covering located between the two layers of the coronary ligament.

biopsy   the removal of a small piece of living tissue for microscopic analysis.

coronary ligaments   left coronary ligament suspends the left lobe of the liver from the diaphragm; right coronary ligament serves as a barrier between the subphrenic space and Morison pouch.

chylous ascites   an accumulation of chyle and emulsified fats in the peritoneal cavity; most commonly associated with an abdominal neoplasm.

crura of the diaphragm   tendinous structure extending downward from the diaphragm to the vertebral column.

exudative ascites   an accumulation of fluid, pus, or serum in the peritoneal cavity; most commonly associated with inflammation or trauma.

fine-needle aspiration   a thin needle and gentle suction is used to obtain tissue samples for pathological testing.

greater omentum   a double-fold of peritoneum attached at the greater curvature of the stomach and superior portion of the duodenum; covers the transverse colon and small intestines.

hemoperitoneum   the presence of extravasated blood in the peritoneal cavity.

hemothorax   an accumulation of blood and fluid in the pleural cavity.

lesser omentum   a portion of peritoneum extending from the portal fissure of the liver to the diaphragm; encloses the lower end of the esophagus.

loculated ascites   the presence of numerous small fluid spaces in the peritoneal cavity.

lymphocele   a collection of lymph from injured lymph vessels.

mesenteric   a double layer of peritoneum suspending the intestine from the posterior abdominal wall.

mesenteric cyst   a congenital thin-walled cyst located between the leaves of the mesentery; most commonly located in the small-bowel mesentery.

paracentesis   a cannula or catheter is passed into the abdominal cavity to allow outflow of fluid into a collecting device for diagnostic or therapeutic purposes.

peritoneum   a serous membrane containing lymphatics, vessels, fat, and nerves.

pleural cavity   a thin space located between the two layers of pleura.

pleural effusion   an accumulation of fluid within the pleural cavity.

pouch of Douglas   a pouch formed by the inferior portion of the parietal peritoneum.

omentum   an extension of the peritoneum surrounding one or more organs adjacent to the stomach.

thoracentesis   a needle is inserted through the chest wall and pleural cavity to aspirate fluid for diagnostic or therapeutic purposes.

transudative ascites   an accumulation of a fluid in the peritoneal cavity containing small protein cells; most commonly associated with cirrhosis or congestive heart failure.

PHYSIOLOGY

FUNCTIONS OF THE PERITONEUM

- Secretes serous fluid to reduce friction between structures.
- Suspends and enfolds organs.

PERITONEUM ANATOMY (Fig. 18-1)

- An extensive serous membrane lining the entire abdominal wall.
- Folds of peritoneum form several potential spaces.
- Suspensory ligaments extend between organs.

GREATER OMENTUM

- A transparent double fold of peritoneum that spreads like an apron inferiorly to cover most of the abdominopelvic cavity.
- In cases of trauma, will often seal hernias and wall off infections.
- Keeps the small intestines warm.

LESSER OMENTUM (GASTROHEPATIC OMENTUM)

- Membranous extension from the portal fissure to the diaphragm.

ORGANS CONTAINED WITHIN THE PERITONEUM INCLUDE

- Duodenal bulb.
- Gallbladder.
- Ileum.
- Jejunum.
- Liver.
- Portions of the small intestines.
- Sigmoid colon.
- Spleen.
- Stomach.
- Transverse colon.
- Uterine body.

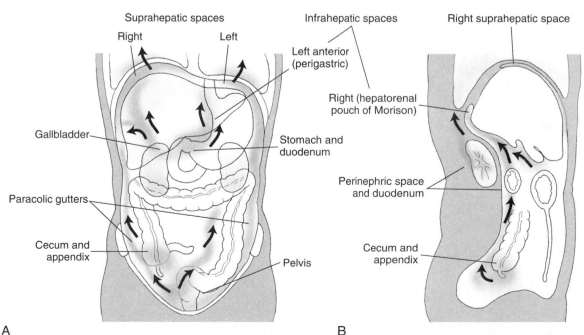

A   B

FIG. 18-1 Peritoneal anatomy.

PERITONEAL SPACES

LESSER SAC (OMENTAL BURSA)

- Separates the pancreas from the stomach.
- Located between the diaphragm and transverse colon.
- Communicates with the subhepatic space through the foramen of Winslow.

MORISON POUCH (HEPATORENAL POUCH)

- Located superior and anterior to the right kidney and posterior to the lateral portion of the right lobe of the liver.
- Unable to communicate with the subphrenic space because of the right coronary ligament (bare area).
- Communicates with the right paracolic gutter.
- Frequent site for fluid to collect.

PARACOLIC GUTTERS

- Located lateral to the colon.
- Serve as conduits for fluid between the deep pelvis and upper abdomen.
- Left paracolic gutter is shallow.
- Right paracolic gutter demonstrates less resistance and is the more common route of fluid extension.

PELVIC SPACES

- Retrovesical pouch is located posterior to the urinary bladder and anterior to the rectum.
- Retrouterine pouch is located posterior to the uterus and anterior to the rectum. Also called posterior cul de sac or pouch of Douglas.
- Vesicouterine pouch is located anterior to the uterus and posterior to the urinary bladder. Also called anterior cul de sac.
- Prevesical or retropubic space is located anterior to the urinary bladder and posterior to the symphysis pubis. Also known as space of Retzius.

Subhepatic Space

- Extends from the inferior border of the liver to a deep recess anterior to the right kidney.
- Most common site for fluid to collect.

Subphrenic Spaces

- Divided into the left and right subphrenic spaces by the falciform ligament.
- Left subphrenic space is located inferior to the diaphragm and superior to the spleen.
- Left subphrenic space includes spaces between the left diaphragm, left lobe of the liver, stomach, and spleen.
- Right subphrenic space is located inferior to the diaphragm and superior to the liver.
- Right subphrenic space extends over several rib spaces to the right coronary ligament (bare area).

LOCATION OF THE PERITONEUM

- Extends from the anterior abdominal wall to the retroperitoneum and paraspinal tissues.
- Extends from the diaphragm to the deep pelvic spaces around the bladder.

ANATOMY OF THE PLEURA

- A delicate serous membrane composed of a visceral and parietal layer.
- Visceral pleura covers the lung and has a low sensitivity to pain.
- Parietal pleura lines the chest wall and has a high sensitivity to pain.
- Pleural cavity is a thin space between the two layers of the pleura.
- Pleural fluid lubricates the pleural surfaces.
- Pleural membrane separates the two lungs.

SONOGRAPHIC APPEARANCE

- Fluid collections are not generally demonstrated in the chest or abdominal cavity.
- A small amount of pelvic fluid may be identified in ovulatory patients.

TECHNIQUE

PREPARATION

- No preparation is necessary to evaluate the peritoneal or pleural cavity.

EXAMINATION TECHNIQUE

- Use the highest-frequency abdominal transducer possible to obtain optimal resolution for penetration depth.
- Ensure proper focal zone and depth placement.
- Use a systemic approach to evaluate and document the entire abdominal and pelvic cavities.
- Use an intercostal approach for noncardiac imaging of the chest.
- Decrease in dynamic range or compression from the abdominal technique.
- Increase in transducer pressure may be necessary in abdominal examinations.
- Patients are typically examined in a supine position when evaluating the peritoneal cavity.
- Patients are typically examined in a sitting position when evaluating the thoracic cavity.
- Oblique, decubitus, or erect positions may also be used.

INDICATIONS FOR PERITONEAL CAVITY EXAMINATION

- Increase in abdominal girth.
- Chronic liver disease.
- Congestive heart failure.
- Ultrasound-guided paracentesis or biopsy.
- Evaluate pathology demonstrated on a previous medical imaging study (e.g., CT).

INDICATIONS FOR PLEURAL CAVITY EXAMINATION

- Shortness of breath.
- Ultrasound-guided thoracentesis.
- Evaluate fluid collection demonstrated on previous medical imaging study (e.g., chest x-ray examination).

LABORATORY VALUES

- Laboratory values will vary with individual cases.
- Decreased hematocrit is suspicious for internal bleeding.
- Leukocytosis is suspicious for infection.

Peritoneal Fluid Collections

FLUID COLLECTION	ETIOLOGY	CLINICAL FINDINGS	SONOGRAPHIC FINDINGS	DIFFERENTIAL CONSIDERATIONS
Abscess	• Infection	• Abdominal pain • Fever • Leukocytosis • Fatigue • Nausea/vomiting	• Complex mass is most common • Thick, irregular wall margins • Displacement of adjacent structures • Nonvascular mass • May demonstrate septations, shadowing (air), or mild acoustic enhancement	• Hematoma • Complex ascites • Lymphadenopathy
Benign ascites	• Congestive heart failure • Cirrhosis • Hypoalbuminemia • Infection • Inflammation • Portal venous obstruction • Postoperative complication	• Abdominal distention • Abdominal pain	• Anechoic fluid accumulation in the peritoneal cavity • Mobility of fluid with patient position change • Bowel may appear "floating" within the fluid • Most commonly located in the subhepatic space followed by the paracolic gutters • Thick-appearing gallbladder wall with adjacent ascites	• Fluid-filled loops of bowel • Abscess • Hemoperitoneum • Lymphocele • Cystic neoplasm
Hemoperitoneum	• Surgery • Ruptured blood vessel • Trauma • Fistulas • Necrotic neoplasm	• Abdominal pain • Decrease in hematocrit • Shock	• Hypoechoic fluid collection(s) • Swirling low-level echoes • Hyperechoic mass(es) within the fluid representing clot formation	• Ascites • Pseudomyxoma peritonei
Lymphocele	• Complication of a renal transplant or vascular, urological, or gynecological surgery	• Asymptomatic • Abdominal pain or discomfort	• Anechoic cystic mass frequently containing septations • Round or oval in shape • Well-defined wall margins • Posterior acoustic enhancement • Usually found medial to a renal transplant	• Seroma • Resolving hematoma • Urinoma • Loculated ascites
Malignant ascites	• Metastasis	• Abdominal distention • Abdominal pain or discomfort	• Anechoic fluid accumulation in the peritoneal cavity • Gallbladder wall measuring 3 mm or less with adjacent ascites • Internal low-level echoes may be demonstrated	• Benign ascites • Pseudomyxoma peritonei
Pseudomyxoma peritonei	• Metastasis • Ruptured mucinous cystadenoma	• Abdominal pain • Abdominal distention • Constipation	• Multiseptated cystic areas in the peritoneal cavity • Internal echoes or echogenic linear strands • Matted bowel loops compressed posteriorly	• Loculated ascites • Hemoperitoneum
Seroma	• Trauma • Surgery	• Asymptomatic • Abdominal pain or discomfort	• Anechoic mass • Smooth wall margins • May conform to the surrounding structures	• Biloma • Urinoma • Lymphocele • Resolving hematoma

Peritoneal Masses

CYSTS	ETIOLOGY	CLINICAL FINDINGS	SONOGRAPHIC FINDINGS	DIFFERENTIAL CONSIDERATIONS
Lymphoma	• Hodgkin or non-Hodgkin	• Superficial abdominal mass	• Mesentery • Superficial mass • Thick, hypoechoic mass that follows the shape of the anterior and lateral abdominal wall	• Lymphadenopathy • Bowel
Mesenteric cyst	• Wolffian or lymphatic duct in origin	• Colicky abdominal pain • Intestinal obstruction	• Cystic structure located in the mesentery • Smooth wall margins • Is not associated with any adjacent structure • Most commonly located in the small-bowel mesentery	• Renal cyst • Ascites • Hematoma • Abscess • Neoplasm
Mesenteric lymphomatous	• Lymphoma	• Found more frequently with non-Hodgkin lymphoma	• Anechoic mass containing a central echogenic target ("sandwich sign")	• Lymphadenopathy • Bowel
Omental cyst	• Congenital failure of the mesentery to fuse • Trauma	• Asymptomatic	• Small cystic structure located adjacent to the stomach or lesser sac • Mass will contour to the bowel margins • Smooth wall margins • Honeycomb appearance	• Renal cyst • Pancreatic pseudocyst • Hematoma • Abscess • Ascites • Neoplasm

Noncardiac Chest Fluid Collections

FLUID COLLECTION	ETIOLOGY	CLINICAL FINDINGS	SONOGRAPHIC FINDINGS	DIFFERENTIAL CONSIDERATIONS
Hemothorax	• Trauma • Necrotic neoplasms • Inflammation	• Shortness of breath • Chest pain • Decrease in hematocrit • Shock	• Hypoechoic fluid collection in the dependent portion of the thorax • Hyperechoic areas within the fluid collection	• Pleural effusion • Subphrenic ascites
Pleural effusion	• Infection • Cardiovascular disease • Trauma	• Shortness of breath • Chest pain • Nonproductive cough	• Anechoic fluid collection in the dependent portion of the thorax	• Subphrenic ascites • Hemothorax • Artifact

INVASIVE PROCEDURES

• A diagnostic or therapeutic technique that requires entry of a body cavity or interruption of normal body function.

TYPES OF INVASIVE PROCEDURES

Biopsy
• A larger core needle is used to remove a small piece of living tissue.
• The excised tissue is examined by a pathologist.

Fine-Needle Aspiration
• A very slender needle along with gentle suction is used to obtain tissue samples.
• Aspirated material is examined by a pathologist.

Paracentesis

- A cannula or catheter is passed into the abdominal cavity to allow outflow of fluid into a collecting device.
- May be for diagnostic or therapeutic purposes.

Thoracentesis

- Perforating the chest wall and pleural cavity with a needle to aspirate fluid.
- May be for diagnostic or therapeutic purposes.

TECHNIQUE

PREPARATION

- Preparation will vary with the type of invasive procedure.

EXAMINATION TECHNIQUE

- A sterile procedure technique should be used.
- A sterile transducer sheath may be necessary to cover the transducer and cord.
- Sterile gel should be used.
- Use the highest-frequency abdominal transducer possible to obtain optimal resolution for penetration depth.
- Ensure proper focal zone and depth placement.
- Localize the area of interest remaining perpendicular to the table or floor.
- Limit the amount of transducer pressure when measuring distance to the fluid collection.
- Visualization of the needle is obtained at a plane parallel with the needle path.
- In paracentesis procedures, the patient is usually in a supine position with the table flat; a pillow may or may not be used.
- In thoracentesis procedures, the patient is in a sitting position leaning slightly forward, with arms resting on a table for stability.

PERITONEUM, NONCARDIAC CHEST, AND INVASIVE PROCEDURES REVIEW

1. A patient arrives by ambulance to the emergency department following a motor vehicle accident. On ultrasound, a large hypoechoic fluid collection is identified in the left subphrenic space. On the basis of the clinical history, this fluid collection most likely represents:
   a. ascites
   b. a lymphocele
   c. pleural effusion
   d. hemoperitoneum
   e. fluid within the stomach

2. Predisposing conditions associated with the development of a pleural effusion may include all of the following EXCEPT:
   a. bronchitis
   b. pneumonia
   c. emphysema
   d. congestive heart failure
   e. portal vein thrombosis

3. Free fluid most commonly accumulates in which of the following peritoneal spaces?
   a. lesser sac
   b. subphrenic space
   c. paracolic gutter
   d. space of Retzius
   e. subhepatic space

4. Which of the following structures lines the abdominal cavity?
   a. mesentery
   b. peritoneum
   c. lesser omentum
   d. retroperitoneum
   e. greater omentum

5. A patient is most commonly placed in which of the following positions during a thoracentesis procedure?
   a. supine
   b. prone
   c. sitting
   d. decubitus
   e. reverse Trendelenburg

6. The lesser sac communicates with the subhepatic space through the foramen of:
   a. Monro
   b. Ovale
   c. Vater
   d. Winslow
   e. Magendie

7. Organs contained within the peritoneum include all of the following EXCEPT:
   a. liver
   b. spleen
   c. pancreas
   d. stomach
   e. gallbladder

8. Chylous ascites is most commonly associated with which of the following abnormalities?
   a. cirrhosis
   b. acute cholecystitis
   c. ectopic pregnancy
   d. abdominal neoplasm
   e. congestive heart failure

9. Which of the following peritoneal spaces is located lateral to the intestines?
   a. lesser sac
   b. retrovesical pouch
   c. subhepatic space
   d. paracolic gutter
   e. subphrenic space

10. Which of the following fluid collections is typically located medial to a renal transplant?
    a. seroma
    b. biloma
    c. urinoma
    d. lymphocele
    e. hematoma

11. Withdrawing fluid from the abdominal cavity is accomplished by which of the following invasive procedures?
    a. fine-needle aspiration
    b. peritoneal biopsy
    c. thoracentesis
    d. laparoscopy
    e. paracentesis

12. Peritoneal ascites is a complication of all of the following conditions EXCEPT:
    a. malignancy
    b. postoperative complication
    c. polycystic disease
    d. chronic liver disease
    e. congestive heart failure

13. A decrease in hematocrit is most consistent with which of the following conditions?
    a. infection
    b. inflammation
    c. malignancy
    d. hemorrhage
    e. thrombosis

14. An apron of peritoneum covering the small intestines describes the:
    a. linea alba
    b. perineum
    c. mesentery
    d. retroperitoneum
    e. greater omentum

15. The peritoneum is described as extending from the:
    a. posterior abdominal wall to the retroperitoneum
    b. diaphragm to the umbilicus
    c. anterior abdominal wall to the diaphragm
    d. diaphragm to the deep pelvic recesses
    e. posterior abdominal wall to the paraspinal tissues

16. Which of the following peritoneal spaces is located anterior to the uterus and posterior to the urinary bladder?
    a. retrouterine
    b. prevesical
    c. vesicouterine
    d. retropubic
    e. retrovesical

17. A delicate serous membrane composed of a visceral and a parietal layer BEST describes the:
    a. pleura
    b. mesentery
    c. omentum
    d. peritoneum
    e. retroperitoneum

18. On ultrasound, visualization of a biopsy needle is obtained in a plane:
    a. perpendicular to the examination table
    b. parallel with the needle path
    c. oblique to the needle path
    d. perpendicular to the needle path
    e. parallel to the examination table

19. Which of the following structures is located within the right coronary ligament?
    a. pleura
    b. bare area
    c. peritoneum
    d. diaphragmatic crura
    e. inferior vena cava

20. A thin needle is used to obtain tissue samples in which of the following invasive procedures?
    a. core biopsy
    b. thoracentesis
    c. paracentesis
    d. amniocentesis
    e. fine-needle aspiration

Using Fig. 18-2, answer question 21.

21. Which of the following peritoneal spaces is most likely identified by the arrow?
    a. lesser sac
    b. pleural space
    c. subphrenic space
    d. Morison pouch
    e. pouch of Douglas

Using Fig. 18-3, answer question 22.

22. Which of the following structures is located within the peritoneal cavity?
    a. aorta
    b. liver
    c. pancreas
    d. right kidney
    e. inferior vena cava

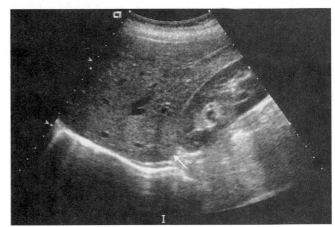

FIG. 18-2 Sagittal sonogram of the right upper quadrant.

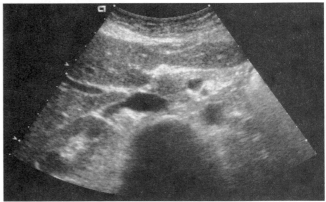

FIG. 18-3 Transverse sonogram of the upper abdomen.

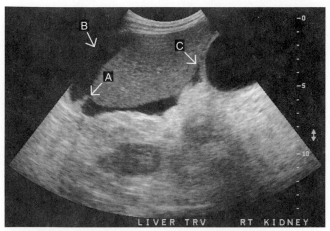

FIG. 18-4   Transverse sonogram of the right upper quadrant.

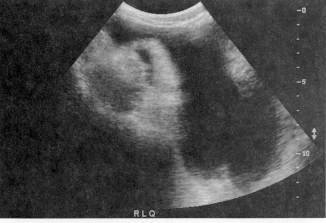

FIG. 18-5   Sonogram of the right lower quadrant.

Using Fig. 18-4, answer questions 23-25.

23. A middle-aged patient presents with a history of cirrhosis and abdominal bloating. Free fluid is identified in the right upper quadrant. Arrow **A** is most likely identifying which of the following structures?
    a. pleura
    b. diaphragm
    c. falciform ligament
    d. coronary ligament
    e. hepatic flexure

24. An anechoic fluid collection is identified by Arrow **B**. This is most consistent with which of the following conditions?
    a. hemothorax
    b. pleural effusion
    c. subphrenic ascites
    d. hemoperitoneum
    e. subhepatic ascites

25. Which of the following peritoneal spaces is identified by Arrow **C**?
    a. lesser sac
    b. subphrenic
    c. Morison pouch
    d. subhepatic space
    e. right paracolic gutter

Using Fig. 18-5, answer question 26.

26. A patient presents with a history of Hepatitis C. Ascites is identified in which of the following peritoneal spaces?
    a. lesser sac
    b. space of Retzius
    c. subhepatic space
    d. paracolic gutter
    e. retrovesical pouch

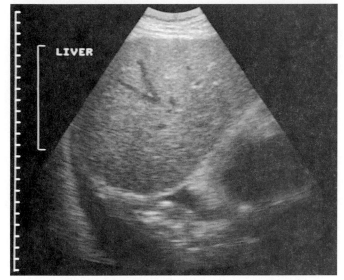

FIG. 18-6   Transverse sonogram of the right upper quadrant.

Using Fig. 18-6, answer question 27.

27. A patient presents with a history of elevated liver function tests and shortness of breath. An anechoic fluid collection is identified in which of the following regions?
    a. lesser sac
    b. pleural space
    c. subhepatic space
    d. subphrenic space
    e. Morison pouch

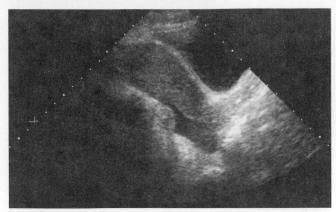

FIG. 18-7 Sagittal sonogram of the female pelvis.

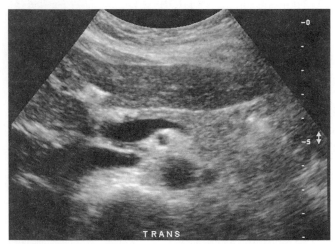

FIG. 18-8 Transverse sonogram of the upper abdomen.

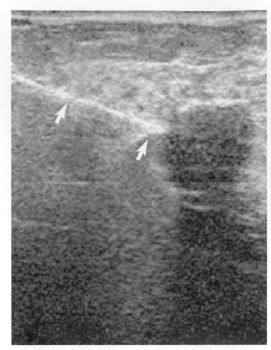

FIG. 18-9 Sonogram of the breast.

Using Fig. 18-9, answer question 30.

30. Which of the following invasive procedures is documented in this sonogram?
    a. angioplasty
    b. cyst aspiration
    c. core-needle biopsy
    d. stent placement
    e. fine-needle aspiration

31. Which of the following functions is considered the responsibility of the peritoneum?
    a. secretion of hormones
    b. production of lymphocytes
    c. production of antibodies
    d. secretion of serous fluid to reduce organ friction
    e. serves as a barrier between the subphrenic and subhepatic spaces

32. The lesser omentum is also known as the:
    a. omental bursa
    b. splenorenal omentum
    c. hepatorenal omentum
    d. gastrohepatic omentum
    e. hepatoduodenal ligament

33. The subphrenic space is divided into right and left sides by the:
    a. lesser sac
    b. coronary ligament
    c. falciform ligament
    d. ligamentum venosum
    e. crura of the diaphragm

Using Fig. 18-7, answer question 28.

28. A 28-year-old female presents to the ultrasound department complaining of left lower quadrant pain. An anechoic area is identified in which of the following regions?
    a. anterior cul de sac
    b. retropubic space
    c. pouch of Douglas
    d. space of Retzius
    e. paracolic gutter

Using Fig. 18-8, answer question 29.

29. Which of the following peritoneal spaces is located in this sonogram?
    a. lesser sac
    b. subhepatic space
    c. pararenal space
    d. subphrenic space
    e. Morison pouch

34. The lungs are separated into hemispheres by which of the following structures?
    a. heart
    b. sternum
    c. pleural cavity
    d. pleural fluid
    e. pleural membrane

35. Which of the following acoustic windows is generally used in noncardiac imaging of the chest?
    a. subcostal
    b. intercostal
    c. substernal
    d. intracostal
    e. suprasternal

36. Omental cysts generally develop adjacent to which of the following structures?
    a. liver and right kidney
    b. pancreas and stomach
    c. spleen and diaphragm
    d. urinary bladder and rectum
    e. umbilicus and urinary bladder

37. Which of the following patient positions is utilized for a paracentesis procedure?
    a. prone
    b. supine
    c. sitting
    d. decubitus
    e. 30° oblique

38. The prevesical space is located in which of the following regions?
    a. pelvis
    b. chest
    c. umbilical
    d. left upper quadrant
    e. right upper quadrant

39. Which of the following terms BEST describes an intraperitoneal collection of anechoic free fluid?
    a. ascites
    b. seroma
    c. abscess
    d. hematoma
    e. lymphocele

40. Which of the following structures has the potential to seal off infections within the peritoneal cavity?
    a. greater omentum
    b. mesentery
    c. peritoneum
    d. lesser omentum
    e. retroperitoneum

41. The inferior portion of the peritoneum is formed by which of the following structures?
    a. pouch of Douglas
    b. space of Retzius
    c. greater omentum
    d. vesicouterine pouch
    e. Morison pouch

42. Which of the following peritoneal spaces serves as a conduit between the upper abdominal cavity and pelvis?
    a. lesser sac
    b. Morison pouch
    c. paracolic gutters
    d. retrovesical pouch
    e. subhepatic space

43. Hemoperitoneum may be associated with all of the following EXCEPT:
    a. trauma
    b. cirrhosis
    c. necrotic neoplasm
    d. ectopic pregnancy
    e. postsurgical complication

44. Failure of the mesentery to fuse is a congenital anomaly associated with development of a(n):
    a. ileus
    b. omental cyst
    c. mesentery cyst
    d. umbilical hernia
    e. Meckel diverticulum

45. Which of the following terms is most likely used to describe the sonographic appearance of mesenteric lymphomatous?
    a. target sign
    b. water lily sign
    c. sandwich sign
    d. keyboard sign
    e. doughnut sign

46. Which of the following structures encloses the inferior esophagus?
    a. lesser sac
    b. mesentery
    c. retroperitoneum
    d. lesser omentum
    e. greater omentum

47. Hemothorax is best described as an accumulation of:
    a. blood in the pericardium
    b. fluid in the pleural cavity
    c. blood in the pleural membrane
    d. fluid and blood in the pleural cavity
    e. blood in the pericardium and pleural cavity

48. An accumulation of fluid and pus in the peritoneal cavity describes:
    a. chylous ascites
    b. peritonitis
    c. exudative ascites
    d. hemoperitoneum
    e. transudative ascites

49. Which of the following invasive procedures removes a small piece of tissue for microscopic analysis?
    a. biopsy
    b. lumpectomy
    c. cyst aspiration
    d. laparoscopy
    e. fine-needle aspiration

50. When localizing a fluid collection for a paracentesis procedure, the sonographer must:
    a. increase transducer pressure
    b. remain parallel to the floor
    c. increase the transducer frequency
    d. remain perpendicular to the floor
    e. decrease the transducer frequency

1. Which of the following structures is used as a sonographic landmark in locating the gallbladder fossa?
   a. main portal vein
   b. ligamentum of Teres
   c. main lobar fissure
   d. intersegmental fissure
   e. ligamentum of venosum

2. Which of the following conditions is the most common cause of acute pancreatitis?
   a. alcohol abuse
   b. biliary disease
   c. hyperlipidemia
   d. parathyroid disease
   e. acute renal failure

3. Gerota fascia provides a protective covering around which of the following organs?
   a. liver
   b. spleen
   c. kidney
   d. prostate
   e. pancreas

4. Increased pressure within the portosplenic venous system will most likely lead to which of the following conditions?
   a. hepatitis
   b. fatty infiltration
   c. intestinal angina
   d. portal hypertension
   e. portal vein thrombosis

5. Normal diameter of the main portal vein should not exceed:
   a. 0.3 cm
   b. 0.5 cm
   c. 1.3 cm
   d. 1.5 cm
   e. 2.0 cm

6. The integrity of which of the following structures is evaluated with the Thompson test?
   a. calf muscles
   b. rotator cuff
   c. Achilles tendon
   d. carpal tunnel nerve
   e. anterior abdominal wall

7. A small hyperechoic pancreas is identified on ultrasound. This is most suspicious for which of the following abnormalities?
   a. islet cell tumor
   b. malignancy
   c. cystic fibrosis
   d. chronic pancreatitis
   e. fatty infiltration

8. All of the following structures are part of the endocrine system EXCEPT:
   a. testes
   b. pancreas
   c. thyroid gland
   d. gallbladder
   e. pituitary gland

9. Which of the following is a sonographic finding of an echinococcal cyst?
   a. target lesions
   b. cystic masses
   c. complex masses
   d. hyperechoic lesions
   e. septated cystic mass

10. Predisposing risk factors associated with the development of cholangiocarcinoma may include all of the following EXCEPT:
    a. male gender
    b. cholangitis
    c. ulcerative colitis
    d. choledochal cyst
    e. cholecystitis

11. A synovial cyst located in the medial popliteal fossa describes a:
    a. Hunter cyst
    b. Baker cyst
    c. Cooper cyst
    d. Caroli cyst
    e. Thompson cyst

12. Normal caliber of the superior mesenteric vein should not exceed:
    a. 0.5 cm
    b. 1.0 cm
    c. 1.5 cm
    d. 2.0 cm
    e. 2.5 cm

13. A patient presents with a history of abdominal pain and lower-extremity edema. An ultrasound is requested to rule out Budd-Chiari syndrome. The sonographer should thoroughly evaluate which of the following organs?
    a. liver
    b. spleen
    c. kidneys
    d. pancreas
    e. adrenal glands

14. Which of the following structures divide the left lobe into two segments?
    a. left portal vein and ligamentum of Teres
    b. middle hepatic vein and main lobar fissure
    c. left hepatic vein and ligamentum of venosum
    d. left hepatic vein and ligamentum of Teres
    e. main portal vein and ligamentum of venosum

15. Cholecystokinin is stimulated once food reaches the:
    a. mouth
    b. cecum
    c. stomach
    d. esophagus
    e. duodenum

16. The gallbladder is located on the posterior surface of the liver and:
    a. lateral to the right kidney
    b. medial to the inferior vena cava
    c. anterior to the main lobar fissure
    d. anterior to the right kidney
    e. superior to the main lobar fissure

17. All of the following are functions of the pancreas EXCEPT:
    a. breaks down fats
    b. breaks down proteins
    c. destroys red blood cells
    d. regulates sugar metabolism
    e. stimulates secretion of bicarbonate

18. A patient presents with a history of severe back pain, weight loss, and painless jaundice. An abnormality in which of the following organs is most likely to correlate with these symptoms?
    a. liver
    b. spleen
    c. kidney
    d. pancreas
    e. adrenal gland

19. The popliteal artery is considered dilated once the diameter exceeds:
    a. 0.5 cm
    b. 1.0 cm
    c. 1.5 cm
    d. 2.0 cm
    e. 3.0 cm

20. Which of the following structures surrounds the liver?
    a. mesentery
    b. Gerota fascia
    c. greater omentum
    d. surgical capsule
    e. Glisson capsule

21. Which of the following conditions is associated with Mirizzi syndrome?
    a. thyroiditis
    b. biliary atresia
    c. pancreatic neoplasm
    d. gallbladder neoplasm
    e. impacted stone in the cystic duct

22. A spaghetti-like echogenic tubular structure within a bile duct is a sonographic finding associated with:
    a. hepatitis
    b. ascariasis
    c. clonorchiasis
    d. hydatid disease
    e. schistosomiasis

23. Gallbladder wall thickening is NOT a sonographic finding in:
    a. cirrhosis
    b. benign ascites
    c. nonfasting patients
    d. hyperalbuminemia
    e. congestive heart failure

24. Congenital anomalies of the gallbladder include all of the following EXCEPT:
    a. agenesis
    b. duplication
    c. ectopic location
    d. hourglass shape
    e. strawberry appearance

25. A fluid collection caused by extravasated bile is termed a:
    a. urinoma
    b. biloma
    c. seroma
    d. hematoma
    e. lymphocele

26. Renal artery stenosis is suggested once the renal artery to aortic ratio exceeds:
    a. 2.0
    b. 2.5
    c. 3.5
    d. 4.0
    e. 5.0

27. All of the following structures are located in the retroperitoneum EXCEPT the:
    a. spleen
    b. kidneys
    c. pancreas
    d. adrenal glands
    e. inferior vena cava

28. Which of the following structures lies within the anterior pararenal space?
    a. aorta
    b. spleen
    c. kidneys
    d. pancreas
    e. adrenal glands

29. The crura of the diaphragm are located:
    a. anterior to the inferior vena cava and abdominal aorta
    b. posterior to the inferior vena cava and abdominal aorta
    c. anterior to the inferior vena cava and posterior to the abdominal aorta
    d. posterior to the inferior vena cava and anterior to the abdominal aorta
    e. medial to the inferior vena cava and lateral to the abdominal aorta

30. Splenomegaly is a consistent finding in which of the following liver pathologies?
    a. polycystic disease
    b. hepatic vein thrombosis
    c. portal hypertension
    d. cavernous hemangioma
    e. hepatocellular carcinoma

31. Carcinoma in which of the following structures can directly extend into the gallbladder?
    a. spleen
    b. lung
    c. kidney
    d. stomach
    e. esophagus

32. Enlargement of the gallbladder caused by obstruction of the common bile duct by a distal external neoplasm is termed:
    a. Bouveret sign
    b. Murphy sign
    c. Mirizzi syndrome
    d. Courvoisier sign
    e. Budd-Chiari syndrome

33. Which of the following structures define the superior and inferior borders of the retroperitoneum?
    a. diaphragm and pelvic rim
    b. pancreas and urinary bladder
    c. crura of the diaphragm and symphysis pubis
    d. posterior peritoneum and the posterior abdominal wall muscles
    e. transversalis fascia and peritoneal portions of the mesentery

34. Elevation in prostatic specific antigen (PSA) is suspicious for:
    a. prostatitis
    b. infertility
    c. hydronephrosis
    d. prostatic carcinoma
    e. benign prostatic hypertrophy

35. Thrombosis involving the hepatic veins describes which of the following conditions?
    a. portal hypertension
    b. biliary obstruction
    c. Caroli disease
    d. Budd-Chiari syndrome
    e. Couinaud syndrome

36. A patient presents with a history of right upper quadrant pain, nausea, and vomiting. A sonogram of the right upper quadrant demonstrates a calculus lodged in the cystic duct. This finding is a predisposing factor for developing:
    a. cholangitis
    b. portal hypertension
    c. acute cholecystitis
    d. adenomyomatosis
    e. portal vein thrombosis

37. Which of the following structures may be mistaken for an extrarenal pelvis?
    a. renal vein
    b. adrenal cyst
    c. dromedary hump
    d. junctional parenchymal defect
    e. hypertrophied column of Bertin

38. A patient presents with a history of intermittent fever, nausea, and elevated alkaline phosphatase. He admits to recently traveling to the Middle East. A complex, solitary mass is identified in the right lobe of the liver. This mass is most suspicious for a(n):
    a. hepatoma
    b. cystadenoma
    c. amebic abscess
    d. cavernous hemangioma
    e. echinococcal cyst

39. Which of the following terms is more commonly used to describe an enlarged or dilated vein?
    a. varix
    b. shunt
    c. venule
    d. aneurysm
    e. perforator

40. The formation of a hepatic abscess is most commonly caused by which of the following conditions?
    a. hepatitis
    b. cholelithiasis
    c. acute pancreatitis
    d. acute cholecystitis
    e. ascending cholangitis

41. Which of the following structures is located in the anterolateral portion of the pancreatic head?
    a. splenic vein
    b. common bile duct
    c. gastroduodenal artery
    d. superior mesenteric artery
    e. portosplenic confluence

42. A patient presents with a palpable neck mass. A sonogram demonstrates an echogenic mass in the superior lobe of the right thyroid gland. A prominent hypoechoic ring surrounds this nodule. This mass is most suspicious for which of the following neoplasms?
    a. goiter
    b. lipoma
    c. adenoma
    d. carcinoma
    e. metastatic lesion

43. Which of the following organs is responsible for manufacturing heparin?
    a. liver
    b. spleen
    c. kidney
    d. thyroid
    e. pancreas

44. The length of a normal adult spleen should not exceed:
    a. 8 cm
    b. 10 cm
    c. 13 cm
    d. 17 cm
    e. 20 cm

45. Which type of aneurysms is most commonly associated with a bacterial infection?
    a. true aneurysm
    b. mycotic aneurysm
    c. ectatic aneurysm
    d. pseudoaneurysm
    e. dissecting aneurysm

46. Which of the following enzymes is produced by the stomach?
    a. lipase
    b. gastrin
    c. pepsin
    d. amylase
    e. cholecystokinin

47. Which of the following conditions is associated with rebound pain at McBurney point?
    a. pancreatitis
    b. cholecystitis
    c. appendicitis
    d. Crohn disease
    e. hydronephrosis

48. A round anechoic mass is identified next to the renal pelvis. This is most suspicious for which of the following?
    a. hydroureter
    b. adrenal cyst
    c. peripelvic cyst
    d. extrarenal pelvis
    e. parapelvic cyst

49. Which of the following is the most common clinical symptom associated with portal vein thrombosis?
    a. jaundice
    b. weight loss
    c. tachycardia
    d. lower-extremity edema
    e. severe abdominal pain

50. The diameter of a transjugular intrahepatic portosystemic shunt (TIPS) should measure a minimum of:
    a. 2-4 mm
    b. 6-8 mm
    c. 8-12 mm
    d. 10-20 mm
    e. 20-25 mm

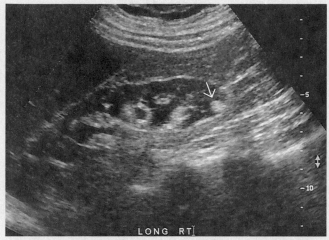

FIG. 1 Longitudinal sonogram of the right kidney.

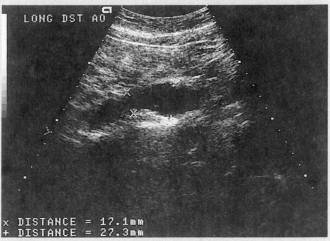

FIG. 2 Sagittal sonogram of the distal abdominal aorta.

Using Fig. 1, answer questions 51 and 52.

51. A retroperitoneal ultrasound is ordered to follow up on previously documented hydronephrosis of the right kidney. The patient is presently asymptomatic. An image of the right kidney demonstrates a small hyperechoic focus in the inferior pole of the kidney. This focus is most suspicious for a renal:
    a. calculus
    b. adenoma
    c. carcinoma
    d. hemangioma
    e. angiomyolipoma

52. In regards to the patient's previous history of hydronephrosis, the sonographer's technical impression on this current image should include:
    a. nephrolithiasis
    b. within normal limits
    c. severe hydronephrosis
    d. multiple peripelvic cysts
    e. mild hydronephrosis

Using Fig. 2, answer question 53.

53. A patient presents with a history of a pulsatile abdominal mass found on a physical examination. The sonogram of the distal abdominal aorta is most consistent with a(n):
    a. pseudoaneurysm
    b. ectatic aneurysm
    c. dissecting aneurysm
    d. intraluminal thrombus
    e. abdominal aortic aneurysm

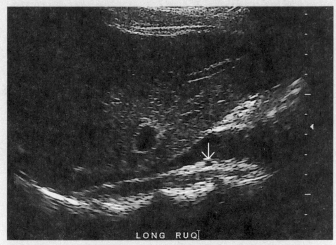

FIG. 3 Longitudinal sonogram of the right upper quadrant.

Using Fig. 3, answer question 54.

54. Which of the following vascular structures does the arrow identify?
    a. lumbar artery
    b. right renal vein
    c. main portal vein
    d. right renal artery
    e. proper hepatic artery

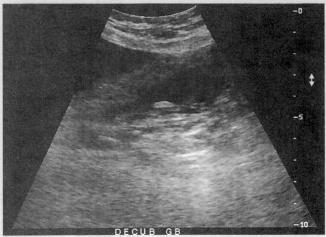

FIG. 4 Sagittal sonogram of the gallbladder.

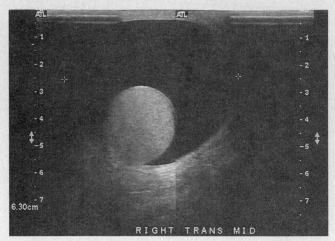

FIG. 5 Transverse sonogram of the scrotum.

Using Fig. 4, answer question 55.

55. A patient presents to the emergency department with severe right upper quadrant pain. Laboratory tests demonstrate leukocytosis and elevation in total bilirubin levels. On the basis of this clinical history, the pathology identified is most suspicious for:
   a. cholangitis
   b. acute pancreatitis
   c. adenomyomatosis
   d. acute cholecystitis
   e. gallbladder carcinoma

Using Fig. 5, answer question 56.

56. A 70-year-old male presents with a history of scrotal enlargement. He denies trauma to the scrotum or groin areas. On the basis of this clinical history, the sonographic finding is most suspicious for a(n):
   a. hydrocele
   b. varicocele
   c. spermatocele
   d. inguinal hernia
   e. epididymal cyst

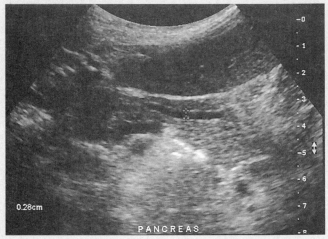

FIG. 6 Transverse sonogram of the pancreas.

Using Fig. 6, answer question 57.

57. A patient presents with a history of elevated liver function tests. An anechoic tubular structure is identified in the body of the pancreas. This structure most likely represents the:
   a. celiac axis
   b. splenic vein
   c. splenic artery
   d. pancreatic duct
   e. common bile duct

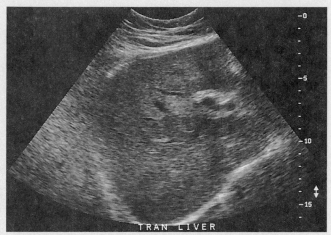

FIG. 7 Transverse sonogram of the liver.

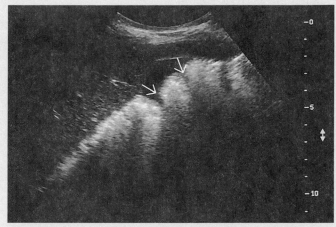

FIG. 8 Sonogram of the transverse colon.

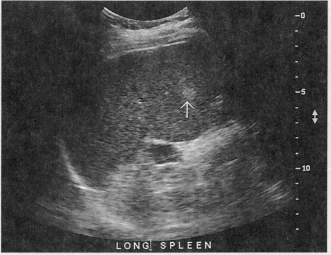

FIG. 9 Longitudinal sonogram of the spleen.

Using Fig. 7, answer question 58.

58. An obese patient presents with a history of elevated liver function tests discovered during a life insurance medical examination. The patient has no complaints. The sonographic findings in this image are most suspicious for:
  a. cirrhosis
  b. hepatoma
  c. fatty infiltration
  d. focal nodular hyperplasia
  e. degenerating hemangioma

Using Fig. 8, answer question 59.

59. Which of the following structures do the arrows identify?
  a. rugae
  b. haustra
  c. ulcers
  d. polyps
  e. diverticulum

Using Fig. 9, answer question 60.

60. A 30-year-old patient presents with a history of right upper quadrant pain. Laboratory tests are within normal limits. An image of the spleen demonstrates an incidental hyperechoic mass. This mass is most suspicious for a(n):
  a. abscess
  b. adenoma
  c. lipoma
  d. metastatic lesion
  e. cavernous hemangioma

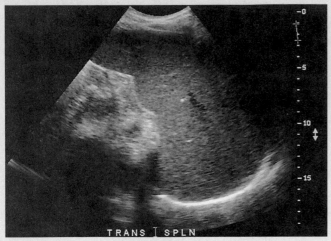

FIG. 10   Transverse sonogram of the left upper quadrant.

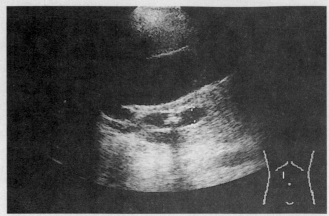

FIG. 11   Sagittal sonogram of the right upper quadrant.

Using Fig. 10, answer questions 61 and 62.

61. A patient presents with a history of alcohol abuse. Which of the following splenic pathologies is most likely identified in this sonogram?
   a. rupture
   b. metastasis
   c. infarction
   d. lymphoma
   e. splenomegaly

62. With this pathological finding, the sonographer should evaluate for:
   a. pancreatitis
   b. appendicitis
   c. cholelithiasis
   d. hydronephrosis
   e. venous collaterals

Using Fig. 11, answer question 63.

63. A patient presents to the emergency department with a history of severe epigastric pain. Laboratory results are pending. An abdominal ultrasound is ordered to rule out biliary disease. Which of the following pathologies is identified in this sonogram of the porta hepatis?
   a. cholangitis
   b. cholelithiasis
   c. choledochal cyst
   d. choledocholithiasis
   e. cholangiocarcinoma

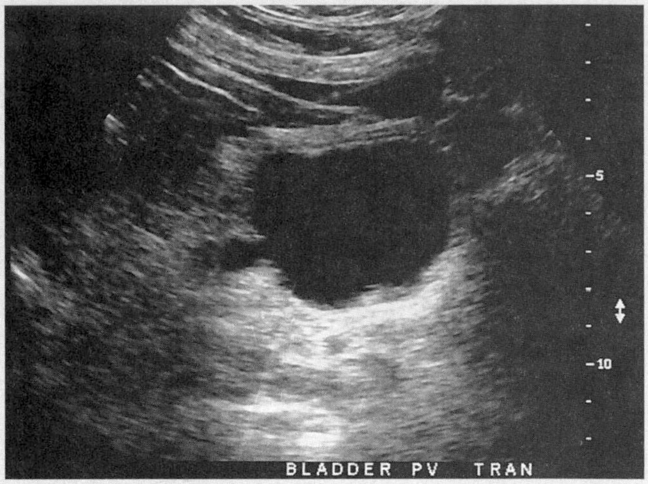

FIG. 12   Transverse sonogram of the urinary bladder.

Using Fig. 12, answer question 64.

64. An elderly patient presents with a history of elevated creatinine and microscopic hematuria. An abnormal finding is identified in this sonogram most consistent with a:
   a. hydroureter
   b. ureterocele
   c. bladder polyp
   d. bladder carcinoma
   e. bladder diverticulum

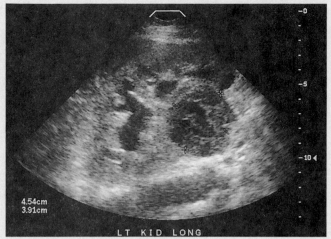

FIG. 13 Longitudinal sonogram of the left kidney.

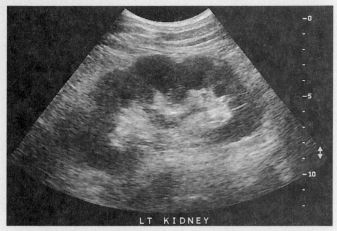

FIG. 14 Sagittal sonogram of the left kidney.

Using Fig. 13, answer questions 65 and 66.

65. A patient presents with a history of uncontrolled hypertension and painless hematuria. A hypervascular complex mass is identified near the renal hilum. On the basis of the clinical history, the mass is most suspicious for a(n):
  a. renal abscess
  b. angiomyolipoma
  c. extrarenal pelvis
  d. dromedary hump
  e. malignant neoplasm

66. Which of the following conditions is also identified in this sonogram?
  a. renal failure
  b. polycystic disease
  c. multicystic disease
  d. mild hydronephrosis
  e. renal vein thrombosis

Using Fig. 14, answer question 67.

67. Which of the following congenital anomalies is identified in this image of the left kidney?
  a. duplication
  b. renal ptosis
  c. fetal lobulation
  d. dromedary hump
  e. junctional parenchymal defect

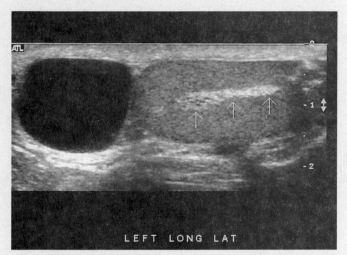

FIG. 15 Sonogram of the left scrotal sac.

Using Fig. 15, answer questions 68 and 69.

68. A 40-year-old patient presents with a palpable left scrotal mass and a previous history of epididymitis. The hyperechoic intratesticular structure is most suspicious for:
  a. orchitis
  b. malignancy
  c. polyorchism
  d. microcalcifications
  e. tubular ectasia of the rete testis

69. A large anechoic structure is demonstrated in the superior portion of the left scrotum. This structure most likely represents a:
  a. hernia
  b. varicocele
  c. hydrocele
  d. testicular cyst
  e. epididymal cyst

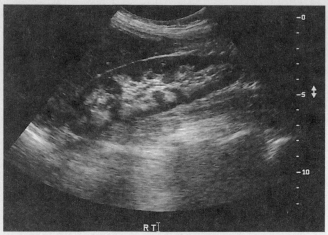

FIG. 16 Sagittal sonogram of the right kidney.

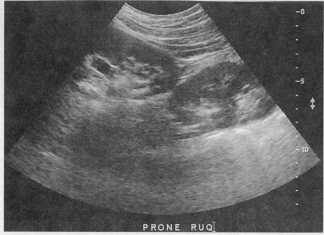

FIG. 17 Sonogram of the right upper quadrant.

Using Fig. 16, answer questions 70 and 71.

70. An elderly patient presents with a history of urinary frequency and elevated creatinine. Which of the following congenital anomalies is most likely identified in this sonogram of the right kidney?
    a. dromedary hump
    b. horseshoe kidney
    c. fetal lobulation
    d. renal duplication
    e. junctional parenchymal defect

71. On the basis of the cortical thickness, which of the following abnormalities is most likely identified in this single image of the right kidney?
    a. pyelonephritis
    b. acute tubular necrosis
    c. chronic renal disease
    d. glomerulonephritis
    e. medullary sponge disease

Using Fig. 17, answer question 72.

72. A 50-year-old patient presents with a history of a palpable right abdominal mass. A sagittal image of the right upper quadrant identifies two contiguous kidneys. The left renal fossa demonstrated normal bowel patterns. Which of the following congenital anomalies is most likely demonstrated in this sonogram?
    a. cake kidney
    b. renal ptosis
    c. pelvic kidney
    d. sigmoid kidney
    e. renal duplication

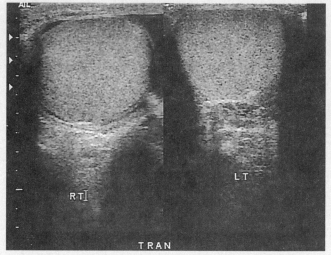

FIG. 18 Transverse sonogram of the scrotum.

Using Fig. 18, answer question 73.

73. A patient presents with acute left scrotal pain. He denies a fever or trauma. Which of the following abnormalities is most likely identified in this transverse sonogram of the scrotum?
    a. right varicocele
    b. torsion of the right testis
    c. hydrocele in the left scrotal sac
    d. inflammation of the left epididymis
    e. tubular ectasia of the left rete testis

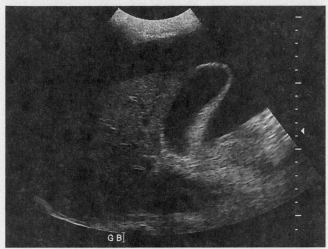

FIG. 19 Sonogram of the right upper quadrant.

Using Fig. 19, answer questions 74 and 75.

74. A patient presents with a history of abdominal distention and elevated liver function tests. Sonographic evaluation of the right upper quadrant demonstrated a negative Murphy sign. Which of the following peritoneal spaces demonstrate a fluid collection?
    a. subphrenic space and Morison pouch
    b. subhepatic space and lesser sac
    c. subphrenic and subhepatic spaces
    d. subphrenic space and lesser sac
    e. subhepatic space and Morison pouch

75. The sonographer's technical impression of the gallbladder should state:
    a. cholelithiasis
    b. acute cholecystitis
    c. hydropic gallbladder
    d. probable nonfunctioning gallbladder
    e. probable noninflammatory wall thickening

76. Which of the following structures separates the caudate lobe from the left lobe of the liver?
    a. left portal vein
    b. main portal vein
    c. falciform ligament
    d. main lobar fissure
    e. ligamentum venosum

77. A questionable mass is identified in the anterior portion of the right lobe of the liver. Which of the following structures border this region?
    a. left portal and main portal veins
    b. left hepatic and right hepatic veins
    c. right portal and right hepatic veins
    d. middle hepatic and right hepatic veins
    e. right hepatic and main portal veins

78. A mass displacing the renal calyces is documented on a recent intravenous pyelogram. A sonogram over this area demonstrates a smooth circular anechoic renal mass. This mass is most suspicious for a(n):
    a. hematoma
    b. simple cyst
    c. cystadenoma
    d. extrarenal pelvis
    e. malignant neoplasm

79. When hydronephrosis is encountered, the sonographer should evaluate the urinary bladder for evidence of a(n):
    a. cyst
    b. infection
    c. obstruction
    d. duplication
    e. inflammation

80. Sonographic characteristics of a neonatal kidney include all of the following EXCEPT:
    a. prominent renal sinus
    b. anechoic medullary pyramid
    c. sparse amount of perinephric fat
    d. moderately echogenic renal cortex
    e. difficulty in distinguishing the renal capsule

81. To aid in demonstrating posterior acoustic shadowing, the sonographer should:
    a. increase the overall gain
    b. decrease the image depth
    c. decrease the dynamic range
    d. increase the transducer frequency
    e. decrease the number of focal zones

82. All of the following patient positions can be used for visualization of the abdominal aorta EXCEPT:
    a. supine
    b. erect
    c. prone
    d. oblique
    e. decubitus

83. Extension of pancreatic inflammation into the surrounding tissues is termed a(n):
    a. abscess
    b. pseudocyst
    c. hemorrhage
    d. phlegmon
    e. gastrinoma

84. Elevation in conjugated bilirubin levels is associated with all of the following conditions **except**:
    a. hepatitis
    b. cirrhosis
    c. choledocholithiasis
    d. liver metastasis
    e. fatty infiltration

85. Which of the following organs is associated with an elevation of aldosterone?
    a. liver
    b. spleen
    c. thyroid
    d. pancreas
    e. adrenal gland

86. An extrarenal pelvis may be mistaken for all of the following structures EXCEPT:
    a. hydroureter
    b. renal cyst
    c. renal vein
    d. renal neoplasm
    e. hypertrophied column of Bertin

87. Which of the following vascular structures is commonly mistaken as the pancreatic duct?
    a. splenic artery
    b. celiac axis
    c. splenic vein
    d. gastric artery
    e. gastroduodenal artery

88. Cortical thickness of the normal adult kidney should measure a minimum of:
    a. 0.5 cm
    b. 0.7 cm
    c. 1.0 cm
    d. 1.5 cm
    e. 2.0 cm

89. Which of the following conditions is associated with a complete failure of the adrenocortical function?
    a. Cushing disease
    b. Addison disease
    c. Caroli disease
    d. Grave disease
    e. Crohn disease

90. The main renal arteries arise from the lateral aspect of the aorta approximately 1.5 cm inferior to the:
    a. celiac axis
    b. portosplenic confluence
    c. caudate lobe of the liver
    d. superior mesenteric artery
    e. uncinate process of the pancreas

91. Splenomegaly can be associated with all of the following conditions EXCEPT:
    a. cirrhosis
    b. hepatitis
    c. cholelithiasis
    d. mononucleosis
    e. congestive heart failure

92. Which of the following is an abnormal flow characteristic of the hepatic veins?
    a. pulsatile
    b. hepatopetal
    c. multiphasic
    d. spontaneous
    e. slow flow velocity

93. Which of the following organs is associated with the "olive sign"?
    a. liver
    b. pancreas
    c. stomach
    d. appendix
    e. gallbladder

94. Sonographic findings associated with acute appendicitis may include all of the following EXCEPT:
    a. hypervascular tubular structure
    b. appendix diameter exceeding 6 mm
    c. compressible tubular structure
    d. appendix wall thickness exceeding 2 mm
    e. rebound pain at McBurney point

95. Which of the following structures is most commonly mistaken as a renal neoplasm?
    a. psoas muscle
    b. extrarenal pelvis
    c. dilated renal vein
    d. junctional parenchymal defect
    e. hypertrophied column of Bertin

96. Which of the following laboratory tests will most likely elevate in cases of nonobstructive jaundice?
    a. serum albumin
    b. indirect bilirubin
    c. alkaline phosphatase
    d. conjugated bilirubin
    e. aspartate aminotransferase

97. Which region of the gallbladder is located most superiorly?
    a. body
    b. neck
    c. fundus
    d. phrygian cap
    e. Hartmann pouch

98. Which of the following conditions is associated with an increased risk in developing a thyroid malignancy?
   a. Graves disease
   b. De Quervain syndrome
   c. Hashimoto disease
   d. Addison disease
   e. Budd-Chiari syndrome

99. Which of the following invasive procedures removes a small piece of living tissue for microscopic analysis?
   a. core biopsy
   b. thoracentesis
   c. paracentesis
   d. fine-needle biopsy
   e. cyst aspiration

100. A pancreatic pseudocyst is most commonly located in which of the following regions?
   a. lesser sac
   b. subphrenic space
   c. pararenal space
   d. paracolic gutter
   e. Morison pouch

101. A patient presents to the emergency department with severe left upper quadrant pain. Laboratory values demonstrate a serum lipase of 670 IU/L. An abdominal ultrasound is ordered to rule out:
   a. cirrhosis
   b. splenomegaly
   c. hydronephrosis
   d. biliary disease
   e. hepatic malignancy

102. Which of the following anatomical variants demonstrates an outward bulge to the lateral renal cortex?
   a. fetal lobulation
   b. dromedary hump
   c. renal duplication
   d. junctional parenchymal defect
   e. hypertrophied column of Bertin

103. A congenital anomaly associated with the fusion of both kidneys within the same body quadrant describes:
   a. a cake kidney
   b. a sigmoid kidney
   c. renal ptosis
   d. a horseshoe kidney
   e. crossed fused ectopia

104. A patient with a recent history of angioplasty presents with a pulsatile inguinal mass. A fluid collection adjacent to the common femoral artery is identified. Color and spectral Doppler demonstrates turbulent blood flow within the fluid collection. On the basis of the clinical history, the sonographic findings are most consistent with a(n):
   a. lipoma
   b. hematoma
   c. pseudoaneurysm
   d. enlarged lymph node
   e. aneurysm of the common femoral artery

105. A 25-year-old patient presents with a nontender palpable breast mass. A hypoechoic, oval-shaped mass demonstrating posterior acoustic enhancement is identified in the breast parenchyma. On the basis of this clinical history, the sonographic finding is most suspicious for a:
   a. lipoma
   b. hamartoma
   c. complex cyst
   d. fibroadenoma
   e. galactocele

106. Which of the following tasks is a function of the spleen?
   a. regulate serum electrolytes
   b. secrete and release hormones
   c. remove foreign material from the blood
   d. convert excess amino acids into glucose
   e. maintain homeostasis of calcium concentration

107. An abnormality of the gallbladder wall exhibiting a "comet tail" artifact describes:
   a. pneumobilia
   b. adenomyomatosis
   c. chronic cholecystitis
   d. porcelain gallbladder
   e. gallbladder carcinoma

108. Clinical findings associated with hypertrophied pyloric stenosis may include all of the following EXCEPT:
   a. weight loss
   b. dehydration
   c. projectile vomiting
   d. lymphadenopathy
   e. palpable upper abdominal mass

109. Which of the following descriptions most accurately portrays the sonographic appearance and location of a Meckel diverticulum?
    a. hyperechoic mass located near the anal canal
    b. isoechoic mass located near the ileocecal valve
    c. anechoic or complex mass, slightly to the right of the umbilicus
    d. complex mass, slightly inferior to the ligamentum venosum
    e. anechoic or complex mass, slightly medial to the falciform ligament

110. Which of the following terms describes a noninflammatory degenerative change in a tendon?
    a. tenalgia
    b. tenesmus
    c. tendonitis
    d. tenodynia
    e. tendinosis

111. Within 5 years, the risk for rupture of an abdominal aortic aneurysm measuring 5 cm in diameter is:
    a. 5%
    b. 15%
    c. 25%
    d. 50%
    e. 75%

112. Prior to the bifurcation, the last major visceral branch of the abdominal aorta is the:
    a. lumbar artery
    b. gonadal artery
    c. hypogastric artery
    d. median sacral artery
    e. inferior mesenteric artery

113. Which of the following abnormalities commonly coexists in patients with a popliteal aneurysm?
    a. synovial cyst
    b. deep vein thrombosis
    c. carotid artery stenosis
    d. congestive heart failure
    e. abdominal aortic aneurysm

114. Which of the following peritoneal spaces is located superior to the liver?
    a. lesser sac
    b. prevesical space
    c. subphrenic space
    d. Morison pouch
    e. pouch of Douglas

115. A patient arrives for an abdominal ultrasound owing to a history of hepatitis B. Which of the following abnormalities is the clinician likely excluding?
    a. cirrhosis
    b. fatty infiltration
    c. biliary obstruction
    d. portal hypertension
    e. hepatocellular carcinoma

116. The majority of metastatic lesions in the liver originate from which of the following sites?
    a. lung
    b. breast
    c. colon
    d. ovarian
    e. pancreas

117. The common bile duct passes through which of the following structures prior to entering the duodenum?
    a. duct of Santorini
    b. ampulla of Oddi
    c. duct of Wirsung
    d. ampulla of Vater
    e. foramen of Winslow

118. Which of the following conditions is the most common cause of hypothyroidism?
    a. Graves disease
    b. De Quervain syndrome
    c. Hashimoto disease
    d. Cushing disease
    e. Bouveret syndrome

119. The pyramidal lobe of the thyroid gland arises from the:
    a. inferior aspect of a thyroid lobe
    b. superior aspect of the isthmus
    c. anterior aspect of the thyroid gland
    d. posterior aspect of the isthmus
    e. superior aspect of the right lobe

120. All of the following structures are located within the renal sinus EXCEPT:
    a. ureter
    b. lymphatics
    c. minor calyces
    d. fibrous tissues
    e. major calyces

121. Which of the following abnormalities involves the distal ureter and the urinary bladder?
    a. simple cyst
    b. ureterocele
    c. diverticulum
    d. urachal sinus
    e. bladder polyp

122. Postvoid residual in a normal adult urinary bladder should not exceed:
    a. 5 mL
    b. 20 mL
    c. 50 mL
    d. 100 mL
    e. 150 mL

123. All of the following sonographic findings are likely associated with portal hypertension EXCEPT:
    a. splenomegaly
    b. acute pancreatitis
    c. intrinsic liver disease
    d. dilated main portal vein
    e. portosystemic collaterals

124. Which of the following vascular structures courses posterior to the superior mesenteric artery?
    a. splenic vein
    b. splenic artery
    c. left renal vein
    d. gastroduodenal artery
    e. superior mesenteric vein

125. On ultrasound, visualization of a needle during an invasive procedure is attained in a plane:
    a. parallel to the needle path
    b. oblique to the needle path
    c. perpendicular to the needle path
    d. posterior to the needle path
    e. perpendicular to the examination

Using Fig. 20, answer questions 126 and 127.

126. A patient presents with a history of elevated liver function tests and malaise. On the basis of this clinical history, the sonographic findings are most suspicious for which of the following abnormalities?
    a. candidiasis
    b. liver metastasis
    c. fatty infiltration
    d. schistosomiasis
    e. focal nodular hyperplasia

127. A round anechoic mass is identified in the medial portion of the liver. Which of the following structures does this anechoic mass most likely represent?
    a. biloma
    b. gallbladder
    c. hepatic cyst
    d. hepatic abscess
    e. choledochal cyst

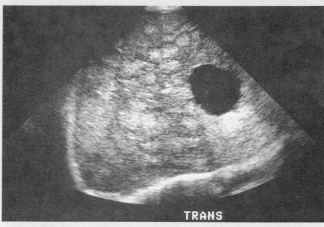

FIG. 20 Transverse sonogram of the liver.

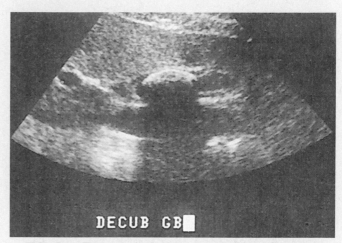

FIG. 21 Transverse sonogram of the gallbladder.

Using Fig. 21, answer question 128.

128. An asymptomatic patient presents with a history of elevated liver function tests. A large hyperechoic focus is identified in the gallbladder fossa. This sonographic finding is characteristic of the:
    a. target sign
    b. WES sign
    c. Murphy sign
    d. water lily sign
    e. McBurney sign

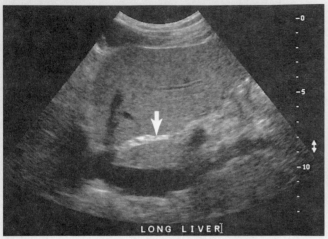

FIG. 22 Sonogram of the liver.

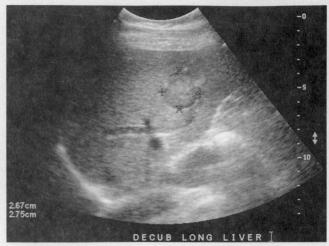

2.67cm
2.75cm

FIG. 23 Sagittal sonogram of the liver.

Using Fig. 22, answer question 129.

129. Which of the following intrahepatic structures does the arrow identify?
a. falciform ligament
b. main lobar fissure
c. ligamentum teres
d. calcified hepatic artery
e. ligamentum venosum

Using Fig. 23, answer question 130.

130. An annual screening examination of the upper abdomen is ordered on an asymptomatic patient with a history of hepatitis B. An intrahepatic lesion is identified and outlined by the calipers. On the basis of the clinical history, this neoplasm is most suspicious for a(n):
a. abscess
b. hepatoma
c. complicated cyst
d. metastatic lesion
e. cavernous hemangioma

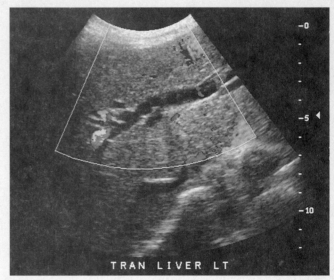

FIG. 24 Transverse sonogram of the liver (see color plate 6).

Using Fig. 24 (and color plate 6), answer question 131.

131. A 40-year-old patient presents with a history of cholecystectomy 10 years prior and a new onset of elevated liver function tests. She complains of abdominal cramping for several weeks. Which of the following conditions is most likely identified in this sonogram of the left biliary tree?
a. Berry syndrome
b. Caroli disease
c. Klatskin disease
d. Budd-Chiari syndrome
e. Courvoisier syndrome

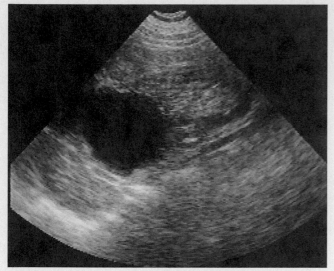

FIG. 25 Sagittal sonogram of the right upper quadrant.

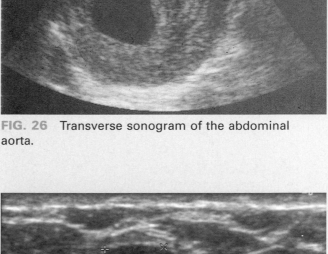

FIG. 26 Transverse sonogram of the abdominal aorta.

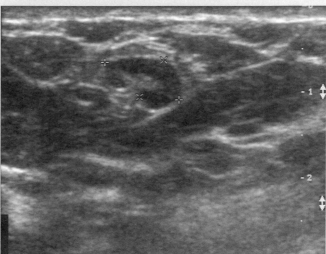

FIG. 27 Sonogram of the axilla.

Using Fig. 25, answer question 132.

132. An elderly patient presents with a history of hypertension and elevated creatinine. A nonvascular mass is identified in the superior pole of the right kidney. The sonographic characteristics of this mass are most consistent with a(n):
   a. abscess
   b. renal cyst
   c. hematoma
   d. adrenal cyst
   e. malignant neoplasm

Using Fig. 26, answer question 133.

133. A patient with a history of an abdominal aortic aneurysm arrives to the emergency department complaining of severe back pain. An ultrasound is requested to rule out a ruptured aneurysm. Which of the following abnormalities is most likely identified in this transverse sonogram of the distal aorta?
   a. aortic rupture
   b. aortic dissection
   c. mycotic aneurysm
   d. aneurysm with intraluminal thrombus
   e. aneurysm with surrounding lymphadenopathy

Using Fig. 27, answer question 134.

134. An ultrasound examination is ordered to evaluate a palpable mass in the upper outer quadrant of the right breast near the axilla. An oval-shaped solid structure is identified between the calibers on ultrasound. Which of the following structures is most consistent with these sonographic findings?
   a. lipoma
   b. lymph node
   c. hamartoma
   d. fibroadenoma
   e. cystosarcoma phyllodes

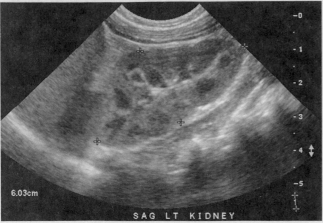

FIG. 28 Sagittal sonogram of a neonatal kidney.

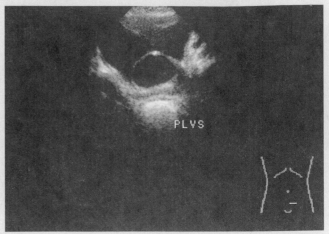

FIG. 29 Transverse sonogram of the urinary bladder.

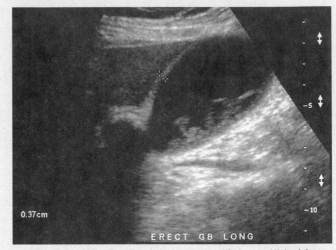

FIG. 30 Longitudinal sonogram of the gallbladder.

Using Fig. 28, answer question 135.

135. A newborn presents with a history of a single
urinary tract infection. A renal sonogram is
requested to evaluate for urinary tract
pathology. An image of the left kidney reveals
which of the following conditions?
   a. pyelonephritis
   b. mild hydronephrosis
   c. infantile polycystic disease
   d. multiple peripelvic cysts
   e. normal neonatal kidney

Using Fig. 29, answer question 136.

136. A toddler presents with a history of several
urinary tract infections. An ultrasound of the
kidneys is requested to rule out pathology. An
incidental finding is identified near the left
ureteric orifice of the urinary bladder. Which of
the following abnormalities does this finding
most likely represent?
   a. polyp
   b. ureterocele
   c. hydroureter
   d. diverticulum
   e. catheter balloon

Using Fig. 30, answer question 137.

137. An elderly patient presents with a history of
epigastric pain, weight loss, and elevated
alkaline phosphatase. A calculus is identified in
the neck of the gallbladder. Irregular echogenic
foci are identified in the posterior wall of the
gallbladder body. On the basis of this clinical
history, the echogenic foci are suspicious for
tumefactive sludge or:
   a. adenomyomatosis
   b. metastatic lesions
   c. porcelain gallbladder
   d. chronic cholecystitis
   e. gallbladder carcinoma

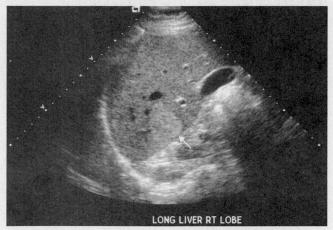

FIG. 31 Longitudinal sonogram of the liver.

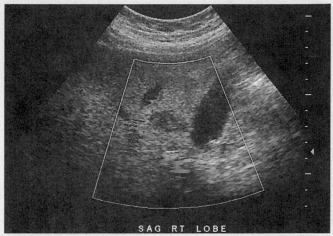

FIG. 32 Sagittal sonogram of the liver.

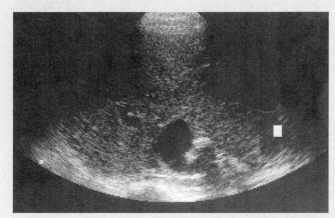

FIG. 33 Transverse sonogram of the gallbladder.

Using Fig. 31, answer question 138.

138. An ultrasound examination of the abdomen is ordered on a thin female patient to evaluate a liver mass demonstrated on a CT scan. The patient is presently asymptomatic with normal laboratory values. A focal hyperechoic mass is identified in the right lobe of the liver. Which of the following pathologies is the arrow most likely identifying?
  a. hepatoma
  b. adenoma
  c. metastatic lesion
  d. cavernous hemangioma
  e. focal area of fatty infiltration

Using Fig. 32, answer question 139.

139. A middle-aged male patient presents with a history of elevated levels with liver function tests. An abdominal ultrasound is requested to evaluate for possible cholelithiasis. A hypoechoic focus is identified in the liver, anterior to the portal vein and lateral to the gallbladder. On the basis of the clinical history, the sonographic findings are most suspicious for which of the following abnormalities?
  a. hepatic abscess
  b. metastatic lesion
  c. hepatic adenoma
  d. portal vein thrombosis
  e. fatty infiltration with a focal area of fat sparing

Using Fig. 33, answer questions 140 and 141.

140. Which of the following structures is (are) demonstrated in the region of the gallbladder neck?
  a. calculi
  b. phrygian cap
  c. surgical clip
  d. junctional fold
  e. Hartmann cap

141. This finding is most likely associated with which of the following?
  a. a decrease in serum creatinine levels
  b. previous history of adenomyomatosis
  c. previous history of an abdominal surgery
  d. increased risk for developing cholelithiasis
  e. increased risk for developing acute cholecystitis

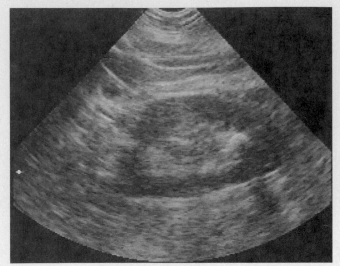

FIG. 34 Sagittal sonogram of the left kidney.

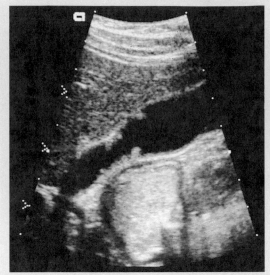

FIG. 35 Supine sonogram of the gallbladder.

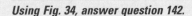

Using Fig. 34, answer question 142.

142. A patient presents with a history of hematuria and left flank pain. A sagittal image of the left kidney reveals which of the following abnormalities?
    a. hamartoma
    b. nephrolithiasis
    c. angiomyolipoma
    d. arterial calcification
    e. medullary sponge disease

Using Fig. 35, answer questions 143 and 144.

143. A patient presents with a history of vague right upper quadrant pain and elevated levels in liver function tests. The sonographic findings in this image are most consistent with which of the following abnormalities?
    a. polyps
    b. cholelithiasis
    c. metastatic lesions
    d. acute cholecystitis
    e. biliary obstruction

144. Which of the following sonographic techniques will be most helpful in narrowing the differential considerations in this case?
    a. deep inspiration
    b. decubitus position
    c. ingestion of a fatty meal
    d. increasing the transducer frequency
    e. increased transducer pressure over the gallbladder

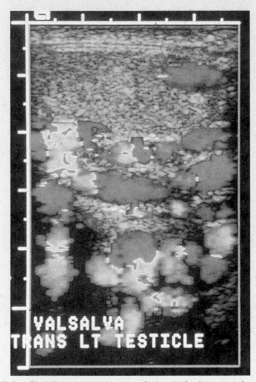

FIG. 36 Duplex sonogram of the inferior portion of the left scrotum (see color plate 7).

Using Fig. 36 (and color plate 7), answer questions 145 and 146.

145. A patient presents with a history of a left scrotal mass and scrotal aching. A duplex image of the inferior portion of the left scrotum is documented during a Valsalva maneuver. The sonographic findings are most suspicious for which of the following pathologies?
    a. orchitis
    b. varicocele
    c. epididymitis
    d. spermatocele
    e. cryptorchidism

286

146. This pathology is a possible etiology for which of the following conditions?

   a. prostatitis
   b. infertility
   c. elevated testosterone
   d. a urinary tract infection
   e. a sexually transmitted disease

Using Fig. 37, answer question 147.

147. An 8-week-old male infant presents with a history of projectile vomiting and a failure to thrive. His last feeding was 3 hours prior. A sonogram of the pyloric wall and canal are imaged and measured. These sonographic findings are most suspicious for which of the following conditions?

   a. ileus
   b. gastritis
   c. peptic ulcer
   d. pyloric stenosis
   e. intussusception

Using Fig. 38, answer question 148.

148. A patient presents to the emergency department with a previous history of gallstones He presently complains of severe upper back pain and a lack of appetite. Laboratory values demonstrate an elevation in direct bilirubin levels. On the basis of this clinical history, the sonographic findings are most suspicious for which of the following abnormalities?

   a. pseudocyst
   b. cystic fibrosis
   c. acute pancreatitis
   d. polycystic disease
   e. malignant neoplasm

Using Fig. 39, answer question 149.

149. A young adult presents with a history of a palpable scrotal mass. He was treated for epididymitis 2 months ago. He denies any recent scrotal pain or trauma. On the basis of this clinical history, the sonographic findings are most suspicious for which of the following pathologies?

   a. hematoma
   b. varicocele
   c. chronic orchitis
   d. malignant neoplasm
   e. tubular ectasia of the rete testis

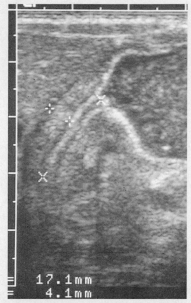

17.1mm
4.1mm

FIG. 37 Transverse sonogram.

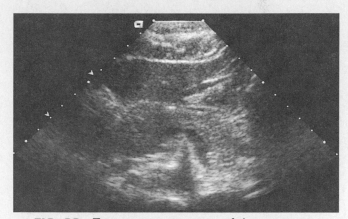

FIG. 38 Transverse sonogram of the pancreas.

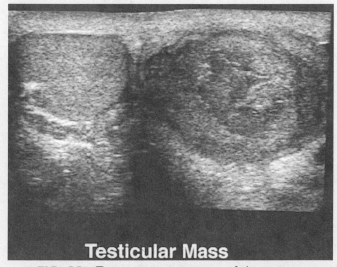

Testicular Mass

FIG. 39 Transverse sonogram of the testes.

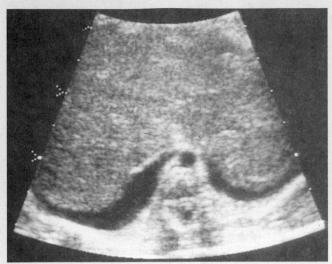

FIG. 40 Transverse sonogram of the upper abdomen.

Using Fig. 40, answer question 150.

150. A toddler presents with pneumonia and abdominal tenderness. A sonogram of the abdomen is requested to rule out pathology. Fluid collections, are identified in which of the following regions?
   a. bilateral pleural spaces
   b. bilateral subphrenic space
   c. bilateral paracolic gutters
   d. subhepatic space and lesser sac
   e. Morison pouch and the left subphrenic space

151. The pyloric canal is considered abnormal when the length exceeds:
   a. 4 mm
   b. 7 mm
   c. 15 mm
   d. 18 mm
   e. 25 mm

152. The Whipple procedure is a surgical resection of which of the following organs?
   a. liver
   b. kidney
   c. spleen
   d. pancreas
   e. gallbladder

153. Which of the following peritoneal spaces most commonly demonstrates ascites?
   a. lesser sac
   b. paracolic gutter
   c. retropubic space
   d. subphrenic space
   e. subhepatic space

154. Which of the following structures is most likely located adjacent to an omental cyst?
   a. stomach
   b. left kidney
   c. umbilicus
   d. gallbladder
   e. sigmoid colon

155. All of the following statements accurately describe the portal veins EXCEPT:
   a. Portal veins are interlobar in location.
   b. The portal veins contain echogenic fibrin.
   c. Nutrient-rich blood is transported through the portal veins.
   d. The majority of the liver's blood supply is through the portal veins.
   e. The main portal vein divides into the right and left portal veins near the hepatic hilum.

156. A patient presents with a mass in the lateral aspect of the neck. An anechoic structure is demonstrated just beneath the jawline. Which of the following cystic structures is most likely identified?
   a. lingual cyst
   b. parotid gland cyst
   c. thyroglossal cyst
   d. brachial cleft cyst
   e. pedunculated thyroid cyst

157. The inferior vena cava is considered enlarged once the diameter exceeds:
   a. 1.7 cm
   b. 2.5 cm
   c. 3.0 cm
   d. 3.7 cm
   e. 4.5 cm

158. A round, homogeneous, solid mass is identified medial to the splenic hilum. The echo texture is similar to the adjacent splenic parenchyma. On the basis of these sonographic findings, the mass is most consistent with which of the following?
   a. gastric neoplasm
   b. accessory spleen
   c. adrenal adenoma
   d. left lobe of the liver
   e. visceral lymph node

159. Which of the following structures is most commonly associated with internal hemorrhage?
   a. platelets
   b. leukocytes
   c. hematocrit
   d. hemoglobin
   e. erythrocytes

160. Which of the following patient positions is typically used during a thoracentesis?
    a. prone
    b. supine
    c. sitting
    d. decubitus
    e. Trendelenburg

161. A transplant kidney is more commonly placed in which of the following regions?
    a. left lower quadrant
    b. periumbilical area
    c. right lower quadrant
    d. left posterior flank
    e. right upper quadrant

162. Peritoneal ascites is associated with all of the following conditions EXCEPT:
    a. pneumonia
    b. recent surgery
    c. chronic liver disease
    d. congestive heart failure
    e. portal venous obstruction

163. Under normal conditions, which of the following arteries supply the majority of blood to the brain?
    a. vertebral arteries
    b. subclavian arteries
    c. external carotid arteries
    d. internal carotid arteries
    e. middle cerebral arteries

164. Malignant neoplasms involving the colon are more commonly located in which of the following regions?
    a. anus
    b. cecum
    c. rectum
    d. sigmoid colon
    e. descending colon

165. The head of the pancreas surrounds the duodenum in which of the following anomalies?
    a. phlegmon
    b. cake pancreas
    c. ectopic pancreas
    d. annular pancreas
    e. pancreas divisum

166. Nonshadowing, low-amplitude echoes layering in the dependent portion of the gallbladder describes:
    a. polyps
    b. gallstones
    c. biliary sludge
    d. adenomyomatosis
    e. tumefactive sludge

167. Which portion of the pancreas is located most superiorly in the abdomen?
    a. tail
    b. head
    c. neck
    d. body
    e. uncinate process

168. Which of the following conditions is an inherited disorder?
    a. biliary atresia
    b. intussusception
    c. hyperaldosteronism
    d. polycystic kidney disease
    e. multicystic renal dysplasia

169. Renal dialysis patients have a predisposing factor for developing a renal:
    a. abscess
    b. lipoma
    c. calculus
    d. hematoma
    e. carcinoma

170. The diameter of a normal common iliac artery should not exceed:
    a. 0.5 cm
    b. 1.0 cm
    c. 1.5 cm
    d. 2.0 cm
    e. 2.5 cm

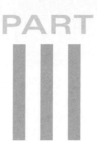

PART

III

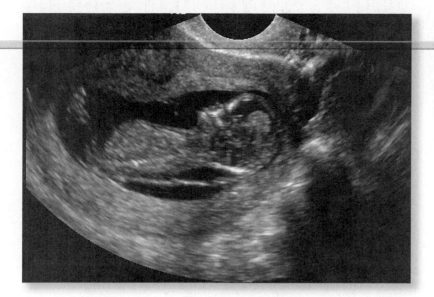

Obstetrics and Gynecology

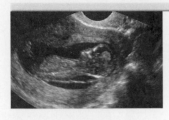

CHAPTER 19

Pelvic Anatomy

KEY TERMS

adnexa region to include the fallopian tube and ovary.

false pelvis region of the pelvis located above the pelvic brim.

fimbriae ovarica the one fimbriae attached to the ovary.

iliopectineal line a bony ridge on the inner surface of the ilium and pubic bones that divides the true and false pelvis.

ligament extension of a double layer of peritoneum between visceral organs.

menarche onset of menstrual cycles.

menopause cessation of menses.

perineum the surface region in both males and females between the pubic symphysis and the coccyx; area below the pelvic floor.

premenarche time before the onset of menstrual cycles.

puberty refers to the process of physical changes by which a child's body becomes an adult body capable of reproduction.

true pelvis region of the pelvis found below the pelvic brim.

PELVIC ANATOMY (Fig. 19-1)

- Pelvis begins at the iliac crests and ends at the symphysis pubis.
- Divided into the true and false pelvis by the iliopectineal line.

TRUE PELVIS

- Also known as pelvic cavity.
- Located below the pelvic brim.
- Muscles and ligaments form a pelvic floor.
- Anterior boundary—symphysis pubis.
- Posterior boundary—sacrum and coccyx.
- Posterolateral wall—piriformis and coccygeus muscles.
- Anterolateral wall—hip bone and obturator internus muscles.
- Lateral boundaries—fused ilium and ischium.
- Pelvic floor—levator ani and coccygeus muscles.
- Contains—female reproductive system, urinary bladder, distal ureters, and bowel.

FALSE PELVIS

- Located above the pelvic brim.
- Anterior boundary—abdominal wall.
- Posterior boundary—flanged portions of the iliac bones and base of the sacrum.
- Lateral boundaries—abdominal wall.
- Contains—loops of bowel.

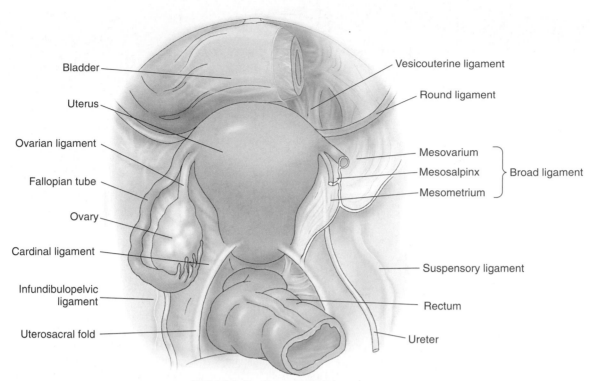

FIG. 19-1 Female pelvic anatomy.

Pelvic Muscles

PELVIC MUSCLE	DESCRIPTION	LOCATION	SONOGRAPHIC APPEARANCE

Levator ani	• Name given to a group of muscles
	  1. puborectalis
	  2. iliococcygeus
	  3. pubococcygeus
	• Forms the pelvic floor along with the piriformis muscles
	• Supports and positions the pelvic organs
		• Medial to the obturator internus muscles
		• Posterior to the vagina and cervix
			• Low-level, mildly curved linear echoes
			• Hypoechoic compared to the normal uterus

Iliopsoas muscles	• Formed by the psoas major and iliacus muscles • Lateral landmark of the true pelvis	• Course anterior and lateral through the false pelvis • Descend until attaching to the lesser trochanter of the femur	• Low-level gray echoes with a distinct central hyperechoic focus
Piriformis muscles	• Arise from the sacrum • Form part of the pelvic floor • Course through the greater sciatic notch	• Posterior to the uterus, ovaries, vagina, and rectum • Anterior to the sacrum • Course diagonally to the obturator internus muscle	• Low-level linear echoes • Hypoechoic compared to the normal uterus
Obturator internus muscles	• Lateral margins of the true pelvis • Surround the obturator foramen	• Posterior and medial to the iliopsoas muscles • Level of the vagina • Lateral to the ovaries	• Low-level linear echoes abutting the lateral walls of the urinary bladder

PELVIC LIGAMENTS

- Not routinely visualized by ultrasound.
- With intraperitoneal fluid collections, ligaments will appear moderately thin and hyperechoic.

Pelvic Ligaments

PELVIC LIGAMENT	DESCRIPTION
Broad	• Wing-like double fold of peritoneum • Drapes over the fallopian tubes, uterus, ovaries, and blood vessels • Extends from the lateral walls of the uterus to the sidewalls of the pelvis • Provides a small amount of support for the uterus • Creates the retrouterine and vesicouterine pouches • Divided into the mesometrium, mesosalpinx, and mesovarium segments
Cardinal	• Continuation of the broad ligament • Extends across the pelvic floor • Firmly supports the cervix
Ovarian	• Extends from the cornua of the uterus to the medial aspect of the ovary
Round	• Arises in the uterine cornua, anterior to the fallopian tubes • Extends from the uterine fundus to the pelvic sidewalls • Helps to maintain anteflexion of the uterine body and fundus • Excessive stretching can permit retroflexion of the uterine body and fundus • Contracts during labor
Suspensory	• Also known as infundibulopelvic ligament • Extends from the lateral portion of the ovary to the pelvic sidewall
Uterosacral	• Extends from the upper cervix to the lateral margins of the sacrum • Firmly supports the cervix

Pelvic Vasculature

VESSEL	LOCATION	INFORMATION
Arcuate vessels	• Prominent vascular structures in the outer one-third of the myometrium	• Branch of the uterine artery • Radial arteries arise from the arcuate arteries • Spiral arteries of the endometrium arise from the radial arteries • Larger-caliber vessels are typically arcuate veins
Internal iliac arteries	• Posterior to the uterus and ovaries • Follows a posterior course and enters the true pelvis near the sacral prominence	• Aka: hypogastric arteries • Supply the bladder, uterus, vagina, and rectum • Give rise to the uterine arteries
Ovarian arteries	• Arise from the lateral margins of the abdominal aorta, slightly inferior to the renal arteries • Course medial within the suspensory ligaments	• Primary blood supply to the ovaries • Connect with the uterine arteries
Ovarian veins	• Course within the suspensory ligaments	• Right ovarian vein empties directly into the inferior vena cava • Left ovarian vein empties into the left renal vein
Uterine arteries	• Medial in the levator ani muscles • Ascend in a tortuous course lateral to the uterus within the broad ligament	• Supply the cervix, vagina, uterus, ovaries, and fallopian tubes • Course lateral and terminate at the confluence with the ovarian artery

PELVIC SPACES

- Not uncommon to visualize a small amount of free fluid in the retrouterine pouch.
- Masses within the space of Retzius will displace the urinary bladder posteriorly.
- Masses within the vesicouterine pouch will displace the urinary bladder anteriorly.

Pelvic Spaces

PELVIC SPACE	LOCATION
Retrouterine Pouch	• Anterior to the rectum
• Posterior cul de sac	• Posterior to the uterus
• Pouch of Douglas	• Most inferior point in the pelvic cavity
Space of Retzius	• Anterior to the urinary bladder
• Retropubic space	• Posterior to the symphysis pubis
• Prevesical space	• Anterior to the uterus
Vesicouterine Pouch	• Posterior to the urinary bladder
• Anterior cul de sac	

FEMALE REPRODUCTIVE SYSTEM (Fig. 19-2)

VAGINA

- Collapsed muscular tube located posterior to the urinary bladder and urethra and anterior to the rectum and anus.
- Extends from the vulva to the cervix.
- Sides of the vagina are enclosed between the levator ani muscles.
- Half of the vagina lies above and the other half below the pelvic brim.
- Supplied by the vaginal and uterine arteries and empties into the internal iliac veins.

FIG. 19-2
Female reproductive anatomy.

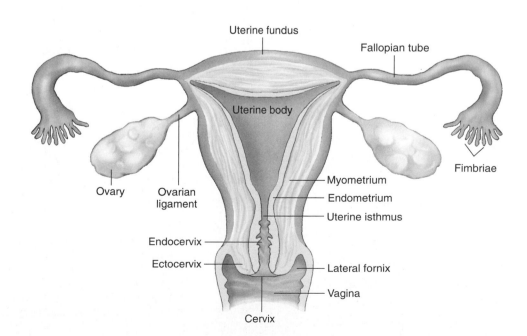

SONOGRAPH APPEARANCE

- Vaginal walls demonstrate low-level homogeneous echoes.
- Vaginal canal demonstrates a central hyperechoic linear echo pattern.

UTERUS

- Hollow, pear-shaped retroperitoneal organ.
- Derived from the fused caudal portion of the paired, hollow müllerian ducts.
- Muscular organ covered by peritoneum, except below the anterior cervical os.
- Supported by the levator ani muscles, cardinal ligaments, and uterosacral ligaments.

TISSUE LAYERS OF THE UTERUS

Perimetrium

- Serosal or external surface.
- Part of the parietal peritoneum.

Myometrium

- Thickest layer of the uterus.
- Composed of thick, smooth muscle supported by connective tissue containing large blood vessels.
- Innermost layer of the myometrium is known as the **junctional zone.**

Endometrium

- Mucous membrane lining the uterine cavity.
- Thickness is related to hormone levels.

Regions of the Uterus	
REGION	**DESCRIPTION**
Body	• Aka: corpus
	• Largest portion of the uterus
	• Thick muscular segment of the uterus
	• Located posterior to the vesicouterine pouch
	• Located anterior to the retrouterine pouch
	• Located medial to the broad ligaments and uterine vessels
Cervix	• Distal portion of the uterus
	• Projects into the vaginal canal
	• More fibrous and less flexible
	• Anchored at the angle of the bladder by the parametrium
	• Located between the vagina and the uterine isthmus
	• Peritoneal reflection is not demonstrated anterior to the cervix
	• Approximately 2.5 cm in length
Cornua	• Lateral funnel-shaped horns of the uterus
	• Located between the uterine fundus and the fallopian tube
Endometrial cavity	• Consists of a superficial functional layer and a deep basal layer
	• Functional layer sheds with menses
	• Basal layer regenerates new endometrium
	• Thickness is dependant on hormone levels
Fundus	• Dome-shaped uppermost portion of the uterus
	• Located superior to the insertion of the fallopian tubes
	• Position may vary with bladder filling
Isthmus	• "Narrow waist" of the uterus
	• Located between the cervix and body of the uterus
	• Termed lower uterine segment during pregnancy

LOCATION OF THE UTERUS

- Positioned in the pelvis, anterior to the rectum and posterior to the urinary bladder.

NORMAL SONOGRAPHIC APPEARANCE OF THE UTERUS

- Homogeneous mid to low gray echoes surrounding a hyperechoic endometrial cavity.
- Uterine arteries demonstrate a high-resistance flow pattern.
- Resistive index of the arcuate arteries range between 0.86 and 0.89.

NORMAL SONOGRAPHIC APPEARANCE OF THE ENDOMETRIUM

- Outer basal layer appears hypoechoic.
- Inner functional layer typically appears hyperechoic.
- Thickness varies with menstrual phase or status but should not exceed 14 mm.

MEASURING THE UTERUS (Fig. 19-3)

- Length is measured from the fundus to the inferior cervix.
- Height (thickness) is measured perpendicular to the length of the widest portion of the uterine body.
- Width is measured at the widest portion of the uterine body in the short axis.

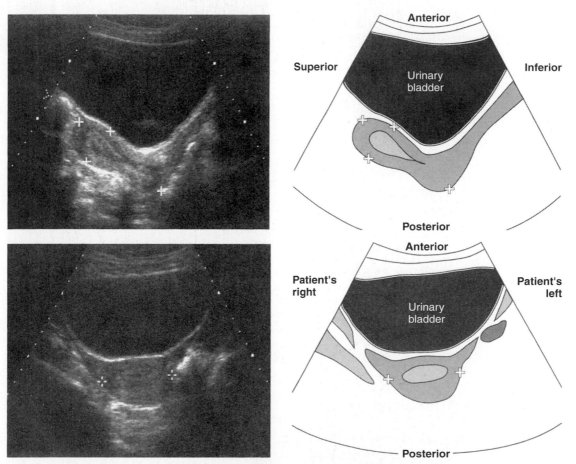

FIG. 19-3 Uterine measurements.

FIG. 19-4
Sonogram endometrium
measurement.

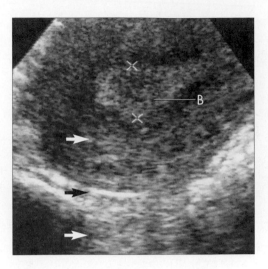

MEASURING THE ENDOMETRIUM (Fig. 19-4)

- Anterior-posterior thickness is measured in the sagittal plane.
- Measure from echogenic interface to echogenic interface (functional layer).
- Thin hypoechoic area (basal layer) is *not* included in the measurement.
- Fluid within the endometrial cavity is *not* included in the measurement.

Uterine Size

MENSTRUAL STATUS	LENGTH (cm)	HEIGHT (cm)	WIDTH (cm)	CERVIX/CORPUS RATIO
Premenarche	• 2.0-4.0	• 0.5-1.0	• 1.0-2.0	• 2:1
Menarche	• 6.0-8.0 nulliparous	• 3.0-5.0 nulliparous	• 3.0-5.0 nulliparous	• 1:2
	• 8.0-10.0 parous	• 5.0-6.0 parous	• 5.0-6.0 parous	
Postmenopausal	• 3.5-7.5	• 2.0-3.0	• 2.0-4.0	• 1:1

Uterine Positions

POSITION	DESCRIPTION
Anteflexion	• Uterine fundus bends upon the cervix
Anteversion	• Uterus bends slightly forward
	• Cervix forms an angle ≤90° with the vaginal canal
	• Most common uterine position
Dextroflexion	• Uterine body is displaced or flexed to the right of the cervix
Levoflexion	• Uterine body is displaced or flexed to the left of the cervix
Retroflexion	• Uterine fundus or body is curved backwards upon the cervix
	• Cervix remains in an anteverted position
Retroversion	• Uterus and cervix display a posterior tilt
	• Cervix forms an angle <90° with the vaginal canal

CONGENITAL UTERINE ANOMALIES

- Congenital anomalies result from improper fusion of the müllerian ducts or incomplete absorption of the septum between them.
- Coexisting renal anomalies occur in 20% to 30% of cases.

Congenital Anomalies of the Uterus

ANOMALY	ETIOLOGY	CLINICAL FINDINGS	SONOGRAPHIC FINDINGS	DIFFERENTIAL CONSIDERATIONS
Agenesis	• Lack of the caudal müllerian ducts to develop • Fallopian tubes are present	• Amenorrhea	• Absent uterus	• Hysterectomy • Unicornuate uterus
Arcuate	• Septum between the müllerian ducts is not completely reabsorbed	• Asymptomatic • Infertility	• Shallow notch in the superior portion of the fundus • "Heart-shaped" fundal contour • Slight separation of the superior endometrium	• Leiomyoma • Synechiae • Endometrial polyp
Bicornuate	• Partial fusion of the müllerian ducts • Two uteri in the superior portion of the uterus • Two superior endometrial cavities	• Asymptomatic • Infertility • Spontaneous abortion	• Deep notch in the fundus • Two distinct endometriums separated by a small amount of myometrium	• Fibroid • Septated uterus
Didelphys	• Complete failure of the müllerian ducts to fuse	• Asymptomatic • Infertility • Spontaneous abortion • Vaginal septation	• Wide separation between two distinct uterine fundi • Two separate cervix • Possible septated vagina	• Pelvic muscles • Pedunculated fibroid
Septae	• Complete fusion of the müllerian ducts with failure to completely reabsorb the septum	• Asymptomatic • High incidence of infertility • Spontaneous abortion	• Normal uterine contour • Thin or wide separation within the endometrial cavity by fibrous tissue or myometrium	• Fibroid • Adenomyosis • Endometrial polyp
Unicornuate	• Unilateral development of the paired müllerian ducts	• Asymptomatic • Hypomenorrhea • Infertility	• Small uterine size • Lateral uterine position • Rudimentary horn may be visualized	• Uterine didelphys

OVARIES

- Paired, almond-shaped endocrine glands located lateral to the uterus.
- Smooth surface in early life, becoming markedly pitted after years of ovulation.
- Without hormone replacement therapy, ovaries decrease in size after menopause.
- Attached to the posterior surface of the broad ligament by the mesovarium.
- The only organs in the abdominopelvic cavity not lined by peritoneum.
- Dual blood supply through the ovarian and uterine arteries.

ANATOMY OF THE OVARIES

- The ovary is composed of an outer cortex and a central medulla.
    - **Cortex** consists of follicles and is covered with the tunica albuginea.
    - **Medulla** is composed of connective tissue and contains nerves, blood, lymph vessels, and smooth muscle at the hilus region.
    - **Tunica albuginea** is surrounded by a thin layer of germinal epithelium.
- Each ovary is connected by:
    - mesovarium ligament to the broad ligament.
    - utero-ovarian ligament to the inferior portion of the uterus.
    - suspensory ligament to the pelvic sidewall.

PHYSIOLOGY OF THE OVARIES

Function
- Produce ova.
- Produce hormones.
  - Estrogen—secreted by the follicle.
  - Progesterone—secreted by the corpus luteum.

LOCATION OF THE OVARIES
- Level of the uterine cornua.
- Medial to the external iliac vessels.
- Anterior to the internal iliac vessels and ureter.

NORMAL SONOGRAPHIC APPEARANCE OF THE OVARY
- Ovoid medium-level echogenic structure.
- Hypoechoic periphery representing the tunica albuginea.
- Anechoic follicle(s) demonstrating posterior enhancement may be present.
- Resistance of the ovarian arteries depends on the menstrual cycle.
- During menses and the early proliferative phases, the ovarian artery demonstrates a high resistance with a low flow velocity.
- Resistive index normally ranges from 0.4 to 0.8.
- Pulsatility index normally ranges from 0.6 to 2.5.

MEASUREMENT OF THE OVARIES (Fig. 19-5)
- Measure the length of the long axis.
- Anteroposterior dimension is measured perpendicular to the length.
- Width is measured in the transverse or coronal plane.

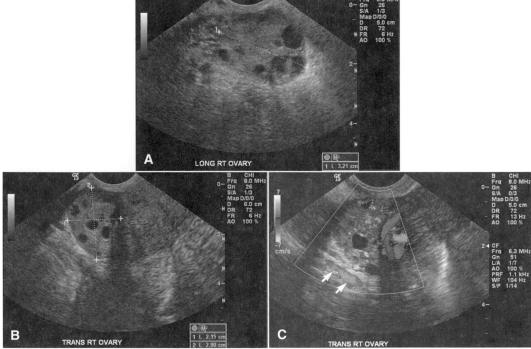

FIG. 19-5

OVARIAN SIZE

Menarche

- 2.5 to 5.0 cm in length.
- 1.5 to 3.0 cm in width.
- 0.6 to 2.2 cm in height.

Ovarian Volume

- Volume varies with age and menstrual status.
- Lowest volume during the luteal phase.
- Highest volume during the periovulatory phase.
- Larger volume at birth a result of maternal hormones.
- Stable volumes up to age 5 years.
- Volume peaks in the third decade.
- Begins to decline in the fifth decade.

Ovarian Volumes	
Premenarche	3.0 cm^3
Menstruating	9.8 cm^3
Postmenopause	5.8 cm^3

$$\text{Ovarian volume (cm}^3) = \frac{\text{Length} \times \text{Width} \times \text{Height}}{2}$$

ANATOMICAL OVARIAN VARIANT

L-Shaped Ovary

- Normal ovarian variant giving the appearance of two "arms."
- Lesions in one "arm" may appear exophytic or extrinsic to the ovary.

CONGENITAL OVARIAN ANOMALIES

Agenesis

- Associated with an abnormal karyotype.

Unilateral Ovary

- Rare occurrence.

FALLOPIAN TUBES (OVIDUCT) (Fig. 19-6)

- Derived from the nonfused cranial portion of the müllerian ducts.
- Contained in the superior portion of the broad ligament and covered by peritoneum.

PHYSIOLOGY OF THE FALLOPIAN TUBES

Function

- Attract and transfer ova from the surface of the ovary to the endometrial cavity.

FIG. 19-6

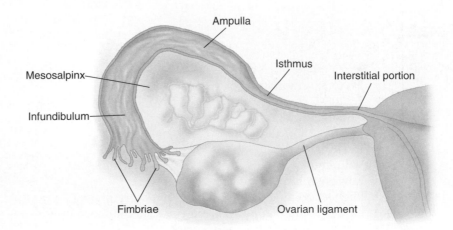

Divisions of the Fallopian Tube

SEGMENT	DESCRIPTION
Interstitial	• Passes through the cornua of the uterus
	• Narrowest portion
Isthmus	• Immediately adjacent to the uterine wall
	• Short, straight, narrow portion of the tube
Ampulla	• Widest, longest, and most coiled portion
	• Region where fertilization most commonly occurs
	• Most common area of ectopic pregnancies
Infundibulum	• Funnel-shaped distal portion of the tube
	• Terminates at the fimbrial processes
	• One fimbriae is attached to the ovary
	• Opens into the peritoneal cavity adjacent to the ovary

LOCATION

- Superior to the utero-ovarian ligaments, round ligaments, and blood vessels.
- Course posterior and lateral from the cornua of the uterus curving over the ovary.

SONOGRAPHIC APPEARANCE OF THE FALLOPIAN TUBE

- Normal fallopian tube is not routinely visualized.
- Interstitial segment appears as a long tenuous structure extending laterally from the uterine wall.

SIZE

- 7- to 12-cm coiled muscular tubes composed of smooth muscle and lined by a mucosa.

URINARY BLADDER

ANATOMY

Apex—superior portion of the bladder.
Neck—inferior portion of the bladder continuous with the urethra.
Trigone—region between the apex and neck of the bladder.
- Normal bladder wall thickness is 3 mm when distended.
- Normal bladder wall thickness is 5 mm when empty.
- Normal bladder wall is thicker in infants than in adults.
- Ureters enter the bladder wall at an oblique angle approximately 5 cm above the bladder outlet.
- Postvoid residual normally should not exceed 20 mL.

NORMAL SONOGRAPHIC APPEARANCE

- Anechoic, fluid-filled structure located in the pelvic midline.
- Ureteric orifices appear as small echogenic protuberances on the posterior aspect of the bladder.
- Bladder wall thickness is dependent on distention of urinary bladder but should not exceed 5 mm.

Congenital Abnormalities of the Urinary Bladder

CONGENITAL ABNORMALITY	ETIOLOGY	CLINICAL FINDINGS	SONOGRAPHIC FINDINGS	DIFFERENTIAL CONSIDERATIONS
Bladder diverticulum	• Bladder wall muscle weakness	• Asymptomatic • Urinary tract infection • Pelvic pain	• Anechoic pedunculation of the urinary bladder • Neck of diverticulum is small • May enlarge when bladder contracts	• Ovarian cyst • Fluid-filled bowel • Ascites
Bladder ureterocele	• Congenital obstruction of the ureteric orifice	• Asymptomatic • Urinary tract infection	• Hyperechoic septation seen within the bladder at the ureteric orifice • Demonstrated when urine enters the bladder	• Artifact • Bladder tumor • Catheter balloon

Pathology of the Urinary Bladder

BLADDER PATHOLOGY	ETIOLOGY	CLINICAL FINDINGS	SONOGRAPHIC FINDINGS	DIFFERENTIAL CONSIDERATIONS
Bladder calculus	• Develops in the bladder • Migrate from the kidney(s)	• Asymptomatic • Hematuria	• Hyperechoic focus within the urinary bladder • Posterior acoustic shadowing • Mobile with patient position change	• Intestinal air • Calcified vessel
Cystitis	• Infection	• Dysuria • Urinary frequency • Leukocytosis	• Increase in bladder wall thickness • Mobile internal echoes	• Bladder sludge • Hematuria
Bladder sludge	• Debris in the bladder	• Asymptomatic	• Homogeneous low-level echoes • Mobile with patient position change	• Cystitis • Hematuria
Bladder malignancy	• Transitional cell carcinoma	• Painless hematuria • Frequent urination • Dysuria	• Echogenic mass • Irregular margins • Immobile with patient position change • Internal vascular blood flow	• Benign tumor • Bladder sludge • Ureterocele
Bladder polyp	• Papilloma	• Asymptomatic • Frequent urination	• Echogenic intraluminal mass • Smooth margins • Immobile with patient position change • Internal vascular flow	• Malignant tumor • Bladder sludge • Ureterocele

PELVIC ANATOMY REVIEW

1. Which pelvic ligament extends from the cornua of the uterus to the medial aspect of the ovary?
   a. round
   b. broad
   c. cardinal
   d. ovarian
   e. suspensory

2. Prominent anechoic structures near the periphery of the uterus most likely represent:
   a. endometriomas
   b. arcuate vessels
   c. nabothian cysts
   d. physiological cysts
   e. submucosal leiomyomas

3. Which of the following muscles abuts the lateral walls of the urinary bladder?
   a. psoas
   b. piriformis
   c. levator ani
   d. rectus abdominus
   e. obturator internus

4. The region including the ovary and fallopian tube is termed the:
   a. oviduct
   b. adnexa
   c. broad ligament
   d. fimbriae ovarica
   e. space of Retzius

5. Which segment of the fallopian tube connects with the uterus?
   a. ampulla
   b. isthmus
   c. interstitial
   d. suspensory
   e. infundibulum

6. The flanged portions of the iliac bones form the:
   a. lateral border of the true pelvis
   b. superior border of the false pelvis
   c. posterior border of the true pelvis
   d. inferior border of the true pelvis
   e. posterior border of the false pelvis

7. Which uterine position displays the fundus of the uterus anterior to the cervix?
   a. anteversion
   b. levoflexion
   c. anteflexion
   d. retroversion
   e. retroflexion

8. When measuring endometrial thickness, calipers are placed from:
   a. superior interface to inferior interface
   b. posterior interface to superior interface
   c. echogenic interface to echogenic interface
   d. echogenic interface to hypoechoic interface
   e. hypoechoic interface to hypoechoic interface

9. The ovary is attached to the pelvic sidewall by the:
   a. broad ligament
   b. round ligament
   c. ovarian ligament
   d. cardinal ligament
   e. suspensory ligament

10. Failure of the müllerian ducts to fuse will most likely result in:
    a. uterine septae
    b. uterine agenesis
    c. bicornuate uterus
    d. uterine didelphys
    e. uterine retroversion

11. Which of the following correctly measures endometrial thickness?
    a. anterior–posterior dimension in the coronal plane
    b. transverse dimension in the coronal plane
    c. anterior–posterior dimension in the sagittal plane
    d. transverse diameter in the transverse plane
    e. anterior–posterior diameter in the transverse plane

12. Which of the following most accurately describes the perimetrium?
    a. The perimetrium lines the uterine cavity.
    b. The perimetrium is composed of smooth muscle.
    c. The serosal surface of the uterus is termed the perimetrium.
    d. The thickest layer of the uterus is termed the perimetrium.
    e. The perimetrium is composed of connective tissue and large blood vessels.

13. Secondary blood supply to the ovaries is through the:
    a. arcuate arteries
    b. uterine arteries
    c. ovarian arteries
    d. hypogastric arteries
    e. external iliac arteries

14. The vesicouterine pouch is located:
    a. posterior to the uterus and anterior to the rectum
    b. anterior to the uterus and posterior to the urinary bladder
    c. anterior to the urinary bladder and posterior to the uterus
    d. posterior to the symphysis pubis and anterior to the uterus
    e. anterior to the symphysis pubis and posterior to the rectus abdominus

15. In premenarche the size of the uterine cervix is expected to be:
    a. half the size of the corpus
    b. equal to the uterine corpus
    c. twice as large as the corpus
    d. equal to the uterine fundus
    e. equal to the width of the fundus

Using Fig. 19-7, answer question 16.

16. This sagittal image of the uterus most likely represents a:
    a. septae uterus
    b. menarche uterus
    c. bicornuate uterus
    d. premenarche uterus
    e. postmenopausal uterus

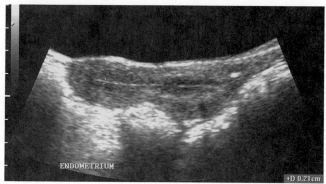

FIG. 19-7 Sagittal sonogram of the uterus (on CD).

Using Fig. 19-8, answer question 17.

17. In this sagittal sonogram, the uterus is lying in which of the following positions?
    a. anteversion
    b. retroflexion
    c. anteflexion
    d. retroversion
    e. dextroflexion

Using Fig. 19-9, answer question 18.

18. Which pelvic muscles are the arrows identifying?
    a. iliopsoas
    b. levator ani
    c. suspensory
    d. uterosacral
    e. obturator internus

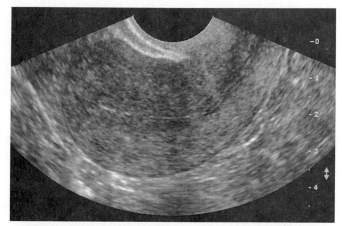

FIG. 19-8 Endovaginal sonogram of the uterus.

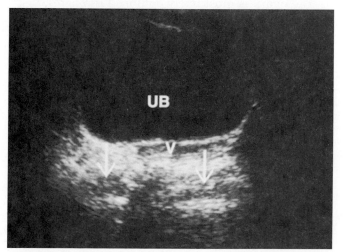

FIG. 19-9 Transverse sonogram at the level of the vagina.

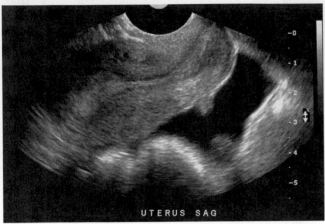

FIG. 19-10 Endovaginal sonogram.

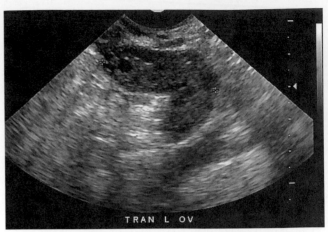

FIG. 19-11 Sonogram of the left ovary.

Using Fig. 19-10, answer questions 19 and 20.

19. A perimenopausal patient presents with a history of pelvic fullness and pain. A sagittal sonogram displays a fluid collection in the:
    a. prevesical space
    b. space of Retzius
    c. Morrison pouch
    d. pouch of Douglas
    e. vesicouterine pouch

20. The position of the uterus is:
    a. anteverted
    b. anteflexed
    c. levoverted
    d. retroflexed
    e. retroverted

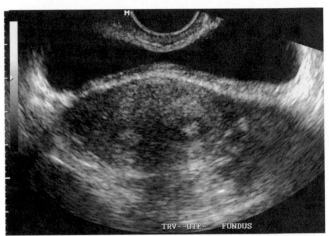

FIG. 19-12 Transverse transabdominal sonogram (on CD).

Using Fig. 19-11, answer question 21.

21. The ovary is most likely demonstrating a(n):
    a. pyosalpinx
    b. parovarian cyst
    c. benign neoplasm
    d. anatomical variant
    e. malignant neoplasm

Using Fig. 19-12, answer question 22.

22. A patient presents with a history of multiple miscarriages. Her last menstrual period was 3 weeks prior. On the basis of this clinical history, the sonogram is **most suspicious** for a(n):
    a. arcuate uterus
    b. septae uterus
    c. uterine didelphys
    d. bicornuate uterus
    e. submucosal leiomyoma

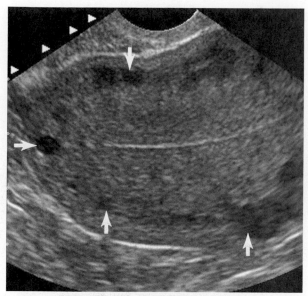

FIG. 19-13   Sagittal sonogram.

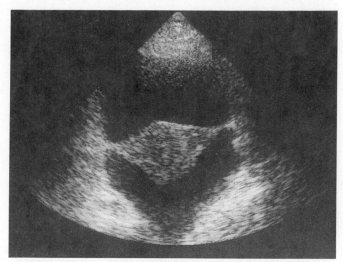

FIG. 19-14   Transverse sonogram of the uterus.

Using Fig. 19-13, answer question 23.

23. A 30-year-old patient presents with a history of dysmenorrhea. The arrows in the sonogram are most likely identifying:
  a. leiomyomas
  b. adenomyosis
  c. arcuate vessels
  d. uterine arteries
  e. endometriomas

Using Fig. 19-14, answer question 24.

24. A patient presents with a history of chronic cirrhosis and abdominal distention. The hyperechoic linear structures lateral to the uterus most likely represent the:
  a. fallopian tubes
  b. broad ligaments
  c. round ligaments
  d. iliopsoas muscles
  e. ovarian ligaments

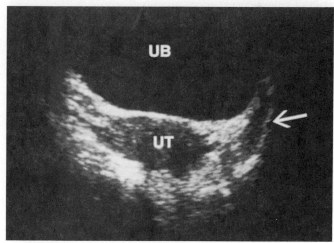

FIG. 19-15   Transverse sonogram of the uterus.

Using Fig. 19-15, answer question 25.

25. The hypoechoic structure identified by the arrow most likely represents the:
  a. ascites
  b. pelvis bone
  c. iliopsoas muscle
  d. piriformis muscle
  e. obturator internus muscle

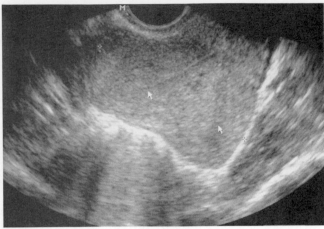

FIG. 19-16 Sagittal sonogram of the uterus.

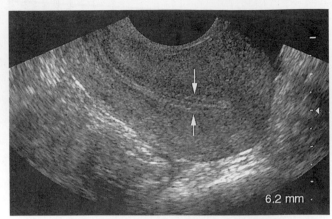

FIG. 19-18 Endovaginal sonogram.

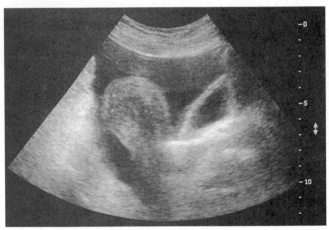

FIG. 19-17 Sagittal sonogram (on CD).

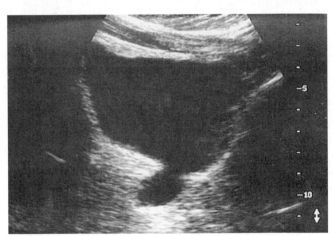

FIG. 19-19 Transverse sonogram of the urinary bladder (on CD).

Using Fig. 19-16, answer question 26.

26. The arrows are most likely identifying:
    a. two subserosal leiomyomas
    b. the lateral horns of the uterus
    c. two individual endometrial cavities
    d. the interstitial portions of the fallopian tubes
    e. the cervix and fundus in a retroverted uterus

Using Fig. 19-17, answer question 27.

27. Identification of free fluid in the pelvis is located in the:
    a. vesicouterine space
    b. prevesical and retrouterine spaces
    c. retrouterine and retropubic spaces
    d. vesicouterine and retrouterine spaces
    e. retrouterine, vesicouterine, and retropubic spaces

Using Fig. 19-18, answer question 28.

28. The position of the uterus in this sagittal sonogram is termed:
    a. anteflexion
    b. anteversion
    c. levoflexion
    d. retroflexion
    e. retroversion

Using Fig. 19-19, answer question 29.

29. An anechoic mass contiguous with the posterior wall of the urinary bladder is most consistent with a(n):
    a. ureterocele
    b. hydroureter
    c. ovarian cyst
    d. hydrosalpinx
    e. bladder diverticulum

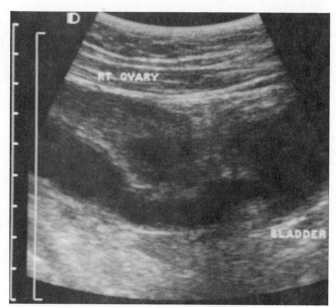

FIG. 19-20 Sagittal sonogram of the right lower quadrant.

Using Fig. 19-20, answer question 30.

30. A sagittal sonogram of the right lower quadrant demonstrates an anechoic tubular structure. This structure most likely represents a(n):
    a. ureterocele
    b. hydroureter
    c. hydrosalpinx
    d. external iliac vein
    e. fluid-filled loop of bowel

31. Which of the following attaches to the ovary?
    a. peritoneum
    b. parametrium
    c. broad ligament
    d. tunica albuginea
    e. ovarian ligament

32. Ovarian volume is lowest during the:
    a. luteal phase
    b. follicular phase
    c. ovulatory phase
    d. menstrual phase
    e. periovulatory phase

33. The fallopian tube divides into which of the following segments?
    a. fimbria, isthmus, cornua, ampulla
    b. isthmus, ampulla, cornua, interstitial
    c. ampulla, infundibulum, fimbria, isthmus
    d. infundibulum, interstitial, fimbria, ampulla
    e. interstitial, isthmus, ampulla, infundibulum

34. Visualization of pelvic ligaments appear on sonography as:
    a. hypoechoic ovoid structures
    b. hyperechoic linear structures
    c. hyperechoic tubular structures
    d. hypoechoic tortuous structures
    e. heterogeneous linear structures

35. The cornua of the uterus is located between the:
    a. corpus and fundus of the uterus
    b. cervix and fundus of the uterus
    c. corpus and cervix of the uterus
    d. uterine fundus and fallopian tube
    e. uterine corpus and fallopian tube

36. The primary blood supply to which of the following pelvic structures is provided by the spiral artery?
    a. cervix
    b. vagina
    c. ovaries
    d. endometrium
    e. fallopian tubes

37. Congenital uterine anomalies are associated with coexisting anomalies of the:
    a. ovaries
    b. kidneys
    c. oviducts
    d. adrenal glands
    e. thyroid glands

38. Which uterine anomaly is most likely to demonstrate a small dimple in the fundus?
    a. septae
    b. arcuate
    c. didelphys
    d. bicornuate
    e. unicornuate

39. It is common to visualize a small amount of free fluid in the:
    a. prevesical space
    b. space of Retzius
    c. retropubic space
    d. retrouterine space
    e. vesicouterine space

40. The section of time prior to the onset of menstruation is termed:
    a. puberty
    b. menarche
    c. premenarche
    d. perimenopause
    e. postmenopause

41. Which of the following is a surface region located below the pelvic floor?
    a. mesentery
    b. omentum
    c. perineum
    d. peritoneum
    e. retroperitoneum

42. Which congenital uterine anomaly does not distort the normal contour of the fundus?
    a. septae
    b. arcuate
    c. didelphys
    d. bicornuate
    e. unicornuate

43. Partial fusion of the caudal müllerian ducts will most likely result in an anomaly of the:
    a. anus
    b. uterus
    c. ovary
    d. vagina
    e. fallopian tube

44. The pelvis is divided into the true and false pelvis by the:
    a. hip bones
    b. iliac bones
    c. broad ligaments
    d. iliopectineal line
    e. iliopsoas muscles

45. The pelvic floor is formed by pelvic:
    a. bones and muscles
    b. bones and ligaments
    c. organs and ligaments
    d. ligaments and muscles
    e. ligaments and blood vessels

46. The uterosacral ligament extends from the lateral margins of the sacrum to the:
    a. cornua
    b. superior cervix
    c. inferior fundus
    d. inferior vagina
    e. superior isthmus

47. The innermost layer of the myometrium is termed the:
    a. basal zone
    b. functional zone
    c. junctional zone
    d. albuginea zone
    e. medullary zone

48. In the menarche patient, the endometrial thickness should not exceed:
    a. 8 mm
    b. 10 mm
    c. 14 mm
    d. 20 mm
    e. 25 mm

49. Which of the following structures is **not** lined by peritoneum?
    a. cervix
    b. uterus
    c. ovary
    d. bowel
    e. oviduct

50. Ovarian volume is the highest during the:
    a. luteal phase
    b. secretory phase
    c. follicular phase
    d. menstrual phase
    e. periovulatory phase

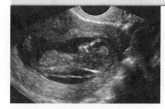

CHAPTER 20

Physiology of the Female Pelvis

KEY TERMS

amenorrhea   absence of menstruation.

corpus albicans   scar from prior corpus luteum.

corpus luteum   a fluid structure formed from the graafian follicle after ovulation; produces progesterone.

cumulus oophorus   protrusion within the graafian follicle containing the oocyte.

dysmenorrhea   painful menses.

estrogen   hormone secreted by the follicle, promoting growth of the endometrium.

follicle   functional or physiological ovulatory cyst consisting of an ovum surrounded by a layer of cells.

follicle-stimulating hormone   hormone that stimulates growth and maturation of the graafian follicle(s).

graafian follicle   mature follicle containing a cumulus mass with a single oocyte.

luteinizing hormone   hormone that stimulates ovulation.

menorrhagia   abnormally heavy or long menses.

menstrual cycle   monthly cyclic changes in the female reproductive system typically 28 days in length.

mittelschmerz   term used to describe pelvic pain proceeding ovulation.

oligomenorrhea   time between monthly menstrual cycles exceeds 35 days.

ovulation   explosive release of an ovum from a ruptured graafian follicle.

polymenorrhea   time between monthly menstrual cycles is less than 21 days.

precocious puberty   an unusually early onset of puberty.

progesterone   hormone that helps to prepare and maintain the endometrium.

NORMAL PHYSIOLOGY

- The onset of menstruation generally occurs between 11 and 13 years of age.
- Cessation of menstruation usually occurs around 50 years of age.
- The length of a menstrual cycle ranges between 21 and 35 days.
- Rupture of a graafian follicle should occur each cycle.
- Menstruation depends on the functional integrity of the hypothalamus, pituitary gland, and ovarian axis.

LABORATORY VALUES

ESTRADIOL

- Normal levels.
  - Follicular: 30 to 100 pg/mL.
  - Ovulatory: 200 to 400 pg/mL.
  - Luteal: 50 to 140 pg/mL.
- Primarily reflects the activity of the ovaries.
- During pregnancy, estradiol levels will steadily rise.
- Small amounts are present in the adrenal cortex and arterial walls.

ESTROGEN

- Normal levels 5-100 μg/24 hr (urine).
- Primary female sex hormone.
- Naturally occurring estrogens include estradiol, estriol, and estrone.
- Primarily produced by developing follicles and the placenta.

- Follicle-stimulating hormone (FSH) and luteinizing hormone (LH) stimulate the production of estrogen in the ovaries.
- Small amount of estrogen is produced by the breasts, liver, and adrenal glands.
- Functions include promotes formation of female secondary sex characteristics, accelerates height growth and metabolism, reduces muscle mass, stimulates endometrial growth, and increases uterine growth.

FOLLICLE-STIMULATING HORMONE

- Normal levels:
  - Premenopause: 4 to 25 mU/mL.
  - Postmenopause: 4 to 30 mU/mL.
- Initiates follicular growth and stimulates the maturation of the graafian follicle(s).
- Secreted by the anterior pituitary gland.
- Levels are normally low in childhood and slightly higher after menopause.
- Levels decline in the late follicular phase and demonstrate a slight increase at the end of the luteal phase.

FOLLICLE-STIMULATING HORMONE–RELEASING FACTOR

- Becomes active before puberty.
- Produced by the hypothalamus.
- Released into the bloodstream, reaching the anterior pituitary gland.

LUTEINIZING HORMONE (LH)

- Normal levels:
  - Follicular: 2 to 10 u/L.
  - Midcycle peak: 15 to 65 u/L.
  - Luteal: 10 to 12 u/L.
  - Postmenopause: 1.3 to 2.1 mg/dL.
- Essential in both males and females for reproduction.
- Secreted by the anterior pituitary gland.
- A surge in LH levels triggers ovulation and initiates the conversion of the residual follicle into a corpus luteum. The corpus luteum produces progesterone to prepare the endometrium for possible implantation.
- LH surge typically lasts only 48 hours.

LUTEINIZING HORMONE–RELEASING FACTOR (LHRF)

- Becomes active prior to puberty.
- Produced by the hypothalamus.
- Released into the bloodstream, reaching the anterior pituitary gland.

PROGESTERONE

- Normal levels:
  - Follicular: 0.1 to 1.5 ng/mL.
  - Luteal: 2.5 to 28.0 ng/mL.
- Levels are low in childhood and postmenopause.
- Produced in the adrenal glands, corpus luteum, brain, and placenta.
- Increasing amounts of progesterone are produced during pregnancy.
- Levels are low during the preovulatory phase, increase after ovulation, and remain elevated during the luteal phase.
- Functions include preparing the endometrium for possible implantation or starting the next menstrual cycle.

ENDOMETRIUM

- Endometrial thickness should not exceed 14 mm.
- Thickness of the postmenopausal endometrium without hormone replacement therapy should not exceed 8 mm and is consistently benign when measuring 5 mm or less.
- Fluid within the endometrial cavity is not included in the measurement of the endometrial thickness.

PREMENARCHE

- Time before the onset of menses.
- Follicular cysts may be present.
- Cervix to corpus ratio is 2:1.

PRECOCIOUS PUBERTY

- Early pubic hair, breast, or genital development may result from natural early maturation or from several other conditions.
- Pubic hair or genital enlargement in boys before 9 years.
- Breast development in boys before appearance of pubic hair and testicular enlargement.
- Pubic hair before 8 years or breast development in girls before 7 years.
- Menstruation in girls before 10 years.
- Elevated hormone levels indicate the possible presence of a hypothalamus, gonad, or adrenal gland neoplasm.
- Induces early bone maturation and reduces eventual adult height.
- Uterus and ovaries enlarge.
- Functional ovarian cysts are often present.

MENARCHE

- Onset of menstruation (Fig. 20-1).

FIG. 20-1
Menstrual phase.

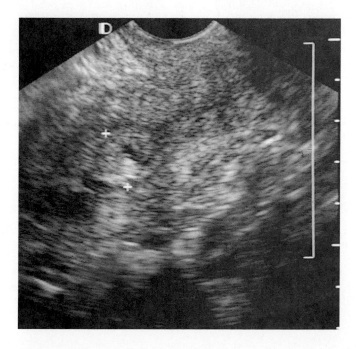

Menstural Phase of the Endometrium

DESCRIPTION	SONOGRAPHIC APPEARANCE
• Menstruation occurs from days 1 to 5 • Functional layer undergoes necrosis from a decrease in hormone levels • Postmenstruation occurs from days 6 to 9	Early Phase • Hypoechoic central line during menstruation measuring 4-8 mm Late Phase • Thin, discrete, hyperechoic line postmenstruation measuring 2-3 mm

Proliferation Phase of the Endometrium

DESCRIPTION	SONOGRAPHIC APPEARANCE
• Proliferation phase overlaps the post menstruation phase and occurs from days 6 to 13 • Increasing estrogen levels regenerates the functional layer • Coincides with the follicular phase of the ovary	Early Phase (Fig. 20-2) • Thin echogenic endometrium in measuring 4-6 mm Late Phase (Fig. 20-3) • A triple-line appearance measuring around 6-10 mm • Thick hypoechoic functional layer and hyperechoic basal layer

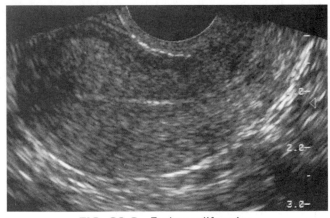

FIG. 20-2   Early proliferation.

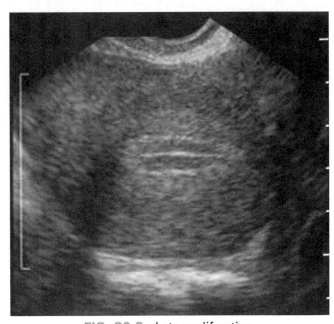

FIG. 20-3   Late proliferation.

Secretory Phase of the Endometrium

DESCRIPTION	SONOGRAPHIC APPEARANCE
• Also known as postovulatory, premenstrual, or luteal phase (Figs. 20-4 and 20-5) • Days 13-28 • Functional layer continues to thicken • Progesterone levels increase	• Functional layer appears hyperechoic • Basal layer appears hypoechoic • May demonstrate posterior acoustic enhancement • Greatest thickness in this phase measuring 7-14 mm

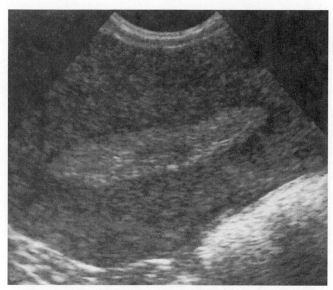

FIG. 20-4   Secretory phase.

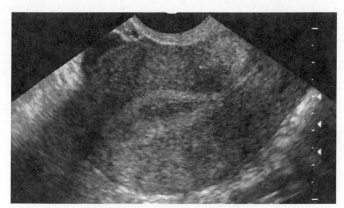

FIG. 20-5   Secretory phase.

OVARIES

- At birth, each ovary contains approximately 200,000 primary follicles.
- Secretion of FSH stimulates follicular development.
- Follicles will fill with fluid and secrete increasing amounts of estrogen.
- Typically, 5 to 11 follicles will begin to develop, with one reaching maturity each cycle.
- 80% of patients will demonstrate a nondominant follicle.
- Visualization of a cumulus oophorus indicates follicular maturity, with ovulation typically occurring within 36 hours.
- Ovulation is regulated by the hypothalamus within the brain.
- LH usually reaches its peak 10 to 12 hours before ovulation.
- A surge in LH accompanied by a smaller FSH surge triggers ovulation.

Follicular Phase of the Ovary

DESCRIPTION	SONOGRAPHIC APPEARANCE
• Begins at the start of menstruation • Ends at ovulation • Variable length but generally 14 days • Between days 5 and 7, a dominant secondary follicle is determined • Dominant follicle will grow 2-3 mm/day • Estrogen levels increase	Early Phase (Fig. 20-6) • Multiple small anechoic functional cysts • 5-11 small follicles typically begin to develop Late Phase (Fig. 20-7) • Graafian follicle reaches 2.0-2.4 cm in diameter prior to ovulation • Visualization of a cumulus oophorus increases the probability that ovulation will occur within the next 36 hours

Ovulatory Phase of the Ovary

DESCRIPTION	SONOGRAPHIC APPEARANCE
• Occurs at the rupture of the graafian follicle (Figs. 20-8 and 20-9) • Pelvic pain increases over the ovulatory ovary (Mittelschmerz)	• Additional nondominant follicles of varying sizes are visualized in 80% of cases • Irregular-shaped cystic structure • Minimal amount of cul de sac fluid

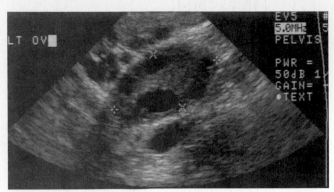

FIG. 20-6   Early follicular.

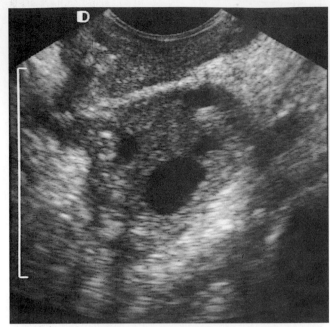

FIG. 20-7   Late follicular.

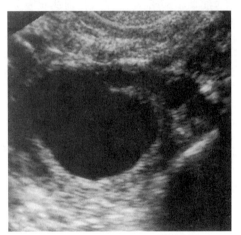

FIG. 20-8   Preovulatory.

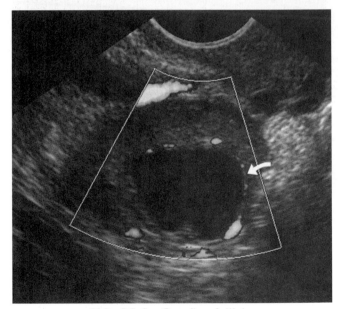

FIG. 20-9   Graafian follicle.

Luteal Phase of the Ovary

DESCRIPTION	SONOGRAPHIC APPEARANCE
• Begins postovulation • Constant 14-day lifespan • Corpus luteum grows for 7-8 days secreting some estrogen and an increasing amount of progesterone • If the ovum is fertilized, the corpus luteum will continue to secrete progesterone • If fertilization does not occur, the corpus luteum regresses and progesterone levels will decrease	• 90% of ruptured follicles will disappear postovulation • Nondominant follicles of varying size • Amount of cul de sac fluid reaches peak volume in the early luteal phase (Fig. 20-10) **Corpus Luteal Cyst** • Small, irregular anechoic structure • Thick, hyperechoic wall margins • May contain internal echoes (hemorrhage) • Cystic mass demonstrates peripheral hypervascularity (ring of fire) (Fig. 20-11)

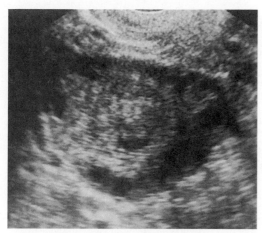

FIG. 20-10 Early luteal.

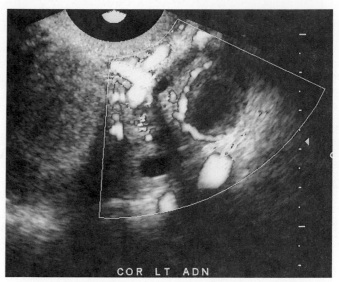

COR LT ADN

FIG. 20-11 Late luteal.

Physiological Ovarian Cysts

NEOPLASM	ETIOLOGY	CLINICAL FINDINGS	SONOGRAPHIC FINDINGS	DIFFERENTIAL CONSIDERATIONS
Corpus luteal cyst	• Formed by the ruptured graafian follicle	• Asymptomatic • Pelvic pain	• Small, irregular cystic ovarian mass • Hyperechoic, thick walls • May contain internal low-level echoes • Hypervascular periphery (ring of fire)	• Ectopic pregnancy
Corpus albicans	• Scar from previous corpus luteum	• Asymptomatic	• Hyperechoic focus within the ovary	• Cystic teratoma
Hemorrhagic cyst	• Rupture of a blood vessel at ovulation	• Severe acute pelvic pain • Nausea/vomiting • Low-grade fever	• Complex echo pattern • Hypoechoic mass • Thin septations may be present	• Ovarian torsion • Cystadenoma • Ectopic pregnancy • Theca lutein cyst
Simple cyst	Premenarche • Follicular in origin resulting from excessive hormones Menarche • Failure of a dominant follicle to rupture Postmenopausal • Follicular in origin	• Asymptomatic • Pelvic pain • Irregular menses	• Anechoic mass • Smooth wall margins • Posterior enhancement • Most measure <5.0 cm and regress with subsequent menses	• Serous cystadenoma • Hydrosalpinx • Bladder diverticulum

POSTMENOPAUSE

- Cessation of menstruation.
- Approximately 15% of cases will demonstrate a simple ovarian cyst.
- Simple ovarian cysts <5.0 cm in diameter are most likely benign.

WITH HORMONE REPLACEMENT THERAPY

- Includes both estrogen and progesterone.
- Endometrium varies in thickness.
- Atrophy of the ovaries is not as prevalent.

WITHOUT HORMONE REPLACEMENT THERAPY

- Uterus generally decreases in length and width.
- Endometrial thickness should not exceed 8 mm.
- Ovaries atrophy and may be difficult to visualize.
- Decreases in estrogen can shorten the vagina and decrease cervical mucus.

CONTRACEPTION

Contraceptive Devices

TYPE OF CONTRACEPTION	DESCRIPTION	SONOGRAPHIC FINDINGS
Oral contraceptives	• Inhibits ovulation and changes endometrial lining and cervical mucus	• Ovulatory phase should not occur • Nondominant follicles may be present • Endometrium appears as a thin echogenic line
Depot-medroxyprogesterone acetate	• Inhibits ovulation and thickens cervical mucus • Intramuscular injection every 3 months	• Ovulatory phase should not occur • Endometrium appears as a thin echogenic line
Levonorgestrel implants	• Inhibits ovulation and thickens cervical mucus • Thin capsule is placed under the skin • Lasts 5 years	• Ovulatory phase should not occur • Endometrium appears as a thin echogenic line
Intrauterine device	• Foreign body is placed in the endometrial cavity at the level of the fundus and superior corpus Risk Factors • Infection • Perforation • Attachment to the basal layer	• Series of hyperechoic linear echoes demonstrating posterior acoustic shadowing • Should be located in the center of the endometrial cavity • Ovulation and formation of a corpus luteum continue

PHYSIOLOGY OF THE FEMALE PELVIS REVIEW

1. Progesterone levels increase in the:
   a. secretory phase
   b. follicular phase
   c. ovulatory phase
   d. menstrual phase
   e. periovulatory phase

2. Which of the following endometrial phases demonstrates the thinnest dimension?
   a. late secretory
   b. early menstrual
   c. early secretory
   d. late proliferation
   e. early proliferation

3. Which of the following hormones reflects the activity of the ovaries?
   a. estriol
   b. estradiol
   c. progesterone
   d. luteinizing hormone
   e. follicle-stimulating hormone

4. An asymptomatic postmenopausal patient displays a 3.0-cm simple ovarian cyst. This finding is considered:
   a. rare
   b. benign
   c. serious
   d. emergent
   e. malignant

5. If fertilization does not occur, the corpus luteum will:
   a. decrease in size and estrogen levels will increase
   b. increase in size and estrogen levels will decrease
   c. increase in size and progesterone levels will increase
   d. decrease in size and progesterone levels will decrease
   e. increase in size and progesterone levels will decrease

6. The endometrium is generally thinnest between days:
   a. 1-5
   b. 6-9
   c. 10-14
   d. 14-21
   e. 21-28

7. A hyperechoic focus within a mature follicle most likely represents a:
   a. morula
   b. follicle
   c. cumulus
   d. blastocyst
   e. corpus albicans

8. Visualization of a corpus luteal cyst indicates:
   a. ovulation is imminent
   b. ovulation has occurred
   c. fertilization has occurred
   d. ovulatory hemorrhage has occurred
   e. an imbalance in reproductive hormones

9. Which ovarian phase has a constant lifespan?
   a. luteal
   b. follicular
   c. menstrual
   d. proliferation
   e. periovulatory

10. Luteinizing hormone is secreted by the:
    a. ovary
    b. hypothalamus
    c. thyroid gland
    d. adrenal gland
    e. pituitary gland

11. Which of the following structures produces small amounts of estrogen?
    a. lung
    b. spleen
    c. kidney
    d. pancreas
    e. adrenal gland

12. Which of the following hormones stimulates ovulation?
    a. estrogen
    b. estradiol
    c. progesterone
    d. luteinizing hormone
    e. follicle-stimulating hormone

13. Fluid within the endometrial cavity is:
    a. produced by the corpus luteum
    b. produced by the granulosa cells
    c. suspicious for endometrial hyperplasia
    d. not included in the endometrial measurement
    e. highly suspicious for endometrial malignancy

14. Mittelschmerz is associated with:
    a. pregnancy
    b. ovulation
    c. hemorrhage
    d. menopause
    e. menstruation

15. Hyperstimulation of the ovaries will likely result in:
    a. theca lutein cysts
    b. polycystic disease
    c. corpus luteal cysts
    d. hemorrhagic cysts
    e. surface epithelial cysts

Using Fig. 20-12, answer questions 16 and 17.

16. A patient presents with a history of intermittent lower quadrant pain. Her last menstrual period was 1 week prior and she denies the use of hormone contraceptives. On the basis of this clinical history, the anechoic areas most likely represent:
    a. simple cysts
    b. corpus albicans
    c. functional cysts
    d. graafian follicles
    e. corpus luteal cysts

17. Hyperechoic foci within the ovary are most suspicious for:
    a. corpus luteum
    b. cystic teratoma
    c. corpus albicans
    d. hemorrhagic cysts
    e. cumulus oophorus

Using Fig. 20-13, answer question 18.

18. Which endometrial phase is most likely demonstrated in this endovaginal sonogram?
    a. luteal
    b. secretory
    c. follicular
    d. menstrual
    e. proliferative

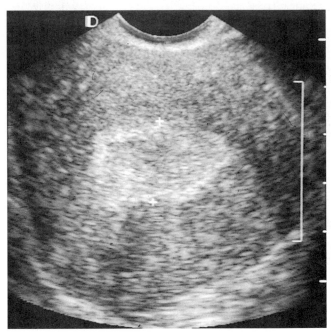

FIG. 20-13 Endovaginal sonogram.

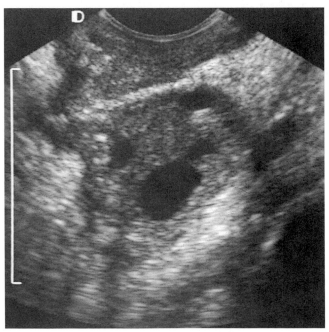

FIG. 20-12 Sonogram of the ovary.

Using Fig. 20-14, answer question 19.

19. A patient presents with a history of right lower quadrant pain. Her last menstrual period was 7 days ago. She denies contraceptive hormone therapy. On the basis of this clinical history, the anechoic mass most likely represents a:
    a. simple cyst
    b. graafian follicle
    c. corpus luteal cyst
    d. serous cystadenoma
    e. peritoneal inclusion cyst

Using Fig. 20-15, answer question 20.

20. The ovaries in this sonogram coincide with which of the following ovarian phases?
    a. ovulatory
    b. late luteal
    c. early luteal
    d. late proliferation
    e. early proliferation

Using Fig. 20-16, answer question 21.

21. Which of the following endometrial phases is most likely displayed in this sagittal sonogram of the uterus?
    a. late secretory
    b. early menstrual
    c. early secretory
    d. late proliferative
    e. early proliferative

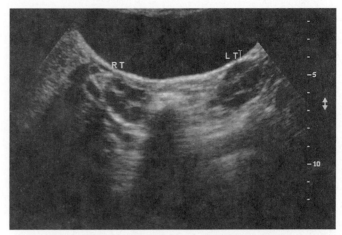

FIG. 20-15   Transabdominal sonogram.

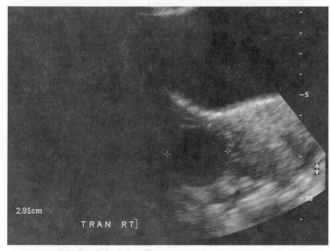

FIG. 20-14   Transverse sonogram.

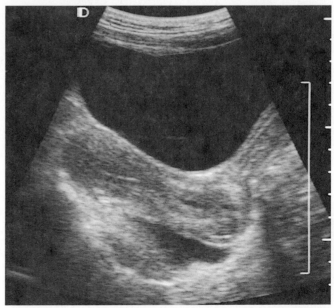

FIG. 20-16   Sagittal sonogram.

322   PART III   Obstetrics and Gynecology

Using Fig. 20-17, answer question 22.

22. A patient presents with a history of irregular menses. A transabdominal sonogram of the uterus demonstrates:
    a. endometritis
    b. Asherman syndrome
    c. the late menstrual phase
    d. endometrial hyperplasia
    e. an intrauterine contraceptive device

Using Fig. 20-18, answer question 23.

23. A patient presents with severe right lower quadrant pain for the last 2 days and a negative pregnancy test. Her last menstrual period was approximately 2 weeks ago. She denies any history of endometriosis. On the basis of this clinical history, the sonographic finding is most suspicious for a(n):
    a. endometrioma
    b. cystic teratoma
    c. graafian follicle
    d. hemorrhagic cyst
    e. serous cystadenoma

Using Fig. 20-19, answer questions 24 and 25.

24. A 25-year-old patient presents with an 18-mm anechoic ovarian mass. This is most consistent with a:
    a. simple cyst
    b. corpus luteum
    c. graafian follicle
    d. corpus albicans
    e. serous cystadenoma

25. The echogenic focus demonstrated on the posterior wall just anterior to the caliper is most suspicious for:
    a. hemorrhage
    b. malignancy
    c. blood vessel
    d. serous debris
    e. cumulus oophorus

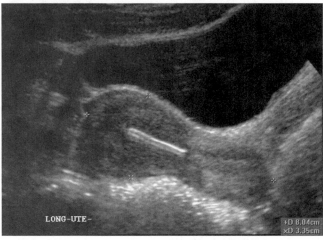

FIG. 20-17   Transabdominal sonogram.

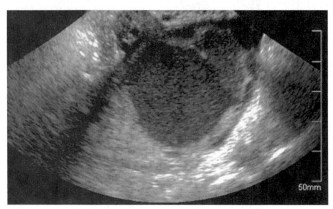

FIG. 20-18   Sagittal sonogram.

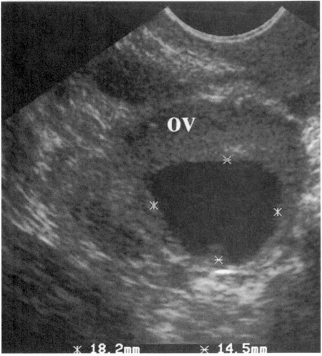

FIG. 20-19   Sonogram of the right ovary.

Using Fig. 20-20, answer questions 26 and 27.

26. Which of the following endometrial phases is most likely displayed in this sagittal sonogram?
    a. early luteal
    b. late secretory
    c. late follicular
    d. early menstrual
    e. late proliferation

27. The sonographic appearance of this endometrium is termed:
    a. shotgun sign
    b. junctional zones
    c. decidual reaction
    d. triple-line pattern
    e. double decidua sign

Using Fig. 20-21 (and color plate 8), answer question 28.

28. A 28-year-old patient presents with a sudden onset of right lower quadrant pain. Her last menstrual period was approximately 3 weeks ago. A duplex sonogram demonstrates a hypoechoic ovarian mass (arrow) with peripheral blood flow. This is most suspicious for a(n):
    a. endometrioma
    b. graafian follicle
    c. ectopic pregnancy
    d. corpus luteal cyst
    e. nondominant follicle

Using Fig. 20-22, answer question 29.

29. A patient presents with a family history of ovarian carcinoma. The endometrial phase in this patient is most consistent with:
    a. late secretory
    b. late menstrual
    c. early secretory
    d. early menstrual
    e. late proliferation

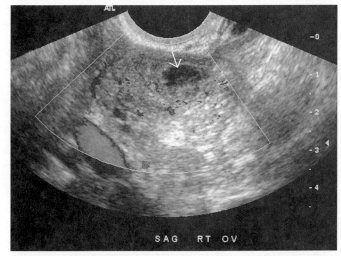

FIG. 20-21 Endovaginal sonogram (see color plate 8).

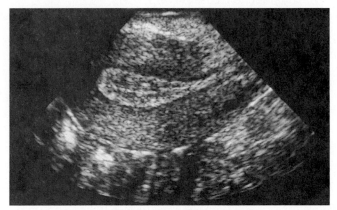

FIG. 20-20 Sagittal sonogram.

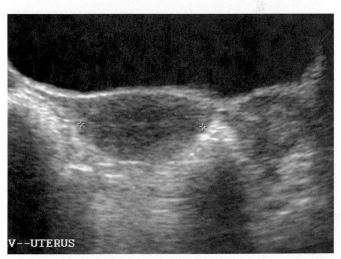

FIG. 20-22 Transverse sonogram.

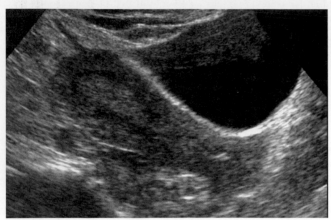

FIG. 20-23   Transabdominal sonogram.

Using Fig. 20-23, answer question 30.

30. Which of the following ovarian masses will most likely coincide with this endometrial phase?
   a. simple cyst
   b. corpus albicans
   c. graafian follicle
   d. theca lutein cyst
   e. corpus luteal cyst

31. A patient complains of heavy menstrual cycles. This is most consistent with:
   a. menoxenia
   b. amenorrhea
   c. dyspareunia
   d. menorrhagia
   e. dysmenorrhea

32. Levels of follicle-stimulating hormone begin declining in the:
   a. late luteal phase
   b. late secretory phase
   c. late follicular phase
   d. early secretory phase
   e. early follicular phase

33. During the ovulatory phase, normal estradiol levels range between:
   a. 10 and 50 pg/mL
   b. 50 and 100 pg/mL
   c. 10 and 200 pg/mL
   d. 100 and 200 pg/mL
   e. 200 and 400 pg/mL

34. Which of the following ovarian phases coincides with the proliferation phase of the endometrium?
   a. luteal
   b. secretory
   c. follicular
   d. ovulatory
   e. menstrual

35. The endometrial cavity in patients using hormone contraceptive therapy appears on ultrasound as a:
   a. thin, anechoic linear structure
   b. thin, echogenic linear structure
   c. thin, hypoechoic linear structure
   d. thick, hypoechoic linear structure
   e. thick, hyperechoic linear structure

36. Thickness of the normal postmenopausal endometrium denying hormone replacement therapy should not exceed:
   a. 2 mm
   b. 4 mm
   c. 8 mm
   d. 10 mm
   e. 14 mm

37. Which of the following hormone levels can be slightly higher after menopause?
   a. estrogen
   b. estradiol
   c. progesterone
   d. luteinizing hormone
   e. follicle-stimulating hormone

38. Which of the following describe the sonographic appearance of the endometrium during the late proliferation phase?
   a. thick, hyperechoic functional layer and a hyperechoic basal layer
   b. thin, hyperechoic functional layer and a hypoechoic basal layer
   c. thin, hypoechoic functional layer and a hyperechoic basal layer
   d. thick, hyperechoic functional layer and a hypoechoic basal layer
   e. thick, hypoechoic functional layer and a hyperechoic basal layer

39. Acute pelvic pain during the periovulatory phase is termed:
   a. Meckel sign
   b. Murphy sign
   c. Mittelschmerz
   d. McBurney sign
   e. Tip of the Iceberg

40. Which of the following hormones help to prepare the endometrium for implantation of the blastocyst?
   a. estrogen
   b. estradiol
   c. testosterone
   d. progesterone
   e. luteinizing hormone

41. Estrogen is primarily secreted by the:
   a. thyroid glands
   b. corpus luteum
   c. pituitary gland
   d. corpus albicans
   e. graafian follicle

42. The length of a normal menstrual cycle ranges between:
   a. 14 and 28 days
   b. 21 and 28 days
   c. 21 and 35 days
   d. 28 and 35 days
   e. 28 and 40 days

43. An early onset of puberty may be the result of a(n):
   a. renal neoplasm
   b. hepatic neoplasm
   c. ovarian neoplasm
   d. thyroid gland neoplasm
   e. pituitary gland neoplasm

44. Regeneration of the endometrium occurs as a result of:
   a. increases in estrogen levels
   b. decreases in estrogen levels
   c. increases in progesterone levels
   d. decreases in progesterone levels
   e. increases in luteinizing hormone

45. The endometrium displays the greatest thickness during the:
   a. follicular phase
   b. secretory phase
   c. menstrual phase
   d. ovulatory phase
   e. proliferation phase

46. An adolescent patient presents with a history of severe acute right lower quadrant pain. Her last menstrual period was 2 to 3 weeks prior. A hypoechoic ovarian mass is identified on ultrasound. On the basis of this clinical history, the sonographic findings are most suspicious for a(n):
   a. endometrioma
   b. cystic teratoma
   c. corpus albicans
   d. graafian follicle
   e. hemorrhagic cyst

47. If fertilization occurs, the corpus luteum will continue to secrete:
   a. estrogen
   b. estradiol
   c. progesterone
   d. luteinizing hormone
   e. human chorionic gonadotropin

48. Which of the following describes the expected appearance of the endometrium in a patient using oral contraceptives?
   a. thin echogenic line
   b. thin hypoechoic line
   c. triple-line appearance
   d. thick and hyperechoic
   e. thick and hypoechoic

49. Approximately 15% of postmenopausal patients will exhibit a(n):
   a. hydrosalpinx
   b. endometrioma
   c. hemorrhagic cyst
   d. simple ovarian cyst
   e. ovarian malignancy

50. Decreases in estrogen in postmenopausal patients can decrease cervical mucus and:
   a. shorten vaginal length
   b. increase cervical length
   c. thicken the vaginal walls
   d. increase the size of the uterus
   e. thicken the endometrial cavity

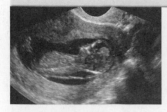

CHAPTER 21

Uterine and
Ovarian Pathology

KEY TERMS

adenomyosis benign invasive growth of endometrium into the myometrium.

Asherman syndrome intrauterine adhesions ablating the endometrial lining.

Gartner duct cyst small cyst within the vagina.

hematocolpos blood accumulation in the vagina.

hematometra blood accumulation in the uterus.

hematometrocolpos blood accumulation in the uterus and vagina.

hyperplasia proliferation of the endometrial lining.

intramural leiomyoma mass distorting the myometrium; most common location.

leiomyoma most common benign tumor of the myometrium.

Meigs syndrome combination of pleural effusion, ascites, and an ovarian mass that resolve after surgery.

submucosal leiomyoma mass distorting the endometrium; least common but most likely to cause symptoms.

subserosal leiomyoma mass found on the serosal surface of the uterus.

tamoxifen antiestrogen medication used in treating breast cancer.

Tip of the Iceberg a term used to describe the sonographic appearance of a dense ovarian dermoid tumor.

Descriptive Terms for Pelvic Pathology

MASS CHARACTERISTIC	DESCRIPTIVE TERMS
Overall composition	• Anechoic, echogenic, complex • Hypoechoic, hyperechoic • Homogenous, heterogeneous
Internal characteristics	• Unilocular, multilocular • Fluid—fluid levels • Mural nodules, internal debris
Wall definition	• Thin, thick • Smooth, irregular • Well defined, ill defined
Doppler characteristics	• Lack of vascular flow • Hypervascular, hypovascular • High resistance, low resistance

UTERINE PATHOLOGY

- Intramural leiomyomas are the most common uterine neoplasm.

Pathology of the Cervix

PATHOLOGY	ETIOLOGY	CLINICAL FINDINGS	SONOGRAPHIC FINDINGS	DIFFERENTIAL CONSIDERATIONS
Carcinoma	• Epithelial neoplasm Risk Factors • Early sexual activity • Multiple sex partners • Herpes simplex II	• Vaginal discharge or bleeding • Palpable mass • Weight loss	• Hypoechoic or heterogeneous retrovesical mass • Irregular margins • Hydroureter • Hydronephrosis	• Leiomyoma • Complex cervical cyst • Ovarian mass
Nabothian cyst	• Obstructed inclusion cyst(s) • Chronic cervicitis	• Asymptomatic	• Round, anechoic structure • Multiple or solitary • Usually <2.0 cm in diameter • May contain internal echoes • Posterior enhancement	• Leiomyoma • Arcuate vessel • Retained products of conception

Pathology of the Uterus

PATHOLOGY	ETIOLOGY	CLINICAL FINDINGS	SONOGRAPHIC FINDINGS	DIFFERENTIAL CONSIDERATIONS
Adenomyosis	• Ectopic endometrial tissue within the myometrium Risk Factors • Multiparity • Elevated estrogen • Aggressive curettage	• Pelvic pain or cramping • Uterine enlargement and tenderness on physical exam • Menorrhagia • Dysmenorrhea	• Diffuse uterine enlargement • Inhomogeneous myometrium • Poorly defined anechoic areas within the myometrium • Endometrium appears normal	• Degenerating fibroid • Endometrial neoplasm
Leiomyoma Also called fibroid **Intramural** • Distorts the myometrium **Pedunculated** • Attached to the uterus by a stalk **Submucosal** • Distorts the endometrium **Subserosal** • Located under the perimetrium	• Benign neoplasm of the uterine myometrium	• Asymptomatic • Menorrhagia • Pelvic pain • Uterine enlargement • Irregular menses • Urinary frequency • Infertility	• Well-defined hypoechoic uterine mass • Range from anechoic to hyperechoic • Heterogeneous with associated necrosis or hemorrhage • Often multiple • Diffuse uterine enlargement • May increase in size with estrogen stimulation • May decrease in size after menopause	• Ovarian neoplasm • Leiomyosarcoma
Leiomyosarcoma	• Derived from the smooth muscle of the uterus	• Asymptomatic • Vaginal bleeding	• Heterogeneous uterine mass • Irregular margins	• Leiomyoma • Endometrial carcinoma

Endometrial Abnormalities

ABNORMALITY	ETIOLOGY	CLINICAL FINDINGS	SONOGRAPHIC FINDINGS	DIFFERENTIAL CONSIDERATIONS
Asherman syndrome	• Adhesions from a prior deep curettage or endometrial infection	• Asymptomatic • Amenorrhea • Dysmenorrhea • Hypomenorrhea • Infertility	• Inability to distinguish an endometrial cavity • Bright echoes within the endometrial cavity	• Normal early proliferative phase • Uterine mass compressing endometrial cavity
Carcinoma	• Unknown • Associated with estrogen stimulation • Adenocarcinoma is most common Risk Factors • Obesity • Diabetes • Nulliparity • Postmenopause	• Abnormal bleeding	• Focal irregularity of the endometrium • Myometrial distortion • Thickened endometrium • Complex endometrial mass	• Endometrial hyperplasia • Endometrial polyp
Endometritis	• Pelvic inflammatory disease • Retained products of conception • Postprocedural complication • Vaginitis	• Pelvic pain • Fever • Leukocytosis	• Normal findings • Thick and irregular endometrium • Pronounced endometrium • Enlarged, inhomogeneous uterus • Hypervascular endometrium and myometrium	• Normal uterus • Adenomyosis • Leiomyoma
Hematometra	• Imperforated hymen • Cervical stenosis • Vagina neoplasm	• Pelvic pain • Amenorrhea • Hypomenorrhea • Pelvic mass	• Large hypoechoic midline uterine mass • Posterior enhancement • Minimal or lack of visible myometrial tissue	• Submucosal leiomyoma • Endometrioma • Retained products of conception
Hyperplasia	• Unopposed estrogen • Tamoxifen therapy	• Abnormal bleeding • Asymptomatic	• Prominent thickening of the endometrium • Premenopausal thickness >14 mm • Postmenopausal thickness >8 mm	• Endometrial carcinoma • Endometrial polyp
Polyp	• Overgrowth of endometrial tissue • Unresponsive to progesterone	• Asymptomatic • Abnormal bleeding • Infertility	• Focal areas of echogenic endometrial thickening • Hypoechoic mass within the endometrial cavity • Round or ovoid echogenic mass within the endometrial cavity	• Endometrial carcinoma • Endometrial hyperplasia • Submucosal leiomyoma
Tamoxifen effect	• Side effects of tamoxifen therapy	• Asymptomatic • Abnormal bleeding	• Normal-appearing endometrium • Thickening of the endometrial cavity • Complex appearance to the endometrial cavity	• Endometrial hyperplasia • Endometrial polyp • Endometrial carcinoma • Submucosal leiomyoma

OVARIAN PATHOLOGY

- The majority of ovarian masses removed from premenopausal patients are benign.
- Cystic teratoma (dermoid) is the most common primary ovarian neoplasm.

Cystic Ovarian Pathology

PATHOLOGY	ETIOLOGY	CLINICAL FINDINGS	SONOGRAPHIC FINDINGS	DIFFERENTIAL CONSIDERATIONS
Cystadenocarcinoma	• Epithelial neoplasm	• Palpable pelvic mass • Unexplained weight gain • Pelvic pain	• Multilocular, complex mass • Ill-defined wall margins • Mural nodules • Ascites	• Cystadenoma • Cystic teratoma • Tubo-ovarian abscess
Cystic teratoma Also called dermoid	• Arises from the wall of a follicle • Germ cell tumor • Contains fat, hair, skin, and teeth	• Asymptomatic • Abdominal pressure • Mild to acute pelvic pain • Palpable pelvic mass	• "Tip of the Iceberg"—solid mass with diffusely bright internal echoes with or without shadowing • Complex mass • Thick, irregular margins • Calcifications • Commonly located superior to the uterine fundus	• Endometrioma • Hemorrhagic cyst • Serous cystadenoma • Ectopic pregnancy
Mucinous cystadenoma	• Epithelial neoplasm	• Pelvic pain • Rapid increase in pelvic mass • Irregular menses	• Multilocular anechoic mass • Thick, smooth wall margins • May contain debris	• Endometrioma • Tubo-ovarian abscess • Theca lutein cyst • Cystadenocarcinoma
Polycystic ovarian disease	• Endocrine imbalance causing chronic anovulation	• Irregular menses • Hirsutism • Infertility • Obesity	• Round, enlarged ovaries • Presence of ten or more follicles per ovary • Multiple, small peripheral cysts	• Functional cysts
Serous cystadenoma	• Epithelial neoplasm	• Rapid increase of a pelvic mass • Pelvic pain • Irregular menses	• Large unilocular or multilocular anechoic mass • Smooth, thin-walled margins • May contain internal debris and septae • Unilateral (70%)	• Hydrosalpinx • Theca lutein cysts
Surface epithelial cyst	• Arise from the cortex of the ovary	• Asymptomatic • Pelvic pain	• Small cluster of cysts	• Polycystic ovarian disease • Cystadenoma
Theca lutein cysts	• High level of hCG	• Asymptomatic • Hyperemesis • Abdominal bloating	• Multilocular cystic structure • Bilateral condition	• Cystadenoma • Hydrosalpinx

Solid Ovarian Neoplasms

NEOPLASM	ETIOLOGY	CLINICAL FINDINGS	SONOGRAPHIC FINDINGS	DIFFERENTIAL CONSIDERATIONS
Brenner tumor	• Benign tumor arising from fibroepithelial tissue • Estrogenic in nature	• Asymptomatic • Unilateral pelvic pain or fullness • Associated with Meigs syndrome	• Small, hyperechoic, solid ovarian mass • Well-defined wall margins • Does *not* demonstrate posterior acoustic enhancement • May demonstrate necrosis	• Fibroma • Pedunculated fibroid • Thecoma

Continued

Solid Ovarian Neoplasms—cont'd

NEOPLASM	ETIOLOGY	CLINICAL FINDINGS	SONOGRAPHIC FINDINGS	DIFFERENTIAL CONSIDERATIONS
Carcinoma	• Epithelial or germ cell neoplasm Risk Factors • High fat diet • Infertility • Nulliparity • Family history of breast or ovarian carcinoma	• Asymptomatic • Vague abdominal pain • Palpable pelvic mass • Elevated CA125 • Vague GI symptoms	• Predominantly solid, hypoechoic ovarian mass • Irregular ovarian margins • May appear complex • Internal blood flow • Resistive index <1.0 suggests malignancy	• Endometrioma • Metastatic lesion • Granulosa cell tumor
Dysgerminoma	• Malignant germ cell neoplasm • Most common ovarian malignancy in childhood	• Asymptomatic • Precocious puberty • Pelvic pain • Palpable pelvic mass • Associated with AFP and hCG levels • Spreads to the lymphatics	• Predominantly solid, homogeneous mass • Irregular margins • May appear complex • Lymphadenopathy • Unilateral (90%)	• Cystadenocarcinoma • Metastatic lesion
Fibroma	• Rare, benign stromal tumor	• Asymptomatic • Pelvic pain or fullness • Urinary or intestinal disturbance • Menopause	• Solid, hyperechoic adnexal mass • Dense mass • May demonstrate posterior shadowing • Ascites • 5-10 cm in size • Unilateral (90%)	• Pedunculated fibroid • Teratoma • Thecoma • Brenner tumor
Granulosa cell tumor	• Hormonal tumor	• Increase in estrogen • Palpable mass • Irregular bleeding	• Solid, homogeneous adnexal mass • May appear complex • Thickening of the endometrium	• Pedunculated fibroid
Thecoma	• Benign stromal tumor	• Pelvic pain or pressure • Menopause	• Hyperechoic mass • Prominent posterior shadowing	• Fibroma • Teratoma • Brenner tumor

Miscellaneous Ovarian Abnormalities

ABNORMALITY	ETIOLOGY	CLINICAL FINDINGS	SONOGRAPHIC FINDINGS	DIFFERENTIAL CONSIDERATIONS
Ovarian torsion	• Partial or complete rotation of the ovary on its pedicle • Commonly associated with an adnexal mass	• Severe or consistent pelvic pain • Nausea/vomiting • Palpable pelvic mass	• Decreased or absent blood flow to the ovary • Large, heterogeneous ovarian mass • Free fluid • Coexisting adnexal mass	• Normal ovary • Hemorrhagic cyst • Cystic teratoma

UTERINE AND OVARIAN PATHOLOGY REVIEW

1. Abnormal accumulation of blood within the vagina is termed:
   a. hydrometra
   b. hematometra
   c. hydrocolpos
   d. hematocolpos
   e. hematometrocolpos

2. Risk factors associated with developing endometrial carcinoma include:
   a. anorexia, multiparity, hypertension
   b. obesity, diabetes mellitus, nulliparity
   c. hypertension, obesity, thyroid disease
   d. oral contraceptives, hypertension, diabetes mellitus
   e. multiparity, thyroid disease, hormone replacement therapy

3. Hypervascularity within the endometrium is a characteristic finding in:
   a. endometritis
   b. adenomyosis
   c. endometriosis
   d. Asherman syndrome
   e. endometrial hyperplasia

4. The most common ovarian malignancy occurring in childhood is a:
   a. fibroma
   b. thecoma
   c. dysgerminoma
   d. Brenner tumor
   e. granulosa cell tumor

5. Which of the following is a common clinical symptom associated with adenomyosis?
   a. amenorrhea
   b. mittelschmerz
   c. lower back pain
   d. urinary frequency
   e. uterine tenderness

6. A 50-year-old patient presents with a history of abdominal distention. In the left adnexa, a 10-cm, multilocular mass is identified. This mass most likely represents:
   a. a cystadenoma
   b. a cystic teratoma
   c. theca lutein cysts
   d. polycystic disease
   e. surface epithelial cysts

7. The most common location for a uterine leiomyoma to develop is:
   a. serosal
   b. subserosal
   c. intramural
   d. submucosal
   e. pedunculated

8. Inability to distinguish the endometrial cavity is an identifiable sonographic finding in:
   a. infertility
   b. endometritis
   c. tamoxifen therapy
   d. Asherman syndrome
   e. polycystic ovarian disease

9. Ovarian torsion is commonly associated with a coexisting:
   a. uterine mass
   b. hydrosalpinx
   c. adnexal mass
   d. nabothian cyst
   e. ectopic pregnancy

10. Tamoxifen therapy is most likely to affect which of the following structures?
    a. cervix
    b. ovaries
    c. myometrium
    d. endometrium
    e. fallopian tubes

11. A reproductive-age patient demonstrates a complex adnexal mass with diffusely bright internal echoes. These sonographic findings most likely describe a:
    a. dysgerminoma
    b. cystic teratoma
    c. hemorrhagic cyst
    d. theca lutein cysts
    e. cystadenocarcinoma

12. The most common location of a cystic teratoma is:
    a. lateral to the cervix
    b. medial to the cornua
    c. anterior to the fundus
    d. superior to the fundus
    e. adjacent to the isthmus

13. Obstruction of an inclusion cyst results in a(n):
    a. nabothian cyst
    b. cystic teratoma
    c. endometrial polyp
    d. corpus luteum cyst
    e. serous cystadenoma

14. Which location is a fibroid most likely to cause irregular uterine bleeding?
    a. cervical
    b. subserosal
    c. intramural
    d. submucosal
    e. pedunculated

15. Polycystic ovarian disease can result from:
    a. high levels of hCG
    b. unopposed estrogen
    c. an endocrine imbalance
    d. unopposed progesterone
    e. follicular hyperstimulation

Using Fig. 21-1, answer question 16.

16. An asymptomatic 60-year-old patient presents with a history of breast cancer. She has been treated with tamoxifen therapy for the last 3 years. On the basis of this clinical history, the sonographic findings are most suspicious for:
    a. a leiomyoma
    b. adenomyosis
    c. endometriosis
    d. Asherman syndrome
    e. an endometrial polyp

Using Fig. 21-2, answer question 17.

17. A premenarcheal 13-year-old presents with a history of abdominal pain and a palpable pelvic mass. On the basis of this clinical history, the sonographic findings are most suspicious for:
    a. adenomyosis
    b. hematometra
    c. hematocolpos
    d. endometrioma
    e. hemorrhagic cyst

Using Fig. 21-3, answer questions 18 and 19.

18. A 35-year-old patient presents with a history of urinary frequency and normal menstrual cycles. She denies any history of urinary tract infection or trauma. A sagittal image of the uterus demonstrates a hypoechoic mass (arrows). On the basis of this clinical history, the mass most likely represents a:
    a. hematoma
    b. leiomyoma
    c. cystic teratoma
    d. bicornuate uterus
    e. mucinous cystadenoma

19. Free fluid is identified in which of the following pelvic recesses?
    a. prevesical space
    b. retropubic space
    c. right colic gutter
    d. retrouterine space
    e. vesicouterine space

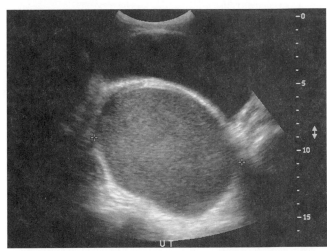

FIG. 21-2 Transabdominal sonogram of the uterus.

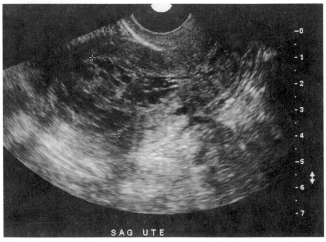

FIG. 21-1 Endovaginal sonogram of the uterus.

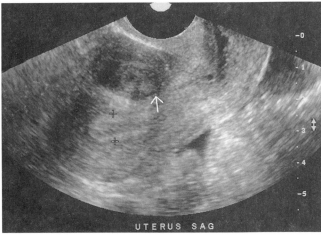

FIG. 21-3 Endovaginal sonogram.

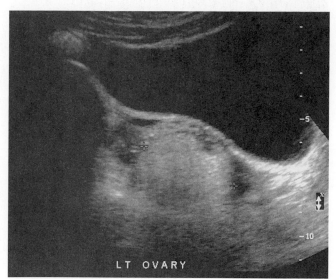

FIG. 21-4 Transabdominal sonogram of the left ovary.

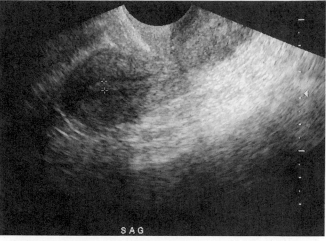

FIG. 21-5 Sagittal sonogram of the uterus.

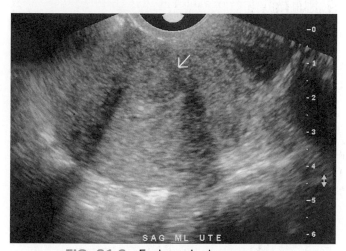

FIG. 21-6 Endovaginal sonogram.

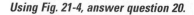

Using Fig. 21-4, answer question 20.

20. A 30-year-old patient presents with a history of mild pelvic pain for the last year. Her last menstrual period was 2 weeks ago. She denies a history of hormone contraceptive therapy or possibility of pregnancy. On the basis of this clinical history, the sonographic findings are most suspicious for:
    a. endometrioma
    b. cystic teratoma
    c. hemorrhagic cyst
    d. ovarian carcinoma
    e. tubo-ovarian abscess

Using Fig. 21-5, answer questions 21 and 22.

21. This sagittal sonogram is most likely displaying:
    a. a cervical mass
    b. a nabothian cyst
    c. uterine didelphys
    d. a bicornuate uterus
    e. endometrial hyperplasia

22. Which of the following is a clinical symptom associated with this finding?
    a. menorrhagia
    b. dysmenorrhea
    c. pelvic fullness
    d. spontaneous abortion
    e. postmenopausal bleeding

Using Fig. 21-6, answer questions 23 and 24.

23. A sagittal image of the uterus reveals a small isoechoic mass identified by the arrow. This mass is most suspicious for:
    a. leiomyoma
    b. adenomyosis
    c. endometrioma
    d. endometrial polyp
    e. endometrial carcinoma

24. Which clinical finding is most likely associated with this pathology?
    a. amenorrhea
    b. menorrhagia
    c. dysmenorrhea
    d. vaginal discharge
    e. postmenopausal bleeding

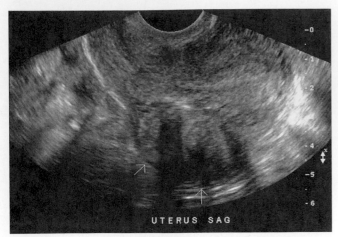

FIG. 21-7 Endovaginal sonogram.

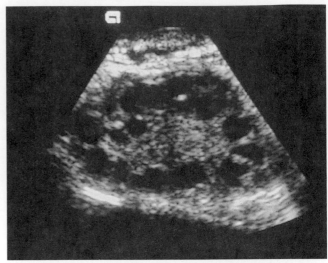

FIG. 21-8 Sonogram of the right ovary.

Using Fig. 21-7, answer questions 25 and 26.

25. An asymptomatic patient presents with a history of an enlarged uterus. On the basis of this clinical history, the pathology demonstrated most likely represents a(n):
    a. endometrioma
    b. ectopic pregnancy
    c. subserosal fibroids
    d. intramural fibroids
    e. submucosal fibroids

26. This abnormality is located on the:
    a. posterior surface of an anteflexed uterus
    b. anterior surface of a retroverted uterus
    c. posterior surface of a retroverted uterus
    d. anterior surface of a retroflexed uterus
    e. posterior surface of an anteverted uterus

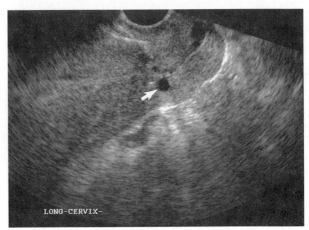

FIG. 21-9 Endovaginal sonogram.

Using Fig. 21-8, answer questions 27 and 28.

27. The sonographic findings are most suspicious for which of the following pathologies?
    a. theca lutein cysts
    b. surface epithelial cysts
    c. polycystic ovarian disease
    d. overstimulation syndrome
    e. normal physiological cysts

28. Which of the following is a common symptom associated with this pathology?
    a. pelvic pain
    b. dysmenorrhea
    c. irregular menses
    d. nausea and vomiting
    e. abdominal distention

Using Fig. 21-9, answer question 29.

29. An asymptomatic patient presents with a history of an enlarged uterus on physical exam. A sagittal image of the uterus is most likely displaying a(n):
    a. abscess
    b. nabothian cyst
    c. endometrial polyp
    d. cervical malignancy
    e. degenerating leiomyoma

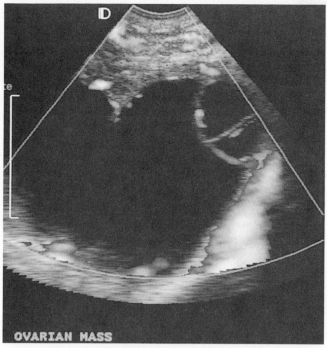

FIG. 21-10 Sonogram of the left adnexa.

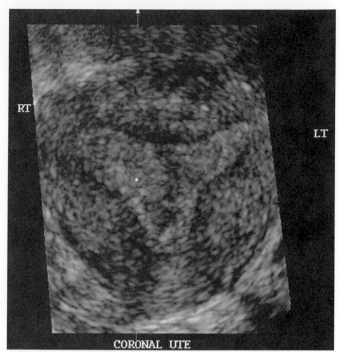

FIG. 21-11 Coronal sonogram of the uterus.

Using Fig. 21-10, answer question 30.

30. A patient presents with a history of irregular menses and a large pelvic mass. On the basis of this clinical history, the sonographic finding is most suspicious for:
a. a cystic teratoma
b. surface epithelial cyst
c. a mucinous cystadenoma
d. polycystic ovarian disease
e. overstimulation syndrome

Using Fig. 21-11, answer question 31.

31. A 35-year-old patient presents with a history of infertility. Her last menstrual period was 3 weeks ago. A coronal image of the uterus reveals a:
a. bicornuate uterus
b. myometrial mass
c. hypoechoic endometrial mass
d. hyperechoic endometrial mass
e. normal-appearing endometrial cavity

32. Which of the following describe the typical sonographic appearance of Asherman syndrome?
a. diffuse uterine enlargement
b. large hypoechoic intrauterine mass
c. discrete hypoechoic myometrial mass
d. inability to distinguish an endometrial cavity
e. hypoechoic irregularity to the endometrial cavity

33. A coexisting adnexal mass is commonly associated with which of the following ovarian pathologies?
a. cystadenoma
b. dysgerminoma
c. cystic teratoma
d. ovarian torsion
e. cystadenocarcinoma

34. Hirsutism is a clinical symptom of:
a. endometriosis
b. hematometrocolpos
c. Asherman syndrome
d. polycystic ovarian disease
e. pelvic inflammatory disease

35. A rapid increasing pelvic mass is most suspicious for a(n):
a. leiomyoma
b. cystadenoma
c. endometrioma
d. dysgerminoma
e. cystic teratoma

36. A small cluster of ovarian cysts is a common sonographic finding associated with:
a. ovarian torsion
b. theca lutein cysts
c. cystadenocarcinoma
d. surface epithelial cysts
e. polycystic ovarian disease

37. Which of the following fibroid locations is most likely to cause menorrhagia?
    a. cornual
    b. intramural
    c. subserosal
    d. submucosal
    e. pedunculated

38. Which of the following structures regulates ovulation?
    a. ovary
    b. thyroid gland
    c. adrenal gland
    d. pituitary gland
    e. hypothalamus

39. The endometrium may demonstrate posterior acoustic enhancement in which of the following phases?
    a. ovulatory
    b. secretory
    c. follicular
    d. menstrual
    e. proliferation

40. Sonographic appearance of ovarian carcinoma is generally described as a(n):
    a. irregular hypoechoic ovarian mass
    b. smooth hyperechoic ovarian mass
    c. irregular hypoechoic adnexal mass
    d. smooth hypoechoic adnexal mass
    e. irregular hyperechoic ovarian mass

41. If a patient displays an endometrial thickness of 2.0 cm, it is considered:
    a. suspicious for adenomyosis
    b. suspicious for endometriosis
    c. within normal limits in a menarche patient
    d. suspicious for proliferation of the endometrium
    e. within normal limits regardless of menstrual status

42. Which of the following ovarian abnormalities may contain skin and hair?
    a. thecoma
    b. dysgerminoma
    c. cystic teratoma
    d. granulosa cell tumor
    e. mucinous cystadenoma

43. Multiparity is a risk factor associated with which of the following abnormalities?
    a. adenomyosis
    b. endometriosis
    c. nabothian cyst
    d. hematometrocolpos
    e. polycystic ovarian disease

44. Which of the following ovarian neoplasms will most likely demonstrate posterior acoustic shadowing?
    a. fibroma
    b. thecoma
    c. dysgerminoma
    d. Brenner tumor
    e. granulosa cell tumor

45. A patient presents with a history of an intramural leiomyoma. An intramural leiomyoma:
    a. alters the perimetrium
    b. distorts the endometrium
    c. distorts the myometrium
    d. extends into the endometrium
    e. extends from the uterine fundus

46. A Garner cyst is located within the:
    a. uterus
    b. ovary
    c. cervix
    d. vagina
    e. oviduct

47. A patient presents with a history of postmenopausal bleeding. A heterogeneous intrauterine mass is identified on sonography. On the basis of the clinical history, the sonographic findings are most suspicious for:
    a. leiomyoma
    b. endometrioma
    c. leiomyosarcoma
    d. hematometrocolpos
    e. endometrial hyperplasia

48. A patient presents with a history of breast cancer and tamoxifen therapy. Which of the following pelvic structures requires additional evaluation?
    a. uterus
    b. ovary
    c. adnexa
    d. endometrium
    e. fallopian tube

49. An ill-defined, multilocular, complex ovarian mass is most suspicious for:
    a. cystadenoma
    b. leiomyosarcoma
    c. theca lutein cysts
    d. cystadenocarcinoma
    e. granulosa cell tumor

50. An ovarian mass combined with a pleural effusion and ascites resolving after surgery is known as:
    a. Meigs syndrome
    b. Turner syndrome
    c. Asherman syndrome
    d. Stein-Leventhal syndrome
    e. Beckwith-Wiedemann syndrome

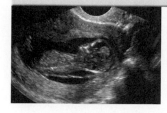

CHAPTER 22

Adnexal Pathology and Infertility

KEY TERMS

endometrioma a collection of extravasated endometrial tissue.

endometriosis a condition occurring when active endometrial tissue invades the peritoneal cavity.

human chorionic gonadotropin (hCG) a substitute for luteinizing hormone used in fertility assistance to trigger ovulation.

hydrosalpinx dilatation of the fallopian tube with fluid.

Meckel diverticulum an anomalous sac protruding from the ileum; caused by an incomplete closure of the yolk stalk.

pelvic inflammatory disease (PID) a general classification for inflammatory conditions of the cervix, uterus, ovaries, fallopian tubes, and peritoneal surfaces.

salpingitis inflammation within the fallopian tube.

synechia scarring caused by previous dilation and curettage or spontaneous abortion; demonstrated as hyperechoic band of echoes within the endometrial cavity.

Adnexal Pathology

PATHOLOGY	ETIOLOGY	CLINICAL FINDINGS	SONOGRAPHIC FINDINGS	DIFFERENTIAL CONSIDERATIONS
Endometriosis	• Ectopic location of functional endometrial tissue • Attaches to the fallopian tubes, ovaries, colon, and bladder	• Asymptomatic • Dysmenorrhea • Pelvic pain • Irregular menses • Dyspareunia • Infertility	• Difficult to visualize with sonography • Obscure organ boundaries • Fixation of the ovaries posterior to the uterus • Endometrioma	• Adhesions • Bowel interference
Endometrioma	• Focal collection of ectopic endometrial tissue • Termed "chocolate cyst"	• Pelvic pain • Palpable pelvic mass • Irregular bleeding • Dyspareunia • Infertility	• Hypoechoic, homogeneous adnexal mass • Thick, well-defined wall margins • Diffuse, low-level echoes with or without solid components • Avascular mass • Fluid/Fluid level • Mass will not regress in size on serial sonograms	• Hemorrhagic cyst • Pedunculated fibroid • Cystic teratoma
Krukenberg tumors	• Metastatic lesions • Primary lesion from gastric carcinoma • Other primary structures may include large intestines, breast, or appendix	• Asymptomatic • Abdominal pain • Bloating	• Bilateral adnexal or ovarian masses • Oval or lobulated margins • Hypoechoic areas within the mass • Posterior enhancement • Ascites • Generally bilateral	• Ovarian carcinoma • Degenerating fibroid • Tubo-ovarian abscess • Cystic teratoma • Endometrioma

Continued

Adnexal Pathology—cont'd

PATHOLOGY	ETIOLOGY	CLINICAL FINDINGS	SONOGRAPHIC FINDINGS	DIFFERENTIAL CONSIDERATIONS
Parovarian cyst	• Mesothelial in origin • Typically located in the broad ligament • Not associated with a history of pelvic inflammation, surgery, or endometriosis	• Asymptomatic • Pelvic pain • Palpable pelvic mass	• Round or ovoid anechoic adnexal mass • Separate from ipsilateral ovary • Thin, smooth wall margins • Stable size on serial sonograms	• Cystadenoma • Hydrosalpinx • Ovarian cyst • Meckel diverticulum • Peritoneal cyst
Pelvic inflammatory disease	• Bacterial infection • Diverticulitis • Appendicitis	• Abdominal pain • Fever • Vaginal discharge • Urinary frequency	• Normal pelvic appearance • Thick and hypervascular endometrium • Complex tubular adnexal mass • Ill-defined multilocular adnexal mass	• Normal pelvis • Loops of bowel • Endometriosis • Ectopic pregnancy
Peritoneal inclusion cyst	• Adhesions trap fluid normally produced by the ovary	• Asymptomatic • Lower abdominal pain • Palpable mass	• Septated fluid collection surrounding an ovary • Vascular flow can be demonstrated in septae • Unilocular peritoneal cyst	• Ascites • Parovarian cyst • Hydrosalpinx

Pathology of the Fallopian Tubes

PATHOLOGY	ETIOLOGY	CLINICAL FINDINGS	SONOGRAPHIC FINDINGS	DIFFERENTIAL CONSIDERATIONS
Carcinoma	• Dysplasia • Carcinoma in situ	• Pelvic pain • Abnormal bleeding • Pelvic mass	• Sausage-shaped complex adnexal mass • Papillary projections	• Tubo-ovarian abscess • Loops of bowel
Hydrosalpinx	• Pelvic inflammatory disease • Endometriosis • Postoperative adhesions	• Asymptomatic • Pelvic fullness • Infertility	• Anechoic tubular adnexal mass • Thin wall margins • Absence of peristalsis	• Fluid-filled loop of bowel • Dilated ureter • External iliac vein • Ovarian cyst • Omental cyst
Pyosalpinx	• Bacterial infection • Diverticulitis • Appendicitis	• Asymptomatic • Low-grade fever • Pelvic fullness	• Complex tubular adnexal mass • Wall thickness ≥5 mm • Irregular wall margins • Mass attenuates the sound	• Bowel loops • Ovarian neoplasm • Iliac vessel • Hydroureter
Salpingitis	• Pelvic infection	• Pelvic pain • Fever • Leukocytosis	• Nodular, thick tubular adnexal mass • Complex adnexal mass • Posterior enhancement	• Loops of bowel • Endometriosis
Tubo-ovarian abscess	• Pelvic infection • Sexually transmitted disease	• Severe pelvic pain • Fever • Leukocytosis	• Complex multilocular adnexal mass • Ill-defined wall margins • Total breakdown of the normal adnexal anatomy	• Endometriosis • Ectopic pregnancy • Hemorrhagic cyst

INFERTILITY

- Infertility is suggested when conception does not occur within 1 year.
- Caused by male or female reproductive abnormalities.
- Most common cause of female infertility is ovulatory disorders.
- Fibroids are responsible for 15% of infertility cases.
- Other causes include oviduct disease, congenital uterine anomalies, endometrial pathology, nutritional factors, metabolic disorders, and synechiae.

METHODS OF FERTILITY ASSISTANCE

- There are several methods of fertility assistance.

OVARIAN INDUCTION THERAPY

- Medications are injected to stimulate follicular development.
- Stimulates the pituitary gland to increase secretion of follicle-stimulating hormone.
- Follicular growth is monitored by periodic ultrasound examinations.
- Estradiol levels are monitored for timing of intramuscular injection of hCG.

IN VITRO FERTILIZATION

- Mature ova are aspirated with ultrasound guidance.
- Fertilization is accomplished in a laboratory setting.
- Endometrium is prepared to accept embryo.
- Embryo(s) are transferred into the endometrium.

GAMETE INTRAFOLLICULAR TRANSFER

- Requires ovulation stimulation and retrieval of oocytes.
- The oocytes are mixed with sperm, then transferred into the fallopian tube.

ZYGOTE INTRAFALLOPIAN TRANSFER

- Zygote is transferred into the fallopian tube.

ULTRASOUND EVALUATION OF THE UTERUS

- Ultrasound is used to assess the structural anatomy of the uterus and endometrium.
- Uterus is evaluated for congenital anomalies or abnormalities.
- A septae uterus has a high incidence of infertility and can be amended with surgery.

ULTRASOUND MONITORING OF THE ENDOMETRIUM

- An endometrial thickness <8 mm is associated with a decrease in fertility.

ULTRASOUND MONITORING OF THE OVARIES

BASELINE STUDY PRIOR TO THERAPY

- Assess for the presence of an ovarian cyst or dominant follicles.

DURING INDUCTION THERAPY

- Monitor the size and number of follicles per ovary.
- Count and measure only the follicles greater than 1.0 cm in diameter.
- Optimal follicle size prior to ovulation is 1.5 to 2.0 cm in diameter.
- Correlate estradiol level with size and number of follicles.

COMPLICATIONS OF FERTILITY ASSISTANCE

ECTOPIC PREGNANCY

- More common in patients with a history of infertility.

MULTIPLE GESTATIONS

- Most common with in vitro technique (25% of cases).

OVARIAN HYPERSTIMULATION SYNDROME

- Caused by high levels of hCG.
- Clinical findings include lower abdominal or back pain, abdominal distention, nausea/vomiting, hypotension, and leg edema.
- Multicystic ovarian enlargement >5 cm in diameter.
- Additional sonographic findings may include ascites and pleural effusion.

ADNEXAL PATHOLOGY AND INFERTILITY REVIEW

1. Krukenberg tumors are a result of:
   a. endometriosis
   b. hyperstimulation
   c. metastatic disease
   d. Asherman syndrome
   e. pelvic inflammatory disease

2. A cystic structure located in the inferior broad ligament is most suspicious for a(n):
   a. hydrosalpinx
   b. endometrioma
   c. parovarian cyst
   d. serous cystadenoma
   e. Meckel diverticulum

3. Which of the following most accurately describes endometriosis?
   a. proliferation of the endometrial lining
   b. collection of ectopic endometrial tissue
   c. inflammation of the endometrial cavity
   d. ectopic endometrial tissue located in the myometrium
   e. active endometrial tissue invades the peritoneal cavity

4. Infertility is suggested when conception does not occur within:
   a. 3 months
   b. 6 months
   c. 9 months
   d. 12 months
   e. 24 months

5. Which of the following complications is commonly associated with in vitro fertilization?
   a. hyperstimulation
   b. ectopic pregnancy
   c. multiple gestations
   d. spontaneous abortion
   e. congenital anomalies

6. A 25-year-old woman presents with high-grade fever, pelvic pain, and leukocytosis. An ill-defined, complex mass is identified in the left adnexa. On the basis of this clinical history, the sonographic finding is most suspicious for:
   a. salpingitis
   b. pyosalpinx
   c. endometritis
   d. hydrosalpinx
   e. tubo-ovarian abscess

7. A patient presents with lower abdominal pain and a palpable pelvic mass. A septated fluid collection surrounds a normal-appearing right ovary. The patient has a previous history of a ruptured appendix. On the basis of this clinic history, the sonographic finding is most suspicious for which of the following pathologies?
   a. salpingitis
   b. endometriosis
   c. tubo-ovarian abscess
   d. mucinous cystadenoma
   e. peritoneal inclusion cyst

8. With the gamete intrafollicular transfer technique, the:
   a. zygotes are transferred to the fallopian tube
   b. embryos are transferred to the endometrial cavity
   c. zygotes are transferred to the endometrial cavity
   d. oocytes and sperm are transferred to the fallopian tube
   e. oocytes and sperm are transferred to the endometrial cavity

9. During ovarian induction therapy, monitoring of this hormone is routine.
   a. estrogen
   b. estradiol
   c. progesterone
   d. luteinizing hormone
   e. follicle-stimulating hormone

10. Metastatic lesions in the adnexa are more commonly associated with a primary malignancy of the:
    a. respiratory system
    b. genitourinary tract
    c. reproductive organs
    d. gastrointestinal tract
    e. musculoskeletal system

11. Which of the following abnormalities is most likely a consequence of pelvic inflammatory disease?
    a. adenomyosis
    b. hydrosalpinx
    c. endometriosis
    d. parovarian cyst
    e. serous cystadenoma

12. A decrease in fertility is suggested when the endometrial thickness does not exceed:
    a. 2 mm
    b. 4 mm
    c. 8 mm
    d. 10 mm
    e. 14 mm

13. Which fertility assistance program inserts oocytes and sperm into the fallopian tube?
    a. in vitro fertilization
    b. follicle-stimulating hormone
    c. zygote intrafallopian transfer
    d. gamete intrafollicular transfer
    e. oocyte and sperm fallopian transfer

14. Which of the following complications is most likely associated with ovulation induction therapy?
    a. ovarian torsion
    b. ectopic pregnancy
    c. multiple gestations
    d. spontaneous abortion
    e. hyperstimulation syndrome

15. A large cystic mass posterior and lateral to the uterus in a patient with a history of a previous pelvic infection is most suspicious for a(n):
    a. salpingitis
    b. hydrosalpinx
    c. endometrioma
    d. parovarian cyst
    e. corpus luteal cyst

Using Fig. 22-1, answer questions 16 and 17.

16. Differential considerations for this pelvic mass would most likely include:
    a. hydrosalpinx vs. simple cyst
    b. simple cyst vs. parovarian cyst
    c. hydrosalpinx vs. endometrioma
    d. simple cyst vs. ectopic pregnancy
    e. parovarian cyst vs. endometrioma

17. Suggested follow-up care on this patient would most likely include:
    a. pregnancy testing
    b. surgical intervention
    c. infertility assessment
    d. sonogram in 6 to 8 weeks
    e. sonogram in 2 to 3 weeks

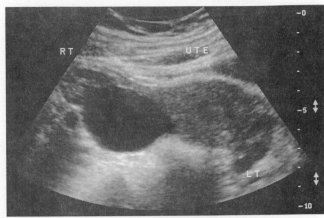

FIG. 22-1 Sonogram of the left adnexa.

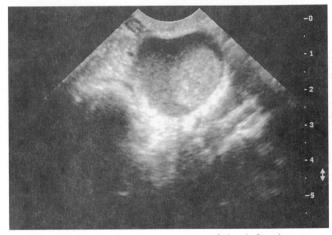

FIG. 22-2 Coronal sonogram of the left adnexa.

Using Fig. 22-2, answer question 18.

18. A patient presents with a history of dyspareunia and irregular menstrual cycles. A complex mass is identified adjacent to a normal-appearing ovary. On the basis of this clinical history, the sonographic finding is **most** suspicious for:
    a. endometrioma
    b. cystic teratoma
    c. hemorrhagic cyst
    d. ectopic pregnancy
    e. pedunculated leiomyoma

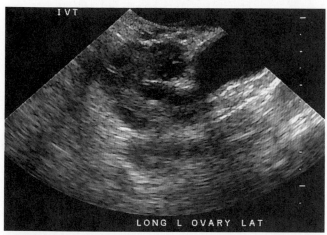

FIG. 22-3   Sagittal sonogram of the left adnexa.

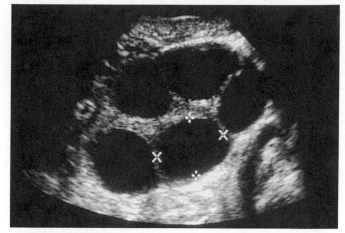

FIG. 22-4   Sonogram of the ovary.

Using Fig. 22-3, answer questions 19 and 20.

19. A patient presents with a history of a palpable pelvic mass. Additional questions revealed a previous history of a pelvic infection following an appendectomy. She denies pelvic pain or fever. The anechoic area in this sonogram is most suspicious for a(n):
   a. hydroureter
   b. hydrosalpinx
   c. parovarian cyst
   d. external iliac vein
   e. bladder diverticulum

20. The ovary is most likely demonstrating a:
   a. multicystic ovary
   b. hemorrhagic cyst
   c. suspicious solid mass
   d. normal anatomic variant
   e. suspicious isoechoic mass

Using Fig. 22-4, answer question 21.

21. The sonogram is most likely demonstrating:
   a. serous cystadenoma
   b. hypostimulation syndrome
   c. normal physiological cysts
   d. polycystic ovarian disease
   e. normal stimulated follicles

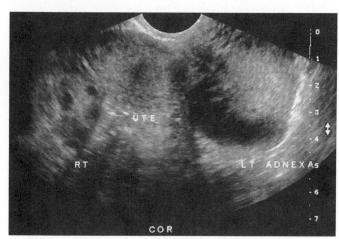

FIG. 22-5   Coronal sonogram.

Using Fig. 22-5, answer questions 22 and 23.

22. A 32-year-old patient presents with a history of endometriosis. Endometriosis is a result of:
   a. previous pelvic inflammatory disease
   b. endometrial tissue within the myometrium
   c. an accumulation of ectopic endometrial tissue
   d. endometrial tissue within the peritoneal cavity
   e. abnormal proliferation of the endometrial lining

23. The adnexal mass is most likely a(n):
   a. endometrioma
   b. cystic teratoma
   c. hemorrhagic cyst
   d. ectopic pregnancy
   e. tubo-ovarian abscess

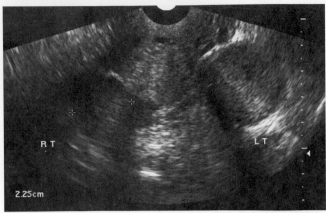

FIG. 22-6 Coronal sonogram.

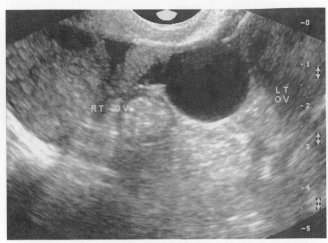

FIG. 22-7 Coronal sonogram.

Using Fig. 22-6, answer question 24.

24. A 55-year-old patient presents with a 6-month history of pelvic fullness. She has a history of breast cancer and a recent diagnosis of metastatic liver disease. On the basis of this clinical history, the sonographic findings are most suspicious for:
    a. endometriomas
    b. ovarian carcinoma
    c. hemorrhagic cysts
    d. Krukenberg tumors
    e. Meckel diverticulum

Using Fig. 22-7, answer question 25.

25. An asymptomatic patient presents with a history of a palpable pelvic mass on physical examination. On the basis of this clinical history, the sonographic findings are most suspicious for a:
    a. hydrosalpinx
    b. corpus luteum
    c. parovarian cyst
    d. fimbriae ovarica
    e. physiological cyst

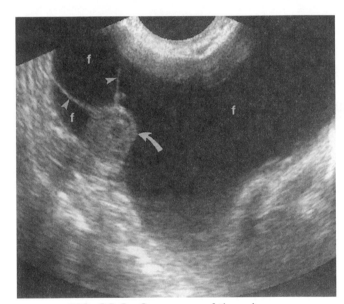

FIG. 22-8 Sonogram of the adnexa.

Using Fig. 22-8, answer question 26.

26. A patient presents with a history of a palpable pelvic mass and last menstrual period 2 weeks prior. On further questioning, the patient admits to prior pelvic surgery for a ruptured appendix. A sonogram demonstrates the ovary (curved arrow) surrounded by anechoic fluid. On the basis of the clinical history, the sonographic findings are most suspicious for a(n):
    a. endometrioma
    b. parovarian cyst
    c. serous cystadenoma
    d. tubo-ovarian abscess
    e. peritoneal inclusion cyst

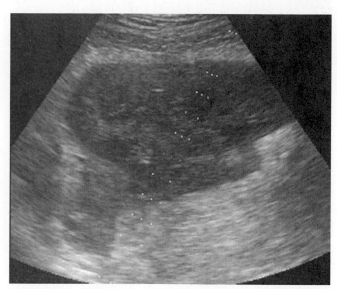

FIG. 22-9 Transverse sonogram of the right adnexa.

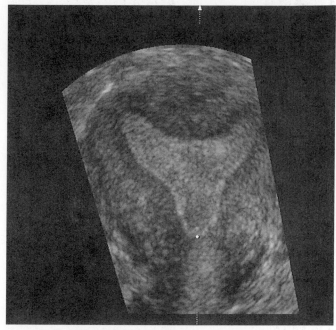

FIG. 22-10 Coronal sonogram.

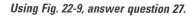

Using Fig. 22-9, answer question 27.

27. A 20-year-old patient presents with a history of severe pelvic pain and fever. Her last menstrual period was 3 weeks prior and urine pregnancy testing produced a negative result. On the basis of this clinical history, the sonographic findings are most suspicious for a(n):
   a. endometrioma
   b. ectopic pregnancy
   c. tubo-ovarian abscess
   d. complicated parovarian cyst
   e. carcinoma of the fallopian tube

Using Fig. 22-10, answer question 28.

28. A patient presents with a history of infertility. The sonographic findings in this coronal sonogram are most suspicious for:
   a. adenomyosis
   b. arcuate uterus
   c. endometriosis
   d. bicornuate uterus
   e. submucosal leiomyoma

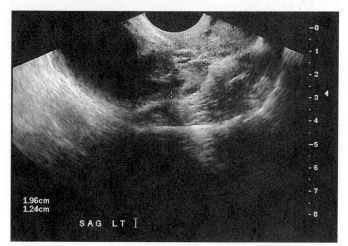

FIG. 22-11 Endovaginal sonogram of the left adnexa.

Using Fig. 22-11, answer question 29.

29. A patient presents with intermittent left lower quadrant pain. Additional questioning reveals a previous history of chlamydia. On the basis of this clinical history, the sonographic findings are most suspicious for a:
   a. hydroureter
   b. hydrosalpinx
   c. tubo-ovarian abscess
   d. hypogastric aneurysm
   e. peritoneal inclusion cyst

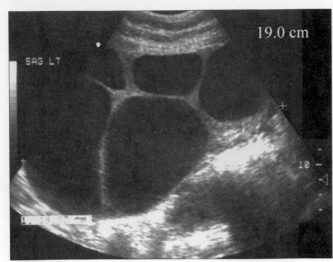

FIG. 22-12 Sonogram of a medically stimulated ovary.

Using Fig. 22-12, answer question 30.

30. An additional sonographic finding commonly associated with this abnormality is:
a. ascites
b. leiomyoma
c. hydrosalpinx
d. endometrioma
e. ectopic pregnancy

31. Pelvic inflammatory disease is best described as a(n):
a. sexually transmitted disease
b. ectopic location of endometrial tissue
c. specific inflammatory process of the ovaries
d. general classification of inflammatory conditions
e. specific inflammatory condition of the fallopian tubes

32. During ovarian induction therapy, follicles are only measured when exceeding:
a. 0.5 cm
b. 1.0 cm
c. 1.5 cm
d. 2.0 cm
e. all follicles are measured

33. Which of the following uterine anomalies is NOT likely to cause infertility?
a. leiomyoma
b. septae uterus
c. nabothian cyst
d. bicornuate uterus
e. endometrial polyp

34. On serial examinations, a parovarian cyst will:
a. slowly resolve
b. remain unchanged
c. rapidly increase in size
d. increase in size after menopause
e. vary according to the ovulatory phase

35. A common symptom of endometriosis is:
a. amenorrhea
b. menorrhagia
c. dysmenorrhea
d. hypomenorrhea
e. urinary frequency

36. Which of the following most accurately describes the sonographic appearance of a peritoneal inclusion cyst?
a. complex ovarian cyst
b. large unilocular adnexal mass
c. small cluster of ovarian cysts
d. anechoic mass between the uterus and ovary
e. septated fluid collection surrounding an ovary

37. A common sonographic finding associated with an endometrioma is a(n):
a. irregular, hypoechoic ovarian mass
b. multilocular cystic adnexal mass
c. well-defined anechoic ovarian mass
d. heterogeneous, complex adnexal mass
e. hypoechoic, homogeneous adnexal mass

38. Inflammation within the fallopian tube is termed:
a. adnexitis
b. salpingitis
c. pyosalpinx
d. hydrosalpinx
e. tubo-ovarian abscess

39. With ovarian induction therapy, intramuscular injection of what hormone triggers ovulation?
a. estradiol
b. progesterone
c. luteinizing hormone
d. follicle-stimulating hormone
e. human chorionic gonadotropin

40. Scarring within the endometrium caused by invasive procedures is termed:
a. albicans
b. synechiae
c. hyperplasia
d. endometritis
e. adenomyosis

41. Fixation of the ovaries posterior to the uterus is a sonographic finding associated with:
    a. pyosalpinx
    b. adenomyosis
    c. endometriosis
    d. tubo-ovarian abscess
    e. pelvic inflammatory disease

42. A total breakdown of the normal adnexal anatomy is a sonographic finding associated with:
    a. pyosalpinx
    b. adenomyosis
    c. endometriosis
    d. Krukenberg tumors
    e. tubo-ovarian abscess

43. Which of the following is an acquired cause of infertility?
    a. endometritis
    b. bicornuate uterus
    c. Meigs' syndrome
    d. uterine didelphys
    e. Gartner's duct cyst

44. Which of the following best describes the sonographic appearance of uterine synechiae?
    a. thick, irregular endometrium
    b. hypoechoic endometrial mass
    c. irregular hypoechoic myometrial masses
    d. hypoechoic, homogeneous adnexal mass
    e. bright band of echoes within the endometrium

45. Assessment for the presence of an ovarian cyst or dominant follicle is scheduled:
    a. prior to in vitro fertilization
    b. after gamete intrafollicular transfer
    c. prior to gamete intrafollicular transfer
    d. after initiating ovarian induction therapy
    e. prior to initiating ovarian induction therapy

46. Which of the following is NOT a sonographic finding in pelvic inflammatory disease?
    a. normal-appearing pelvis
    b. complex tubular adnexal mass
    c. focal hypoechoic adnexal mass
    d. thick and hypervascular endometrium
    e. ill-defined multilocular adnexal mass

47. Which of the following most accurately describes an endometrioma?
    a. overgrowth of endometrial tissue
    b. a collection of ectopic endometrial tissue
    c. ectopic location of active endometrial tissue
    d. benign neoplasm of the uterine myometrium
    e. ectopic endometrial tissue within the myometrium

48. A patient presents with a history of a leiomyoma. Which location will most likely cause infertility?
    a. serosal
    b. subserosal
    c. intramural
    d. submucosal
    e. pedunculated

49. A nodular tubular adnexal mass demonstrating posterior acoustic enhancement is most suspicious for:
    a. salpingitis
    b. pyosalpinx
    c. hydrosalpinx
    d. endometrioma
    e. peritoneal inclusion cyst

50. A large multicystic ovarian mass, in an ovarian-stimulated patient, is most suspicious for:
    a. a corpus luteum
    b. a corpus albicans
    c. polycystic ovarian disease
    d. multicystic ovarian disease
    e. ovarian hyperstimulation syndrome

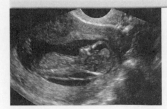

CHAPTER 23

Assessment of the First Trimester

KEY TERMS

amnion extra-embryonic membrane that lines the chorion and contains the fetus and amniotic fluid.

blastocyst consists of an outer trophoblast and an inner cell mass.

bradycardia fetal heart rate below 90 beats per minute.

chorion outermost of the fetal membranes; ultimately shrinks and is obliterated by the amnion between 12 and 16 weeks.

decidua name applied to the endometrium during pregnancy.

decidua basalis portion of the endometrium on which the implanted conceptus rests.

decidua capsularis decidua that covers the surface of the implanted conceptus.

decidua parietalis decidua exclusive of the area occupied by the implanted conceptus; aka decidua vera.

double decidua sign composed of the decidua capsularis and decidua parietalis; thick hyperechoic rim surrounding a sonolucency; indicative of an intrauterine pregnancy.

embryo term used for a developing zygote through the tenth week of gestation.

embryonic phase gestational weeks 6 through 10.

empty amnion sign visualization of the amniotic cavity without the presence of an embryo.

gestational age length of time calculated from the first day of the last menstrual period.

gestational sac fluid-filled structure normally found in the uterus, containing the pregnancy.

intrauterine pregnancy (IUP) pregnancy located within the uterus.

morula solid mass of cells formed by cleavage of a fertilized ovum.

nuchal translucency the sonographic appearance of subcutaneous accumulation of fluid behind the fetal neck in the first trimester of pregnancy; increases associated with chromosomal and other abnormalities.

pseudogestational sac centrally located endometrial fluid collection demonstrated with a coexisting ectopic pregnancy.

tachycardia fetal heart rate exceeding 170 beats per minute.

yolk sac provides nutrients to the embryo and is the initial site of alpha-fetoprotein.

EARLY EMBRYOLOGY (Fig. 23-1)

- Fertilization to implantation—approximately 5 to 7 days.
  - Ovum and sperm join in the distal fallopian tube, forming a zygote.
  - Cells of the zygote multiply, forming a cluster termed the morula.
  - Fluid rapidly enters the morula, forming a blastocyst.
  - The blastocyst implants into the endometrium.
- After implantation—trophoblastic growth continues.
  - Maternal vessels erode, establishing a circulation on the maternal side of the forming placenta (chorion basalis).
  - Trophoblastic tissue covers the entire embryo, developing into the fetal side of the forming placenta (chorion frondosum).
  - Human chorionic gonadotropin (hCG) is secreted by the trophoblastic tissue.
  - Organogenesis is generally completed by the tenth gestational week.

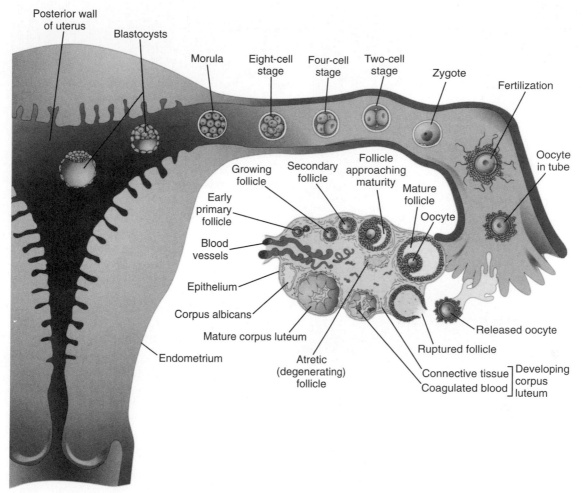

FIG. 23-1 Early embryology.

BLASTOCYST DEVELOPMENT (Fig. 23-2)

- Amnion begins.
- Secondary yolk sac begins.
- Chorionic villi evenly surround the blastocyst.
- Embryo is located between the amnion and yolk sac (Fig. 23-2, *A*).
- Embryo folds into the amnion.
- Amnion attaches to the anterior portion of the embryo.
- Yolk sac becomes "pinched" near the embryo, forming the body stalk.
- Chorionic villi become more prolific near the implantation site (Fig. 23-2, *B*).
- Amnion begins to fill more of the chorionic cavity.
- Yolk sac is pushed into the chorionic cavity.
- Umbilical cord begins to develop about the seventh to eighth gestational week.
- Areas of the chorion away from the implantation site becomes smooth (Fig. 23-2, *C*).
- Amnion fuses to the smooth chorion.
- Embryo or fetus lies within the amniotic cavity.
- Chorionic villi and decidua basalis have formed a placenta (Fig. 23-2, *D*).

FIG. 23-2
Blastocyst development.

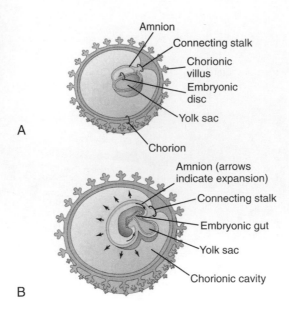

A

Amnion
Connecting stalk
Chorionic villus
Embryonic disc
Yolk sac
Chorion

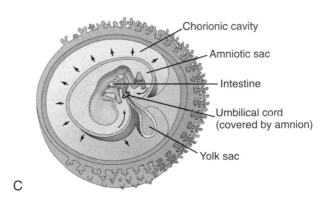

B

Amnion (arrows indicate expansion)
Connecting stalk
Embryonic gut
Yolk sac
Chorionic cavity

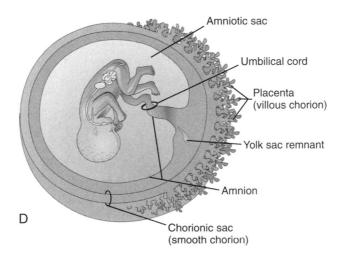

C

Chorionic cavity
Amniotic sac
Intestine
Umbilical cord (covered by amnion)
Yolk sac

D

Amniotic sac
Umbilical cord
Placenta (villous chorion)
Yolk sac remnant
Amnion
Chorionic sac (smooth chorion)

ANATOMY

First-Trimester Anatomy

STRUCTURE	DESCRIPTION	NORMAL SONOGRAPHIC FINDINGS
Abdominal wall	• Physiological herniation of the fetal bowel into the umbilical cord • Bowel returns into abdomen and herniation resolves by the 11th gestational week	• Umbilical herniation contiguous with the umbilical cord • Abnormal if persists after 12 weeks' gestation
Cardiovascular system	• First system to function in the embryo • Four heart chambers are formed by the ninth gestational week	• Cardiac motion as early as 5.5 weeks
Cranium	• Prosencephalon—forebrain • Mesencephalon—midbrain • Rhombencephalon—hindbrain	• Prominent cystic space in the posterior portion of the brain (rhombencephalon)
Skeletal system	• Vertebral bodies and ribs are forming at 6 weeks • Arms and legs are forming at 7 weeks • Ossification of the vertebral bodies and rib cartilage at 9 weeks • Long bones form during the tenth week	• Spine appears as parallel echogenic linear structures in the center of the embryo or fetus • Long bones appear as hyperechoic linear structure(s) within the soft tissue of the extremities

LABORATORY VALUES

HUMAN CHORIONIC GONADOTROPIN (hCG)

- Produced by the trophoblastic cells of the developing chorionic villi.
- Normally doubles every 30 to 48 hours.
- Peaks at the tenth gestational week (100,000 mIU/mL).
- Declines after the tenth week and levels out about 18 weeks (5,000 mIU/mL).
- Gestational sac should be identified transvaginally once the hCG levels reaches 1000 mIU/mL and as early as 500 mIU/mL.

FIRST-TRIMESTER MEASUREMENTS

MEAN SAC DIAMETER (MSD)

- Establishes gestational age prior to visualization of an embryonic disc.
- Measure the length, height, and width of the inner to outer borders of the gestational sac.

$$MSD\,(mm) = \frac{Length\,(mm) + Height\,(mm) + Width\,(mm)}{3}$$

CROWN–RUMP LENGTH (CRL)

- Measured until the 12th gestational week.
- Most accurate method of dating a pregnancy.
- Sagittal measurement of the embryo or fetus from the top of the head to the bottom of the rump.
- Lower extremities are not included in the measurement.

NUCHAL TRANSLUCENCY

- The gestation should be 11 weeks 0 days to 13 weeks 6 days and the crown–rump length (CRL) should be a minimum of 45 mm and a maximum of 84 mm.

- Mid-sagittal section of the fetus should be in a neutral position.
- Only the fetal head and upper thorax should be included in the image.
- Maximum thickness of the subcutaneous translucency between the skin and soft tissue overlying the cervical spine is measured.
- Calipers are placed on the hyperechoic lines, *not* in the nuchal fluid.
- More than one measurement must be taken and the maximum one is to be recorded.
- Nuchal translucency exceeding 3 mm is abnormal.

FIRST-TRIMESTER PROTOCOL

EVALUATE AND DOCUMENT THE FOLLOWING:

- Location and gestational age of pregnancy.
- Presence or absence of viability.
- Fetal number.
- Evaluation of the uterus and adnexal structures.

INDICATIONS FOR SONOGRAPHIC EVALUATION

- Confirm intrauterine pregnancy.
- Confirm viability.
- Define vaginal bleeding.
- Rule out ectopic pregnancy.
- Estimate gestational age.
- Evaluate pelvic mass or pain.
- Abnormal serial hCG levels.

Sonographic Findings in the First Trimester

GESTATIONAL FINDING	DESCRIPTION	NORMAL SONOGRAPHIC FINDINGS	ABNORMAL SONOGRAPHIC FINDINGS
Gestational sac (GS)	• Fluid-filled structure normally found in the uterus, containing the developing embryo • First definitive sonographic finding to suggest early pregnancy • Anechoic structure represents the chorionic cavity • Echogenic rim represents decidual tissue and the developing chorionic villi • Beta hCG of 1000 mIU/mL should demonstrate a GS transvaginally	• Round anechoic structure • Surrounded by a thick hyperechoic rim (2 mm) • Located in the mid to upper portion of the uterus • Eccentric location within the endometrium Transabdominal • 5 mm mean sac diameter (MSD) about 5-6 weeks • Double decidual sign evident with an MSD of 10 mm Transvaginal • 2-3 mm about 4-5 weeks	• Irregular or distorted GS • Large GS without evidence of YS • Abnormal uterine location • Visualization of amnion without concomitant embryo Transabdominal • Failure to identify a YS with an MSD ≥20 mm • Failure to identify an embryo in a GS ≥25 mm Transvaginal • Failure to identify a YS with an MSD ≥8 mm • Failure to identify an embryo in a GS ≥16 mm

Sonographic Findings in the First Trimester—cont'd

GESTATIONAL FINDING	DESCRIPTION	NORMAL SONOGRAPHIC FINDINGS	ABNORMAL SONOGRAPHIC FINDINGS
Yolk sac (YS)	• Located in the chorionic cavity • Provides nutrition to the embryo • Earliest structure visualized in the gestational sac • Attached to the embryo by the vitelline duct • Used as a landmark to locate the embryonic disc and early cardiac activity • Ultimately detaches from the embryo and remains within the chorionic cavity	• Hyperechoic ring within the gestational sac • Round or oval in shape • Diameter should not exceed 6 mm Transabdominal • Evident within an MSD of 20 mm Transvaginal • Evident within an MSD of 8 mm	• YS diameter exceeding 8 mm
Embryo	• Embryonic period extends from the sixth through the tenth gestational weeks	• Initially a local thickening adjacent to the yolk sac • Echogenic focus adjacent to the yolk sac Transabdominal • Usually detected within an MSD of 25 mm Transvaginal • Usually detected in an MSD of 13-18 mm	• Embryo too small for gestational sac • No cardiac activity in an embryo exceeding 7 mm
Amnion	• Initially surrounds the newly formed amniotic cavity • Attaches to the embryo at the umbilical cord insertion • Expands with accumulation of amniotic fluid and growth of the embryo • Obliterates the chorionic cavity by the 16th week	• Thin hyperechoic line between the embryo and the yolk sac (chorion)	• Visualization of the amnion without an embryo • Thick hyperechoic amnion • Large amniotic cavity compared with the size of the embryo
Cardiac activity	• First system to function in the embryo	• Cardiac activity should be identified by 6 weeks and as early as 5.5 weeks • 100-115 beats per minute before 6 weeks • 120-160 beats per minute after 6 weeks Transabdominal • Should be evident with an MSD of 25 mm Transvaginal • Should be evident with an MSD of 16 mm *or* • Crown–rump length (CRL) exceeding 5 mm	• Heart rates below 85 beats per minute are associated with poor outcomes Transabdominal • No cardiac activity in an embryo ≥9 mm • Failure to identify cardiac activity in a GS ≥25 mm Transvaginal • No cardiac activity in an embryo ≥7 mm • Failure to identify cardiac activity in a GS ≥16 mm

Weekly Findings During the Normal First Trimester

GESTATIONAL WEEK	SONOGRAPHIC FINDINGS
Fourth	• Thickening of the endometrium • Mean sac diameter (MSD) = 2-3 mm
Fifth	• MSD = 10 mm • Yolk sac seen with vaginal imaging • May visualize embryonic disc • May visualize cardiac activity
Sixth	• 15-20 mm gestational sac • Yolk sac visualized • C-shaped embryo measuring approximately 5 mm • Cardiac activity should be present
Seventh	• MSD = 30 mm • Crown–rump length (CRL) = 1.0 cm • Cardiac activity should be present • Head constitutes one-half of the embryo • Limb buds appear
Eighth	• CRL = 2.0 cm • Embryo unfolds • Head becomes dominant • Midgut has herniated into the base of the umbilical cord • Placenta location may be identified • Spine may be visualized
Ninth	• CRL = 3.0 cm • Can differentiate the cerebral hemispheres • Visualization of limb buds • Early ossifications may be seen
Tenth	• CRL approaches 4.0 cm • Muscular movement has begun • Hyperechoic choroid plexuses • Cystic rhombencephalon demonstrated in the posterior fossa
Twelfth	• CRL reaches 7.0 cm • Yolk sac no longer visualized • Midgut has returned to the abdominal cavity • Amnion is now abutting the chorion • Fetus demonstrates a skeletal body • Fluid is displayed in the fetal stomach

Abnormal First-Trimester Pregnancy

ABNORMALITY	DESCRIPTION	CLINICAL FINDINGS	SONOGRAPHIC FINDINGS	DIFFERENTIAL CONSIDERATIONS
Anembryonic	• Zygote develops into a blastocyst, but the inner cell mass fails to develop • Blighted ovum	• Asymptomatic • Serial beta hCG levels may remain normal • Small for dates • No fetal heart tones	• Large gestational sac • Absent yolk sac, amnion, and embryo	• Missed abortion • Pseudogestational sac
Complete abortion	• Miscarriage	• Bleeding • Cramping • Rapid decline in serial beta hCG levels	• No evidence of intrauterine pregnancy • No adnexal masses	• Ectopic pregnancy • Early intrauterine pregnancy

Abnormal First-Trimester Pregnancy—cont'd

ABNORMALITY	DESCRIPTION	CLINICAL FINDINGS	SONOGRAPHIC FINDINGS	DIFFERENTIAL CONSIDERATIONS
Ectopic risk factors • **Pelvic infection** • **Intrauterine device** • **Oviduct surgery** • **Infertility treatment** • **Previous ectopic pregnancy**	• Pregnancy in an abnormal location • 95% are located in the fallopian tube • Other areas may include ovary, cervix, peritoneum, broad ligament, and cornua of the uterus	• Pelvic pain • Bleeding • Palpable mass • Abnormal rise in serial beta hCG levels • Hypotension	• No intrauterine pregnancy • Centrally located endometrial fluid collection Fallopian tube • Complex adnexal mass • Cul de sac fluid • May display an extrauterine gestational sac with or without embryo Cornual • Laterally placed gestational sac • Myometrium incompletely surrounds the gestational sac • Highly vascular location	• Early intrauterine pregnancy with a corpus luteal cyst • Pregnancy in one horn of a bicornuate uterus
Embryonic or fetal demise	• Evidence of a nonliving embryo or fetus	• Small for dates • No fetal heart tones • Spotting	• Presence of an embryo or fetus • No cardiac activity • No fetal movement • Overlapping of cranial bones	• Incorrect dates
Gestational trophoblastic disease	• Proliferative disease of the trophoblast • Hydatid swelling in a blighted ovum • Trophoblastic changes in retained placental tissue	• Bleeding • Hyperemesis • Dramatically elevated beta hCG levels • Large for dates • No fetal heart tones • Low maternal AFP • Preeclampsia	• Moderately echogenic soft tissue uterine mass • Small cystic structures within the mass • Demonstrates vascular flow • Theca lutein cysts	• Incomplete abortion • Degenerating fibroid • Adenomyosis
Heterotopic pregnancy	• Extrauterine and intrauterine pregnancies • Dizygotic pregnancy • 1:30,000	• Pelvic pain • Cramping • Bleeding • Hypotension	• Intrauterine pregnancy • Complex adnexal mass • Cul de sac fluid	• Pregnancy in both horns of a bicornuate uterus • Intrauterine pregnancy with coexisting complex corpus luteal cyst
Incomplete abortion	• Retained products of conception	• Asymptomatic • Bleeding • Cramping • Abnormal rise in serial beta hCG levels	• Thick, complex endometrium • Intact gestational sac with nonviable embryo • Collapsed gestational sac	• Endometrial dysplasia • Ectopic pregnancy
Pseudocyesis	• False pregnancy • Psychological condition	• Nausea/vomiting • Abdominal distention • Amenorrhea • Negative pregnancy test	• Normal nongravid uterus • Normal adnexa	• Recent miscarriage
Subchorionic hemorrhage	• Low-pressure bleed from implantation of blastocyst	• Asymptomatic • Spotting	• Echogenic fluid collection between the gestational sac and uterine wall • Becomes more anechoic with time • Avascular mass • Variable size • Resolves over time	• Nonviable twin pregnancy • Incomplete abortion • Placenta abruption

Pelvic Masses During Early Pregnancy

MASS	DESCRIPTION	CLINICAL FINDINGS	SONOGRAPHIC FINDINGS	DIFFERENTIAL CONSIDERATIONS
Corpus luteum	• Secretes progesterone prior to placental circulation	• Asymptomatic • Pelvic pain	• Anechoic ovarian mass • Hyperechoic, thick wall margins • May contain internal low-level echoes • Hypervascular periphery (ring of fire)	• Ectopic pregnancy • Endometrioma
Leiomyoma	• Benign neoplasm of the uterine myometrium • May increase in size with increases in hormones	• Asymptomatic • Pelvic pain	• Well-defined hypoechoic uterine mass • May appear complex or heterogeneous • Relationship to the cervix and placenta must be documented	• Subchorionic hemorrhage • Uterine contraction

ASSESSMENT OF THE FIRST TRIMESTER REVIEW

1. Ectopic pregnancies are commonly located in the:
   a. ovary
   b. cervix
   c. fallopian tube
   d. uterine cornua
   e. broad ligament

2. Which of the following structures implants into the endometrium?
   a. zygote
   b. morula
   c. embryo
   d. blastocyst
   e. trophoblast

3. Which of the following structures secretes human chorionic gonadotropin?
   a. yolk sac
   b. decidua basalis
   c. chorionic cavity
   d. decidua parietalis
   e. trophoblastic tissue

4. The optimal gestational age for measuring fetal nuchal translucency is from:
   a. 11 weeks 0 days to 13 weeks 6 days
   b. 10 weeks 0 days to 12 weeks 0 days
   c. 11 weeks 6 days to 13 weeks 0 days
   d. 11 weeks 0 days to 12 weeks 6 days
   e. 10 weeks 0 days to 12 weeks 6 days

5. Which area of the embryo attaches to the amnion?
   a. calvaria
   b. nuchal fold
   c. thoracic cavity
   d. umbilical insertion
   e. none of the above

6. The mean sac diameter (MSD) measures gestational age prior to visualization of the:
   a. amnion
   b. embryo
   c. yolk sac
   d. placenta
   e. fetal heart

7. Gestational weeks 6 through 10 constitute the:
   a. fetal phase
   b. first trimester
   c. conceptus phase
   d. embryonic phase
   e. chorionic period

8. The decidua capsularis and decidua parietalis produce the:
   a. blastocyst
   b. decidua basalis
   c. empty amnion sign
   d. double decidua sign
   e. pseudogestational sac

9. A rapid decline in serial hCG levels will most likely correlate with a(n):
   a. ectopic pregnancy
   b. spontaneous abortion
   c. anembryonic pregnancy
   d. heterotopic pregnancy
   e. normal intrauterine pregnancy

10. Which of the following is an abnormal finding in a first-trimester pregnancy?
   a. prominent cystic structure in the posterior brain
   b. visualization of the amnion without an embryo
   c. fetal heart rate of 100 beats per minute
   d. yolk sac measuring 5 mm in diameter
   e. herniation of the fetal bowel into the umbilical cord

11. Subchorionic hemorrhage is a common consequence of:
   a. fertilization of the ovum
   b. implantation of the conceptus
   c. the amniotic cavity expanding
   d. an ectopic location of the conceptus
   e. the obliteration of the chorionic cavity

12. Pseudocyesis is a condition associated with:
   a. endometriosis
   b. false pregnancy
   c. embryonic demise
   d. heterotopic pregnancy
   e. gestational trophoblastic disease

13. Which of the following formulas calculates the mean sac diameter of the gestational sac?
   a. Length × Height × Width
   b. Length + Height + Width
   c. $\frac{Length + Width}{Height}$
   d. $\frac{Length + Height + Width}{3}$
   e. $\frac{Length \times Height \times Width}{3}$

14. Normally, by how many gestational weeks should the chorionic cavity no longer be visible?
    a. 10
    b. 12
    c. 16
    d. 20
    e. 24

15. Hyperemesis is a common clinical finding associated with:
    a. ectopic pregnancy
    b. embryonic demise
    c. trophoblastic disease
    d. heterotopic pregnancy
    e. subchorionic hemorrhage

Using Fig. 23-3, answer questions 16 and 17.

16. A patient presents with a history of pelvic pain, vaginal bleeding, and a positive urine pregnancy test. Her last menstrual period was 4 weeks ago. On the basis of this clinical history, the sonogram is most suspicious for a(n):
    a. ovarian torsion
    b. ectopic pregnancy
    c. incomplete abortion
    d. tubo-ovarian abscess
    e. anembryonic pregnancy

17. The hypoechoic areas in the anterior and posterior portions of the right adnexa are most suspicious for:
    a. pyosalpinx
    b. iliac vessels
    c. tissue edema
    d. hydrosalpinx
    e. hemoperitoneum

Using Fig. 23-4, answer question 18.

18. A transvaginal sonogram of the superior uterus demonstrates a(n):
    a. embryonic demise
    b. pseudogestational sac
    c. anembryonic pregnancy
    d. amnion in an intrauterine pregnancy
    e. yolk sac in an intrauterine pregnancy

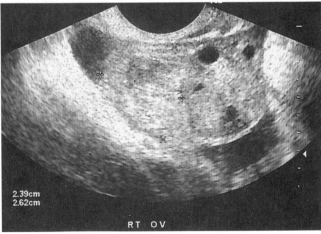

FIG. 23-3 Transvaginal sonogram.

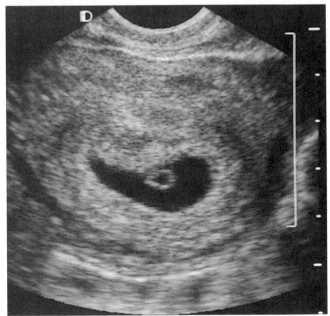

FIG. 23-4 Transvaginal sonogram.

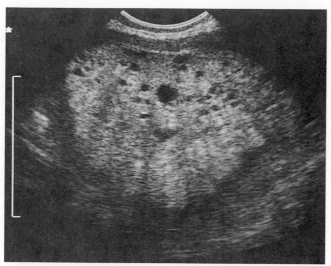

FIG. 23-5   Transabdominal sonogram of the uterus.

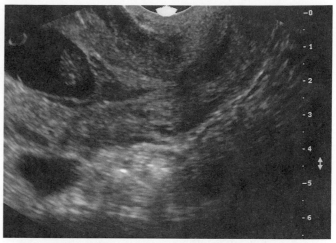

FIG. 23-6   First trimester sonogram.

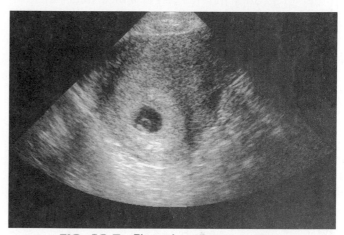

FIG. 23-7   First trimester sonogram.

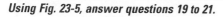

Using Fig. 23-5, answer questions 19 to 21.

19. A patient presents with a history of rapidly increasing hCG levels. On the basis of this clinical history, the sonogram is most suspicious for:
  a. pseudocyesis
  b. heterotopic pregnancy
  c. subchorionic hemorrhage
  d. retained products of conception
  e. gestational trophoblastic disease

20. With this abnormality, the adnexa are most likely to demonstrate:
  a. theca lutein cysts
  b. corpus luteal cysts
  c. solid ovarian masses
  d. anechoic tubular masses
  e. complex adnexal masses

21. The most common clinical symptom associated with this abnormality is:
  a. hyperemesis
  b. vaginal spotting
  c. pelvic cramping
  d. shortness of breath
  e. lower-extremity swelling

Using Fig. 23-6, answer question 22.

22. The sonogram is most likely demonstrating a(n):
  a. cornual pregnancy
  b. incompetent cervix
  c. pseudogestational sac
  d. subchorionic hemorrhage
  e. pregnancy in one horn of a bicornuate uterus

Using Fig. 23-7, answer question 23.

23. This sonogram is most consistent with a(n):
  a. cornual pregnancy
  b. incomplete abortion
  c. intrauterine pregnancy
  d. anembryonic pregnancy
  e. subchorionic hemorrhage

Using Fig. 23-8, answer question 24.

24. This gestational sac is demonstrating a(n):
    a. large complex yolk sac
    b. embryo and the amnion
    c. abnormal twin gestation
    d. subchorionic hemorrhage
    e. embryo and large yolk sac

Using Fig. 23-9, answer questions 25 and 26.

25. What is the most likely diagnosis of this transvaginal sonogram?
    a. appendicitis
    b. corpus luteal cyst
    c. ectopic pregnancy
    d. incomplete abortion
    e. pregnancy in one horn of a bicornuate uterus

26. Which clinical presentation is most likely associated with this diagnosis?
    a. leukocytosis
    b. elevated progesterone
    c. decreasing hCG levels
    d. slowly rising hCG levels
    e. normal serial hCG levels

Using Fig. 23-10, answer question 27.

27. An asymptomatic patient presents for an obstetrical ultrasound for gestational dating. She has a positive urine pregnancy test and is unsure of her last menstrual period. On the basis of this clinical history, the sonogram is most suspicious for a(n):
    a. fetal demise
    b. pseudogestational sac
    c. anembryonic pregnancy
    d. normal intrauterine pregnancy
    e. gestational trophoblastic disease

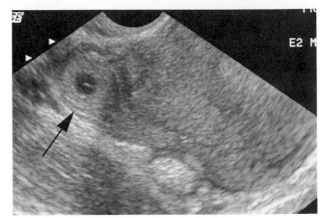

FIG. 23-9 Transvaginal sonogram.

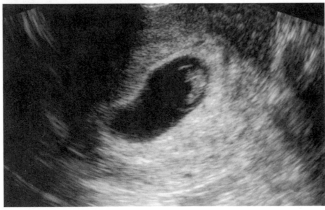

FIG. 23-8 Transvaginal sonogram.

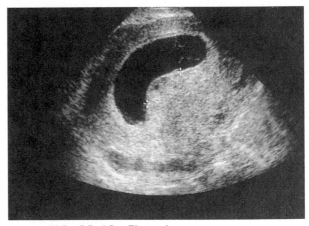

FIG. 23-10 First trimester sonogram.

Using Fig. 23-11, answer question 28.

28. A patient presents with a history of a therapeutic abortion 2 weeks prior. She complains of continued vaginal spotting since the procedure. She denies pelvic pain or fever. On the basis of this clinical history, the sonogram is most suspicious for:
    a. endometritis
    b. pseudogestational sac
    c. endometrial carcinoma
    d. degenerating leiomyoma
    e. retained products of conception

Using Fig. 23-12, answer question 29.

29. A well-defined cystic area is displayed in the posterior portion of the fetal head. This is most suspicious for a:
    a. cystic hygroma
    b. subarachnoid cyst
    c. Dandy-Walker cyst
    d. normal prosencephalon
    e. normal rhombencephalon

Using Fig. 23-13, answer question 30.

30. A hyperechoic linear structure located posterior to the fetus is most likely:
    a. a cystic hygroma
    b. the normal amnion
    c. a uterine synechia
    d. a Dandy-Walker cyst
    e. a subchorionic hemorrhage

31. Subcutaneous accumulation of fluid behind the fetal neck measuring 3 mm in thickness is a(n):
    a. normal finding in the late first trimester
    b. abnormal finding in the late first trimester
    c. normal finding in the late second trimester
    d. abnormal finding in the early first trimester
    e. abnormal finding regardless of gestational age

32. A patient presents with a positive pregnancy test and an hCG level of 750 mIU/mL. On the basis of this clinical history, which of the following best describes the expected sonographic findings?
    a. small gestational sac on transabdominal imaging
    b. possible small gestational sac on transvaginal imaging
    c. yolk sac within a gestational sac on transvaginal imaging
    d. gestational sac with viable embryo on transvaginal imaging
    e. yolk sac within a gestational sac on transabdominal imaging

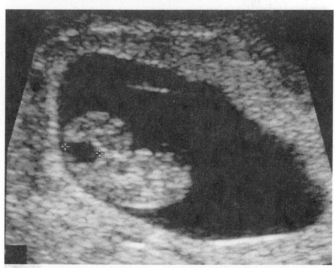

FIG. 23-12   First trimester sonogram.

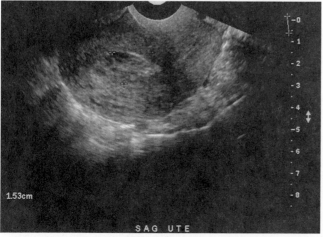

FIG. 23-11

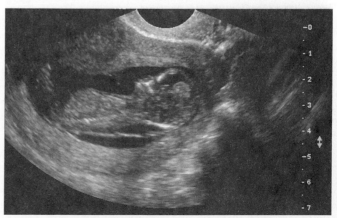

FIG. 23-13   First trimester sonogram.

33. Normal human chorionic gonadotropin levels should:
    a. double every 24 hours
    b. double every 30-48 hours
    c. peak about the 20th gestational week
    d. continue to increase throughout the pregnancy
    e. decrease and level out after the 12th gestational week

34. On transvaginal imaging, in a normal pregnancy, cardiac activity must be identified within a gestational sac with a mean sac diameter of:
    a. 7 mm
    b. 10 mm
    c. 16 mm
    d. 20 mm
    e. 25 mm

35. Presence of an embryo without visualization of the amnion is considered:
    a. a normal finding
    b. suspicious for fetal demise
    c. a precursor of an impending abortion
    d. suspicious for amniotic band syndrome
    e. a precursor of an abdominal wall defect

36. Which of the following is an abnormal sonographic finding during the first trimester of pregnancy?
    a. failure to visualize an amnion adjacent to an embryo
    b. failure to demonstrate cardiac activity by 5 gestational weeks when utilizing a transabdominal approach
    c. failure to demonstrate a yolk sac within a mean sac diameter of 10 mm when using the transvaginal approach
    d. failure to demonstrate a yolk sac within a mean sac diameter of 15 mm when using the transabdominal approach
    e. failure to demonstrate an embryo within a mean sac diameter of 20 mm when using a transabdominal approach

37. Indications for a first-trimester sonogram include all of the following EXCEPT:
    a. unsure dates
    b. vaginal bleeding
    c. confirm viability
    d. gender determination
    e. palpable pelvic mass

38. The secondary yolk sac:
    a. has no specific function
    b. is located in the chorionic cavity
    c. is visualized after the embryonic disc
    d. represents the developing chorionic villi
    e. secretes human chorionic gonadotropin

39. Initial visualization of the hyperechoic choroid plexuses is expected near the:
    a. 6th gestational week
    b. 8th gestational week
    c. 10th gestational week
    d. 14th gestational week
    e. 18th gestational week

40. Which of the following ectopic locations is most life threatening to the patient?
    a. ovarian
    b. cervical
    c. ampullary
    d. interstitial
    e. peritoneal

41. Retained products of conception can be a contributing factor of:
    a. an ectopic pregnancy
    b. trophoblastic disease
    c. a heterotopic pregnancy
    d. polycystic ovarian disease
    e. ovarian hyperstimulation syndrome

42. An extrauterine and intrauterine pregnancy is termed a(n):
    a. mirror pregnancy
    b. manifold pregnancy
    c. interstitial pregnancy
    d. bicornuate pregnancy
    e. heterotopic pregnancy

43. Which of the following lines the chorion and contains the fetus?
    a. amnion
    b. yolk sac
    c. decidua basalis
    d. chorion frondosum
    e. trophoblastic tissue

44. The term *embryo* is used to describe a developing zygote through the:
    a. 4th gestational week
    b. 8th gestational week
    c. 10th gestational week
    d. 13th gestational week
    e. 16th gestational week

45. A solid mass of cells formed by proliferation of a fertilized ovum is termed the:
    a. zygote
    b. morula
    c. graafian
    d. blastocyst
    e. trophoblast

46. Chorionic villi are more prolific:
   a. near the amnion
   b. adjacent to the yolk sac
   c. opposite the cervical os
   d. near the implantation site
   e. adjacent to the uterine fundus

47. Which of the following is the first system to function in the developing embryo?
   a. biliary
   b. respiratory
   c. genitourinary
   d. cardiovascular
   e. gastrointestinal

48. A corpus luteum is most likely misdiagnosed as a(n):
   a. hydrosalpinx
   b. ovarian torsion
   c. missed abortion
   d. ectopic pregnancy
   e. anembryonic pregnancy

49. Human chorionic gonadotropin peaks at the:
   a. 10th gestational week
   b. 12th gestational week
   c. 14th gestational week
   d. 16th gestational week
   e. 18th gestational week

50. Which of the following is the most accurate method of measuring gestational age?
   a. yolk sac diameter
   b. mean sac diameter
   c. crown–rump length
   d. biparietal diameter
   e. nuchal translucency

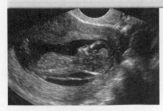

CHAPTER 24

Assessment of the Second Trimester

KEY TERMS

cavum septum pellucidi the space between the leaves of the septum pellucidum.

cephalic index a ratio of the cranium derived to determine the normality of the fetal head shape.

brachycephalic round shape to the fetal cranium; cephalic index 85%.

dolichocephalic elongated shape to the fetal cranium; cephalic index <70%.

falx cerebri a sickle-shaped fold of dura mater separating the two hemispheres of the cerebrum.

maternal alpha-fetoprotein a blood test to assist in diagnosing certain fetal anomalies.

meconium a material that collects in the intestines of the fetus and forms the first stool of a newborn.

railway sign term describing the sonographic appearance of the fetal spine.

tentorium "tent" structure in the posterior fossa that separates the cerebellum from the cerebrum.

thalamus one of a pair of large oval nervous structures forming most of the lateral walls of the third ventricle of the brain and part of the diencephalon.

vermis cerebelli narrow median part of the cerebellum between the two lateral hemispheres.

SECOND TRIMESTER BIOMETRIC MEASUREMENTS

BIPARIETAL DIAMETER

- Two-dimensional measurement.
- Accurate predictor of gestational age before 20 weeks.
- Measured in a plane that passes through the third ventricle and thalami.
- Transverse axial plane is most common and includes the following landmarks:
  - Falx cerebri.
  - Third ventricle.
  - Thalamic nuclei.
  - Cavum septi pellucidi.
  - Atrium of each lateral ventricle.
- Measure perpendicular to the falx placing calipers from the outer margin of the upper cranium to the inner margin of the lower cranium.
- Measurement of the biparietal diameter (BPD) can be obtained from the head circumference plane.

HEAD CIRCUMFERENCE

- Three-dimensional measurement.
- Reliable measurement independent of cranial shape.
- Measure in plane that must include the cavum septum pellucidi and the tentorial hiatus.

364

- Measured parallel to the base of the skull, placing the calipers on the outer margins of the cranium.
- Measurement of the head circumference cannot always be obtained from the BPD plane.

CEPHALIC INDEX

- Three-dimensional measurement.
- Devised to determine the normality of the fetal head shape.
- Normal cephalic index is approximately 78%.
- Abnormal when less than 74% or greater than 83%.

ABDOMINAL CIRCUMFERENCE

- Three-dimensional measurement.
- Predictor of fetal growth, not gestational age.
- Most difficult measurement to obtain.
- Cross-sectional measurement slightly superior to the cord insertion at the junction of the left and right portal veins (hockey stick) or demonstrates a short length of the umbilical vein and the left portal vein.
- Place calipers on the outer margins of the skin edge.
- Measured at a level to include the liver.

FEMUR LENGTH

- One-dimensional measurement.
- Long bone of choice due to ease of measurement.
- Normal femur demonstrates a straight lateral border and a curved medial border.
- Measure parallel to the femoral shaft placing calipers at the level of the femoral head cartilage and the distal femoral condyle.

LABORATORY VALUES

ALPHA-FETOPROTEIN

- Produced by the fetus.
- Found in the amniotic fluid and maternal serum.
- Normal values vary with gestational age.

Causes of High Alpha-fetoprotein

- Underestimated gestational age.
- Multiple gestations.
- Open neural tube defect.
- Abdominal wall defect.
- Cystic hygroma.
- Fetal death.

Causes of Low Alpha-fetoprotein

- Overestimated gestational age.
- Chromosomal abnormalities.
- Trophoblastic disease.
- Long-standing fetal demise.
- Chronic maternal hypertension or diabetes.

SECOND-TRIMESTER PROTOCOL

ASSESSMENT OF FETAL AGE

- Biparietal diameter.
- Head circumference.
- Abdominal circumference.
- Femur length.

Second Trimester—Fetal Survelliance

REGION	EVALUATE AND DOCUMENT
Cranial	• Face
	• Falx
	• Cerebellum
	• Cisterna magna
	• Cavum septi pellucidi
	• Atrium of the lateral ventricle
Thorax	• Four-chamber view of the heart
	• Left ventricular outflow tract
	• Right ventricular outflow tract
	• Motion mode tracing to include beats per minute
	• Diaphragm
Abdomen	• Stomach
	• Kidneys
	• Bladder
Spine	• Cervical, thoracic, lumbar, and sacral portions of the spine in the sagittal and transverse planes
Extremities	• Four extremities
Placenta	• Echogenicity
	• Location
	• Relationship to the cervix
Umbilical cord	• Insertion
	• Number of vessels
Cervical os	• Length
	• Relationship to the placenta
Amniotic fluid	• Volume
Fetal position	• Presentation of fetus in relationship to maternal anatomical planes
Pelvic structures	• Uterus and ovaries
	• Maternal urinary bladder

FETAL ANATOMY

FETAL CIRCULATION

- Oxygenated blood leaves the placenta and enters the fetus through the umbilical vein.
- After entering the abdomen, blood courses through the ductus venosum reaching the right atrium of the heart.
- Blood travels from the right to left atrium through the foramen ovale.
- From the left atrium to the left ventricle, blood ascends the aorta distributing blood to the fetal tissues.
- Approximately half of the blood leaves through the umbilical arteries, back to the placenta for reoxygenation.

Normal Cranial Anatomy

STRUCTURE	INFORMATION	SONOGRAPHIC APPEARANCE
Atrium of the lateral ventricle	• Junction of the anterior, occipital, and temporal horns • Located slightly inferior to the level of the biparietal diameter (BPD) • Evaluates for ventricular enlargement	• Hyperechoic thin ventricle wall • Hyperechoic choroid plexus • Measure perpendicular to the ventricle walls from the glomus of the choroid plexus to the lateral ventricular wall • Measures between 6 and 10 mm throughout pregnancy
Cavum septi pellucidi	• Presence excludes almost every subtle midline brain malformation • Filled with cerebrospinal fluid • Found at the level of the BPD • Located inferior to the anterior horns of the lateral ventricles • Closes by 2 years of age	• Small anechoic box located in the midline portion of the anterior brain
Cerebellum	• Consists of a vermis and two lateral horns • Located in the posterior fossa	• Dumb-bell–shaped echogenic structure located in the midline of the posterior fossa
Choroid plexus	• Echogenic cluster of cells • Important in the production of cerebrospinal fluid • Not located in the anterior or occipital horns • Choroid plexus cyst(s) will normally regress by 23 gestational weeks	• Hyperechoic structures located within each lateral ventricle • Lie along the atrium of the lateral ventricle • Cysts may be displayed within choroid
Cisterna magna	• Fluid-filled space located between the undersurface of the cerebellum and medulla oblongata	• Anterior–posterior diameter ≤10 mm • Measure from the cerebellar vermis to the calvaria
Falx cerebri	• Intrahemisphere fissure • Separates the cerebral hemispheres	• Echogenic midline linear structure
Nuchal thickness	• Soft-tissue thickness between the calvaria and posterior skin line • Measured in the axial plane at a level to include the cerebellum, cistern magnum, and cavum septum pellucidi • Accurate up to 20 gestational weeks • Thickening associated with aneuploidy	• Thickness ≤6 mm

Normal Thoracic Anatomy

STRUCTURE	INFORMATION	SONOGRAPHIC APPEARANCE
Diaphragm	• Muscle separating the thorax and abdominal cavities • Courses anterior to posterior	• Curvilinear hypoechoic structure • Abdominal contents lie inferior • Chest contents lie superior
Heart	• Apex points toward the left side of the body at about a 45° angle • Right ventricle lies most anterior • Left atrium lies most posterior	• Lies midline in the chest • Hyperechoic ventricular and atrial septums • 120-160 beats per min • Hyperechoic focus within the ventricle is most likely the papillary muscle
Lungs	• Serve as lateral borders to the heart • Lie superior to the diaphragm	• Moderately echogenic • Homogeneous • Increases in echogenicity as gestation progresses

Normal Abdominal Anatomy

STRUCTURE	INFORMATION	SONOGRAPHIC APPEARANCE
Bladder	• Signifies genitourinary system is working • The bladder fills and empties approximately every 30-60 minutes	• Round anechoic structure located centrally in the inferior pelvis
Bowel	• Meconium begins to accumulate in the small bowel • Small bowel becomes visible in the late second trimester • Large bowel becomes visible in the third trimester	Small Bowel • Moderately echogenic • Hyperechoic compared to the normal liver • Hypoechoic compared to bone Large Bowel • Hypoechoic to the small bowel
Gallbladder	• Visualization peaks around 20-32 gestational weeks • Signifies the presence of the biliary tree	• Elongated fluid-filled structure • Located inferior and to the right of the umbilical vein

Kidneys	• Urine formation begins near the end of the first trimester
	• May be identified as early as 15 weeks
	• Consistently identified by 20 weeks
		• Isoechoic or hypoechoic structures located on each side of the spine
		• Bilateral elliptical structures in the sagittal plane
		• Bilateral circular structures in the transverse plane
		• Renal pelvis contains a small amount of fluid
		  ○ ≤4 mm up to 33 weeks
		  ○ ≤7 mm from 33 weeks to term

Liver	• Largest organ in the fetal torso • Reflects changes in fetal growth	• Moderately echogenic structure • Left lobe is larger than the right lobe • Occupies most of the upper abdomen
Stomach	• Reliably visualized by 13 gestational weeks • Signifies normal swallowing sequence	• Anechoic structure located in the left upper quadrant • Size and shape will vary with recent swallowing • Echogenic debris within the stomach
Umbilical cord insertion	• Placental insertion generally located in the mid portion of the placenta	• Smooth abdominal wall at umbilical insertion • Umbilical vein courses superiorly toward the liver • Umbilical arteries arise from the hypogastric arteries on each side of the fetal bladder

Normal Musculoskeletal Anatomy

STRUCTURE	INFORMATION	SONOGRAPHIC APPEARANCE

Facial structures	• Sagittal view (profile) is useful in determining:
	  1. Relationship of the nose to lips
	  2. Frontal bossing
	  3. Chin formation
	• Coronal view is useful for visualizing:
	  1. Orbital rings
	  2. Maxilla
	  3. Mandible
	  4. Nasal septum
	  5. Parietal bones
	  6. Zygomatic bones
	• Tangential view is useful in determining:
	  1. Craniofacial abnormalities
		• The segments containing the forehead, eyes and nose, and the mouth and chin each form one-third of the face

Spine	• The spine widens near the base of the skull and tapers near the sacrum
	• When evaluating the spine, the transducer must remain perpendicular to the spinous elements
		• Coronal plane
		  1. Three parallel hyperechoic lines
		• Sagittal plane
		  1. Two ossification centers
		  2. Two curvilinear hyperechoic lines
		• Transverse plane
		  1. Three equidistant ossification centers surrounding the neural canal
		  2. Spinal column appears as a closed circle
		• Skin line
		  1. Echogenic smooth line posterior to the spine

Placenta and Umbilical Cord

STRUCTURE	INFORMATION	SONOGRAPHIC APPEARANCE
Amniotic fluid (AF)	• Surrounds and protects the fetus • Provides important information on fetal renal and placental function • Fetus becomes the major producer of AF through swallowing and urine production after 16 weeks	• Anechoic fluid surrounds the fetus • Swirling of fine echogenic particles (vernix)
Cervical os	• Length of cervix determines competence • Length is measured between the internal and external cervical os • Normal length varies between 2.5 and 4.0 cm	• Echogenic linear structure • Hyperechoic central echoes
Placenta	• Communication organ between the fetus and mother • Supplies nutrition and products of metabolism to the fetus	• Echogenic disc-shaped mass of tissue • Hyperechoic compared to the myometrium • Smooth and tapered margins • Thickness <5 cm
Umbilical cord	• Connecting lifeline between the fetus and placenta • Consists of one vein and two arteries • Umbilical vein enters the left portal vein • Umbilical arteries arise from the internal iliac (hypogastric) arteries • Normally inserts into the mid portion of the placenta • Bathed in Wharton jelly	• Solid, coiled structure containing three anechoic vessels • Twisting of the cord is normal Umbilical Artery • Low resistance near the fetal insertion • High resistance near the placental insertion Umbilical Vein • Continuous low flow through systole and diastole • Flow is directed from the placenta to the fetus

ASSESSMENT OF THE SECOND TRIMESTER REVIEW

1. Which portion of the fetal heart is located closest to the spine?
   a. left atrium
   b. right atrium
   c. left ventricle
   d. right ventricle
   e. intraventricular septum

2. Abdominal circumference is measured at the level of the:
   a. liver
   b. spleen
   c. kidneys
   d. hypogastric arteries
   e. umbilical cord insertion

3. Cavum septum pellucidi is located in the:
   a. anterior portion of the fetal brain
   b. posterior portion of the fetal brain
   c. anterior portion of the fetal chest
   d. posterior portion of the fetal chest
   e. anterior abdominal wall of the fetus

4. In the late second trimester, anterior–posterior diameter of the normal renal pelvis should not exceed:
   a. 1 mm
   b. 4 mm
   c. 7 mm
   d. 10 mm
   e. 13 mm

5. Which of the following structures is NOT identified in the biparietal diameter?
   a. falx cerebri
   b. thalami nuclei
   c. fourth ventricle
   d. cavum septum pellucidi
   e. atrium of the lateral ventricle

6. The umbilical arteries arise from which of the following vessels?
   a. spiral arteries
   b. abdominal aorta
   c. internal iliac arteries
   d. external iliac arteries
   e. common iliac arteries

7. Visualization of the fetal gallbladder signifies:
   a. fetal swallowing
   b. normal liver function
   c. a normal fetal karyotype
   d. the presence of the pancreas
   e. the presence of a biliary tree

8. Which of the following best describes the intention of the cephalic index?
   a. Gestational weight is determined by the cephalic index.
   b. The cephalic index primarily determines gestational age.
   c. The cephalic index helps determine the date of conception.
   d. Intrauterine growth restriction is determined by the cephalic index.
   e. The cephalic index helps to determine the normalcy of the fetal head shape.

9. Which of the following measurements is most widely used when determining gestational age in the second trimester?
   a. long bone length
   b. crown–rump length
   c. biparietal diameter
   d. cerebellar dimension
   e. abdominal circumference

10. Choroid plexus cysts will normally regress by:
    a. 12 weeks
    b. 18 weeks
    c. 23 weeks
    d. 28 weeks
    e. 32 weeks

11. Which of the following planes demonstrate the normal fetal spine as three parallel hyperechoic lines on ultrasound?
    a. axial
    b. sagittal
    c. coronal
    d. transverse
    e. tangential

12. The normal length of the cervical os will vary, but measures a minimum of:
    a. 2.0 cm
    b. 2.5 cm
    c. 3.0 cm
    d. 3.5 cm
    e. 4.0 cm

13. The anterior posterior diameter of the cisterna magna should not exceed:
    a. 6 mm
    b. 10 mm
    c. 15 mm
    d. 20 mm
    e. 25 mm

14. Measurement of the nuchal thickness is accurate up to:
    a. 13 weeks
    b. 15 weeks
    c. 20 weeks
    d. 23 weeks
    e. 27 weeks

15. Ventriculomegaly is suspected when the lateral ventricle measurement exceeds:
    a. 6 mm
    b. 10 mm
    c. 15 mm
    d. 23 mm
    e. 25 mm

Using Fig. 24-1, answer question 16.

16. The arrow in this sonogram is identifying the:
    a. thalami
    b. falx cerebri
    c. third ventricle
    d. sylvian fissure
    e. cavum septum pellucidi

Using Fig. 24-2, answer question 17.

17. This coronal sonogram of a 26-week fetus is most likely demonstrating a(n):
    a. abnormal thorax
    b. normal diaphragm
    c. abnormal stomach
    d. normal nuchal thickness
    e. abnormal bowel pattern

Using Fig. 24-3, answer question 18.

18. An asymptomatic patient presents for a second-trimester fetal screening examination. The arrow is identifying which of the following structures?
    a. hydroureter
    b. gallbladder
    c. left portal vein
    d. umbilical vein
    e. right portal vein

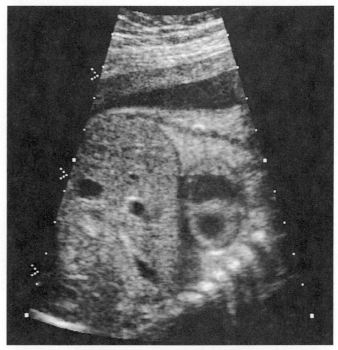

FIG. 24-2 Coronal sonogram.

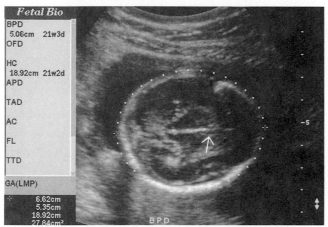

FIG. 24-1 Biparietal diameter.

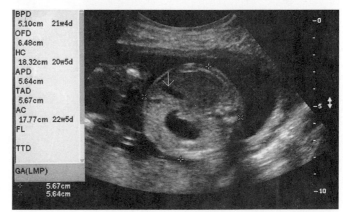

FIG. 24-3 Cross-sectional sonogram of the fetal abdomen.

Using Fig. 24-4, answer questions 19 and 20.

19. Arrow **A** is identifying the:
    a. vermis
    b. cerebellum
    c. sylvian fissure
    d. thalami nuclei
    e. cisterna magna

20. Arrow **B** is identifying the:
    a. cerebellum
    b. nuchal fold
    c. cisterna magna
    d. fourth ventricle
    e. cavum septum pellucidi

Using Fig. 24-5, answer question 21.

21. A sagittal image of the fetal abdomen identifies a structure most consistent with a:
    a. normal right kidney
    b. normal left kidney
    c. left adrenal hemorrhage
    d. right adrenal hemorrhage
    e. normal left adrenal gland

Using Fig. 24-6, answer questions 22 and 23.

22. An obstetrical patient presents with a history of large for dates. A sagittal sonogram reveals several sonolucent structures. Which of the following fetal structures is the arrow most likely identifying?
    a. ovarian cyst
    b. urinary bladder
    c. umbilical varix
    d. hypogastric artery
    e. fluid-filled bowel loop

23. The echogenic focus within the fetal stomach is considered:
    a. a normal incidental finding
    b. suspicious for a malignant tumor
    c. suspicious for Turner's syndrome
    d. a precursor to meconium peritonitis
    e. a consistent finding in Patau syndrome

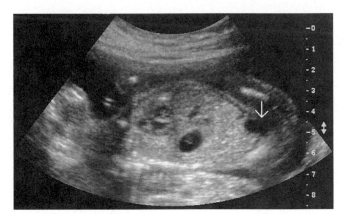

FIG. 24-6   Sagittal sonogram of the fetal body.

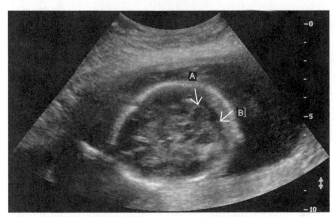

FIG. 24-4   Sonogram of the fetal head.

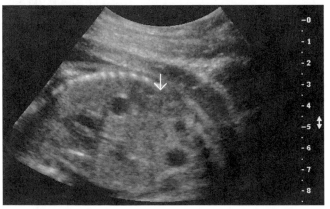

FIG. 24-5   Sonogram of the fetal abdomen.

Using Fig. 24-7, answer question 24.

24. The sonogram displays which of the following cardiac structures?
   a. aortic arch
   b. mitral valve
   c. foramen ovale
   d. left ventricular outflow tract
   e. right ventricular outflow tract

Using Fig. 24-8, answer question 25.

25. The calipers are measuring the:
   a. nuchal fold
   b. cerebellum
   c. cisterna magna
   d. ocular distance
   e. lateral ventricle

Using Fig. 24-9, answer questions 26 and 27.

26. The relationship of the placenta to the internal cervical os is termed:
   a. low-lying placenta
   b. within normal limits
   c. marginal placenta previa
   d. complete placenta previa
   e. incomplete placenta previa

27. This image displays the location of the placenta as:
   a. fundal
   b. anterior
   c. posterior
   d. right lateral
   e. complete previa

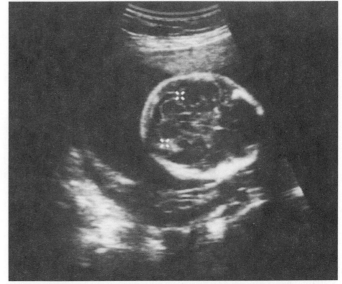
FIG. 24-8 Sonogram of the fetal head.

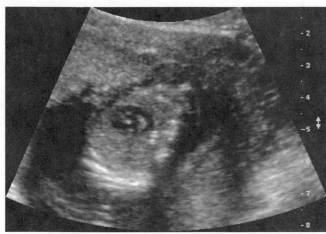
FIG. 24-7 Sonogram of the fetal chest.

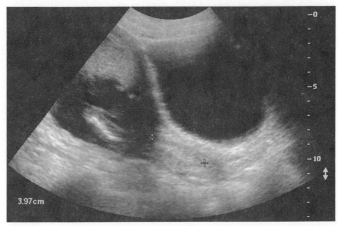
FIG. 24-9 Sagittal sonogram.

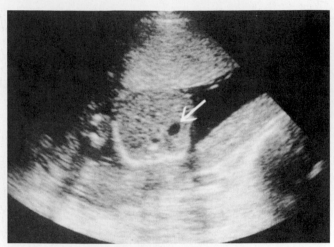

FIG. 24-10 Sonogram of the fetal abdomen.

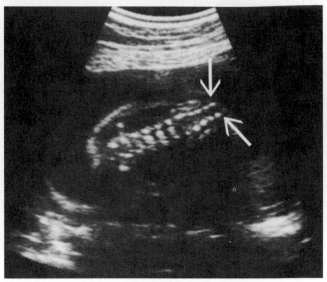

FIG. 24-11 Sonogram of the fetal spine.

Using Fig. 24-10, answer question 28.

28. The arrow is identifying which of the following structures?
a. stomach
b. renal cyst
c. gallbladder
d. renal pelvis
e. umbilical vein varix

Using Fig. 24-11, answer question 29.

29. The arrows in this sonogram are demonstrating a:
a. coronal view of a sacral defect
b. sagittal view of a normal coccyx
c. coronal view of a normal sacrum
d. sagittal view of a normal sacrum
e. coronal view of a normal coccyx

30. In the transverse plane, the normal fetal spine appears on ultrasound as:
a. two ossification centers lateral to the spinal canal
b. three parallel hyperechoic lines surrounding the neural canal
c. three parallel ossification centers surrounding the neural canal
d. four equidistant ossification centers surrounding the spinal canal
e. three equidistant ossification centers surrounding the spinal canal

31. Which landmark localizes the appropriate level for measuring the abdominal circumference?
a. stomach
b. gallbladder
c. cord insertion
d. hypogastric arteries
e. junction of the left and right portal veins

32. Which of the following is a possible cause for elevated maternal alpha-fetoprotein?
a. trophoblastic disease
b. abdominal wall defect
c. chromosomal abnormalities
d. overestimation gestational age
e. chronic maternal hypertension

33. The biparietal diameter measurement is taken at the level of the:
a. cerebellum
b. falx cerebri
c. third ventricle
d. cisterna magna
e. corpus callosum

34. Left ventricular outflow tract denotes the:
a. foramen ovale
b. ascending aorta
c. papillary muscle
d. descending aorta
e. pulmonary artery

35. Which of the following provides important information about fetal renal function?
a. renal size
b. bladder volume
c. placenta maturity
d. renal pelviectasis
e. amniotic fluid volume

36. Normal measurement of the lateral ventricle atria should not exceed:
a. 5 mm
b. 7 mm
c. 10 mm
d. 12 mm
e. 15 mm

37. If the maternal alpha-fetoprotein level is decreased, the sonographer should carefully evaluate for:
    a. neural tube defects
    b. abdominal wall defects
    c. chromosomal abnormalities
    d. genitourinary abnormalities
    e. cardiovascular abnormalities

38. A small echogenic focus within the left ventricle of the fetal heart is mostly likely the:
    a. mitral valve
    b. atrial septum
    c. foramen ovale
    d. pulmonary vein
    e. papillary muscle

39. Insertion of the umbilical cord into the abdominal wall of the fetus is located at a level:
    a. superior to the liver
    b. inferior to the sacrum
    c. superior to the bladder
    d. superior to the adrenal glands
    e. inferior to the hypogastric arteries

40. Which imaging plane is optimal for evaluating the fetus for facial cleft?
    a. profile
    b. sagittal
    c. coronal
    d. tangential
    e. transverse

41. Assessment of gestational age in the second trimester routinely uses all of the following measurements EXCEPT:
    a. femur length
    b. biparietal diameter
    c. crown–rump length
    d. head circumference
    e. abdominal circumference

42. Oxygenated blood enters the fetus through the:
    a. placenta
    b. umbilical vein
    c. chorionic villi
    d. ductus venosum
    e. umbilical arteries

43. Nuchal thickness is measured in a plane to include the:
    a. thalamic cerebri, falx cerebri, third ventricle
    b. cerebellum, cisterna magna, cavum septum pellucidi
    c. lateral ventricle atria, third ventricle, corpus callosum
    d. cisterna magna, lateral ventricle atria, thalamic cerebri
    e. thalamic cerebri, third ventricle, cavum septum pellucidi

44. Sonographic appearance of a normal small bowel during the second trimester is described as:
    a. hyperechoic compared to bone
    b. hyperechoic compared to the liver
    c. hypoechoic compared to the spleen
    d. hyperechoic compared to the rib cage
    e. hypoechoic compared to the large bowel

45. Echogenic debris swirling within the amniotic cavity is:
    a. consistent with fetal demise
    b. a normal sonographic finding
    c. consistent with polyhydramnios
    d. suspicious for chromosomal anomalies
    e. suspicious for anterior abdominal wall defects

46. The fetus becomes the major producer of amniotic fluid in the:
    a. late first trimester
    b. early second trimester
    c. late second trimester
    d. early third trimester
    e. late third trimester

47. Visualization of which brain structure excludes most midline brain abnormalities?
    a. falx cerebri
    b. third ventricle
    c. corpus callosum
    d. thalamic cerebri
    e. cavum septum pellucidi

48. The material collecting in the fetal intestines is termed:
    a. bile
    b. sludge
    c. vernix
    d. vermis
    e. meconium

49. Head circumference is measured at a level to include the:
    a. cerebellum and sylvian fissure
    b. third ventricle and cisterna magna
    c. cavum septum pellucidi and tentorium
    d. peduncles and cavum septum pellucidi
    e. atrium of the lateral ventricle and cerebellum

50. Which of the following measurements is a good predictor of fetal growth?
    a. femur length
    b. humerus length
    c. biparietal diameter
    d. head circumference
    e. abdominal circumference

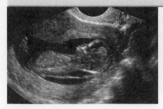

CHAPTER 25

Assessment of the Third Trimester

KEY TERMS

asymmetric intrauterine growth restriction most common type of growth abnormality demonstrating normal cranial growth and a decrease in abdominal growth.

biophysical profile objective means for assessing fetal well-being.

hypertension A systolic pressure ≥140 mmHg or a diastolic pressure ≥90 mmHg.

oligohydramnios amniotic fluid below the normal range for gestational age.

polyhydramnios amniotic fluid above the normal range for gestational age.

postterm pregnancy gestation greater than 42 weeks.

macrosomia a condition in which accelerated fetal growth results in an infant with a birth weight over 4000 g; associated with birth asphyxia and trauma.

symmetric intrauterine growth restriction fetal growth abnormality resulting in a proportionally small fetus.

vernix caseosa fatty material found on the fetal skin and amniotic fluid late in pregnancy.

THIRD TRIMESTER

- The fetus has grown to approximately 15 in. in length and 1000-1400 g in weight by the beginning of the third trimester.
- Lungs, organs, and vessels are maturing in preparation for birth.

THIRD-TRIMESTER MEASUREMENTS

- Biparietal diameter (BPD).
- Head circumference (HC).
- Abdominal circumference (AC).
- Femur length.
- Amniotic fluid volume.
- Head circumference-to-abdominal circumference ratio (HC/AC).
  - During the early third trimester the head circumference is slightly larger than the circumference of the abdomen.
  - During the late third trimester, with the increase of fetal body fat, the abdominal circumference is typically equal to or slightly larger than the head circumference.
- Estimated fetal weight.
  - Most commonly calculated using the biparietal diameter, femur length, and abdominal circumference.
  - Overall accuracy falls within 18% of the fetal actual weight in 95% of the cases.

FETAL GROWTH

- Interval fetal growth can be determined with ultrasound examinations a minimum of 3 weeks apart.
- In the last 3 months of pregnancy, the fetus will grow an additional 4 in. in length and gain an additional 2000-2800 g in weight at 100-200 g per week.

- Distal femoral epiphysis (DFE) is visualized around 32 gestational weeks.
- Proximal tibial epiphysis (PTE) is visualized around 35 gestational weeks.

DECREASE IN FETAL GROWTH

Small for Gestational Age

- Covers both normal and subnormal fetal growth.
- May be a result of incorrect dates or oligohydramnios.

Intrauterine Growth Restriction

- Results from insufficient fetal nutrition.
- Defined as a fetal weight at or below the 10th percentile for gestational age.
- No single reliable criterion is available to diagnose intrauterine growth restriction.
- Associated with maternal hypertension.
- Evaluation of the amniotic fluid volume, estimated fetal weight, and maternal blood pressure results in the most accurate diagnosis.
- Maternal hypertension increases the risk of intrauterine growth restriction by 25%.
- The liver is one of the most severely affected fetal organs.
- Decrease in liver size results in a decrease in abdominal circumference.

Intrauterine Growth Restriction

TYPE	ETIOLOGY	CLINICAL FINDINGS	SONOGRAPHIC FINDINGS	DIFFERENTIAL CONSIDERATIONS
Asymmetric	• Placental insufficiency • Chromosomal abnormality • Infection Maternal Risk Factors • Hypertension • Poor nutrition • Alcohol and drug abuse	• Small for dates • Low maternal weight gain • Hypertension	• Lack of fetal growth on serial sonograms • Decrease in abdominal circumference • Normal head circumference and femur length • Decrease in amniotic fluid volume • Increase in HC/AC ratio • Placentomalacia Umbilical Artery • Systolic–diastolic ratio of umbilical artery >3.0 after 30 weeks • Absence of diastolic flow • Reversal of diastolic flow is considered critical Umbilical Vein • Decrease in flow volume	• Normal small fetus • Skeletal dysplasia
Symmetric	• Result of embryologic insult	• Small for dates	• Symmetrically small head and abdomen circumference • Oligohydramnios	• Incorrect menstrual dates • Normal small fetus • Skeletal dysplasia

INCREASE IN FETAL GROWTH

Large for Gestational Age

- Covers both normal and increased fetal growth.
- May be a result of incorrect dates, macrosomia, or polyhydramnios.

Macrosomia

- Fetal weight above 4000 g or above the 90th percentile for gestational age.
- Fetuses of diabetic mothers are likely to display organomegaly whereas fetuses of nondiabetic mothers will demonstrate normal growth.
- Fetuses of diabetic mothers demonstrate a higher mortality rate.

Macrosomia

CONDITION	ETIOLOGY	CLINICAL FINDINGS	SONOGRAPHIC FINDINGS	DIFFERENTIAL CONSIDERATIONS
Macrosomia	• Maternal diabetes mellitus • Maternal obesity • Postterm pregnancy	• Large for dates	• Large abdominal circumference • Decreased HC/AC ratio • Estimated fetal weight >4000 g • Polyhydramnios • Placentomegaly	• Normal large fetus • Suboptimal fetal measurements

AMNIOTIC FLUID

- Normal volume of amniotic fluid varies with gestational age.
- Early in gestation, the major source of amniotic fluid is the amniotic membrane.
- As the embryo and placenta develop, fluid is produced by the placenta and fetus.
- After 16 gestational weeks, the fetus is the major producer of amniotic fluid.

AMNIOTIC FLUID VOLUME

- Normal volume of amniotic fluid increases progressively until about 33 gestational weeks.
- During the late second and early third trimester, the amniotic fluid volume appears to surround the fetus.
- By the late third trimester, the amniotic fluid displays as isolated fluid pockets.
- Regulated by the production of fluid, swallowing of fluid (removal), fluid exchange within the lungs, membranes, and cord.
- Normal lung development depends on the exchange of amniotic fluid within the lungs.
- Oligohydramnios increases risk of fetal death and neonatal morbidity.

FUNCTIONS OF THE AMNIOTIC FLUID

- Maintains intrauterine temperature.
- Allows fetus free movement within the amniotic cavity.
- Protects the developing fetus from injury.
- Prevents adherence of the amnion to the fetus.
- Allows symmetric growth.

MEASURING AMNIOTIC FLUID VOLUME

- Transducer must remain perpendicular to the maternal coronal plane and parallel to the maternal sagittal plane.
- Fluid pocket must be free of umbilical cord or any fetal part.

Methods of Assessing Amniotic Fluid Volume

METHOD	DESCRIPTION	NORMAL SONOGRAPHIC FINDINGS	ABNORMAL SONOGRAPHIC FINDINGS
Amniotic fluid index (AFI)	• Determined by dividing the uterus into four equal parts • Measure deepest unobstructed pocket in each quadrant • AFI is equal to the sum of all four quadrants	• AFI greater than 5 cm and less than 20 cm	• AFI less than or equal to 5 cm or greater than 20 cm
Single deepest pocket	• Maximum vertical depth of any amniotic fluid pocket	• Largest pocket greater than 2 cm and less than 8 cm	• Largest pocket less than 1 cm or greater than 8 cm
Subjective assessment	• Observing the amount of amniotic fluid during real-time examination • Experience increases accuracy	• Amount of amniotic fluid appears within normal limits for gestation	• Amniotic fluid appears greater or less than expected for the gestational age

Abnormal Amniotic Fluid Volume

ABNORMALITY	ETIOLOGY	SONOGRAPHIC FINDINGS	DIFFERENTIAL CONSIDERATIONS

Oligohydramnios	• Fetal
	  ○ Genitourinary tract abnormality
	  ○ Intrauterine growth restriction
	• Maternal
	  ○ Poor nutrition
	  ○ Placenta insufficiency
	  ○ Premature rupture of membranes
		• AFI below 5 cm
		• Below the 5th percentile for gestational age
		• Largest single pocket below 1 cm
		• Poor fetal–fluid interface
			• Lower limits of normal
			• Premature rupture of membranes

Polyhydramnios	• Fetal Anomalies
	  ○ Central nervous system
	  ○ Gastrointestinal tract
	  ○ Abdominal wall defects
	  ○ Cardiac defects
	• Maternal
	  ○ Diabetes mellitus
	  ○ Cardiac disease
	  ○ Preeclampsia
	• Idiopathic
		• AFI above 20 cm
		• Volume exceeding 2000 mL
		• Above the 95th percentile for gestational age
		• Fetal anatomy is easy to visualize
		• AFI above 24 cm associated with fetal anomalies
			• Upper limits of normal

FETAL WELL-BEING

BIOPHYSICAL PROFILE

- Indirectly tests for fetal hypoxia.
- Nonstress test findings, fetal tone, breathing, and body movements are markers of acute fetal hypoxia.
- Amniotic fluid volume is a marker of chronic fetal hypoxia.

Biophysical Profile

	DESCRIPTION	NORMAL FINDINGS	ABNORMAL FINDINGS

Biophysical profile	• Objective means for assessing fetal well-being
	• Fetus is observed for 30 minutes
	• Five parameters are evaluated:
	  1. Fetal tone
	  2. Fetal movement
	  3. Fetal breathing movement
	  4. Amniotic fluid volume
	  5. Nonstress test or placenta grade
	• Scoring of the parameters:
	  0 = does not exhibit
	  1 = partially exhibits
	  2 = exhibits fully
		1. Fetal Tone
		  • One complete episode of flexion to extension and back to flexion
		2. Fetal Movement
		  • Three separate fetal movements within 30 minutes
		3. Fetal Breathing Movement
		  • Movement of the diaphragm ≥30 seconds
		4. Amniotic Fluid Volume
		  • Amniotic pocket >2 cm
		  or
		  • Amniotic fluid index >5 cm
		5. Nonstress Test
		  • Exhibits two fetal heart accelerations within 20 minutes
		  or
		  • Placental grade ≥2
		  • Total Points ≥8
			1. Fetal Tone
			  • Incomplete or lack of flexion to extension and back to flexion
			2. Fetal Movement
			  • Two or fewer separate fetal movements within 30 minutes
			3. Fetal Breathing Movement
			  • No movement of the diaphragm or duration <30 seconds
			4. Amniotic Fluid Volume
			  • An amniotic pocket <2 cm
			  or
			  • Amniotic fluid index ≤5 cm
			5. Nonstress Test
			  • Exhibits two or fewer fetal heart accelerations within 40 minutes
			  or
			  • Placental grade = 3
			  • Total Points <6

FETAL PRESENTATION

- Relationship of the fetal head with the internal cervical os.
- Fetal position changes less frequently after 34 gestational weeks.
- Nonvertex fetal position after 34 weeks may be predictive of positional or placental problems.

CEPHALIC OR VERTEX

- Fetal head lies most inferior, closest to the cervical os.

TRANSVERSE

- Fetal head and body lie across the maternal abdomen.
- Check for signs of placenta previa.

OBLIQUE

- Fetal head and body are lying at a 45° angle to the maternal sagittal plane.
- Document location of the fetal head.

BREECH

- Fetal head is located in the superior portion of the uterus.
- Presenting part should be determined after 36 weeks' gestation.

Frank Breech

- Fetal buttocks are presenting with the feet near head.
- Most common.

Complete Breech

- Fetal buttocks are presenting with the knees bent and feet down.
- Least common.

Incomplete Breech

- Footling breech.
- Fetal foot is the presenting part.
- One or both legs are extended.
- Greatest risk for prolapsed cord.

ASSESSMENT OF THE THIRD TRIMESTER REVIEW

1. The most common maternal factor associated with intrauterine growth restriction is:
   a. obesity
   b. hypertension
   c. hyperlipidemia
   d. diabetes mellitus
   e. oligohydramnios

2. Polyhydramnios demonstrates an amniotic volume index greater than:
   a. 5 cm
   b. 10 cm
   c. 15 cm
   d. 20 cm
   e. 28 cm

3. The distal femoral epiphysis is consistently visualized by:
   a. 20 weeks
   b. 28 weeks
   c. 32 weeks
   d. 35 weeks
   e. 38 weeks

4. Oligohydramnios in the third trimester is most likely a result of:
   a. anencephaly
   b. duodenal atresia
   c. diaphragmatic hernia
   d. infantile polycystic disease
   e. cystic adenomatoid malformation

5. The most common maternal cause of macrosomia is:
   a. anemia
   b. proteinuria
   c. hypertension
   d. diabetes mellitus
   e. cigarette smoking

6. Which portion of the biophysical profile study is a chronic marker of fetal hypoxia?
   a. fetal tone
   b. nonstress test
   c. fetal movement
   d. amniotic fluid volume
   e. maturity of the placenta

7. When measuring amniotic fluid volume, the transducer must remain:
   a. parallel to both the maternal sagittal and coronal planes
   b. perpendicular to both the maternal sagittal and coronal planes
   c. parallel with the maternal coronal plane and perpendicular to the sagittal plane
   d. perpendicular to the maternal coronal plane and parallel to the maternal sagittal plane
   e. parallel with the maternal transverse plane and perpendicular to the sagittal plane

8. A pregnancy is postterm when the:
   a. fetus weighs more than 3000 g
   b. pregnancy is longer than 40 weeks
   c. fetus weighs more than 4000 g
   d. pregnancy is longer than 42 weeks
   e. fetus weighs more than 4500 g

9. Symmetric intrauterine growth restriction is more commonly a result of:
   a. maternal diabetes
   b. first trimester insult
   c. maternal hypertension
   d. placental insufficiency
   e. second trimester insult

10. Doppler of the umbilical artery evaluates fetal well-being using the:
    a. resistive index
    b. pulsatility index
    c. peak systolic velocity
    d. end diastolic velocity
    e. systolic–diastolic ratio

11. Macrosomia is defined as a newborn weight exceeding:
    a. 1000 g
    b. 2500 g
    c. 4000 g
    d. 5500 g
    e. 6000 g

12. In a biophysical profile, which of the following will document fetal tone?
    a. fetal swallowing or urination
    b. movement of the fetal diaphragm
    c. three separate fetal movements in 30 seconds
    d. two fetal heart accelerations within 20 minutes
    e. complete episode of flexion to extension and back to flexion

13. Documentation of fetal position demonstrates a frank breech presentation. This means the fetal head is located in the superior portion of the uterus and the:
   a. buttocks are down with one foot presenting
   b. fetal foot is presenting with one leg extended
   c. fetal feet are presenting with both legs extended
   d. buttocks are presenting with the feet near the head
   e. buttocks are presenting with the knees bent and feet down

14. Maternal hypertension is defined as a systolic pressure above:
   a. 90 mmHg
   b. 100 mmHg
   c. 140 mmHg
   d. 175 mmHg
   e. 180 mmHg

15. Oligohydramnios is defined as an amniotic fluid index below:
   a. 2 cm
   b. 5 cm
   c. 10 cm
   d. 18 cm
   e. 24 cm

Using Fig. 25-1, answer question 16.

16. This third-trimester image is most suspicious for:
   a. macrosomia
   b. polyhydramnios
   c. oligohydramnios
   d. stuck twin syndrome
   e. gastrointestinal distress

Using Fig. 25-2, answer question 17.

17. Determine the fetal lie in this sonogram of the transverse gravid uterus:
   a. breech
   b. cephalic
   c. transverse head to maternal left
   d. transverse head to maternal right
   e. position cannot be determined by a single image

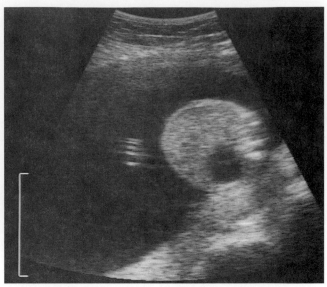

FIG. 25-1   Third trimester sonogram.

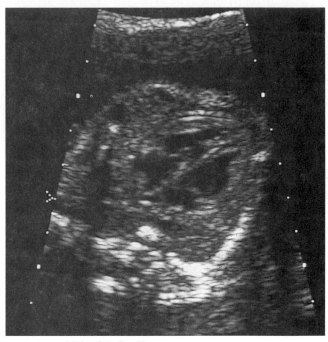

FIG. 25-2   Transverse sonogram.

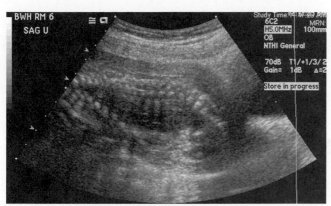

FIG. 25-3   Third trimester sonogram.

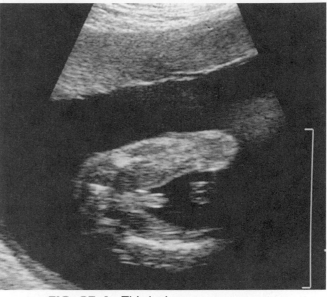

FIG. 25-4   Third trimester sonogram.

Using Fig. 25-3, answer questions 18 and 19.

18. What is this third trimester sonogram demonstrating?
   a. chorioangioma
   b. oligohydramnios
   c. trophoblastic disease
   d. diaphragmatic hernia
   e. cystic adenomatoid malformation

19. Which of the following is the most likely cause of this diagnosis?
   a. fetal hydrops
   b. duodenal atresia
   c. multicystic renal dysplasia
   d. premature rupture of membrane
   e. proliferation of the chorionic villi

Using Fig. 25-4, answer questions 20 and 21.

20. In addition to the gender of the fetus, this image reveals a(n):
   a. anterior placenta
   b. myelomeningocele
   c. skeletal dysplasia
   d. succenturiate placenta
   e. abnormal cord insertion

21. The fluid volume in this image is suspicious for:
   a. polyhydramnios
   b. oligohydramnios
   c. neural tube defects
   d. intrauterine infection
   e. chromosomal anomalies

22. Overall accuracy in sonographic estimation of fetal weight during the third trimester is:
   a. 25%
   b. 50%
   c. 65%
   d. 75%
   e. 95%

23. Comparison of the abdominal circumference to the head circumference during the early third trimester demonstrates a(n):
   a. equal head circumference compared to abdominal circumference
   b. abdominal circumference twice as large as the head circumference
   c. head circumference slightly larger than the abdominal circumference
   d. abdominal circumference slightly larger than the head circumference
   e. head circumference approximately one third of the abdominal circumference

24. Asymmetric intrauterine growth restriction is usually a result of:
   a. preeclampsia
   b. maternal obesity
   c. gestational diabetes
   d. multifetal gestations
   e. placental insufficiency

25. Estimated fetal weight is most commonly calculated using which biometric parameters?
   a. femur length and abdominal circumference
   b. abdominal circumference, femur length, biparietal diameter
   c. head circumference, abdominal circumference, femur length
   d. biparietal diameter, head circumference, abdominal circumference
   e. biparietal diameter, head circumference-to-abdominal circumference ratio, femur length

26. Intrauterine growth restriction most severely affects which fetal body organ?
    a. heart
    b. liver
    c. brain
    d. kidney
    e. stomach

27. Assessing the total amount of amniotic fluid within the gestational sac using the sum of four equal quadrants is termed:
    a. pocket index
    b. total uterine volume
    c. amniotic fluid index
    d. amniotic fluid volume
    e. maximum pocket index

28. The single most sensitive indicator of intrauterine growth restriction is:
    a. femur length
    b. biparietal diameter
    c. head circumference
    d. abdominal circumference
    e. head circumference-to-abdominal circumference ratio

29. Which of the following conditions increases fetal risk of injury during vaginal delivery?
    a. macrosomia
    b. microcephaly
    c. cephalic presentation
    d. lateral placental placement
    e. intrauterine growth restriction

30. Which technique is both valid and reproducible when assessing amniotic fluid volume?
    a. uterine volume
    b. amniotic fluid index
    c. single vertical pocket
    d. subjective assessment
    e. maximum vertical pocket

31. Macrosomia and polyhydramnios encountered in the third trimester should raise suspicion of maternal:
    a. proteinuria
    b. preeclampsia
    c. hypertension
    d. diabetes mellitus
    e. drug or alcohol abuse

32. A biophysical profile examination of a 35-week fetus demonstrates a complete extension and flexion of lower extremities, four separate fetal movements, amniotic fluid volume of 10 cm, and a normal stress test. Fetal diaphragm or breathing motion is not identified. On the basis of these sonographic findings, the biophysical profile score would be:
    a. 2
    b. 5
    c. 8
    d. 10
    e. 15

33. What is the most common cause of painless vaginal bleeding during the third trimester?
    a. preterm labor
    b. placenta previa
    c. placenta accreta
    d. placenta abruption
    e. incompetent cervix

34. Which of the following correctly describes the expected sonographic findings with asymmetric intrauterine growth restriction?
    a. decrease in head circumference and femur length
    b. decrease in abdominal circumference and femur length
    c. normal head circumference and decrease in abdominal circumference
    d. normal abdominal circumference and decrease in head circumference
    e. increase in head circumference and decrease in abdominal circumference

35. Intrauterine growth restriction is defined as a fetal weight:
    a. below the 5th percentile for gestational age
    b. below the 10th percentile for gestational age
    c. at or below the 5th percentile for gestational age
    d. at or below the 10th percentile for gestational age
    e. at or below the 2nd percentile for gestational age

36. The best diagnostic accuracy of intrauterine growth restriction is offered when evaluating the:
    a. amniotic fluid volume, head circumference, and abdominal circumference
    b. placental maturity, umbilical artery, and amniotic fluid volume
    c. head circumference, abdominal circumference, and femur length
    d. cephalic index, abdominal circumference, and placental maturity
    e. amniotic fluid volume, estimated fetal weight, and maternal blood pressure

37. A transverse fetal position in the late third trimester of pregnancy is most likely associated with:
    a. macrosomia
    b. fetal hypoxia
    c. placenta previa
    d. polyhydramnios
    e. intrauterine growth restriction

38. Which of the following fetal positions is at most risk for cord prolapse?
    a. vertex
    b. oblique
    c. transverse
    d. frank breech
    e. incomplete breech

39. The biophysical profile is a sonographic method of evaluating fetal:
    a. age
    b. weight
    c. movement
    d. well-being
    e. swallowing

40. A fetus presents with multicystic dysplastic renal disease. The amniotic fluid volume is expected to appear:
    a. above normal
    b. below normal
    c. slightly lower than normal
    d. slightly higher than normal
    e. normal

41. Which of the following maternal conditions is most likely to result in a growth-restricted fetus?
    a. obesity
    b. diabetes
    c. drug abuse
    d. hypotension
    e. deep vein thrombosis

42. Interval fetal growth can be determined with sonographic examinations performed a minimum of how many weeks apart?
    a. 1
    b. 3
    c. 5
    d. 7
    e. 8

43. Which of the following is NOT a function of the amniotic fluid?
    a. protects fetus from injury
    b. allows free fetal movement
    c. stores protein, calcium, and iron
    d. allows symmetric fetal growth
    e. maintains intrauterine temperature

44. Which of the following is a sonographic finding in cases of asymmetric intrauterine growth restriction?
    a. placentomegaly
    b. polyhydramnios
    c. short femur length
    d. normal biparietal diameter
    e. normal abdominal circumference

45. A systolic-to-diastolic ratio of the umbilical artery can be used to evaluate fetal well-being:
    a. any time during the pregnancy
    b. after the 30th week of gestation
    c. after the first trimester of pregnancy
    d. beginning the 20th week of gestation
    e. beginning the third trimester of pregnancy

46. The single most useful biometric parameter to assess fetal growth is the:
    a. femur length
    b. cerebellar width
    c. biparietal diameter
    d. head circumference
    e. abdominal circumference

47. This term indicates the fetal head is located in the uterine fundus:
    a. vertex
    b. breech
    c. oblique
    d. cephalic
    e. transverse

48. A fetus presenting in the breech position during the third trimester may demonstrate a cranial shape termed:
    a. lemon sign
    b. clover-leaf
    c. dolichocephalic
    d. brachycephalic
    e. strawberry sign

49. If a fetus is lying perpendicular to the maternal sagittal plane, the fetal presentation is:
    a. vertex
    b. breech
    c. oblique
    d. cephalic
    e. transverse

50. Visualization of the proximal tibial epiphysis first occurs around:
    a. 20 weeks' gestation
    b. 24 weeks' gestation
    c. 30 weeks' gestation
    d. 35 weeks' gestation
    e. 38 weeks' gestation

CHAPTER 26

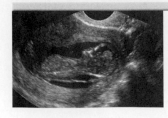

Fetal Abnormalities

KEY TERMS

acromelia   shortening of the bones of the hands or feet.

banana sign   crescent shape to the cerebellum displayed with a coexisting neural tube defect.

bladder exstrophy   protrusion of the posterior bladder wall through a defect in the lower abdominal wall and anterior wall of the urinary bladder.

corpus callosum   band of white matter tissue connecting the cerebral hemispheres; serves a function in both learning and memory.

frontal bossing   protrusion or bulging of the forehead associated with hydrocephalus.

hydrocephalus   overt enlargement of the lateral ventricles.

hypertelorism   abnormally widespread position of the orbits.

hypotelorism   abnormally close position of the orbits.

keyhole sign   appearance of the dilated bladder superior to the obstructed male urethra.

lemon sign   concavity to the front bones of the fetal cranium; associated with spina bifida.

macroglossia   an excessively large tongue.

mesomelia   shortening of the middle portion of a limb.

micromelia   shortening of all portions of a limb.

myelomeningocele   a developmental defect of the central nervous system in which a hernial sac containing a portion of the spinal cord, its meninges, and cerebrospinal fluid protrudes through a congenital cleft in the vertebral column.

nuchal thickness   distance between the calvaria and posterior skin line.

rhizomelia   shortening of the proximal portion of a limb.

steer sign   enlargement and upper displacement of the third ventricle associated with agenesis of the corpus callosum.

vermis   structure located between the hemispheres of the cerebellum.

Cranial Abnormalities

ABNORMALITY	INFORMATION	SONOGRAPHIC FINDINGS	DIFFERENTIAL CONSIDERATIONS
Acrania	• Abnormal migration of mesenchymal tissues • Coexisting spinal defects, clubfoot, cleft lip and palate	• Lack of hyperechoic bony calvaria • Brain tissue development • Prominent sulcal markings	• Anencephaly • Osteogenesis imperfecta
Agenesis of the corpus callosum	• Failure of callosal fibers to form a normal connection • Associated with multiple anomalies	• Dilation of the third ventricle • Outward angling of the frontal and lateral horns (steer sign) • Dilation of the occipital horn • Absent cavum septum pellucidi	• Holoprosencephaly
Arachnoid cyst	• Congenital abnormality of the pia-arachnoid layer • A result of trauma, infarction, or infection	• Splaying of cerebellum hemispheres • Normal vermis	• Dandy-Walker cyst • Prominent cistern magna • Vein of Galen aneurysm • Improper technique
Dandy-Walker syndrome	• Malformation of the cerebellum with associated maldevelopment of the 4th ventricle • Result of alcohol abuse, autosomal recessive disorder, or viral infection	• Enlarged posterior fossa • Splaying of the cerebellar hemispheres • Complete or partial agenesis of the vermis • Cistern magnum >1.0 cm in diameter	• Prominent posterior fossa • Arachnoid cyst • Vein of Galen aneurysm • Artifact

386

Cranial Abnormalities—cont'd

ABNORMALITY	INFORMATION	SONOGRAPHIC FINDINGS	DIFFERENTIAL CONSIDERATIONS
Hydranencephaly	• Destruction of the cerebral cortex resulting from vascular compromise or congenital infection • Brain tissue is replaced by cerebrospinal fluid	• Anechoic brain tissue • Presence of the falx cerebri • Brain stem usually spared • Choroid plexus may be displayed	• Severe hydrocephalus • Holoprosencephaly
Hydrocephalus	• Increase in ventricular volume • Occipital horn dilates first	• Ventriculomegaly is generally symmetrical Mild enlargement • Lateral ventricle measuring 10-15 mm Severe enlargement • Lateral ventricle measuring >15 mm • Dangling of the choroid plexus • Echogenic rim of solid brain tissue	• Hydranencephaly • Holoprosencephaly • Improper technique
Holoprosencephaly	• Group of disorders arising from abnormal development of the forebrain Alobar • Monoventricular cavity • Mostsevere form Semilobar • Monoventricular cavity • Milder form Lobar • Mildest form • Two large lateral ventricles	Alobar • Large central single ventricle • Fused thalami • Absence of cavum septum pellucidi, falx cerebri, corpus callosum, and third ventricle • Normal cerebellum • Hypotelorism • Cyclopia • Proboscis	• Severe hydrocephalus • Hydranencephaly
Microcephaly	• Overall reduction in brain size • Chromosomal aberration • Difficult to detect prior to 24 weeks	• Small BPD and HC • Decreased HC/AC ratio • Sloping forehead	• Anencephaly • Encephalocele
Prosencephaly	• A result of infarction or hemorrhage of the brain	• Anechoic mass within an area of brain tissue • Midline brain shift	• Cystic leukomalacia

Neural Tube Defect

DEFECT	INFORMATION	SONOGRAPHIC FINDINGS	DIFFERENTIAL CONSIDERATIONS
Anencephaly	• Failure of the cephalic end of the neural tube to close completely • Most common neural tube defect • Elevated alpha-fetoprotein (AFP) levels • Associated with malformations of the spine, face, feet, and abdominal wall	• Absence of the cranial vault • Bulging eyes • Rudimentary brain tissue herniating from the defect • Polyhydramnios • Increase in fetal activity	• Severe microcephaly • Acrania • Encephalocele • Amniotic band syndrome
Caudal regression	• Structural abnormality of the caudal end of the neural tube • More common in patients with diabetes	• Absent sacrum • Fused pelvis • Short femurs	• Skeletal dysplasia
Encephalocele	• Normal AFP level • Presence of brain in a cranial protrusion • More commonly arises in the occipital region	• Spherical fluid-filled or brain-filled sac extending from the calvaria • Bony calvarial defect	• Cystic hygroma • Clover-leaf skull deformity • Amniotic band syndrome • Microcephaly
Spina bifida	• Failure of the neural tube to completely close Occulta • Defect is covered by normal soft tissue • Normal AFP level • Rarely diagnosed with ultrasound Aperta • Defect is uncovered • Elevated AFP level • Associated with cleft lip and palate, cardiac defects, encephalocele gastrointestinal anomalies, and clubfoot	Coronal • Disappearance of the middle hyperechoic line • Widening of the external hyperechoic lines Sagittal • Posterior hyperechoic line and overlying soft tissues are absent Transverse • Outward splaying of the lateral posterior ossification centers • Cystic or complex mass protruding from spinal defect • Cerebellum takes on a crescent shape • Frontal bones are concaved	• Sacrococcygeal teratoma

Facial Abnormalities

ABNORMALITY	INFORMATION	SONOGRAPHIC FINDINGS	DIFFERENTIAL CONSIDERATIONS
Facial cleft	• Defect of the upper lip	• Anechoic defect between the upper lip and nostrils • Polyhydramnios	• Technical error
Macroglossia	• Associated with Beckwith-Wiedemann and Down syndromes	• Persistent protrusion of the fetal tongue • Polyhydramnios	• Normal tongue • Umbilical cord
Micrognathia	• Trisomy 18	• Small receding chin and lower lip • Polyhydramnios	• Technical error • Normal chin

Neck Abnormalities

ABNORMALITY	INFORMATION	SONOGRAPHIC FINDINGS	DIFFERENTIAL CONSIDERATIONS
Cystic hygroma	• Developmental defect of the lymphatic system • Associated with chromosomal abnormalities and fetal heart failure	• Multilocular cervical mass • Thin surrounding membrane • No cranial defect • Continuous with abnormal skin and subcutaneous tissues	• Encephalocele • Cystic teratoma • Normal umbilical cord • Thyroglossal cyst • Nuchal edema
Nuchal edema	• Thickening of the nuchal fold • Associated with chromosomal abnormalities	• Anechoic posterior cervical mass • Midline septum	• Cystic hygroma

Chest Abnormalities

ABNORMALITY	INFORMATION	SONOGRAPHIC FINDINGS	DIFFERENTIAL CONSIDERATIONS
Cystic adenomatoid malformation	• Abnormal formation of the bronchial tree • Replacement of normal pulmonary tissues with cysts • May be associated with renal or gastrointestinal abnormalities	• Simple or multiloculated cystic chest mass • Mediastinal shift • Diaphragm is visible and intact • Fetal hydrops • Polyhydramnios • Usually unilateral	• Diaphragmatic hernia • Pleural effusion • Pericardial fluid
Ectopia cordis	• Partial or complete displacement of the heart outside of the thorax	• Heart located outside of the thorax • Extrathoracic pulsating mass	• Acardiac twin • Diaphragmatic hernia
Diaphragmatic hernia	• Diaphragm fails to close allowing herniation of the abdominal cavity • Associated with cardiac, renal, chromosomal, and central nervous system anomalies	• Stomach or liver located in the thorax • Inability to visualize normal diaphragm • Mediastinal shift • Small abdominal circumference • Polyhydramnios • Usually unilateral • Left-sided defect more common	• Cystic adenomatoid malformation
Pleural effusion	• Most commonly a malformation of the thoracic duct • Associated with hydrops, infection, Turner syndrome, and chromosomal and cardiac abnormalities	• Anechoic fluid collection in the fetal chest • Fluid contours to surrounding lung and diaphragm • Lung tissue appears echogenic	• Diaphragmatic hernia • Fetal hydrops

Abnormalities of the Gastrointestinal Tract

ABNORMALITY	INFORMATION	SONOGRAPHIC FINDINGS	DIFFERENTIAL CONSIDERATIONS
Bowel atresia	• Obstruction usually occurring in the inferior small bowel • May be associated with meconium ileus and cystic fibrosis	• Multiple anechoic structures within the fetal abdomen • Polyhydramnios	• Normal prominent loops of bowel • Multicystic kidney
Duodenal atresia	• Blockage of the duodenum • Normal alpha-fetoprotein (AFP) level • Associated with Trisomy 21, cardiac, urinary, and GI anomalies	• Dilated stomach and proximal duodenum (double bubble) • Polyhydramnios	• Normal fluid-filled stomach • Fluid-filled loop of bowel
Esophageal atresia	• Congenital malformation of the foregut	• Absence of stomach • Small stomach on serial exams • Polyhydramnios	• Normal esophagus
Hyperechoic bowel	• Associated with cystic fibrosis, infection, intrauterine growth retardation, and chromosomal abnormalities • If isolated, normal fetal outcome	• Echogenicity of the bowel is equal to bone	• Meconium ileus
Meconium ileus	• Impaction of thick meconium in the distal ileum • Frequently associated with cystic fibrosis	• Dilated ileum • Ileum filled with echogenic material • Colon is small and empty	• Normal echogenic bowel
Meconium peritonitis	• Bowel perforation caused by bowel atresia or meconium ileus	• Abdominal calcification • Bowel dilation • Polyhydramnios	• Gallstone • Splenic calcification • Congenital infection • Hepatic necrosis

Abnormalities of the Genitourinary System

ABNORMALITY	INFORMATION	SONOGRAPHIC FINDINGS	DIFFERENTIAL CONSIDERATIONS
Hydronephrosis	• Urinary tract obstruction	• Pelviectasis ≥10 mm • Ratio of the renal pelvis diameter to the anterior–posterior renal diameter >50%	• Prominent renal pelvis • Renal cyst
Infantile polycystic disease	• Bilateral renal disease • Autosomal recessive • Lethal condition	• Hyperechoic enlarged kidneys • Extreme oligohydramnios • No visible fetal bladder	• Hyperechoic bowel • Premature rupture of membranes
Multicystic dysplastic kidney	• Kidney tissue is replaced by cysts • Additional renal anomalies occur in up to 40% of cases	• Renal tissue is replaced by multiple cysts • Variable size • Usually unilateral	• Fluid-filled bowel loops • Hydronephrosis
Posterior urethral valve obstruction	• Occurs in males • Presence of urethral valves • Urine is unable to pass through the urethra • Results in overdistention of the urinary bladder	• Dilated bladder • Dilated posterior urethra (keyhole) • Hydroureter • Hydronephrosis • Oligohydramnios	• Normal fetal bladder • Ureterovesical obstruction
Renal agenesis	• Absence of one or both kidneys • Pulmonary hyperplasia secondary to oligohydramnios	Unilateral agenesis • Absence of one kidney • Enlarged contralateral kidney • Fetal bladder visualized • Normal amniotic fluid volume Bilateral agenesis • Absence of both kidneys • No evidence of fetal bladder • Extreme oligohydramnios	• Infantile polycystic renal disease
Renal cyst	• Rare finding	• Anechoic renal mass • Round or oval • Smooth, thin wall margins • Posterior acoustic enhancement	• Hydronephrosis • Multicystic dysplastic kidney
Ureteropelvic junction obstruction	• Results from an abnormal bend or kink in the ureter • Obstruction of the proximal ureter	• Hydronephrosis • Normal fetal bladder • Normal amniotic fluid volume level • Unilateral	• Renal cyst • Loop of bowel
Ureterovesical junction	• Results from a urethral defect • Ureterocele • Ureter stenosis	• Dilated ureter (megaureter) • Possible hydronephrosis	• Ureteropelvic junction obstruction • Loop of bowel
Wilms tumor	• Malignant mass	• Echogenic solid renal mass	• Adrenal hemorrhage

Fetal Body Wall Abnormalities

ABNORMALITY	INFORMATION	SONOGRAPHIC FINDINGS	DIFFERENTIAL CONSIDERATIONS
Gastroschisis	• Defect involves all layers of the abdominal wall • Markedly elevated alpha-fetoprotein (AFP) levels • Not associated with other anomalies	• Paraumbilical wall defect • Typically to the right of a normal umbilical cord insertion • Normal cord insertion • Free-floating herniated small bowel within the amniotic cavity • Bowel loops may appear thick and dilated • Possible polyhydramnios	• Ruptured omphalocele • Normal umbilical cord
Omphalocele	• Midline defect covered by the amnion and peritoneum • Normal or elevated AFP level • Associated with cardiac and chromosomal abnormalities	• Midline anterior abdominal wall mass • Mass contains herniated viscera • Umbilical cord enters mass	• Umbilical hernia • Fetal position
Sacrococcygeal teratoma	• Benign neoplasm protruding from the posterior wall of the sacrum • Possible increase in AFP level • Mass may extend into the pelvis and abdomen • Female prevalence	• Solid or complex mass protruding from the fetal rump • Calcifications (bone fragments) • Normal spine • Bladder displacement • Hydronephrosis • Polyhydramnios	• Myelomeningocele
Umbilical hernia	• Less serious than omphalocele	• Small anterior abdominal wall defect • Normal cord insertion • Typically contains peritoneum • Rarely contains omentum or bowel	• Omphalocele • Fetal position

Skeletal Abnormalities

ABNORMALITY	INFORMATION	SONOGRAPHIC FINDINGS	DIFFERENTIAL CONSIDERATIONS
Achondrogenesis	• Lethal short limb dysplasia Type I • Autosomal recessive • 20% of cases • Thin ribs Type II • Autosomal dominant • 80% of cases • Ribs appear thicker	• Severe micromelia • Bowing of long bones • Short trunk • Protruding abdomen and forehead • Poor vertebral and cranial ossifications • Small pelvis	• Achondroplasia • Osteogenesis imperfecta
Achondroplasia	• Abnormal cartilage deposits at the long bone epiphysis • Most common form	• Macrocrania • Micromelia • Frontal bossing • Hypoplastic thorax • Ventriculomegaly	• Achondrogenesis • Osteogenesis imperfecta
Clubfoot	• Developmental defect • Abnormal relationship of the tarsal bones and the calcaneus • 55% of cases are bilateral • Polynesian and Middle Eastern descent prevalence	• Forefoot is oriented in the same plane as the lower leg • Persistent abnormal inversion of the foot at an angle perpendicular to the lower leg	• Normal mobility of the fetal foot

Continued

Skeletal Abnormalities—cont'd

ABNORMALITY	INFORMATION	SONOGRAPHIC FINDINGS	DIFFERENTIAL CONSIDERATION
Osteogenesis imperfecta	• Disorder of collagen production leading to brittle bones • Types I-IV • Type II is most lethal • Before 24 weeks, demineralization of the bone or abnormal limb length or shape may not be yet apparent	Type I • Bowing of long bones • May demonstrate fractures • Thick bones having a wrinkled appearance • Head is of normal size Type II • Hypomineralization • Significant bone shortening • Bell-shaped chest • Multiple fractures of long bones, ribs, and spine • Thin cranium Type III • Occasional rib fractures • Thin cranium • Mild leg bowing Type IV • Bowing of limbs • Occasional rib and limb fractures • Head is of normal size	• Achondroplasia • Achondrogenesis
Rocker bottom foot	• Trisomy 18 • Other chromosomal abnormalities • Fetal syndromes	• Prominent heel • Convex sole	• Normal foot
Thanatophoric dysplasia	• Lethal skeletal dysplasia • Male dominance	• Severe rhizomelia • Micromelia • Bowing of limbs • Clover-leaf skull deformity • Macrocephaly • Frontal bossing • Depressed nasal bridge • Hypertelorism • Ventriculomegaly • Thick soft tissue • Narrow, bell-shaped chest • Protuberant abdomen • Narrow spinal canal • Small hands • Polyhydramnios	• Achondroplasia • Osteogenesis imperfecta

FETAL ABNORMALITIES REVIEW

1. Echogenic debris within the fetal stomach is commonly associated with:
   a. fetal distress
   b. Down syndrome
   c. normal fetal swallowing
   d. tracheoesophageal fistula
   e. Beckwith-Wiedemann syndrome

2. Demonstration of multiple unilateral renal cysts is most suspicious for:
   a. hydronephrosis
   b. infantile polycystic disease
   c. multicystic dysplastic kidney
   d. cystic adenomatoid malformation
   e. ureteropelvic junction obstruction

3. "Double bubble" is a sonographic sign associated with:
   a. spina bifida
   b. hydronephrosis
   c. duodenal atresia
   d. hydranencephaly
   e. agenesis of the corpus callosum

4. Which of the following sonographic findings helps to differentiate Dandy-Walker syndrome from an arachnoid cyst?
   a. ventriculomegaly
   b. presence of a normal vermis
   c. absence of the third ventricle
   d. agenesis of the corpus callosum
   e. splaying of the cerebellar hemispheres

5. Dilation of the third ventricle is a sonographic finding associated with:
   a. anencephaly
   b. prosencephaly
   c. hydranencephaly
   d. holoprosencephaly
   e. agenesis of the corpus callosum

6. Maternal alpha-fetoprotein levels in a pregnancy with gastroschisis will:
   a. markedly increase
   b. mildly increase
   c. remain normal
   d. mildly decrease
   e. markedly decrease

7. Which skeletal abnormality is most likely to demonstrate a clover-leaf skull?
   a. rhizomelia
   b. achondroplasia
   c. achondrogenesis
   d. osteogenesis imperfecta
   e. thanatophoric dysplasia

8. A crescent shape appearance to the cerebellum should signal the sonographer to give additional attention to which of the following fetal structures?
   a. heart
   b. lungs
   c. spine
   d. kidneys
   e. abdominal wall

9. Peritoneal calcifications with associated dilated loops of bowel and polyhydramnios visualized in a 30-week fetus most likely represents:
   a. cholelithiasis
   b. intussusception
   c. arteriosclerosis
   d. hyperechoic bowel
   e. meconium peritonitis

10. Which of the following abnormalities is the most common neural tube defect?
    a. spina bifida
    b. anencephaly
    c. encephalocele
    d. cystic hygroma
    e. caudal regression

11. Which of the following conditions is most likely associated with frontal bossing?
    a. anencephaly
    b. encephalocele
    c. hydrocephalus
    d. cystic hygroma
    e. caudal regression

12. Which of the following abnormalities demonstrates a cranial defect?
    a. encephalocele
    b. cystic hygroma
    c. hydranencephaly
    d. holoprosencephaly
    e. agenesis of the corpus callosum

13. Which of the following is a common sonographic finding with fetal facial abnormalities?
    a. duodenal atresia
    b. polyhydramnios
    c. pleural effusion
    d. diaphragmatic hernia
    e. ventricular septal defect

14. Demonstration of fetal bone fractures raises suspicion for which skeletal abnormality?
    a. achondroplasia
    b. achondrogenesis
    c. thanatophoric dysplasia
    d. osteogenesis imperfecta
    e. sacrococcygeal teratoma

15. A large single ventricular cavity is most suspicious for:
    a. microcephaly
    b. macrocephaly
    c. hydranencephaly
    d. holoprosencephaly
    e. agenesis of the corpus callosum

Using Fig. 26-1, answer question 16.

16. The sonographic finding in this image is most suspicious for:
    a. hydranencephaly
    b. ventriculomegaly
    c. holoprosencephaly
    d. Dandy-Walker syndrome
    e. agenesis of the corpus callosum

Using Fig. 26-2, answer questions 17 and 18.

17. An asymptomatic patient arrives for a second-trimester fetal surveillance examination. A sagittal image of the fetal body is most suspicious for:
    a. gastroschisis
    b. encephalocele
    c. myelomeningocele
    d. diaphragmatic hernia
    e. sacrococcygeal teratoma

18. Associated findings with this abnormality include:
    a. spinal defect
    b. cranial defect
    c. hydronephrosis
    d. polyhydramnios
    e. hypoplastic chest

Using Fig. 26-3, answer questions 19 and 20.

19. During a late second-trimester screening examination, this image of the fetal abdomen is most likely revealing:
    a. renal agenesis
    b. multicystic dysplasia
    c. infantile polycystic disease
    d. bilateral adrenal hemorrhage
    e. thrombosis of the umbilical vein

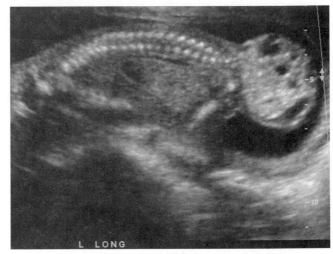

FIG. 26-2

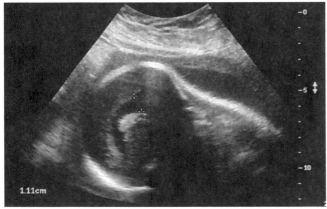

FIG. 26-1

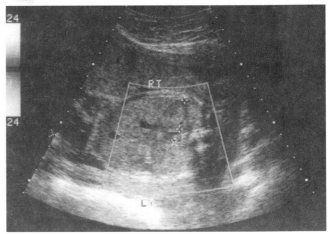

FIG. 26-3

20. Which of the following conditions will likely occur because of this abnormality?
    a. fetal hypoxia
    b. placentomegaly
    c. polyhydramnios
    d. oligohydramnios
    e. none of the above

Using Fig. 26-4, answer question 21.

21. A sagittal image of the fetal abdomen is most likely demonstrating:
    a. renal cyst
    b. hydronephrosis
    c. duodenal atresia
    d. diaphragmatic hernia
    e. multicystic dysplastic kidney

Using Fig. 26-5, answer question 22.

22. A patient arrives for an early second-trimester sonogram for gestational dating. An endovaginal image demonstrates a fetal abnormality **most** suspicious for:
    a. acrania
    b. anencephaly
    c. encephalocele
    d. hydranencephaly
    e. holoprosencephaly

Using Fig. 26-6, answer question 23.

23. A sagittal image of the lower spine is most suspicious for:
    a. spina bifida
    b. encephalocele
    c. umbilical cord
    d. cystic hygroma
    e. caudal regression

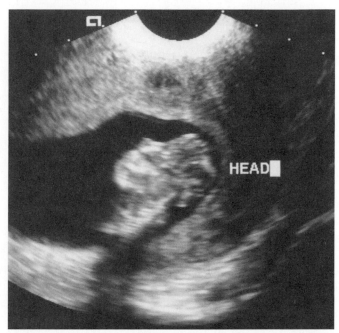

FIG. 26-5

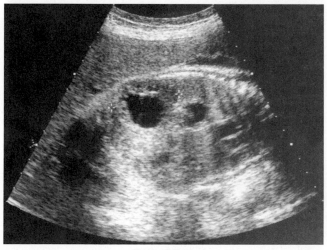

FIG. 26-4

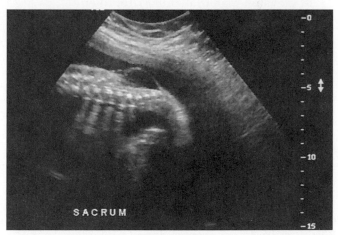

FIG. 26-6

Using Fig. 26-7, answer questions 24 and 25.

24. What abnormality is most likely present in this cross-sectional image of the cranium?
    a. encephalocele
    b. nuchal edema
    c. cystic hygroma
    d. myelomeningocele
    e. amniotic band syndrome

25. The etiology of this abnormality is typically:
    a. idiopathic
    b. Rh sensitivity
    c. autosomal recessive
    d. chromosomal
    e. maternal diabetes mellitus

Using Fig. 26-8, answer questions 26 and 27.

26. A patient presents for an ultrasound to determine gestational age. An image of this early second-trimester fetus is most suspicious for:
    a. acrania
    b. anencephaly
    c. microcephaly
    d. caudal regression
    e. holoprosencephaly

27. Which of the following is most likely associated with this finding?
    a. fetal demise
    b. preeclampsia
    c. gestational diabetes
    d. maternal hypertension
    e. elevated maternal alpha-fetoprotein

Using Fig. 26-9, answer question 28.

28. A patient arrives for a second-trimester screening sonogram. A sagittal image of the fetus is most suspicious for which of the following pathologies?
    a. fetal hydrops
    b. pericardial effusion
    c. diaphragmatic hernia
    d. loculated pleural effusions
    e. cystic adenomatoid malformation

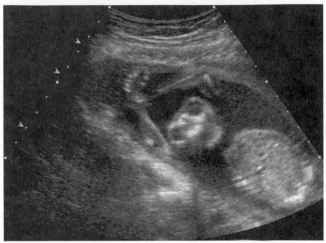

FIG. 26-8

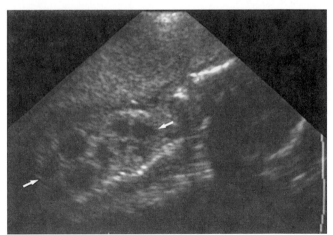

FIG. 26-9

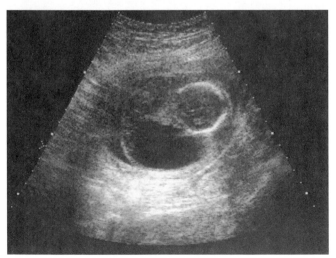

FIG. 26-7

Using Fig. 26-10, answer question 29.

29. This sonogram of an early second-trimester cranium is most suspicious for:
    a. anencephaly
    b. hydrocephalus
    c. hydranencephaly
    d. holoprosencephaly
    e. agenesis of the corpus callosum

Using Fig. 26-11, answer question 30.

30. An oblique sonogram of the fetal abdomen is most likely demonstrating:
    a. hydronephrosis
    b. duodenal atresia
    c. adrenal hemorrhage
    d. infantile polycystic disease
    e. multicystic dysplastic kidney

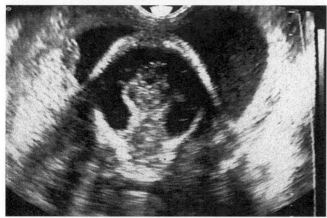

FIG. 26-10

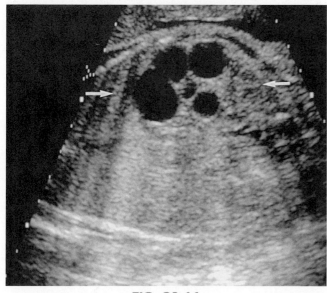

FIG. 26-11

31. Lateral ventricular enlargement is ventriculomegaly once the diameter exceeds:
    a. 4 mm
    b. 6 mm
    c. 8 mm
    d. 10 mm
    e. 12 mm

32. Caudal regression syndrome is more commonly found in patients with:
    a. proteinuria
    b. hypertension
    c. systemic lupus
    d. hyperlipidemia
    e. diabetes mellitus

33. Which of the following is the most common fetal neck mass?
    a. goiter
    b. hemangioma
    c. nuchal edema
    d. cystic hygroma
    e. myelomeningocele

34. Which of the following abnormalities is more commonly associated with proboscis?
    a. spina bifida
    b. hydranencephaly
    c. ventriculomegaly
    d. holoprosencephaly
    e. diaphragmatic hernia

35. Which of the following abnormalities is not associated with pulmonary hypoplasia?
    a. renal agenesis
    b. duodenal atresia
    c. skeletal dysplasia
    d. diaphragmatic hernia
    e. infantile polycystic renal disease

36. A diagnosis of clubfoot may be made with persistent abnormal inversion of the:
    a. foot
    b. ankle
    c. lower leg
    d. foot parallel to the lower leg
    e. foot perpendicular to the lower leg

37. Opening in the layers of the abdominal wall with evisceration of the bowel describes a(n):
    a. gastroschisis
    b. omphalocele
    c. umbilical hernia
    d. intussusceptions
    e. meconium peritonitis

38. Which of the following is the most common **non-lethal** skeletal dysplasia?
    a. achondroplasia
    b. achondrogenesis
    c. diastrophic dysplasia
    d. thanatophoric dysplasia
    e. osteogenesis imperfecta

39. Hydronephrosis in utero is most commonly caused by an obstruction:
    a. in the urethra
    b. in the distal ureter
    c. at the bladder inlet
    d. within the renal calyces
    e. at the ureteropelvic junction

40. Herniated contents of an omphalocele are covered by a membrane consisting of:
    a. chorion and amnion
    b. amnion and peritoneum
    c. peritoneum and chorion
    d. Wharton jelly and amnion
    e. peritoneum and Wharton jelly

41. The presence of a posterior fossa cyst and agenesis of the cerebellar vermis are characteristic findings of:
    a. arachnoid cyst
    b. hydranencephaly
    c. holoprosencephaly
    d. Dandy-Walker malformation
    e. agenesis of the corpus callosum

42. Which of the following is NOT associated with hydrocephalus?
    a. spina bifida
    b. encephalocele
    c. myelomeningocele
    d. choroid plexus cysts
    e. agenesis of corpus callosum

43. Anechoic regions within brain tissue are most suspicious for:
    a. arachnoid cyst
    b. ventriculomegaly
    c. hydranencephaly
    d. holoprosencephaly
    e. choroid plexus cysts

44. Outward angling of the frontal and lateral horn of the lateral ventricles is a sonographic finding in:
    a. ventriculomegaly
    b. hydranencephaly
    c. holoprosencephaly
    d. Dandy-Walker syndrome
    e. agenesis of the corpus callosum

45. The renal pelvis in a third-trimester fetus demonstrates an anterior–posterior diameter of 10 mm. This is considered:
    a. a megaureter
    b. a lethal condition
    c. mild hydronephrosis
    d. within normal limits
    e. moderate hydronephrosis

46. In the late second trimester, which sonographic finding consistently displays with renal agenesis?
    a. facial cleft
    b. omphalocele
    c. oligohydramnios
    d. skeletal dysplasia
    e. diaphragmatic hernia

47. The most common sonographic finding associated with multicystic renal dysplasia is:
    a. unilateral multicystic kidney
    b. bilateral multicystic kidneys
    c. unilateral enlarged hyperechoic kidney
    d. bilateral enlarged hyperechoic kidneys
    e. none of the above

48. Sonographic findings associated with osteogenesis imperfecta may not be apparent before:
    a. 12 weeks' gestation
    b. 18 weeks' gestation
    c. 24 weeks' gestation
    d. 28 weeks' gestation
    e. 32 weeks' gestation

49. Which classification of osteogenesis imperfecta is most severe?
    a. type I
    b. type II
    c. type III
    d. type IV
    e. type V

50. A consistently small fetal stomach on serial sonograms is most suspicious for which abnormality?
    a. gastroschisis
    b. omphalocele
    c. duodenal atresia
    d. esophageal atresia
    e. diaphragmatic hernia

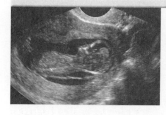

CHAPTER 27

Complications in Pregnancy

KEY TERMS

anasarca   severe generalized massive edema often seen with hydrops fetalis.

clinodactyly   inward curving of the fifth finger associated with Down syndrome.

cubitus valgus   abnormal outward bending or twisting of the elbow.

eclampsia   gravest form of pregnancy-induced maternal hypertension characterized by seizures, coma, proteinuria, and edema.

ectopia cordis   a condition in which the ventral wall of the chest fails to close and the heart develops outside of the chest.

fetus papyraceous   demise of a twin that is too large to reabsorb.

micrognathia   underdevelopment of the jaw, especially the mandible.

microphthalmia   abnormal smallness of one or both eyes.

polydactyly   congenital anomaly characterized by the presence of more than the normal number of digits.

preeclampsia   an abnormal condition characterized by the onset of acute hypertension after 24 weeks' gestation. Classic triad includes maternal edema, proteinuria, and hypertension.

preterm labor   onset of labor prior to 37 weeks' gestation.

Rh disease   caused when the mother forms a corresponding antibody to the fetal blood, resulting in destruction of fetal red blood cells.

sandal toe deformity   Increased distance between the first and second toes associated with Down syndrome.

Spaulding sign   overlapping of the cranial bones associated with fetal demise.

syndactyly   congenital anomaly characterized by the fusion of the fingers or toes.

twin–twin transfusion   the arterial blood of the donor twin pumps into the venous system of the receiving twin.

CHROMOSOMAL ABNORMALITIES

- Found in 1 of 180 live births.

Chromosomal Abnormalities

ANOMALY	INFORMATION	SONOGRAPHIC FINDINGS	DIFFERENTIAL CONSIDERATIONS
Edward syndrome	• Trisomy 18 • 80% of cases display a clenched fist • Decrease in AFP • 1:8000 live births • Overall poor prognosis • 95% spontaneously abort • Female prevalence	• Heart defects • Choroid plexus cysts • Clenched hands • Micrognathia • Clubbed or rocker bottom feet • Renal anomalies • Cleft lip and palate • Omphalocele • Enlargement of the cistern magnum • Microcephaly • Small placenta • Two-vessel cord • Intrauterine growth restriction (IUGR)	• Trisomy 13 • Triploidy

Continued

399

Chromosomal Abnormalities—cont'd

ANOMALY	INFORMATION	SONOGRAPHIC FINDINGS	DIFFERENTIAL CONSIDERATIONS
Down syndrome	• Trisomy 21 • Decrease in alpha-fetoprotein (AFP) levels • 1:800 live births • Coexisting anomalies dictate overall prognosis • Approximately 30% of cases demonstrate duodenal atresia	• Subtle anomalies • Nuchal fold ≥6 mm • Ventricular septal defect • Duodenal atresia • Brachycephaly • Hyperechoic cardiac focus • Macroglossia • Hyperechoic bowel • Sandal toe deformity • Clinodactyly • Low-set ears • Short stature	• Beckwith-Wiedemann syndrome
Patau syndrome	• Trisomy 13 • 90% of cases display cardiac defects • Syndrome of midline defects • 1:25,000 live births • Overall poor prognosis • Multiple anomalies, many involving the brain	• Holoprosencephaly • Microcephaly • Cystic hygroma • Absent or small eyes • Facial clefts • Cardiac defects • Omphalocele • Polycystic kidneys • Clubfoot • Polydactyly • IUGR • Polyhydramnios	• Meckel-Gruber syndrome
Triploidy	• Three complete sets of chromosomes • Most will abort spontaneously • 1:5000 live births	• Early onset IUGR • Holoprosencephaly • Hypertelorism • Micrognathia • Microphthalmia • Ventriculomegaly • Oligohydramnios • Clubfeet • Syndactyly	• Trisomy 13 • Trisomy 18
Turner syndrome	• 45 chromosomes, including a single X chromosome • Elevated AFP levels • Female fetus • 1:5000 live births	• Cystic hygroma • Cardiac defects • Renal anomalies • Cubitus valgus • Short femurs • General lymph edema	• Cephalocele • Trisomy 13 • Hydrops fetalis

FETAL SYNDROMES

- Demonstrate normal karyotype.
- *Malformation* refers to a defect of an organ that results from an intrinsically abnormal development process.
- *Deformation* refers to an abnormal form, shape, or position of a part caused by mechanical forces antenatally.
- *Disruption* is a defect of an organ resulting from the breakdown of previously normal tissue.
- *Sequence* refers to a pattern of multiple anomalies that result from a single anomaly or mechanical factor.

Fetal Syndromes

SYNDROME	INFORMATION	SONOGRAPHIC FINDINGS	DIFFERENTIAL CONSIDERATIONS
Amniotic band syndrome	• Ruptured amnion sticks and entangles fetal parts • Associated with fetal abnormalities and amputations	• Thin hyperechoic linear structure floating within the amniotic cavity • Fetal abnormalities	• Synechia • Amniotic chorionic separation • Placental shelf • Down syndrome
Beckwith-Wiedemann syndrome	• Classic triad of macrosomia, omphalocele, and macroglossia • Normal karyotype • Increases risk of developing Wilms tumor, hemihypertrophy, renal anomalies, and hepatosplenomegaly	• Hemihypertrophy • Macroglossia • Omphalocele	
Eagle-Barrett syndrome	• Prune belly syndrome • Hypotonic abdominal wall muscles • Associated with dilated fetal bladder, small thorax, and imperforate anus	• Hydronephrosis • Megaureter • Oligohydramnios • Small thorax • Large abdomen • Cryptorchidism • Hip dislocation • Scoliosis	• Urinary obstruction • Urethral atresia
Meckel-Gruber syndrome	• Lethal condition • Occurs equally in males and females • Autosomal recessive	• Encephalocele • Infantile polycystic renals • Oligohydramnios • Bladder not visualized • Polydactyly	• Trisomy 13 • Infantile polycystic disease

Pentalogy of Cantrell	• Congenital disorder characterized by two major defects
	  1. ectopia cordis
	  2. abdominal wall defect
		• Pulsating mass outside of the chest cavity
		• Omphalocele
		• Gastroschisis
			• Beckwith-Wiedemann syndrome
			• Acardiac twin

HYDROPS FETALIS

- An abnormal interstitial accumulation of fluid in the body cavities and soft tissues.
- Fluid accumulation may result in anasarca, ascites, pericardial effusion, pleural effusion, placentomegaly, and polyhydramnios.
- Hydrops may result from antibodies in the maternal circulation that destroy the fetal red blood cells (immune) or without evidence of blood group incompatibility (nonimmune).
- Sonography cannot differentiate immune from nonimmune hydrops.

Fetal Hydrops

HYDROPS	CLINICAL FINDINGS	SONOGRAPHIC FINDINGS	DIFFERENTIAL CONSIDERATIONS
Immune	• Rh sensitivity	• Scalp edema • Pleural effusion • Pericardial effusion • Polyhydramnios • Placentomegaly	• Nonimmune hydrops • Pleural effusion

Continued

Fetal Hydrops—cont'd

HYDROPS	CLINICAL FINDINGS	SONOGRAPHIC FINDINGS	DIFFERENTIAL CONSIDERATIONS

Nonimmune	• Large for dates	• Anasarca
		• Edema or fluid accumulation in at least two fetal sites
		  ○ Ascites
		  ○ Scalp edema
		  ○ Pleural effusion
		  ○ Pericardial effusion
		• Polyhydramnios
		• Placentomegaly
		• Fetal tachycardia 200-240 bpm
			• Immune hydrops
			• Pleural effusion

MULTIFETAL GESTATIONS

- Seventy percent of pregnancies beginning with twins will deliver a singleton pregnancy.
- Monozygotic twins result from a single fertilized ovum.
- Dizygotic twins result from two separate ova.
- Majority of pregnancies are dizygotic.
- Dizygotic pregnancies are always dichorionic/diamniotic.

Monozygotic Multifetal Gestations

TYPE	DESCRIPTION	SONOGRAPHIC FINDINGS	DIFFERENTIAL CONSIDERATIONS
Dichorionic/Diamniotic	• Zygote splits within 5 days of fertilization • Four-layered membrane	• Two or more individual gestational sacs • Thick membrane	• Mirror-image artifact
Monochorionic/Diamniotic	• Zygote splits 5-10 days after fertilization • Three-layer membrane	• Two or more individual gestational sacs • Moderately thick membrane	• Mirror-image artifact
Monochorionic/Monoamniotic	• Zygote splits 10-14 days postfertilization	• Two or more fetuses • Single gestational sac • No membrane	• Technical difficulty in locating membrane

Multifetal Gestational Abnormalities

ABNORMALITY	DESCRIPTION	SONOGRAPHIC FINDINGS	DIFFERENTIAL CONSIDERATIONS
Acardiac twin	<ul><li>Diamniotic/monochorionic twin pregnancy</li><li>Rare anomaly</li><li>Blood is shunted through a vein to vein and artery to artery anastomoses from the normal or pump twin to the acardiac twin</li><li>Places a large cardiovascular burden on the normal twin</li></ul>	<ul><li>Partially imaged normal fetus and a large perfused tissue mass lacking an upper body</li></ul>Acardiac twin<ul><li>Poorly developed upper body</li><li>Anencephaly</li><li>Absent or rudimentary heart</li><li>Limbs may be present but truncated</li></ul>Normal twin<ul><li>May develop<ul><li>Hydrops</li><li>Polyhydramnios</li><li>Cardiac failure</li></ul></li></ul>	<ul><li>Twin–twin transfusion</li></ul>
Conjoined twins	<ul><li>Monozygotic</li><li>Fusion of twin fetuses</li><li>Usually anterior and one body part</li></ul>	<ul><li>Inseparable fetal bodies and skin contours</li><li>Limited or no fetal position change</li><li>No membrane</li></ul>	<ul><li>Acardiac twin</li><li>Normal twin pregnancy</li></ul>
Stuck twin	<ul><li>Poli-Oli sequence</li><li>Monochorionic/diamniotic</li><li>Usually manifests between 16 and 26 gestational weeks</li></ul>	<ul><li>One twin displays polyhydramnios</li><li>One twin displays oligohydramnios</li></ul>	<ul><li>Acardiac twin</li><li>Twin–twin transfusion</li></ul>
Twin–twin transfusion	<ul><li>Same-sex fetuses</li><li>Single placenta</li><li>The arterial blood of the donor twin pumps into the venous system of the recipient twin</li><li>Recipient twin ultimately receives too much blood</li></ul>	<ul><li>Fetal weight discordance of ≥20%</li><li>Donor twin may display intrauterine growth restriction and oligohydramnios</li><li>Receiving twin may acquire hydrops fetalis and polyhydramnios</li><li>Thin membrane</li></ul>	<ul><li>Acardiac twin</li><li>Poli-Oli syndrome</li></ul>
Vanishing twin	<ul><li>Early fetal demise of one embryo</li></ul>	<ul><li>Twin pregnancy</li><li>Demised twin resolves</li><li>Becomes singleton pregnancy</li></ul>	<ul><li>Succenturiate placenta</li></ul>

Genetic Testing

TESTING	DESCRIPTION	SONOGRAPHY CONTRIBUTION
Amniocentesis	<ul><li>Used to analyze fetal chromosomes in early pregnancy</li><li>Typically between 15 and 18 gestational weeks</li><li>Can be performed as early as 12 gestational weeks</li></ul>	<ul><li>Fetal survey to exclude congenital anomalies</li><li>Assist in locating the optimal collection site away from:<ul><li>fetus</li><li>umbilical cord</li><li>central placenta</li><li>uterine vessels</li></ul></li><li>Recheck fetal well-being after procedure</li></ul>
Chorionic villi sampling	<ul><li>Performed between 10 and 12 gestational weeks</li><li>Results available in 1 week</li></ul>	<ul><li>Direct the biopsy</li><li>Determine the relationship between the lie of the uterus and cervix and the path of the catheter route</li><li>Assess fetal viability and location</li><li>Identify uterine masses</li><li>Assess the fetus postprocedure</li></ul>
Cordocentesis	<ul><li>Used to analyze fetal chromosomes</li><li>Fetal blood is aspirated through the umbilical cord</li></ul>	<ul><li>Guide aspiration procedure</li><li>Assess the fetus postprocedure</li></ul>
Embryoscopy	<ul><li>Permits direct viewing of the developing fetus</li></ul>	<ul><li>Assess the fetus postprocedure</li></ul>

COMPLICATIONS IN PREGNANCY REVIEW

1. A clenched fetal fist is commonly associated with which of the following syndromes?
   a. Patau
   b. Down
   c. Edward
   d. Eagle-Barrett
   e. Meckel-Gruber

2. Anasarca is a condition often seen in cases of:
   a. triploidy
   b. macrosomia
   c. fetal hydrops
   d. amniotic band syndrome
   e. intrauterine growth restriction

3. Which of the following is a sonographic finding associated with Beckwith-Wiedemann syndrome?
   a. megaureter
   b. micrognathia
   c. encephalocele
   d. macroglossia
   e. cystic hygroma

4. Megaureter and oligohydramnios are sonographic findings associated with which fetal syndrome?
   a. trisomy 13
   b. trisomy 18
   c. Eagle-Barrett
   d. Meckel-Gruber
   e. Beckwith-Wiedemann

5. Twin–twin transfusion generally demonstrates:
   a. fetal hydrops in the donor twin
   b. a minimum fetal weight discordance of 50%
   c. polyhydramnios in the amniotic cavity of the donor twin
   d. a minimum fetal weight discordance of 20%
   e. oligohydramnios in the amniotic cavity of the receiving twin

6. Duodenal atresia is typically documented in one-third of cases of:
   a. fetal hydrops
   b. Down syndrome
   c. Edward syndrome
   d. twin–twin transfusion
   e. Eagle-Barrett syndrome

7. Fetal papyraceus is a term used to describe:
   a. Rh disease
   b. twin–twin transfusion
   c. vanishing twin phenomenon
   d. Beckwith-Wiedemann syndrome
   e. demise of a twin too large to resolve

8. Which of the following most accurately describes twin–twin transfusion?
   a. Venous blood from the donor twin is pumped into the arterial system of the receiving twin.
   b. Arterial blood from the donor twin is pumped into the arterial blood of the receiving twin.
   c. Venous blood of the receiving twin is pumped into the venous system of the donor twin.
   d. Arterial blood from the donor twin is pumped into the venous system of the receiving twin.
   e. Arterial blood of the receiving twin is pumped into the venous system of the donor twin.

9. Fusion of the fingers or toes is termed:
   a. talipes
   b. syndactyly
   c. polydactyly
   d. microdactyly
   e. clinodactyly

10. Which of the following sonographic findings is NOT associated with Meckel-Gruber syndrome?
    a. polydactyly
    b. anencephaly
    c. oligohydramnios
    d. infantile polycystic disease
    e. nonvisualization of the fetal bladder

11. Which of the following sonographic findings differentiates immune from nonimmune fetal hydrops?
    a. ascites
    b. anasarca
    c. pleural effusion
    d. pericardial effusion
    e. none of the above

12. What percentage of twin gestations will generally result in a singleton pregnancy at term?
    a. 5%
    b. 10%
    c. 25%
    d. 50%
    e. 70%

13. Which of the following syndromes is more commonly associated with clinodactyly?
    a. Patau
    b. Down
    c. Turner
    d. Edward
    e. Meckel-Gruber

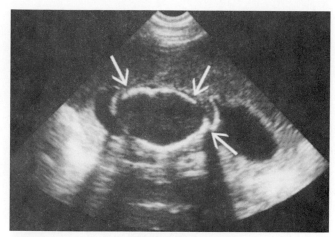

FIG. 27-1

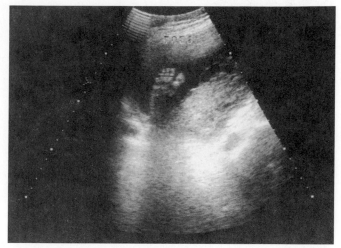

FIG. 27-2

14. Amniocentesis for genetic testing is typically performed between:
    a. 8 and 10 weeks
    b. 8 and 12 weeks
    c. 12 and 15 weeks
    d. 15 and 18 weeks
    e. 20 and 26 weeks

15. Trisomy 13 is also known as:
    a. triploidy
    b. Patau syndrome
    c. Down syndrome
    d. Turner syndrome
    e. Edward syndrome

Using Fig. 27-1, answer question 16

16. What is the most likely cause of the cranial shape on this sonogram?
    a. scalp edema
    b. fetal demise
    c. skeletal dysplasia
    d. neural tube defect
    e. breech presentation

Using Fig. 27-2, answer questions 17 and 18.

17. A plantar image of the fetal foot reveals a sonographic finding termed:
    a. clubfoot
    b. sandal toe
    c. thumb toe
    d. rocker foot
    e. hammer toe

18. This sonographic finding is associated with:
    a. trisomy 13
    b. trisomy 18
    c. trisomy 21
    d. Turner syndrome
    e. Eagle-Barrett syndrome

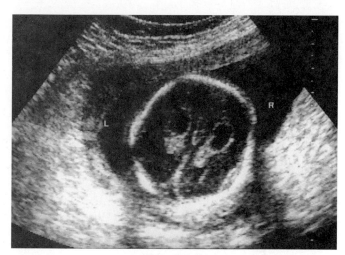

FIG. 27-3

Using Fig. 27-3, answer questions 19 and 20.

19. A second-trimester fetus is demonstrating which of the following abnormalities?
    a. hydranencephaly
    b. holoprosencephaly
    c. Dandy-Walker cysts
    d. bilateral hydrocephalus
    e. bilateral choroid plexus cysts

20. This can be associated with which of the following?
    a. trisomy 13
    b. trisomy 18
    c. trisomy 21
    d. Turner syndrome
    e. Meckel-Gruber syndrome

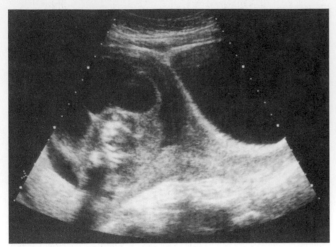

FIG. 27-4

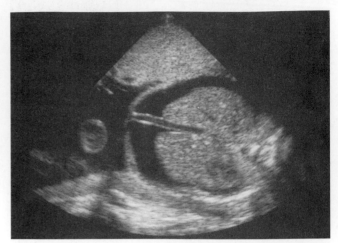

FIG. 27-5

Using Fig. 27-4, answer questions 21 and 22.

21. An early second-trimester obstetrical patient presents with a history of elevated alpha-fetoprotein level. A cross-sectional sonogram at the level of the fetal neck documents which of the following abnormalities?
    a. encephalocele
    b. fetal hydrops
    c. nuchal edema
    d. vanishing twin
    e. cystic hygroma

22. This is a common sonographic finding associated with which chromosomal abnormality?
    a. trisomy 13
    b. trisomy 21
    c. Turner syndrome
    d. Edward syndrome
    e. Meckel-Gruber syndrome

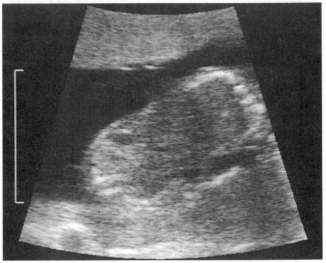

FIG. 27-6

Using Fig. 27-5, answer question 23.

23. The sonographic findings are most suspicious for:
    a. macrosomia
    b. gastroschisis
    c. omphalocele
    d. fetal hydrops
    e. pseudoascites

Using Fig. 27-6, answer question 24.

24. A patient presents for an early second-trimester sonogram. A cross-sectional image reveals two fetal abdomens. This image is most suspicious for:
    a. acardiac twin
    b. vanishing twin
    c. conjoined twins
    d. Poli-Oli sequence
    e. twin–twin transfusion

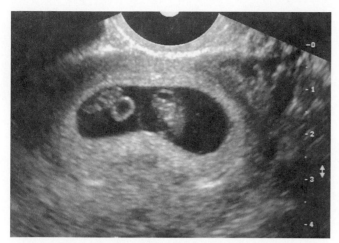

FIG. 27-7

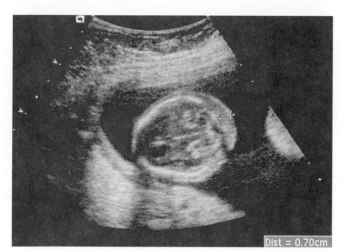

FIG. 27-8

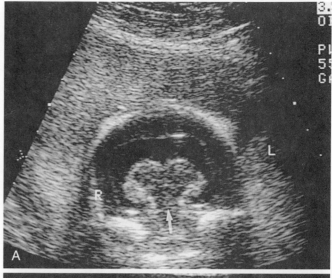

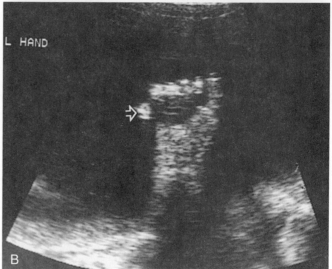

FIG. 27-9

Using Fig. 27-7, answer question 25.

25. A first-trimester sonogram is demonstrating:
  a. triplets
  b. diamniotic twins
  c. dichorionic twins
  d. monoamniotic twins
  e. monochorionic twins

Using Fig. 27-8, answer questions 26 and 27.

26. The abnormality present in this 18-week gestation is most suspicious for which chromosomal anomaly?
  a. triploidy
  b. trisomy 13
  c. trisomy 18
  d. trisomy 21
  e. Turner syndrome

27. Which of the following abnormalities is associated with this syndrome?
  a. omphalocele
  b. microcephaly
  c. cystic hygroma
  d. duodenal atresia
  e. oligohydramnios

Using Fig. 27-9, answer question 28.

28. What is the most likely chromosomal anomaly associated with this second-trimester fetus?
  a. triploidy
  b. trisomy 13
  c. trisomy 18
  d. trisomy 21
  e. Turner syndrome

29. Which of the following extremity malformations is associated with this condition?
    a. amputation
    b. rocker bottom feet
    c. long bone fractures
    d. hypomineralization
    e. sandal toe deformity

30. Preeclampsia is a complication of pregnancy demonstrating:
    a. fetal ascites, pleural effusion, and scalp edema
    b. maternal hypertension, proteinuria, and edema
    c. macrosomia, polyhydramnios, and fetal hydrops
    d. gestational diabetes, hematuria, and hypertension
    e. maternal hypertension, grand mal seizures, and coma

31. Preterm labor is defined as the onset of labor prior to:
    a. estimated due date
    b. 40 weeks' gestation
    c. 39 weeks' gestation
    d. 38 weeks' gestation
    e. 37 weeks' gestation

32. Which of the following is likely to occur if a single zygote divides 7 days after fertilization?
    a. two individual placentas
    b. one amnion and one chorion
    c. two amnion and two chorion
    d. one amnion and two chorion
    e. two amnion and one chorion

33. Arteriovenous shunting within the placenta occurs with:
    a. vanishing twin
    b. conjoined twins
    c. fetal papyraceus
    d. twin–twin transfusion
    e. acardiac twin pregnancy

34. With twin–twin transfusion syndrome, the recipient twin is likely to acquire:
    a. macrosomia
    b. hydrops fetalis
    c. placentomalacia
    d. skeletal dysplasia
    e. trophoblastic disease

35. What sonographic finding confirms the presence of a diamniotic pregnancy?
    a. two embryos
    b. two yolk sacs
    c. two placentas
    d. two allantoic ducts
    e. two gestational sacs

36. Which of the following is NOT a sonographic finding in fetal hydrops?
    a. anasarca
    b. scalp edema
    c. pleural effusion
    d. abdominal ascites
    e. umbilical vein varix

37. Fetal hydrops resulting from fetal tachycardia most commonly demonstrates a fetal heart rate of:
    a. 90-120 beats per minute
    b. 120-200 beats per minute
    c. 160-180 beats per minute
    d. 200-240 beats per minute
    e. 250-300 beats per minute

38. Twin gestation arising from two separate fertilized ova is termed:
    a. zygotic twins
    b. identical twins
    c. dizygotic twins
    d. diamniotic twins
    e. monochorionic twins

39. Which of the following abnormalities increases the risk of fetal injury?
    a. uterine shelf
    b. amniotic bands
    c. amniotic sheets
    d. uterine synechiae
    e. amniochorionic separation

40. Amniotic band syndrome may result in:
    a. macrosomia
    b. polyhydramnios
    c. placenta accreta
    d. an acardiac twin
    e. fetal amputation

41. Which of the following syndromes demonstrates a normal karyotype and is associated with hemihypertrophy?
    a. Down syndrome
    b. Turner syndrome
    c. Eagle-Barrett syndrome
    d. Meckel-Gruber syndrome
    e. Beckwith-Wiedemann syndrome

42. A dizygotic gestation is expected to be:
    a. dichorionic/diamniotic
    b. monochorionic/diamniotic
    c. dichorionic/monoamniotic
    d. monochorionic/monoamniotic
    e. none of the above

43. The gravest form of pregnancy-induced maternal hypertension is termed:
    a. anasarca
    b. epilepsy
    c. eclampsia
    d. preeclampsia
    e. gestational hypertension

44. Sonographic appearance of fetal hydrops in Rh sensitization includes all of the following EXCEPT:
    a. anasarca
    b. pleural effusion
    c. placentomalacia
    d. polyhydramnios
    e. pericardial effusion

45. A monochorionic twin pregnancy in which one develops without an upper body is termed:
    a. acardiac twin
    b. fraternal twin
    c. vanishing twin
    d. conjoined twin
    e. ectopia cordis

46. Which of the following syndromes is manifested by dilatation of the renal collecting system?
    a. Patau syndrome
    b. Edward syndrome
    c. Pentalogy of Cantrell
    d. Eagle-Barrett syndrome
    e. Meckel-Gruber syndrome

47. Which of the following twin abnormalities demonstrates a venous-to-venous anastomosis?
    a. acardiac twin
    b. conjoined twin
    c. vanishing twin
    d. Poli-Oli sequence
    e. twin–twin transfusion

48. Which of the following is a common abnormality associated with trisomy 13?
    a. clinodactyly
    b. macrocephaly
    c. macroglossia
    d. holoprosencephaly
    e. hyperechoic bowel

49. Which of the following conditions displays ectopia cordis and gastroschisis?
    a. Patau syndrome
    b. Down syndrome
    c. Pentalogy of Cantrell
    d. Meckel-Gruber syndrome
    e. Beckwith-Wiedemann syndrome

50. Inward curving of the fifth finger is a clinical finding associated with:
    a. Patau syndrome
    b. Down syndrome
    c. Turner syndrome
    d. Pentalogy of Cantrell
    e. Meckel-Gruber syndrome

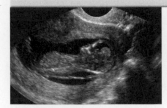

CHAPTER 28

Placenta and
Umbilical Cord

KEY TERMS

abruptio placentae   premature detachment of the placenta from the maternal wall.

allantoic duct   elongated duct that contributes to the development of the umbilical cord.

basal plate   maternal surface of the placenta.

battledore placenta   cord insertion into the margin of the placenta.

Braxton-Hicks contraction   spontaneous uterine contraction occurring throughout pregnancy.

chorion frondosum   the portion of the chorion that develops into the fetal portion of the placenta.

chorionic leave   chorion around the gestational sac on the opposite side of implantation.

chorionic plate   fetal surface of the placenta.

chorionic villi   vascular projections from the chorion at the implantation and placental site.

circumvallate placenta   a placental condition in which the chorionic plate of the placenta is smaller than the basal plate.

nuchal cord   occurs when the cord is completely wrapped around the fetal neck at a minimum of two times.

molar pregnancy   abnormal proliferation of the trophoblastic cells in the first trimester.

placental abruption   premature separation of the normally implanted placenta from the uterus.

placenta accreta   growth of the chorionic villi superficially into the myometrium.

placenta increta   growth of the chorionic villi deep into the myometrium.

placenta percreta   growth of the chorionic villi through the myometrium.

placenta previa   placenta completely covers the internal cervical os.

placental migration   as the uterus enlarges and stretches, the attached placenta appears to "move" further from the lower uterine segment.

retroplacental complex   area behind the placenta composed of the decidua, myometrium, and uteroplacental vessels.

succenturiate placenta   additional placenta tissue (lobes) connected to the body of the placenta by blood vessels.

umbilical herniation   failure of the anterior abdominal wall to close completely at the level of the umbilicus.

vasa previa   occurs when the intramembranous vessels course across the cervical os.

Wharton jelly   mucoid connective tissue that surrounds the vessels within the umbilical cord.

PLACENTA

ANATOMY (Fig. 28-1)

- Formed by the decidua basalis and decidua frondosum.
- Separated from the uterine myometrium by the retroplacental complex.

PHYSIOLOGY

- Vital support organ for the developing fetus.
- Chorionic villus is the major functioning unit of the placenta and contains the intervillous spaces.
- Maternal blood enters the intervillous spaces.

FUNCTIONS

RESPIRATION

- Oxygen in maternal blood passes through the placenta into the fetal blood.
- Carbon dioxide returns through the placenta to the maternal blood.

410

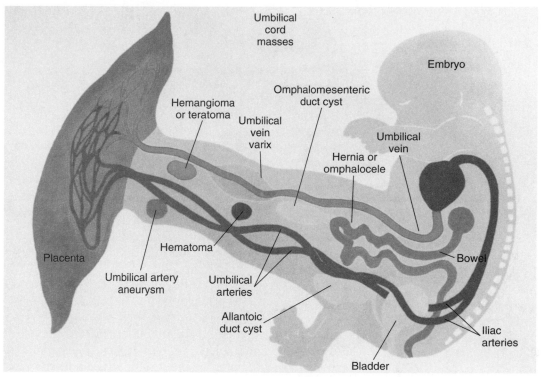

FIG. 28-1 Placental anatomy.

NUTRITION

- Nutrients pass from the maternal blood through the placenta to the fetal blood.

EXCRETION

- Waste products cross from the fetal blood through the placenta to the maternal blood.

PROTECTION

- Provides a barrier between the mother and fetus, protecting the fetus from maternal immune rejection.

STORAGE

- Carbohydrates, proteins, calcium, and iron are stored in the placenta and released into the fetal circulation.

HORMONE PRODUCTION

- Produces human chorionic gonadotropin, estrogens, and progesterone.

SIZE

- Varies with gestational age.
- Generally measures 2 to 3 cm in greatest thickness.
- Maximum thickness should not exceed 4.0 cm.

NORMAL SONOGRAPHIC APPEARANCE

FIRST TRIMESTER

- Thickened area of the hyperechoic gestational sac.

SECOND AND THIRD TRIMESTERS

- Solid, homogeneous medium-gray structure.
- Smooth edges and borders.
- Hyperechoic chorionic plate.
- Cystic areas directly behind chorionic plate (fetal vessels).
- Anechoic or hypoechoic sonolucent areas within placenta (placental lakes) are insignificant and commonly displayed after 25 weeks.
- Hypoechoic retroplacental complex.
- Myometrium appears as a thin hypoechoic layer posterior to the retroplacental complex.

PLACENTAL POSITION

- The blastocyst may implant into any portion of the decidua (endometrium).
- The placenta may be located anterior, posterior, fundal, right lateral, or left lateral.
- The placenta may be implanted over or near the cervical os (previa).

PLACENTA PREVIA

- Placental placement in front of the fetus relative to the birth canal.
- Primary cause of painless vaginal bleeding in the third trimester.
- Risk factors include advanced maternal age, multiparity, and prior cesarean section or abortion.
- Complications of placenta previa include premature delivery, life-threatening maternal hemorrhage, and increased risk of placenta accreta, stillbirth, and intrauterine growth restriction.
- Only 5% of cases diagnosed with placenta previa in the second trimester remain at term, a result of placental migration.

Placenta Previa

TYPE	CLINICAL FINDINGS	SONOGRAPHIC FINDINGS	DIFFERENTIAL CONSIDERATIONS
Complete	• Painless vaginal bleeding	• Placenta covers the entire cervical os	• Myometrial contraction • Overdistention of the urinary bladder • Uterine leiomyoma • Improper technique
Incomplete	• Painless vaginal bleeding	• Placenta covers one side of the cervical os	• Myometrial contraction • Overdistention of the urinary bladder • Uterine leiomyoma • Improper technique
Marginal	• Asymptomatic • Painless vaginal bleeding	• Edge of the placenta abuts the cervical os	• Myometrial contraction • Overdistention of the urinary bladder • Uterine leiomyoma • Low-lying placenta
Low-lying	• Asymptomatic	• Edge of the placenta lies close but does not abut the cervical os • Within 2 cm of the internal os	• Myometrial contraction • Overdistention of the urinary bladder • Uterine leiomyoma • Marginal previa
Vasa previa	• Bleeding • Cord compression • Prolapsed cord • Transverse fetal lie	• Fetal vessels cross over the internal os	• Normal free-floating cord • Velamentous cord • Succenturiate placenta • Myometrial contraction

Placental Abnormalities

ABNORMALITY	INFORMATION	SONOGRAPHIC FINDINGS	DIFFERENTIAL CONSIDERATIONS
Abruption	• Premature placental detachment • Clinical findings include severe pelvic pain and vaginal bleeding • Risk factors include maternal hypertension, smoking, diabetes, and trauma	• Hypoechoic retroplacental mass • Placental thickening • Well-defined margins • Elevation of placental edges • Subamniotic or preplacental locations are rare	• Normal retroplacental complex • Amniochorionic separation • Myometrial contraction • Uterine leiomyoma
Accreta	Accreta • Chorionic villi of the placenta are in direct contact with the uterine myometrium • Attributed to complete or partial absence of the decidua basalis • Risk factors include multiparity, placenta previa, and previous cesarean section • Increta—placenta invades the uterine myometrium • Percreta—placental vessels invade the uterine serosa or urinary bladder	Accreta • Obscured or absent retroplacental complex • Numerous placental lakes Increta • Extension of villi into the myometrium Percreta • Extension of villi outside of the uterus	• Adenomyosis • Myometrial contraction • Uterine leiomyoma
Amniochorionic separation	• Amnion can be separated from the fetal surface of the placenta but cannot be separated from the umbilical insertion site • Chorion can be separated from the endometrial lining but cannot be separated from the placental edge	• Localized fluid between the fetal side of the placenta and the amniotic membrane • Membrane may move	• Placental abruption • Normal venous lakes
Battledore placenta	• Cord inserts into the end margin of the placenta	• Insertion of the cord into the end margin of the placenta	• Normal cord lying adjacent to the placental margin • Velamentous cord
Calcifications	• Sign of maturing placenta • Associated with maternal cigarette smoking or thrombotic disorders	• Hyperechoic focus within the placental tissue • Posterior acoustic shadowing	• Molar pregnancy
Circumvallate placenta	• Abnormal placental shape in which the membranes insert away from the placental edge toward the center • Increases risk for abruption, intrauterine growth restriction, premature labor, and perinatal death	• Rolled up placental edge • Irregular fold or thickening of the placenta • Upturn placental edge contains hypoechoic or cystic spaces • Thick placental cord insertion	• Abruption • Amniotic shelf • Synechiae
Fibrin deposits	• More commonly located along the subchorionic region of the placenta • Attributed to the regulation of intervillous circulation	• Hypoechoic area beneath the chorionic plate of the placenta	• Venous lake • Subchorionic hematoma
Intervillous thrombosis	• Presence of thrombus within the intervillous spaces • Occurs in one-third of pregnancies • Little risk to fetus	• Anechoic or hypoechoic intraplacental mass • Nonvascular	• Chorioangioma • Placental lakes
Placental infarct	• Result of ischemic necrosis • Occurs in 25% of pregnancies • No clinical risk when small	• Hypoechoic focal placental mass • Calcification may occur	• Intervillous thrombosis • Placental lake
Placental lakes	• Also called venous lakes	• Anechoic or hypoechoic area within the placenta • Internal blood flow	• Intervillous thrombosis • Placental infarct

Continued

Placental Abnormalities—cont'd

ABNORMALITY	INFORMATION	SONOGRAPHIC FINDINGS	DIFFERENTIAL CONSIDERATIONS
Placentomalacia	• Small placenta • Intrauterine growth restriction • Intrauterine infection • Chromosomal abnormality	• Small overall placental size • Placental thinning	• Succenturiate placenta • Myometrial contraction • Normal placenta with marked polyhydramnios
Placentomegaly	• Primary causes include maternal diabetes mellitus and Rh sensitivity • Associated with maternal anemia, twin–twin transfusion, fetal anomalies, and intrauterine infection	• Maximum thickness >5.0 cm • Heterogeneous texture associated with triploidy, molar pregnancy, or hemorrhage • Homogeneous texture associated with anemia, fetal hydrops, and Rh sensitivity	• Myometrial contraction • Uterine leiomyoma • Succenturiate placenta • Placental abruption
Succenturiate placenta	• A result of the lack of the adjacent chorionic villi to atrophy • Approximately 5% of pregnancies • Increased risk of velamentous cord and vasa previa	• Additional placental tissue adjacent to the main placenta • Connected to the body of the placenta by blood vessels	• Myometrial contraction • Leiomyoma

Placenta Neoplasms

NEOPLASM	INFORMATION	SONOGRAPHIC FINDINGS	DIFFERENTIAL CONSIDERATIONS
Chorioangioma	• Placental hemangioma • Arises from the amniotic surface of the placenta • Fetus demonstrates distress owing to vascular shunting from the normal placenta to the hemangioma	• Enlarged placenta • Circular, solid hypoechoic mass protruding from the chorionic plate • Polyhydramnios • Fetal hydrops • Intrauterine growth restriction	• Myometrial contraction • Uterine leiomyoma
Choriocarcinoma	• Malignant form of trophoblastic disease • 50% are preceded by a molar pregnancy	• Hypoechoic intraplacental mass	• Myometrial contraction • Uterine leiomyoma
Gestational trophoblastic disease	• Molar pregnancy • Complete molar pregnancy may develop into choriocarcinoma • Partial mole carries little malignant potential	• Inhomogeneous uterine texture • Various-sized cystic structures within the placenta • No identifiable fetal parts when complete molar pregnancy • Coexisting fetus with a decrease in amniotic fluid volume	• Intraplacental hemorrhage • Degenerating uterine leiomyoma • Prominent maternal venous lakes

UMBILICAL CORD

- Essential link to the placenta.
- Normally inserts into the center of the placenta and midline portion of the anterior abdominal wall of the fetus (umbilicus).
- Umbilical vein carries oxygenated blood.
- Umbilical arteries return venous blood back to the placenta.

UMBILICAL CORD ANATOMY

- Formed by the fusion of the yolk stalk and body stalk (allantoic ducts).
- Amniotic membrane covers the umbilical cord and blends into the fetal skin at the umbilicus.
- Composed of one vein and two arteries surrounded by myxomatous connective tissue (Wharton jelly).

UMBILICAL VEIN

- Formed by the confluence of the chorionic veins of the placenta.
- Enters the umbilicus and joins the left portal vein of the fetal liver.
- Carries oxygenated blood to the fetus.

UMBILICAL ARTERIES

- Umbilical arteries are contiguous with the hypogastric arteries on each side of the fetal urinary bladder.
- Exit at the umbilicus.
- Return venous blood from the fetus back to the placenta.

SIZE

- Length of the umbilical cord is equal to the crown–rump length during the first trimester and continues to have the same length as the fetus throughout pregnancy.
- 40 to 60 cm in length during the second and third trimesters.
- Diameter of the umbilical cord usually measures <2.0 cm.
- Umbilical vein diameter normally measures <9 mm.
- Coiling of the umbilical cord is normal and thought to aid in resistance to compression.
- More commonly coiled toward the left than toward the right, developing approximately 40 spiral turns.

Abnormalities of the Umbilical Cord

ABNORMALITY	INFORMATION	SONOGRAPHIC FINDINGS	DIFFERENTIAL CONSIDERATIONS
Cyst	• Normal finding in the first trimester • 50% of cases associated with fetal anomalies in the second and third trimesters	• Nonvascular anechoic enlargement of the umbilical cord	• True or false cord knot
False knots of the cord	• Coiling of the blood vessels, giving the appearance of knots	• Blood vessels folding over on themselves mimicking umbilical nodules	• Normal coiling of the cord • True cord knots
Long cord	• Cord length >80 cm • Associated with nuchal cord	• Nuchal cord • Polyhydramnios • True umbilical cord knots	• Gastroschisis • Normal cord with polyhydramnios
Nuchal cord	• Cord completely surrounds fetal neck with more than one loop • Significant finding at term • Fetus will turn in and out of the umbilical cord throughout the pregnancy	• Two or more complete loops of cord around the fetal neck	• One complete loop around the neck • Prolapsed cord
Prolapsed cord	• Cord precedes the fetus in the birthing process	• Presence of the cord before the presenting fetal part	• Vasa previa • Nuchal cord

Continued

Abnormalities of the Umbilical Cord—cont'd

ABNORMALITY	INFORMATION	SONOGRAPHIC FINDINGS	DIFFERENTIAL CONSIDERATIONS
Short cord	• Cord length <35 cm	• Limited fetal movement • Inadequate fetal descent • Cord compression • Oligohydramnios	• Normal cord length
Single umbilical artery	• More common in multifetal gestations • Umbilical cord may demonstrate both single and double umbilical arteries within the same cord • Increases risk of associated fetal anomalies by 30% to 60% • Associated with malformations of all major organ systems, chromosomal abnormalities • Increases risk of intrauterine growth restriction	• Two vessels of similar size within the umbilical cord • Umbilical artery transverse diameter >4 mm • Straight, noncoiled umbilical cord	• Normal three-vessel cord
Thrombosis of the umbilical vessels	• Primarily the umbilical vein • Results from both primary and secondary causes • Higher incidence in diabetic mothers	• Absent or abnormal blood flow • Hypoechoic enlargement of one or more umbilical vessels	• Two-vessel cord
Varix of the umbilical vein	• Focal dilatation of the umbilical vein • Nearly always intra-abdominal • Associated with normal outcomes	• Intra-abdominal focal dilatation of the umbilical vein • Located between the anterior abdominal wall and the fetal liver	• Gallbladder • Technical error
Velamentous cord insertion	• Umbilical cord inserts into the membranes before entering the placenta • Associated with preterm labor, abnormal fetal heart pattern, low Apgar scores, low birth weight, and intrauterine growth restriction	• Insertion of the umbilical cord into the membranes adjacent to the edge of the placental margin	• Battledore placenta • Normal cord adjacent to the placenta • Succenturiate placenta

CERVICAL OS

- Cylindrical portion of the uterus, which enters the vagina and lies at right angles to it.
- Measures between 2 and 4 cm in length.
- Cervical canal extends from the internal os to the uterus; external os extends to the vagina.

Abnormality of the Cervix

ABNORMALITY	INFORMATION	SONOGRAPHIC FINDINGS	DIFFERENTIAL CONSIDERATIONS
Incompetent cervix	• Cervical shortening • Generally painless • Decrease in cervical length of ≥6 mm on serial examinations increases risk of preterm labor	• Cervical length less than 2.0 cm • Dilating of the cervical os greater than 3 to 6 mm • Funneling of amniotic fluid into the cervical canal	• Myometrial contraction • Improper technique

PLACENTA AND UMBILICAL CORD REVIEW

1. Growth of the placenta into the superficial myometrium is termed placenta:
   a. previa
   b. increta
   c. accreta
   d. percreta
   e. abruptio

2. Placement of the placental margin within 2 cm of the internal cervical os is termed:
   a. low lying placenta
   b. circumvallate placenta
   c. succenturiate placenta
   d. marginal placenta previa
   e. incomplete placenta previa

3. The location of an umbilical vein varix is most frequently within the:
   a. placenta
   b. fetal liver
   c. fetal pelvis
   d. fetal abdomen
   e. umbilical cord

4. The umbilical cord is covered by which of the following?
   a. amnion
   b. chorion
   c. vernix
   d. meconium
   e. Wharton jelly

5. Insertion of the umbilical cord into the end margin of the placenta is termed:
   a. a battledore placenta
   b. placental migration
   c. a velamentous placenta
   d. a membranous placenta
   e. a circumvallate placenta

6. Placenta accreta can be ruled out by observing a normal:
   a. cord insertion
   b. chorionic plate
   c. retroplacental complex
   d. maternal urinary bladder
   e. homogeneous echo pattern

7. A single umbilical artery is associated with a diameter greater than:
   a. 2 mm
   b. 4 mm
   c. 8 mm
   d. 10 mm
   e. 15 mm

8. During the first trimester, the length of the normal umbilical cord is equal to the:
   a. gestational weeks
   b. mean sac diameter
   c. crown–rump length
   d. biparietal diameter
   e. width of the gestational sac

9. Classic symptoms of placental abruption include:
   a. painless vaginal bleeding
   b. severe pelvic pain and vaginal bleeding
   c. mild abdominal pain and vaginal spotting
   d. severe pelvic pain without vaginal bleeding
   e. mild to severe lower back pain and tender cervix

10. Identification of arterial flow on each side of the fetal bladder verifies which of the following?
    a. normal renal function
    b. two umbilical arteries
    c. normal femoral arteries
    d. normal aortic bifurcation
    e. duplicated hypogastric arteries

11. Extension of an anterior placenta into the maternal urinary bladder is a sonographic finding associated with:
    a. adenomyosis
    b. endometriosis
    c. placenta increta
    d. placenta previa
    e. placenta percreta

12. Which portion of the gestational sac develops into the fetal side of the placenta?
    a. chorion leave
    b. chorionic villi
    c. chorion basalis
    d. chorion parietalis
    e. chorion frondosum

13. Which of the following describes a condition where the chorionic plate of the placenta is smaller than the basal plate?
    a. vasa previa
    b. abruptio placentae
    c. battledore placenta
    d. succenturiate placenta
    e. circumvallate placenta

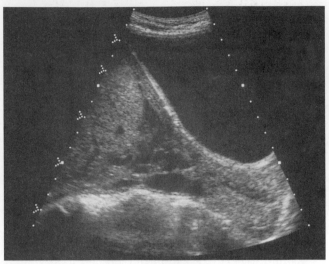

FIG. 28-2   Sagittal sonogram.

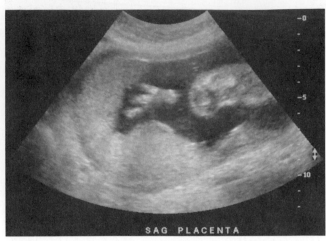

FIG. 28-3   Sagittal sonogram.

14. A true nuchal cord is defined as:
    a. one complete loop of the umbilical cord near the fetal neck
    b. one complete loop of the umbilical cord around the fetal neck
    c. two or more complete loops of the umbilical cord near the fetal neck
    d. two or more complete loops of the umbilical cord around the fetal neck
    e. thickening of the nuchal fold coexisting with one complete loop of the umbilical cord around the fetal neck

15. A placenta located immediately adjacent to the cervix is termed a(n):
    a. low-lying placenta
    b. battledore placenta
    c. succenturiate placenta
    d. marginal placenta previa
    e. incomplete placenta previa

Using Fig. 28-2, answer questions 16 and 17.

16. Which of the following conditions is most likely identified in this sagittal sonogram of the cervix?
    a. vasa previa
    b. placenta previa
    c. placenta accreta
    d. incompetent cervix
    e. velamentous cord insertion

17. Which clinical finding is more commonly associated with this condition?
    a. fetal tachycardia
    b. cephalic fetal lie
    c. small for gestational age
    d. painless vaginal bleeding
    e. premature rupture of membranes

Using Fig. 28-3, answer question 18.

18. Which of the following is the most accurate placental location?
    a. fundal
    b. anterior
    c. posterior
    d. left lateral
    e. right lateral

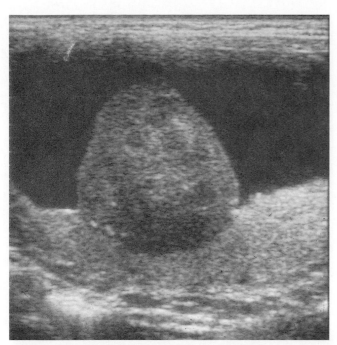

FIG. 28-4   Transverse sonogram.

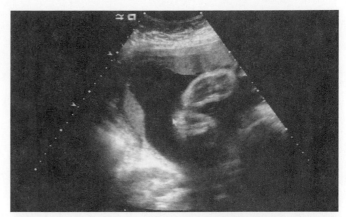

FIG. 28-5   Transverse sonogram.

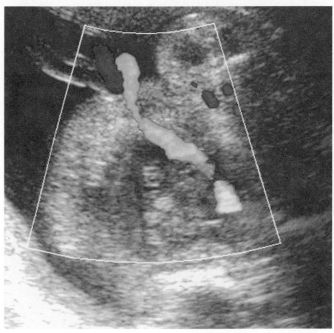

FIG. 28-6   (See color plate 9).

Using Fig. 28-4, answer question 19.

19. The sonogram is most likely identifying which of the following?
  a. chorioangioma
  b. fetal papyraceus
  c. uterine leiomyoma
  d. battledore placenta
  e. myometrial contraction

Using Fig. 28-5, answer question 20.

20. This transverse image of the uterus is most likely demonstrating:
  a. polyhydramnios
  b. battledore placenta
  c. succenturiate placenta
  d. myometrial contraction
  e. vanishing twin syndrome

Using Fig. 28-6 (and color plate 9), answer questions 21 and 22.

21. This duplex image is identifying which of the following structures?
  a. umbilical varix
  b. battledore cord
  c. velamentous cord
  d. single umbilical artery
  e. thrombosis of an umbilical artery

22. This finding is associated with:
  a. fetal demise
  b. macrosomia
  c. premature labor
  d. multifetal gestations
  e. maternal diabetes mellitus

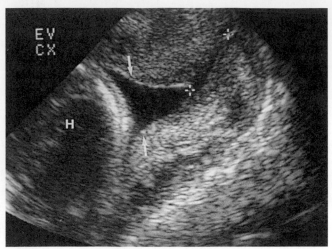

FIG. 28-7　Sagittal sonogram.

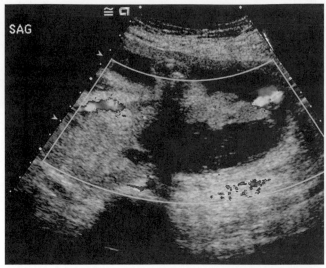

FIG. 28-8

Using Fig. 28-7, answer question 23.

23. The lower uterine segment in this sonogram is consistent with a(n):
    a. prolapsed cord
    b. placenta previa
    c. placenta accreta
    d. velamentous cord
    e. incompetent cervix

Using Fig. 28-8, answer question 24.

24. A patient presents with severe lower abdominal pain and vaginal spotting. A sonogram of the placenta demonstrates a nonvascular hypoechoic mass. On the basis of the clinical history, the sonographic findings are most suspicious for:
    a. chorioangioma
    b. placenta accreta
    c. placenta abruption
    d. circumvallate placenta
    e. amniochorionic separation

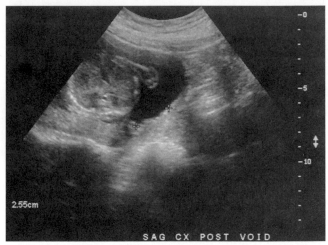

FIG. 28-9　Sagittal sonogram.

Using Fig. 28-9, answer question 25.

25. This postvoid transabdominal image of the cervix demonstrates:
    a. a low-lying placenta
    b. a cervix free of placenta
    c. marginal placenta previa
    d. complete placenta previa
    e. incomplete placenta previa

Using Fig. 28-10, answer questions 26 and 27.

26. A sagittal image of the cervix in a late second-trimester pregnancy is demonstrating:
    a. placenta previa
    b. placental abruption
    c. an incompetent cervix
    d. a left lateral placenta
    e. Braxton-Hicks contraction

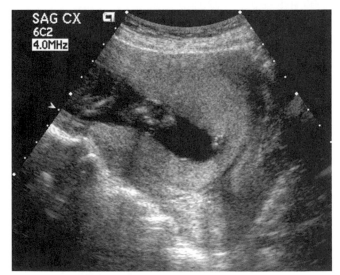

FIG. 28-10　Sagittal sonogram.

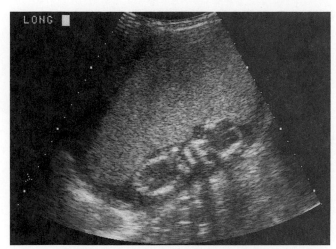

FIG. 28-11   Transverse sonogram.

27. This patient most likely presents with:
   a. mild pelvic pain
   b. urinary frequency
   c. severe pelvic pain
   d. abdominal cramping
   e. painless vaginal bleeding

Using Fig. 28-11, answer questions 28 and 29.

28. An image of an early second-trimester pregnancy is demonstrating:
   a. placenta previa
   b. placentomegaly
   c. placentomalacia
   d. battledore placenta
   e. circumvallate placenta

29. Maternal causes for this abnormality include:
   a. hypertension
   b. diabetes mellitus
   c. pelvic inflammatory disease
   d. previous cesarean section
   e. previous therapeutic abortions

30. Membranous insertion of the umbilical cord is termed a(n):
   a. vasa previa
   b. allantois cord
   c. Wharton cord
   d. velamentous cord
   e. battledore placenta

31. Fusion of the amnion and chorion should occur by:
   a. 10 weeks' gestation
   b. 12 weeks' gestation
   c. 16 weeks' gestation
   d. 20 weeks' gestation
   e. 24 weeks' gestation

32. An eccentric insertion of the umbilical cord into the placenta is termed a:
   a. vasa previa
   b. placenta percreta
   c. velamentous cord
   d. battledore placenta
   e. circumvallate placenta

33. Placental implantation encroaching upon the internal cervical os is termed:
   a. placenta increta
   b. marginal previa
   c. placenta accreta
   d. complete previa
   e. low-lying placenta

34. The vascular projections arising from the chorion are termed:
   a. allantoic ducts
   b. chorionic villi
   c. chorionic leave
   d. chorionic venules
   e. myxomatous tissue

35. Which of the following conditions demonstrates extension of the chorionic villi into the wall of the maternal urinary bladder?
   a. placenta increta
   b. placentomalacia
   c. placenta accreta
   d. placenta percreta
   e. battledore placenta

36. Coiling of the umbilical cord is associated with:
   a. a long cord
   b. a short cord
   c. a normal fetus
   d. premature labor
   e. chromosomal abnormalities

37. Which of the following is the most common placental location for deposits of fibrin to collect?
   a. basal plate
   b. subchorionic
   c. within a placental lake
   d. within a placental neoplasm
   e. within the retroplacental complex

38. The primary cause of placentomegaly is:
   a. maternal hypertension
   b. twin–twin transfusion
   c. succenturiate placenta
   d. maternal diabetes mellitus
   e. intrauterine growth restriction

39. Complications of placenta previa include all of the following EXCEPT:
    a. stillbirth
    b. macrosomia
    c. placenta accreta
    d. premature delivery
    e. maternal hemorrhage

40. The presence of additional placental tissue adjacent to the main placenta is termed a(n):
    a. placenta accreta
    b. accessory placenta
    c. battledore placenta
    d. velamentous placenta
    e. circumvallate placenta

41. Which placenta is most likely to demonstrate an overall abnormal contour?
    a. placenta previa
    b. battledore placenta
    c. velamentous placenta
    d. succenturiate placenta
    e. circumvallate placenta

42. Placentomegaly may result from all of the following conditions EXCEPT:
    a. Rh sensitivity
    b. fetal anomalies
    c. maternal anemia
    d. twin–twin transfusion
    e. intrauterine growth restriction

43. The maternal side of the placenta is formed by the decidua:
    a. villi
    b. leave
    c. basalis
    d. parietalis
    e. frondosum

44. Placental thickness will vary with gestational age but generally measures:
    a. 1-2 cm
    b. 2-3 cm
    c. 4-5 cm
    d. 5-6 cm
    e. 6-7 cm

45. Which of the following conditions is most likely to demonstrate a small placenta?
    a. macrosomia
    b. Rh sensitivity
    c. maternal anemia
    d. maternal diabetes
    e. chromosomal anomalies

46. Which of the following occurs when intramembranous vessels course across the internal cervical os?
    a. vasa previa
    b. placenta previa
    c. placenta accreta
    d. battledore placenta
    e. circumvallate placenta

47. Which of the following is associated with a nuchal cord?
    a. long cord
    b. short cord
    c. velamentous cord
    d. true knots of the cord
    e. false knots of the cord

48. Which of the following describes a prolapsed umbilical cord?
    a. focal dilatation of an umbilical vessel
    b. the cord precedes the fetus in the birthing process
    c. the intramembranous vessels of the fetus precede the fetus
    d. the cord completely surrounds the fetal neck with one loop
    e. the cord completely surrounds the fetal neck with more than one loop

49. A succenturiate placenta is at an increased risk for which of the following?
    a. placenta increta
    b. velamentous cord
    c. placental abruption
    d. intervillous thrombosis
    e. amniochorionic separation

50. Coiling of the umbilical cord is generally:
    a. toward the left
    b. toward the right
    c. associated with a long cord
    d. associated with fetal anomalies
    e. associated with premature labor

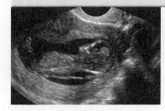

CHAPTER 29

Patient Care and Technique

KEY TERMS

accountability being required to answer for one's actions.

advance directive a legal document describing your health care wishes if you are unable to communicate them.

Agency for Healthcare Research and Quality (AHRQ) a government agency looking to improve the quality, safety, efficiency, and effectiveness of American health care.

autonomy the right to make our own independent decisions.

beneficence bringing about good by maximizing benefits and minimizing possible harm.

code of conduct the moral code, which guides professional conduct of duties and obligations.

ethics systems of valued behaviors and beliefs that govern proper conduct to ensure protection of individual's rights.

glutaraldehyde a powerful solution used to disinfect transducers.

gynecology medical specialty that deals with the reproductive system of the nongravid uterus.

Health Insurance Portability and Accountability Act (HIPAA) federal agency overseeing many health care functions, the primary being patient confidentiality.

integrity adherence to moral and ethical principles.

The Joint Commission (TJC) formerly the Joint Commission on Accreditation of Healthcare Organizations (JCAHO), an organization of health care institutions devoted to improving, regulating, and accrediting its member institutions, with the goal of providing safe and efficient patient care.

morality the protection of cherished values that relate to how persons interact and live in peace.

obstetrics medical specialty that deals with the reproductive system of the gravid uterus.

patient care partnership new standard describing patient's health care rights.

veracity truthfulness; honesty.

PATIENT CARE

- Patient health care rights include:
  - High-quality medical care.
  - A clean and safe environment.
  - Involvement in his or her own care.
  - Ability to express autonomy.
  - Privacy protection of health care information.

SONOGRAPHER RESPONSIBILITIES

- Keep conversations low and private.
- Set screensavers to the lowest setting.
- Keep patient records private and out of public view.
- Maintain privacy of patient information from nonproviding personnel.
- Remove patient identification from images used in publications or presentations.

Examination Responsibilities

TIME FRAME	RESPONSIBILITY
Prior to examination	• Review medical order • Verify proper examination is scheduled • Review prior diagnostic studies, if available • Review institution's examination protocol, if needed • Address patient by their first and last name • Introduce yourself to the patient and family • Explain examination requested by their physician prior to beginning the scan • Obtain patient history, including possible medication or latex allergies in a private environment
During examination	• Maintain patient modesty and privacy • Alleviate and address patient's concerns • Expand on examination protocol as needed
After examination	• Explained expected time frame for the patient's physician to receive a report • Clean transducer(s) and keyboard • Write technical impression of real-time examination

PATIENT HISTORY

- Patient history may be provided by the referring clinician or hospital chart.
- The sonographer often needs to obtain additional patient history for the interpreting physician.

Gynecology History

SUBJECT	QUESTIONS
Menstrual cycle	Date of last menstrual period Menstrual irregularities or abnormalities
Medications	Contraceptive Follicular stimulating Postmenopausal
Pelvic pain	Location Severity Acute or chronic Associated with menstruation or ovulation
Pelvic surgery	Uterus and/or ovaries Tubal ligation Caesarian section Appendectomy Endometriosis
Prior pregnancy	Total number of pregnancies Number of live births Number of miscarriages

Obstetric History

SUBJECT	QUESTIONS
Laboratory results	hCG levels Alpha-fetoprotein Amniocentesis
Maternal health history	Hypertension Diabetes mellitus Fertility assistance

Obstetric History—cont'd	
SUBJECT	QUESTIONS
Menstrual cycle	Last menstrual period
	Estimated delivery date
Pelvic pain	Location
	Severity
	Duration
Previous pregnancy	Grava–Para
	Fetal abnormalities
	Multiple gestations
Vaginal discharge	Bleeding
	Spotting
	Clear fluid

TRANSABDOMINAL EXAMINATION

- Should be the first examination performed.
- Urinary bladder and iliac vessels are imaging landmarks.
- Allows a wider field of view visualizing the entire pelvis and superficial structures.
- Allows better visualization of structures remote from the vagina.
- Requires a lower-frequency transducer to visualize deep pelvic structures.
- Decreased resolution with uterine retroversion or retroflexion.
- Body habitus and bowel gas can affect resolution of the pelvic structures.

PURPOSE OF BLADDER DISTENTION

- Displaces uterus posteriorly and bowel laterally.
- Provides an acoustic window to visualize pelvic structures.
- Provides an anatomical and anechoic reference point.

Optimal Bladder Distention

- Extends past the most superior portion of the uterus.
- Well-distended bladder demonstrates an elongated shape (not circular).

Underdistention

- May still provide an overview of the pelvic structures.

Overdistention

- Compresses and distorts pelvic anatomy.
- Displaces structures out of the field of view.
- Incorrect diagnosis of placenta previa.

ORIENTATION (Fig. 29-1)

TECHNIQUE

Adult Preparation

- Drink 28 to 32 oz of water 1 hour prior to examination.
- If catheterized, fill bladder to 375 mL.
- Maintain full bladder for entire examination.

Child Preparation

- Adjust fluid intake according to age and weight.

GYNECOLOGICAL EXAMINATION TECHNIQUE

- Unless contraindicated, a complete gynecological examination includes transabdominal and transvaginal imaging.

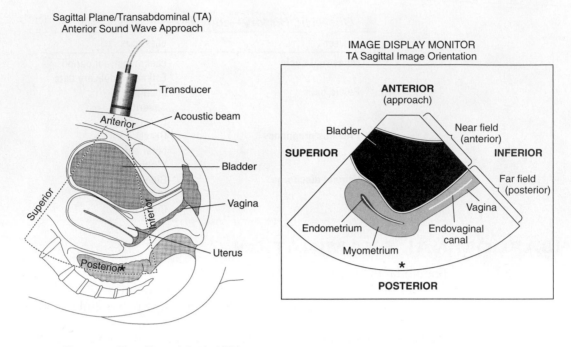

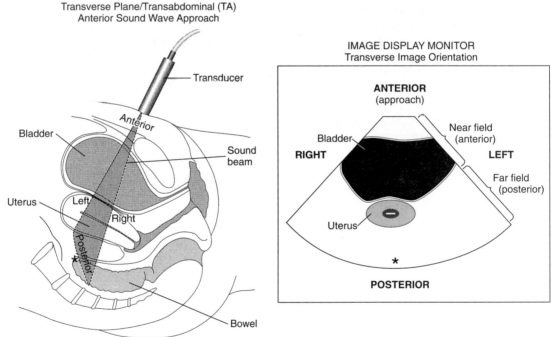

FIG. 29-1   Transabdominal examination orientation.

- Use the highest-frequency transducer possible to obtain optimal resolution and penetration depth.
- Ensure proper focal zone and depth placement to include the posterior cul de sac.
- Gain settings should demonstrate the urinary bladder as an anechoic structure.
- Use a systematic approach to evaluate and document the entire pelvis in both the longitudinal and transverse planes.
- Document and measure the length, height, and width of the uterus.
- Evaluate, document, and measure the endometrium.
- Document and measure the length, height, and width of each ovary.
- Document the adnexal area bilaterally.
- Evaluate the urinary bladder for incidental abnormalities.

- Use color Doppler imaging to evaluate vascular flow within and surrounding the reproductive structures.
- Document and measure in two imaging planes any abnormality that should be included.
- Document and evaluate both kidneys for associated hydronephrosis when encountering a pelvic mass.

INDICATIONS

- Pelvic pain.
- Pelvic mass.
- Menorrhagia.
- Dysmenorrhea.
- Enlarged uterus.
- Postmenopausal bleeding.

OBSTETRIC EXAMINATION TECHNIQUE

- Use the lowest acoustic power possible.
- Use the highest-frequency transducer possible to obtain optimal resolution and penetration depth.
- Ensure proper focal zone and depth placement.
- Note that documentation of an intrauterine pregnancy will vary with gestational age but generally includes fetal number, fetal viability, gestational age measurements, and fetal assessment.
- Document and evaluate the uterus and both ovaries.
- Assessment of fetal growth can be determined with examinations a minimum of 3 weeks apart.

INDICATIONS

- Small for dates.
- Large for dates.
- Fetal surveillance.
- Check for viability.
- Vagina bleeding.
- Rule out ectopic pregnancy.
- Placenta or fetal position.

TRANSVAGINAL EXAMINATION

- Minimally invasive procedure used as a complement to the transabdominal examination.
- Uterine and iliac vessels are imaging landmarks.
- Bypasses the attenuating factors of imaging through the abdominal wall.
- Uses a high-frequency transducer, increasing resolution of the pelvic structures.
- Advantageous with obese patients and uterine retroflexion and retroversion.
- Limited penetration depth and field of view.
- Decreased penetration when encountering highly attenuating structures.
- Contraindicated in premenarche and virgin patients.
- Excellent method of measuring cervical length in the gravid patient.

ORIENTATION (Fig. 29-2)
TECHNIQUE

Preparation

- Empty urinary bladder places the pelvic structures within the field of view.
- Transvaginal transducer is covered with a protective barrier.

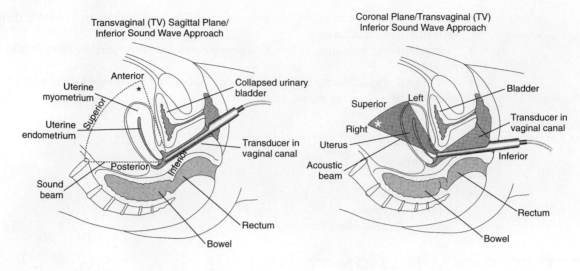

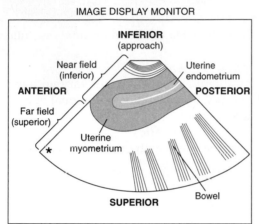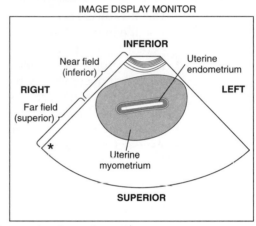

FIG. 29-2 Transvaginal examination orientation.

- Explain the examination to the patient.
- Prior to continuing, the patient must consent to the procedure.
- Patient is placed in a lithotomy position.
- Transducer is inserted into the vaginal canal.

Gynecological Examination Technique

- In both sagittal and coronal planes, document and evaluate the uterus, ovaries, bilateral adnexa, and posterior cul de sac.
- Measure the anterior–posterior endometrial thickness.
- Document and measure the length, height, and width of the uterus and ovaries.
- Document and measure any abnormality in two imaging planes.

Obstetrical Examination Technique

- Document and evaluate the pregnancy location.
- Document and evaluate the fetal number.
- Document and evaluate fetal viability.
- Document and measure the gestational age.
- Document and evaluate both ovaries and adnexa.
- Document the cervical length.

FIG. 29-3
Translabial examination orientation.

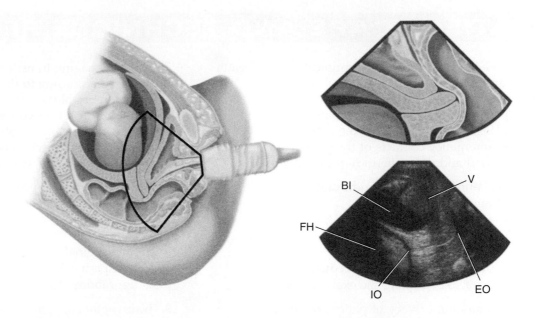

TRANSLABIAL EXAMINATION

- Alternative to the transvaginal approach.
- Vagina and urinary bladder are imaging landmarks.
- Enhances resolution of the cervix and distal vagina.
- Not as accurate as transvaginal imaging in measuring cervical length.

ORIENTATION (Fig. 29-3)

TECHNIQUE

Preparation

- Empty or partially filled urinary bladder.
- Examination is explained to the patient.
- Consent should be given prior to examination.
- Elevate patient's hips with several towels.
- Cover transducer with a protective barrier.

Gynecological and Obstetrical Examination Technique

- Use the highest frequency possible to achieve visualization of target structure.
- Transducer is placed on the perineum or vaginal opening.
- Pivoting or angling the transducer allows visualization of various pelvic structures.
- Scanning challenges include bowel gas and pelvic bones.

Indications

- Cervical mass.
- Vaginal spotting.
- Placental location.

TRANSDUCER CARE

- Following the manufacturer's recommendation, clean and disinfect transducers after each use.
- Probe covers are essential with transvaginal and translabial imaging.
- Do not use heat sterilization technique to disinfect transducer or assembly.

PATIENT CARE AND TECHNIQUE REVIEW

1. An advance directive communicates to all health care providers the:
   a. medical history of the patient
   b. health care wishes of the patient
   c. insurance coverage of the patient
   d. emergency contacts of the patient
   e. food and drug allergies of the patient

2. Explaining the ultrasound examination is accomplished:
   a. after the examination
   b. during the examination
   c. when the patient inquires
   d. prior to an invasive procedure
   e. prior to beginning the examination

3. Maintaining privacy of patient medical information is a primary goal of the:
   a. Patient Care Partnership
   b. Joint Review Committee
   c. Agency for Healthcare Research and Quality
   d. Health Insurance Portability and Accountability Act
   e. The Joint Commission

4. Which of the following is NOT a responsibility of the sonographer?
   a. Keep conversations low and private
   b. Give technical report to the patient
   c. Set screensavers to the lowest setting
   d. Keep patient records out of public view
   e. Remove patient identification from images used in publication

5. Which of the following is NOT a patient health care right?
   a. high-quality medical care
   b. clean and safe environment
   c. subjugation of self-sufficiency
   d. protection of private information
   e. involvement in his or her own medical care

6. Upon completion of the examination, the sonographer should:
   a. introduce himself or herself to the patient
   b. explain the examination to the patient
   c. obtain clinical information from the patient
   d. review institution's protocol for examination
   e. inform patient of expected time frame for examination results

7. Medical imaging transducers are cleaned and sterilized according to the:
   a. preference of the patient
   b. manufacturer's recommendations
   c. supervising sonographer's preference
   d. institution's infection control department
   e. Occupational Safety and Health Administration

8. The sonographic approach recommended for all pelvic examinations is:
   a. translabial
   b. transrectal
   c. transvaginal
   d. transperineal
   e. transabdominal

9. Transvaginal imaging uses which of the following structures as a landmark?
   a. ovary
   b. uterus
   c. vagina
   d. rectum
   e. bladder

10. The translabial approach evaluates which of the following structures?
    a. ovary
    b. uterus
    c. cervix
    d. fallopian tube
    e. endometrial lining

11. Overdistention of the urinary bladder:
    a. displaces the uterus anteriorly
    b. places the bowel within the true pelvis
    c. increases resolution of the pelvic structures
    d. may result in a misdiagnosis of placenta previa
    e. allows a more accurate measurement of the uterine height

12. Which of the following is a contraindication for transvaginal imaging?
    a. geriatric patient
    b. vaginal bleeding
    c. ectopic pregnancy
    d. premenarche patient
    e. bladder incontinence

13. Transabdominal imaging resolution is limited by the patient's:
    a. age
    b. body habitus
    c. clinical history
    d. menstrual status
    e. hormone intake

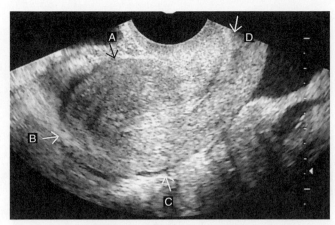

FIG. 29-4   Sagittal sonogram.

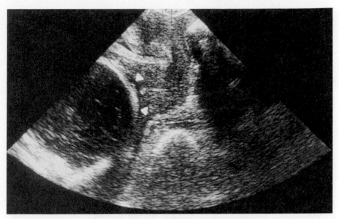

FIG. 29-5   Sagittal sonogram.

14. Optimal bladder distention is determined by the:
    a. referring physician
    b. ability of the patient
    c. location of the ovaries
    d. total number of pregnancies
    e. superior portion of the uterus

15. Which of the following structures is best evaluated with transperineal imaging?
    a. ovary
    b. vagina
    c. peritoneum
    d. fallopian tube
    e. endometrial cavity

16. Which approach is the best method for evaluating superficial structures?
    a. translabial
    b. transrectal
    c. endovaginal
    d. transperineal
    e. transabdominal

Using Fig. 29-4, answer questions 17 to 21.

17. Which of the following accurately describe this sonogram?
    a. endovaginal image of an anteverted uterus
    b. transabdominal image of a retroflexed uterus
    c. transperineal image of an anteflexed uterus
    d. transvaginal image of a retroflexed uterus
    e. transabdominal image of an anteverted uterus

18. With this imaging approach and orientation, label **A** designates which surface of the uterus?
    a. right
    b. anterior
    c. inferior
    d. superior
    e. posterior

19. Which uterine surface is label **B** identifying?
    a. left
    b. right
    c. anterior
    d. inferior
    e. superior

20. Label **C** is identifying which of the following uterine surfaces?
    a. lateral
    b. medial
    c. anterior
    d. inferior
    e. posterior

21. Label **D** designates which uterine surface?
    a. left
    b. inferior
    c. anterior
    d. superior
    e. posterior

Using Fig. 29-5, answer question 22.

22. Which of the following sonographic approaches is used in this sonogram?
    a. transrectal
    b. endovaginal
    c. transperineal
    d. transvaginal
    e. transabdominal

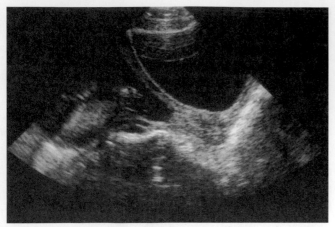

FIG. 29-6 Sagittal sonogram.

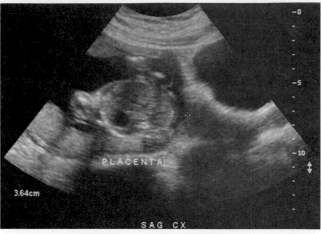

FIG. 29-8 Sagittal sonogram.

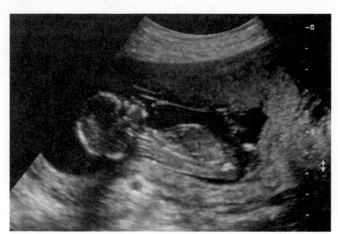

FIG. 29-7

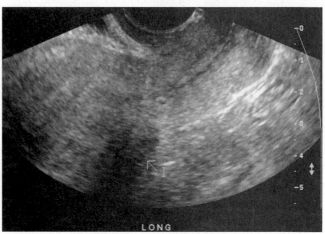

FIG. 29-9 Sagittal sonogram.

Using Fig. 29-6, answer question 23.

23. Which of the following techniques will aid in evaluating the placental margin?
    a. decrease the output power
    b. increase overall gain control
    c. decrease the number of focal zones
    d. increase the transducer frequency
    e. decrease urinary bladder volume

Using Fig. 29-7, answer question 24.

24. Which of the following techniques will improve this sonogram?
    a. raise focal zone
    b. increase output gain
    c. increase penetration depth
    d. decrease transducer frequency
    e. increase the number of focal zones

Using Fig. 29-8, answer questions 25 and 26.

25. The right side of the screen represents the:
    a. lateral portion of the patient
    b. inferior portion of the patient
    c. anterior portion of the patient
    d. superior portion of the patient
    e. posterior portion of the patient

26. The left side of the screen represents the:
    a. caudal portion of the patient
    b. anterior portion of the patient
    c. inferior portion of the patient
    d. superior portion of the patient
    e. posterior portion of the patient

Using Fig. 29-9, answer question 27.

27. The arrow in this image is pointing to the:
    a. anterior surface of an anteverted uterus
    b. inferior surface of an anteflexed uterus
    c. anterior surface of a retroflexed uterus
    d. superior surface of a retroverted uterus
    e. posterior surface of an anteverted uterus

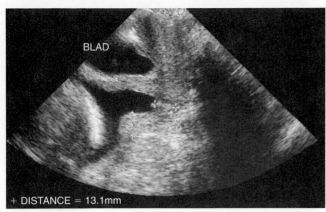

BLAD

+ DISTANCE = 13.1mm

FIG. 29-10

Using Fig. 29-10, answer question 28.

28. Which of the following accurately describes the approach and imaging plane of this sonogram?
    a. transrectal; sagittal
    b. translabial; coronal
    c. endovaginal; sagittal
    d. transvaginal; coronal
    e. transperineal; sagittal

29. The sonographer is responsible for explaining to the patient:
    a. abnormal laboratory results
    b. the results of the ultrasound examination
    c. the reason their doctor ordered the sonogram
    d. the ultrasound examination ordered by their doctor
    e. results of their previous medical imaging examinations

30. Knowledge of the patient's last menstrual period could explain the:
    a. overall size of the uterus
    b. position of the uterine fundus
    c. fullness of the urinary bladder
    d. appearance of the endometrium
    e. appearance of the large intestines

31. Endometrial thickness is measured between which of the following borders?
    a. cephalic to caudal
    b. anterior to posterior
    c. medial to lateral
    d. inferior to superior
    e. coronal to transverse

32. Which of the following is an indication for a transperineal ultrasound?
    a. evaluate adnexal mass
    b. document fetal gender
    c. evaluate placental location
    d. rule out ectopic pregnancy
    e. evaluate for multifetal gestation

33. Which of the following governs proper conduct?
    a. ethics
    b. justice
    c. autonomy
    d. accountability
    e. confidentiality

34. What refers to a person's capacity to formulate, express, and carry out value-based preferences?
    a. ethics
    b. autonomy
    c. beneficence
    d. accountability
    e. nonmaleficence

35. A code of ethics for sonographers has been developed adopted by the:
    a. American Medical Association
    b. Society of Diagnostic Medical Sonographers
    c. American Registry in Diagnostic Medical Sonographers
    d. Joint Review Committee for Diagnostic Medical Sonography
    e. Commission on Accreditation of Allied Health Educational Programs

36. Obstetrical ultrasound examinations allow the clinician to assess all of the following EXCEPT:
    a. fetal gender
    b. gestational age
    c. fetal well-being
    d. amniotic fluid volume
    e. atrial septum competence

37. Overdistention of the maternal urinary bladder may result in a false impression of:
    a. fetal well-being
    b. cervical funneling
    c. umbilical herniation
    d. cervical competence
    e. amniotic band syndrome

38. The purpose for certification in diagnostic medical sonography is to assure the public the sonographer has the necessary:
    a. knowledge of human anatomy
    b. skills to work the system controls
    c. education to perform the examination
    d. experience to perform the examination
    e. all of the above

39. What is the best imaging technique for measuring cervical length?
    a. translabial
    b. transrectal
    c. transvaginal
    d. transperineal
    e. transabdominal

40. What is the best imaging technique to evaluate for the presence of placenta previa?
    a. transvaginal with a full maternal bladder
    b. transperineal with a full maternal bladder
    c. translabial with an empty maternal bladder
    d. transabdominal with a partially full maternal bladder
    e. transabdominal with an overdistended maternal bladder

41. In which imaging plane is spina bifida best recognized?
    a. sagittal
    b. oblique
    c. coronal
    d. transverse
    e. tangential

42. A health care professional's duty to protect the privacy of patient information is termed:
    a. ethics
    b. morality
    c. integrity
    d. beneficence
    e. confidentiality

43. A sonographer can minimize the thermal effects of diagnostic ultrasound by:
    a. scanning over fetal bone
    b. increasing acoustic output
    c. using one acoustic window
    d. increasing examination time
    e. extending the focus as deep as possible

44. In a gynecological examination, depth placement must include the:
    a. cervix
    b. vagina
    c. urinary bladder
    d. anterior cul de sac
    e. posterior cul de sac

45. Which of the following is a mandatory requirement prior to performing a transvaginal examination?
    a. patient consent
    b. radiologist approval
    c. insurance verification
    d. distended urinary bladder
    e. transabdominal examination

46. When a pelvic mass is encountered, the sonographer should evaluate the:
    a. iliac artery for stenosis
    b. iliac vein for thrombosis
    c. appendix for inflammation
    d. kidneys for hydronephrosis
    e. paracolic gutters for ascites

47. In a transvaginal examination, in which position is the patient placed?
    a. prone
    b. lithotomy
    c. Trendelenburg
    d. posterior oblique
    e. reverse Trendelenburg

48. Which of the following is an advantage of transvaginal imaging?
    a. ability to visualize the entire pelvis
    b. ability to visualize superficial structures
    c. increase in resolution in an anteflexed uterus
    d. increase in resolution of deep pelvic structures
    e. increase in resolution of the pelvic structures in obese patients

49. Serial assessment of fetal growth is evaluated a minimum of:
    a. 2 days apart
    b. 5 days apart
    c. 1 week apart
    d. 2 weeks apart
    e. 3 weeks apart

50. Which of the following pelvic preparations is appropriate for a 9-year-old girl?
    a. maintain adult preparation
    b. children are always catheterized
    c. no preparation is necessary for children
    d. adjust fluid intake according to child's weight
    e. maintain adult preparation finishing water 15 minutes before examination

1. A clover-leaf-shaped cranium in a second trimester fetus is characteristic of:
   a. acrania
   b. anencephaly
   c. fetal demise
   d. oligohydramnios
   e. skeletal dysplasia

2. Which genitourinary abnormality depends on fetal gender?
   a. renal agenesis
   b. infantile polycystic disease
   c. multicystic dysplastic kidney
   d. ureteropelvic junction obstruction
   e. posterior urethral valve obstruction

3. Which pelvic structure contains the uterine blood vessels and nerves?
   a. psoas muscles
   b. broad ligament
   c. ovarian ligaments
   d. suspensory ligaments
   e. obturator internus muscles

4. When the vascular space between the placenta and myometrium is absent, the sonographer should suspect:
   a. vasa previa
   b. placenta accreta
   c. placenta abruptio
   d. circumvallate placenta
   e. umbilical vein thrombosis

5. Measurement of the biparietal diameter is taken at a level to include the:
   a. cerebellum
   b. falx cerebri
   c. cisterna magna
   d. fourth ventricle
   e. thalamic cerebri

6. The best measuring method for evaluating gestational age is the:
   a. femur length
   b. mean sac diameter
   c. biparietal diameter
   d. crown–rump length
   e. head circumference

7. Bilateral symmetric pelvic masses are most likely:
   a. iliac vessels
   b. pelvic muscles
   c. follicular cysts
   d. theca lutein cysts
   e. uterine leiomyomas

8. A localized hypoechoic adnexal mass is present on serial sonograms. Physiological ovarian cysts of varying size are present bilaterally. Based on this clinical history, the adnexal mass is most suspicious for a(n):
   a. dermoid cyst
   b. endometrioma
   c. dysgerminoma
   d. parovarian cyst
   e. hemorrhagic cyst

9. Maintaining privacy of a patient's medical and personal information is a primary concern of the:
   a. Patient Care Partnership
   b. Joint Review Committee
   c. Agency for Healthcare Research and Quality
   d. Health Insurance Portability and Accountability Act
   e. The Joint Commission

10. Which of the following is NOT evaluated during a fetal biophysical profile?
    a. fetal tone
    b. nonstress test
    c. fetal swallowing
    d. diaphragm movement
    e. amniotic fluid volume

11. An echogenic endometrium with posterior acoustic enhancement is present during which of the following phases?
    a. follicular
    b. secretory
    c. ovulatory
    d. menstrual
    e. proliferative

12. Normal serum maternal alpha-fetoprotein levels vary with:
    a. fetal weight
    b. fetal gender
    c. maternal age
    d. gestational age
    e. placenta location

13. A diamniotic/monochorionic multifetal pregnancy will demonstrate:
    a. one placenta and one gestational sac
    b. two placentas and one gestational sac
    c. one placenta and two gestational sacs
    d. two placentas and two gestational sacs
    e. two placentas and three gestational sacs

14. Symmetrical intrauterine growth restriction is most likely a result of:
    a. first-trimester insult
    b. placental insufficiency
    c. maternal hypertension
    d. chromosomal abnormality
    e. second-trimester infection

15. Which of the following structures shunts blood away from the fetal lungs?
    a. foramen ovale
    b. pulmonary vein
    c. coronary artery
    d. ductus venosus
    e. ductus arteriosus

16. Which of the following abnormalities demonstrates an arteriovenous anastomosis?
    a. macrosomia
    b. acardiac twin
    c. twin–twin transfusion
    d. succenturiate placenta
    e. intrauterine growth restriction

17. Which rare benign ovarian neoplasm occurs most often in postmenopausal women?
    a. dermoid
    b. thecoma
    c. dysgerminoma
    d. Brenner tumor
    e. granulosa cell tumor

18. Hydranencephaly is an abnormality of the:
    a. vein of Galen
    b. third ventricle
    c. cerebral cortex
    d. cisterna magna
    e. lateral ventricle

19. Common sonographic findings associated with Dandy-Walker syndrome include:
    a. macroglossia and omphalocele
    b. megaureter and oligohydramnios
    c. ectopia cordis and polyhydramnios
    d. infantile polycystic disease and oligohydramnios
    e. enlarged posterior fossa and absence of the cerebellar vermis

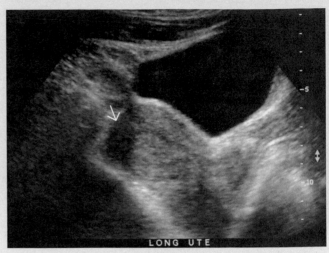

FIG. 1

20. A menarche patient presents with a history of dysmenorrhea and uterine tenderness during a physical examination. Her last menstrual period was 2 weeks prior. The uterine myometrium appears diffusely inhomogeneous on ultrasound. Based on this clinical history, the sonographic presentation is most suspicious for:
    a. endometritis
    b. adenomyosis
    c. endometriosis
    d. subserosal fibroid
    e. Asherman syndrome

Using Fig. 1, answer question 21.

21. Which of the following is the arrow identifying?
    a. adenomyosis
    b. endometriosis
    c. refraction artifact
    d. pedunculating fibroid
    e. overdistention of the urinary bladder

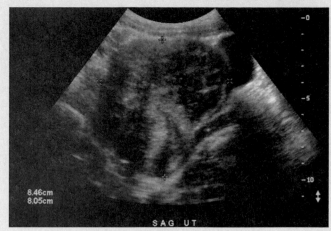

FIG. 2

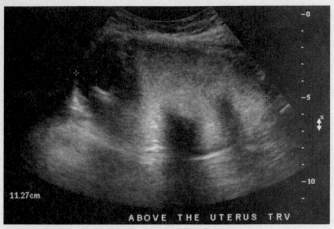

FIG. 3 Transverse sonogram.

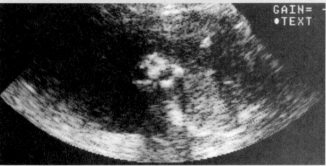

FIG. 4

Using Fig. 2, answer question 22.

22. A menarche patient presents with a history of menorrhagia and an enlarged uterus on physical examination. Based on this clinical history, differential considerations for this sonogram would include:
    a. leiomyomas or leiomyosarcomas
    b. cystic teratomas or endometriosis
    c. ovarian torsion or ectopic pregnancy
    d. endometrial hyperplasia or hematometra
    e. Asherman syndrome or Stein-Leventhal disease

Using Fig. 3, answer question 23.

23. A menarche patient presents with a history of mild pelvic pain. Her menstrual cycles have been normal, with a last menstrual period 3 weeks ago. Only one ovary is identified with certainty. Based on this clinical history, the sonogram is most likely identifying a(n):
    a. appendicitis
    b. endometrioma
    c. cystic teratoma
    d. hemorrhagic cyst
    e. ectopic pregnancy

Using Fig. 4, answer question 24.

24. A 20-year-old patient presents to the emergency room with pelvic cramping and vaginal spotting. The emergency department physician orders a sonogram to verify fetal viability. Based on this clinical history, the sonogram is most suspicious for:
    a. acrania
    b. anencephaly
    c. microcephaly
    d. prosencephaly
    e. hydranencephaly

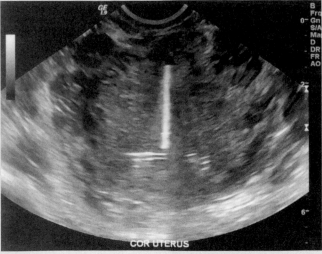

FIG. 5 Endovaginal sonogram.

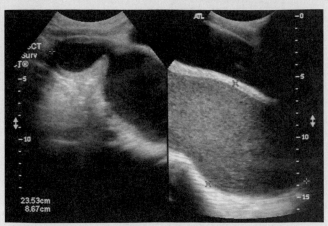

FIG. 7 Sonogram of the pelvic midline.

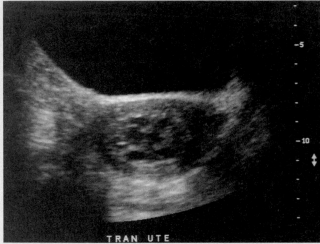

FIG. 6 Transverse sonogram of the uterus.

Using Fig. 5, answer question 25.

25. This coronal image of the uterus is documenting:
    a. chronic endometritis
    b. Asherman syndrome
    c. an intrauterine device
    d. endometrial hyperplasia
    e. intrauterine vascular calcifications

Using Fig. 6, answer question 26.

26. An asymptomatic postmenopausal patient presents with a history of breast cancer and tamoxifen therapy. Based on this clinical history, the sonographic findings are most suspicious for:
    a. endometritis
    b. adenomyosis
    c. cystic teratoma
    d. endometrial polyp
    e. degenerating fibroid

Using Fig. 7, answer question 27.

27. A 15-year-old presents with a history of amenorrhea and pelvic fullness. Based on this clinical history, the sagittal sonogram is most suspicious for:
    a. dermoid
    b. hematometra
    c. endometrioma
    d. tubo-ovarian abscess
    e. mucinous cystadenoma

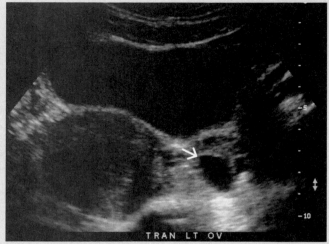

FIG. 8   Sonogram of the left ovary.

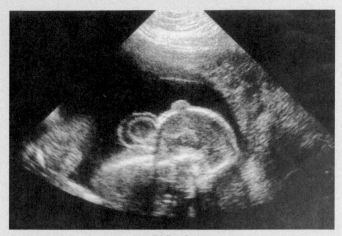

FIG. 9

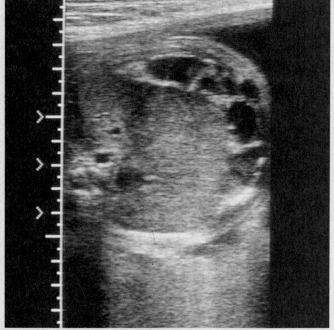

FIG. 10

Using Fig. 8, answer question 28.

28. A menarche patient presents with a history of intermittent left lower quadrant pain over the last 7 days. She states her last menstrual cycle was 2 or 3 weeks ago. Based on this clinical history, the arrow is identifying a:
   a. simple cyst
   b. corpus albicans
   c. parovarian cyst
   d. graafian follicle
   e. corpus luteal cyst

Using Fig. 9, answer question 29.

29. A patient presents in the early second trimester with a history of large for gestational age. A sonogram reveals a twin pregnancy. The sagittal image of the presenting twin is most suspicious for which of the following abnormalities?
   a. anencephaly
   b. nuchal edema
   c. encephaloceles
   d. prolapsed cord
   e. cystic hygroma

Using Fig. 10, answer question 30.

30. This third-trimester cross-sectional image of the fetal abdomen is suspicious for:
   a. megaureter
   b. fetal hydrops
   c. duodenal atresia
   d. meconium peritonitis
   e. multicystic dysplastic kidney

31. Which phase of the endometrium demonstrates the thinnest diameter?
   a. late secretory
   b. early secretory
   c. late menstrual
   d. early menstrual
   e. late proliferative

32. Normal embryonic herniation of the bowel permits development of the:
   a. diaphragm
   b. sexual organs
   c. thoracic cavity
   d. umbilical cord
   e. abdominal organs

33. Which classification of osteogenesis imperfecta is most lethal?
    a. Type I
    b. Type II
    c. Type III
    d. Type IV
    e. Type V

34. Which leiomyoma location is most likely to cause heavy irregular uterine bleeding?
    a. serosal
    b. intramural
    c. subserosal
    d. submucosal
    e. pedunculated

35. The landmark used to localize the correct level for measuring abdominal circumference is:
    a. kidneys
    b. stomach
    c. cord insertion
    d. adrenal glands
    e. left portal vein

36. Which portion of the fetal heart lies closest to the anterior chest wall?
    a. left atrium
    b. right atrium
    c. left ventricle
    d. right ventricle
    e. right and left atrium

37. Normal nuchal translucency does not exceed:
    a. 2 mm
    b. 3 mm
    c. 5 mm
    d. 8 mm
    e. 10 mm

38. Which obstetrical condition is an indication for immediate delivery?
    a. vasa previa
    b. placenta previa
    c. placenta accreta
    d. placental abruption
    e. incompetent cervix

39. At what gestational age are chorionic villus sampling procedures commonly performed?
    a. 5 to 7 weeks
    b. 7 to 9 weeks
    c. 10 to 12 weeks
    d. 15 to 18 weeks
    e. 18 to 20 weeks

40. Which structure would you evaluate if a patient presents with a history of a Gartner cyst?
    a. ovary
    b. cervix
    c. vagina
    d. endometrium
    e. fallopian tube

41. Brightly echogenic bowel in a second trimester is most likely associated with which abnormality?
    a. bowel atresia
    b. meconium ileus
    c. Down syndrome
    d. meconium peritonitis
    e. Pentalogy of Cantrell

42. Clinodactyly refers to:
    a. the fusion of digits
    b. the absence of digits
    c. wide-spread digits
    d. the increased number of digits
    e. the inward curvature of digits

43. In postmenopausal women, endometrial thickness is consistently benign when measuring less than:
    a. 5 mm
    b. 8 mm
    c. 10 mm
    d. 12 mm
    e. 15 mm

44. Fluid within the endometrial cavity is:
    a. a pathological finding
    b. characteristic of an endometrial polyp
    c. a consistent finding in tamoxifen effect
    d. not included in the endometrial measurement
    e. a sonographic finding in Asherman syndrome

45. The cervix-to-corpus ratio of a premenarche uterus is:
    a. 1:2
    b. 3:1
    c. 1:1
    d. 2:1
    e. 1:3

46. Enlargement of the third ventricle is a finding associated with:
    a. hydranencephaly
    b. immune fetal hydrops
    c. Dandy-Walker syndrome
    d. agenesis of the corpus callosum
    e. Beckwith-Wiedemann syndrome

47. Which segment of the fallopian tube is potentially the most life threatening in a ruptured ectopic pregnancy?
   a. isthmus
   b. ampulla
   c. fimbriae
   d. interstitial
   e. infundibulum

48. If the fluid-filled fetal stomach is not visualized on serial sonograms, the sonographer should suspect:
   a. ectopia cordis
   b. duodenal atresia
   c. esophageal atresia
   d. diaphragmatic hernia
   e. meconium peritonitis

49. The yolk sac is abnormal once the diameter exceeds:
   a. 5 mm
   b. 8 mm
   c. 10 mm
   d. 12 mm
   e. 15 mm

50. In relation to the ovaries, the external iliac vessels are located:
   a. medial
   b. lateral
   c. inferior
   d. superior
   e. posterior

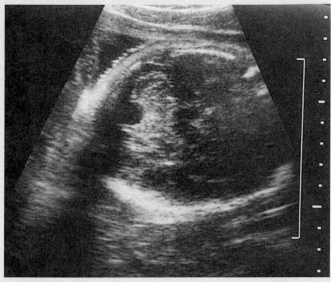

FIG. 11

___

Using Fig. 11, answer question 51.

51. This late second-trimester sonogram of the fetal cranium is most suspicious for which of the following abnormalities?
   a. arachnoid cyst
   b. hydrocephalus
   c. cystic hygroma
   d. coexisting spina bifida
   e. Dandy-Walker syndrome

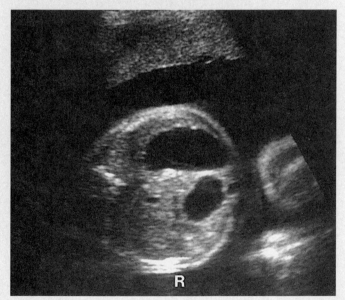

FIG. 12

___

Using Fig. 12, answer questions 52 and 53.

52. This cross-sectional abdominal image of a second-trimester fetus reveals an abnormality most suspicious for:
   a. omental cyst
   b. umbilical varix
   c. meconium ileus
   d. hydronephrosis
   e. duodenal atresia

53. Which of the following most likely coexists with this abnormality?
   a. macrosomia
   b. fetal hydrops
   c. polyhydramnios
   d. intrauterine growth restriction
   e. ureteropelvic junction obstruction

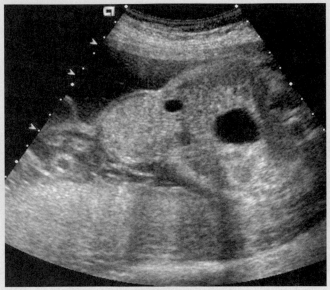

FIG. 13

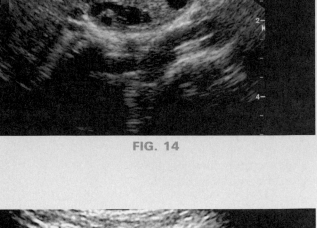

FIG. 14

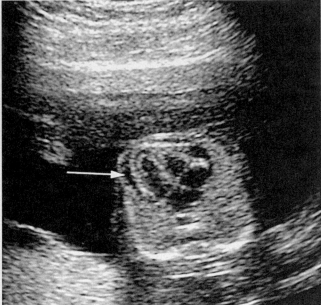

FIG. 15

Using Fig. 13, answer questions 54 and 55.

54. This image of the fetal abdomen is most likely identifying which of the following abnormalities?
   a. gastroschisis
   b. omphalocele
   c. conjoined twins
   d. umbilical hernia
   e. abdominal teratoma

55. With this finding, maternal serum alpha-fetoprotein levels are expected to demonstrate a:
   a. significant decrease
   b. significant elevation
   c. normal or slightly elevated level
   d. normal or markedly elevated level
   e. normal or minimally decreased level

Using Fig. 14, answer question 56.

56. A 30-year-old patient presents with a history of infertility. Based on this history, the sonogram of the right ovary most likely displays which of the following abnormalities?
   a. ovarian torsion
   b. theca lutein cysts
   c. dilated ovarian vessels
   d. polycystic ovarian disease
   e. ovarian hyperstimulation syndrome

Using Fig. 15, answer question 57.

57. The arrow in this cross-sectional image of the fetal chest is identifying which of the following?
   a. ectopia cordis
   b. pleural effusion
   c. pericardial effusion
   d. diaphragmatic hernia
   e. transposition of the great vessels

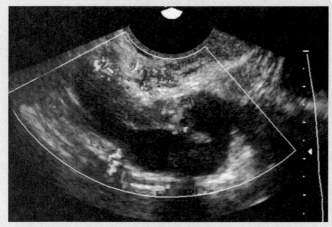

FIG. 16

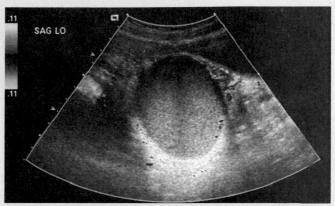

FIG. 17   Sonogram of the adnexa (see color plate 10).

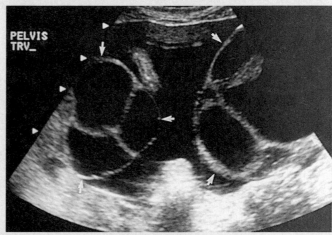

FIG. 18

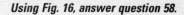

Using Fig. 16, answer question 58.

58. An asymptomatic patient presents with a previous history of pelvic infection. Her last menstrual period was 2 weeks ago. On the basis of this clinical history, the sonogram is most suspicious for:
   a. pyosalpinx
   b. hydrosalpinx
   c. ovarian torsion
   d. tubo-ovarian abscess
   e. ruptured ectopic pregnancy

Using Fig. 17 (and color plate 10), answer question 59.

59. A 30-year-old patient presents with a history of left pelvic fullness. Her last menstrual period was 5 days ago. Bilateral ovaries appear within normal limits. Based on this clinical history, this sonogram of the left adnexa is most suspicious for:
   a. endometrioma
   b. cystic teratoma
   c. ovarian carcinoma
   d. granulosa cell tumor
   e. tubo-ovarian abscess

Using Fig. 18, answer questions 60 and 61.

60. A patient undergoing ovulation induction therapy presents with a history of increased abdominal girth. This transverse sonogram of the pelvis demonstrates which of the following?
   a. heterotopic gestation
   b. bilateral hydrosalpinx
   c. bilateral cystadenomas
   d. polycystic ovarian syndrome
   e. ovarian hyperstimulation syndrome

61. With this diagnosis, the sonographer should also evaluate the:
   a. kidneys for nephrolithiasis
   b. right upper quadrant for ascites
   c. urinary bladder for obstruction
   d. right lower quadrant for appendicitis
   e. right upper quadrant for biliary obstruction

62. Ovulation usually occurs when the diameter of the dominant follicle measures:
   a. 10 mm
   b. 15 mm
   c. 18 mm
   d. 25 mm
   e. 30 mm

63. What adnexal pathology is associated with trophoblastic disease?
    a. hydrosalpinx
    b. endometriosis
    c. theca lutein cysts
    d. ovarian carcinoma
    e. tubo-ovarian abscess

64. Placenta previa is ruled out when the placental edge is located a minimum of what distance from the internal os?
    a. 1.0 cm
    b. 1.5 cm
    c. 2.0 cm
    d. 3.0 cm
    e. 4.0 cm

65. Dangling of the choroid plexus is associated with:
    a. arachnoid cyst
    b. hydranencephaly
    c. ventriculomegaly
    d. holoprosencephaly
    e. agenesis of the corpus callosum

66. A defect of the fetal lymphatic system typically results in development of a(n):
    a. facial cleft
    b. nuchal cord
    c. arachnoid cyst
    d. cystic hygroma
    e. diaphragmatic hernia

67. In a menarche patient, a multilayered appearance is present during which endometrial phase?
    a. late secretory phase
    b. late menstrual phase
    c. early menstrual phase
    d. late proliferation phase
    e. rly proliferation phase

68. Which vessel provides the best imaging landmark for locating the ovaries?
    a. internal iliac artery
    b. external iliac artery
    c. common iliac artery
    d. distal abdominal aorta
    e. common femoral artery

69. Which pelvic muscle is most frequently mistaken for the ovary?
    a. iliopsoas
    b. piriformis
    c. levator ani
    d. pubococcygeus
    e. obturator internus

70. Proliferation of the endometrium is a result of:
    a. estrogen
    b. progesterone
    c. luteinizing hormone
    d. follicle-stimulating hormone
    e. human chorionic gondadotropin

71. The most common cause for postmenopausal bleeding is:
    a. endometritis
    b. adenomyosis
    c. cervical carcinoma
    d. benign hyperplasia
    e. endometrial carcinoma

72. An extrauterine mass most commonly develops on which of the following structures?
    a. ovary
    b. psoas muscle
    c. fallopian tube
    d. large intestines
    e. broad ligament

73. A mature physiological cyst is termed a:
    a. corpus luteum
    b. graafian follicle
    c. corpus albicans
    d. theca lutein cyst
    e. cumulus oophorus

74. The levator ani muscles are at the level of the:
    a. vagina
    b. ovaries
    c. iliac vessels
    d. uterine corpus
    e. cornua of the uterus

75. Which of the following is not physiological in origin?
    a. follicular cyst
    b. nabothian cyst
    c. corpus albicans
    d. theca lutein cyst
    e. corpus lutein cyst

76. Encephaloceles are typically located in which region of the calvaria?
    a. frontal
    b. parietal
    c. temporal
    d. occipital
    e. supraorbital

77. Which of the following is most likely to mimic anencephaly?
    a. acrania
    b. encephalocele
    c. arachnoid cyst
    d. cystic hygroma
    e. holoprosencephaly

78. The most common neural tube defect is:
    a. anencephaly
    b. encephalocele
    c. caudal regression
    d. spina bifida aperta
    e. spina bifida occulta

79. Holoprosencephaly is most often associated with which of the following syndromes?
    a. Patau
    b. Down
    c. Turner
    d. Edward
    e. Noonan

80. Which of the following is the result of a cranial defect?
    a. omphalocele
    b. prosencephaly
    c. encephalocele
    d. cystic hygroma
    e. Dandy-Walker malformation

81. Maternal serum alpha-fetoprotein (MSAFP) will be elevated with all of the following EXCEPT:
    a. anencephaly
    b. encephalocele
    c. spina bifida aperta
    d. multifetal gestation
    e. trophoblastic disease

Using Fig. 19, answer question 82.

82. What anomaly is present in this axial image of the fetal chest?
    a. ectopia cordis
    b. acardiac twin
    c. pericardial effusion
    d. diaphragmatic hernia
    e. cystic adenomatoid malformation

Using Fig. 20, answer question 83.

83. The arrow in this sonogram is identifying which of the following?
    a. uterine fibroid
    b. battledore placenta
    c. trophoblastic disease
    d. succenturiate placenta
    e. myometrial contraction

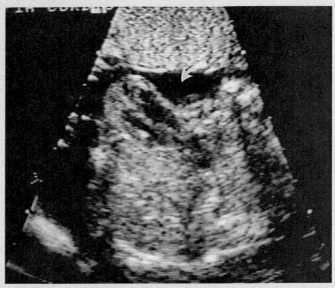

FIG. 19

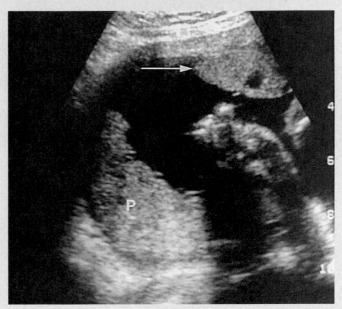

FIG. 20

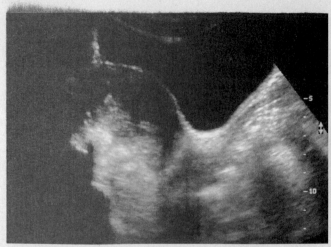

FIG. 21

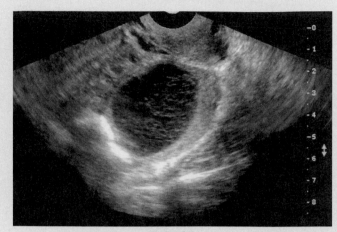

FIG. 22

BLAD W HYPO[

FIG. 23

Using Fig. 21, answer questions 84 and 85.

84. This sonogram most likely displays which of the following pathologies?
    a. adenomyosis
    b. endometriosis
    c. intramural fibroid
    d. submucosal fibroid
    e. myometrial contraction

85. Which clinical finding is most likely associated with this pathology?
    a. asymptomatic
    b. dyspareunia
    c. menorrhagia
    d. pelvic cramping
    e. uterine tenderness

Using Fig. 22, answer question 86.

86. A patient presents with a history of acute left lower quadrant pain. Her last menstrual period was approximately 3 weeks prior. Based on this clinical history, the sonogram is most suspicious for:
    a. endometrioma
    b. cystic teratoma
    c. theca lutein cyst
    d. hemorrhagic cyst
    e. ectopic pregnancy

Using Fig. 23, answer question 87.

87. This duplex image of the fetal pelvis is most suspicious for:
    a. an ovarian cyst
    b. the keyhole sign
    c. the umbilical vein
    d. hyperechoic bowel
    e. one umbilical artery

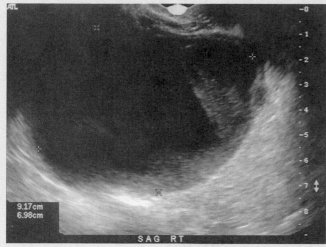

FIG. 24

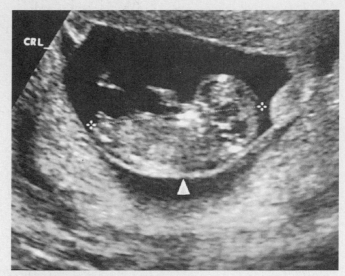

FIG. 26

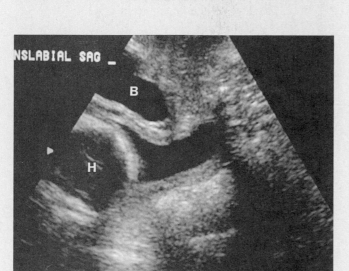

FIG. 25

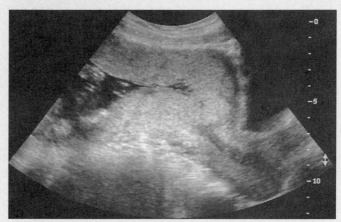

FIG. 27

Using Fig. 24, answer question 88.

88. A patient presents with a history of pelvic pain and irregular menstrual cycles. The sagittal image of the right adnexa is most suspicious for a:
    a. hematometra
    b. cystic teratoma
    c. theca lutein cyst
    d. serous cystadenoma
    e. polycystic ovarian disease

Using Fig. 25, answer question 89.

89. Which of the following abnormalities is most likely displayed in this third-trimester sonogram?
    a. urachal sinus
    b. urethral fistula
    c. prolapsed cord
    d. placenta accreta
    e. incompetent cervix

Using Fig. 26, answer question 90.

90. The arrowhead is most likely identifying a(n):
    a. normal amnion
    b. normal chorion
    c. abnormal amnion
    d. normal nuchal translucency
    e. abnormal nuchal translucency

Using Fig. 27, answer question 91.

91. An asymptomatic patient presents for a second-trimester fetal surveillance examination. This sonogram is most likely demonstrating:
    a. vasa previa
    b. placenta previa
    c. trophoblastic disease
    d. succenturiate placenta
    e. circumvallate placenta

92. Normal maximum placental thickness in a third-trimester pregnancy should not exceed:
   a. 2 cm
   b. 3 cm
   c. 4 cm
   d. 5 cm
   e. 6 cm

93. Which of the following is LEAST likely to be associated with polyhydramnios?
   a. facial cleft
   b. anencephaly
   c. duodenal atresia
   d. diaphragmatic hernia
   e. intrauterine growth restriction

94. Which accurately describes the anatomical relationship between the ureter, ovary, and iliac vessels?
   a. The ureter and iliac vessels lie anterior to the ovary.
   b. The ureter and iliac vessels lie posterior to the ovary.
   c. The ureter lies lateral and the iliac vessels lie medial to the ovary.
   d. The ureter lies posterior and the iliac vessels lie anterior to the ovary.
   e. The ureter lies anterior and the iliac vessels lie posterior to the ovary.

95. Which of the following fetal abnormalities is more commonly associated with diabetic patients?
   a. anencephaly
   b. encephalocele
   c. caudal regression
   d. spina bifida aperta
   e. spina bifida occulta

96. Which hormone is responsible for inducing ovulation during a normal menstrual cycle?
   a. estrogen
   b. progesterone
   c. alpha-fetoprotein
   d. luteinizing hormone
   e. follicle-stimulating hormone

97. A cystic hygroma is often associated with which of the following?
   a. cranial defect
   b. maternal hypertension
   c. placental insufficiency
   d. maternal diabetes mellitus
   e. chromosomal abnormality

98. Nabothian cysts are located in the:
   a. cervix
   b. vagina
   c. perineum
   d. fallopian tube
   e. broad ligament

99. Which portion of the fetal brain demonstrates ventriculomegaly first?
   a. third ventricle
   b. fourth ventricle
   c. frontal horn of the lateral ventricle
   d. occipital horn of the lateral ventricle
   e. temporal horn of the lateral ventricle

100. Which abnormality is associated with trophoblastic disease?
   a. corpus albicans
   b. cystic teratomas
   c. theca lutein cysts
   d. mucinous cystadenomas
   e. polycystic ovarian disease

101. Which of the following is unique to the luteal phase?
   a. pelvic pain
   b. increases in estrogen levels
   c. visualization of the cumulus oophorus
   d. occurs at the rupture of the mature follicle
   e. demonstrates a constant 14-day lifespan

102. A thin septation within the endometrial cavity is consistent with which congenital uterine anomaly?
   a. septae uterus
   b. arcuate uterus
   c. bicornuate uterus
   d. unicornuate uterus
   e. uterine didelphys

103. Thickness of the endometrium is dependent on:
   a. hormone levels
   b. the patient's age
   c. the dominant follicle
   d. total number of pregnancies
   e. the number of days between menses

104. A "chocolate cyst" is a term used to describe which of the following?
   a. dermoid cyst
   b. endometrioma
   c. corpus luteal cyst
   d. hemorrhagic cyst
   e. tubo-ovarian abscess

105. Diffuse uterine enlargement demonstrating diffuse myometrial anechoic areas are sonographic findings consistent with:
    a. endometritis
    b. adenomyosis
    c. endometriosis
    d. intramural fibroid
    e. Asherman syndrome

106. Transvaginally, in a sagittal plane, the urinary bladder should display on which portion of the screen?
    a. bottom
    b. left lower
    c. right lower
    d. left upper
    e. right upper

107. Which laboratory value determines when the ovary is ready to ovulate?
    a. estrogen
    b. estradiol
    c. progesterone
    d. luteinizing hormone
    e. follicle-stimulating hormone

108. A 30-year-old patient with normal menses presents for an ultrasound on the 10th day of her cycle. The endometrial stripe is expected to demonstrate:
    a. thin, hyperechoic functional and basal layers
    b. a thick, hypoechoic functional and basal layers
    c. a thick, hypoechoic functional layer and a hyperechoic basal layer
    d. a thin, hypoechoic functional layer and a thick, hyperechoic basal layer
    e. a thick, hyperechoic functional layer and a thin, hypoechoic basal layer

109. Which of the following statements is true for a postmenopausal patient not receiving hormone replacement therapy?
    a. Ovarian size remains the same.
    b. Ovarian cysts are a common finding.
    c. Endometrial thickness increases with age.
    d. Decreases in estrogen can shorten the vagina.
    e. Endometrial carcinoma is the most common cause of postmenopausal bleeding.

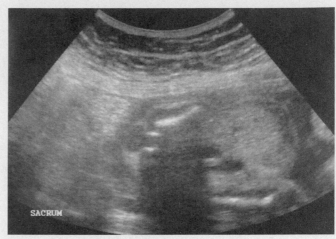

SACRUM

FIG. 28

110. Which portion of the uterus is indistinct in the nongravid state?
    a. cervix
    b. vagina
    c. corpus
    d. fundus
    e. isthmus

111. The suspensory ligament attaches the:
    a. cervix to the sacrum
    b. ovary to the pelvic sidewall
    c. fallopian tube to the uterus
    d. uterus to the pelvic sidewall
    e. ovary to the cornua of the uterus

112. An anechoic tubular adnexal mass posterior and lateral to the uterus in an asymptomatic patient is most likely the:
    a. hydrosalpinx
    b. cystadenoma
    c. endometrioma
    d. parovarian cyst
    e. tubo-ovarian abscess

Using Fig. 28, answer question 113.

113. This image of a second trimester sacrum is most likely demonstrating which of the following?
    a. spina bifida
    b. caudal regression
    c. bladders exstrophy
    d. sacrococcygeal teratoma
    e. prolapsed umbilical cord

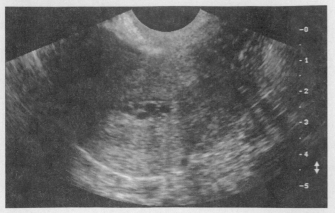

FIG. 29

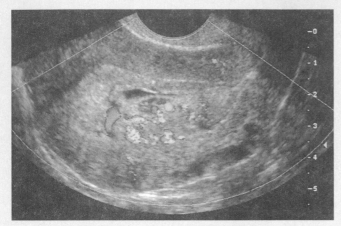

FIG. 30   (See color plate 11).

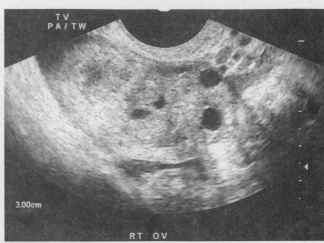

FIG. 31

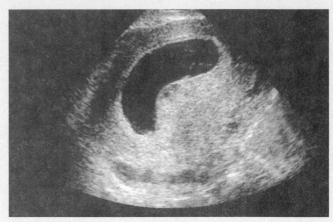

FIG. 32

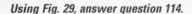

Using Fig. 29, answer question 114.

114. A patient presents with a history of breast carcinoma and tamoxifen therapy. The endovaginal image of the uterus is most suspicious for which of the following abnormalities?
a. adenomyosis
b. endometriosis
c. endometrial polyp
d. degenerating fibroid
e. endometrial hyperplasia

Using Fig. 30 (and color plate 11), answer question 115.

115. A patient presents with a history of pelvic pain and vaginal spotting since a therapeutic abortion 3 weeks prior. The transvaginal sonogram of the uterus is most suspicious for:
a. endometritis
b. trophoblastic disease
c. a pseudogestational sac
d. anembryonic pregnancy
e. a normal intrauterine pregnancy

Using Fig. 31, answer question 116.

116. A patient presents from the emergency department with a last menstrual period 5 weeks ago, a positive urine pregnancy test, and a history of vaginal spotting. This sonogram of the right adnexa is most suspicious for a(n):
a. appendicitis
b. dermoid cyst
c. endometrioma
d. ectopic pregnancy
e. hemorrhagic corpus luteum

Using Fig. 32, answer question 117.

117. A patient presents with a positive pregnancy test and an unsure last menstrual period. This sonogram of the uterus most likely reveals a(n):
a. molar pregnancy
b. ectopic pregnancy
c. pseudogestational sac
d. anembryonic pregnancy
e. amniochorionic separation

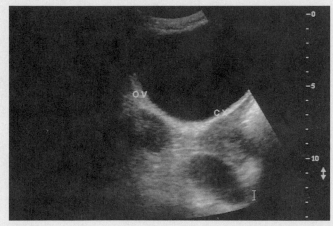

FIG. 33

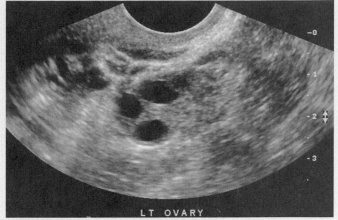

LT OVARY

FIG. 34

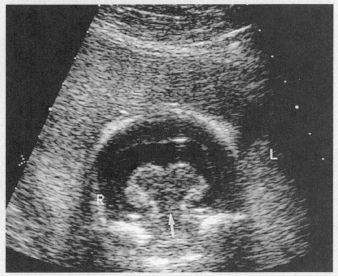

FIG. 35

Using Fig. 33, answer question 118.

118. In which of the following pelvic spaces is the mass located?
  a. space of Retzius
  b. retropubic space
  c. Morison pouch
  d. pouch of Douglas
  e. vesicouterine space

Using Fig. 34, answer question 119.

119. This image of the left ovary is displaying:
  a. theca lutein cysts
  b. corpus luteal cysts
  c. normal functional cysts
  d. ovarian hyperstimulation
  e. polycystic ovarian disease

Using Fig. 35, answer questions 120 and 121.

120. The arrow in this sonogram is identifying:
  a. single choroid plexus
  b. fused thalamic cerebri
  c. stenosis of the fourth ventricle
  d. agenesis of the cerebellar vermis
  e. compressed echogenic brain tissue

121. This abnormality is commonly associated with which of the following syndromes.
  a. Meigs
  b. Down
  c. Patau
  d. Turner
  e. Eagle-Barrett

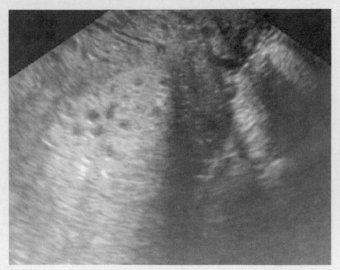

FIG. 36

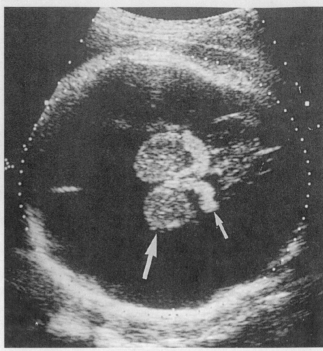

FIG. 37

Using Fig. 36, answer question 122.

122. A patient presents in the first trimester of pregnancy with a history of hyperemesis and small for dates. Based on this clinical history, the sonogram is most likely displaying a(n):
    a. molar pregnancy
    b. endometrial polyp
    c. incomplete abortion
    d. degenerating fibroid
    e. anembryonic pregnancy

Using Fig. 37, answer question 123.

123. This sonogram of a third-trimester fetus is most suspicious for which of the following abnormalities?
    a. hydranencephaly
    b. ventriculomegaly
    c. holoprosencephaly
    d. aqueductal stenosis
    e. Dandy-Walker malformation

124. A cystic teratoma is most commonly located:
    a. lateral to the cervix
    b. in the lateral adnexa
    c. inferior near the cervix
    d. lateral to the uterine isthmus
    e. superior to the uterine fundus

125. Fetuses of diabetic mothers have an increased risk of developing:
    a. macrosomia
    b. fetal hydrops
    c. nuchal edema
    d. ventriculomegaly
    e. hyperechoic bowel

126. Cases of heterotopic pregnancy occur approximately in:
    a. 1:10
    b. 1:800
    c. 1:5000
    d. 1:30,000
    e. 1:100,000

127. Which of the following syndromes is associated with an extra set of chromosomes?
    a. Patau
    b. Turner
    c. Edward
    d. triploidy
    e. Arnold-Chiari

128. Visualization of a fractured fetal femur is most suspicious for:
    a. achondroplasia
    b. achondrogenesis
    c. diastrophic dysplasia
    d. osteogenesis imperfecta
    e. thanatophoric dysplasia

129. All of the following are possible symptoms of uterine leiomyomas EXCEPT:
   a. pelvic pain
   b. menorrhagia
   c. dysmenorrhea
   d. hypomenorrhea
   e. urinary frequency

130. Second-trimester ultrasound examinations are best in determining fetal:
   a. age
   b. viability
   c. position
   d. anatomy
   e. birth weight

131. Which of the following structures allow communication between the right and left atria?
   a. mitral valve
   b. atrial septum
   c. foramen ovale
   d. ductus venosus
   e. ductus arteriosus

132. Precocious puberty may indicate the possible presence of a mass of the:
   a. liver, kidneys, or pituitary gland
   b. gonads, kidneys, or thyroid gland
   c. pituitary gland, kidneys, or gonads
   d. hypothalamus, gonads, or adrenal gland
   e. thyroid gland, pancreas, or adrenal gland

133. A unilocular thin-walled cystic structure is identified adjacent to a normal-appearing ovary. This mass is most suspicious for a(n):
   a. cystadenoma
   b. hydrosalpinx
   c. endometrioma
   d. cystic teratoma
   e. parovarian cyst

134. The most common gynecological malignancy in the United States involves the:
   a. ovary
   b. cervix
   c. vagina
   d. endometrium
   e. fallopian tube

135. A bicornuate uterus is a congenital anomaly resulting from a(n):
   a. septum between the müllerian ducts
   b. absence of the caudal müllerian ducts
   c. incomplete fusion of the müllerian ducts
   d. unilateral development of the müllerian ducts
   e. complete failure of the müllerian ducts to fuse

136. In ectopic pregnancy, serial human chorionic gonadotropin levels are expected to:
   a. increase rapidly
   b. decrease rapidly
   c. abnormally increase
   d. abnormally decrease
   e. double every 36 hours

137. Ovulation typically occurs within how many hours of visualizing a cumulus oophorus?
   a. 6
   b. 12
   c. 36
   d. 48
   e. 72

138. Which endometrial phase demonstrates the greatest dimension?
   a. early secretory
   b. late menstrual
   c. early menstrual
   d. late proliferative
   e. early proliferative

139. Fertilization of the ovum occurs in the:
   a. peritoneum
   b. endometrium
   c. uterine cornua
   d. distal fallopian tube
   e. proximal fallopian tube

140. Which of the following structures is responsible for the secretion of follicle-stimulating hormone?
   a. ovary
   b. hypothalamus
   c. thyroid gland
   d. adrenal gland
   e. pituitary gland

141. The normal endometrium of a postmenopausal patient not receiving hormone replacement therapy is expected to appear:
   a. complex
   b. multilayered
   c. thin and echogenic
   d. thick and echogenic
   e. thick and hypoechoic

142. Cystic structures located within the choroid plexus:
   a. are a precursor of ventriculomegaly
   b. are associated with skeletal dysplasia
   c. are associated with Dandy-Walker syndrome
   d. normally regress by 23 weeks' gestation
   e. are always associated with chromosomal abnormalities

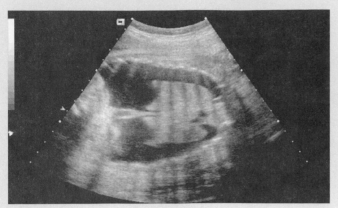

FIG. 38

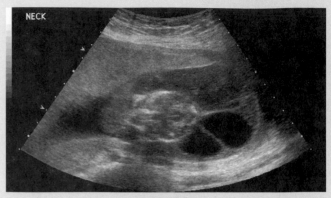

FIG. 39

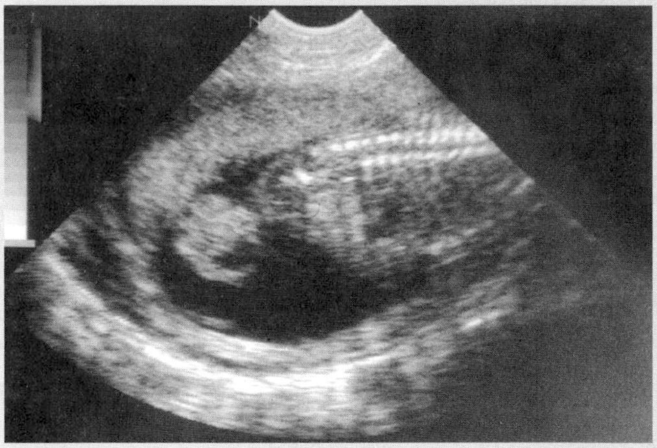

143. Which biometric parameter is most widely used to determine gestational age in the early second trimester?
- **a.** long bone length
- **b.** crown–rump length
- **c.** biparietal diameter
- **d.** head circumference
- **e.** abdominal circumference

144. Which of the following neoplasms is most likely associated with Meigs syndrome?
- **a.** fibroma
- **b.** endometrioma
- **c.** cystic teratoma
- **d.** theca lutein cysts
- **e.** polycystic ovarian disease

Using Fig. 38, answer question 145.

145. This coronal sonogram of the fetal chest is most suspicious for which of the following?
- **a.** pleural effusion
- **b.** esophageal atresia
- **c.** hypoplastic thorax
- **d.** diaphragmatic hernia
- **e.** cystic adenomatoid malformation

Using Fig. 39, answer question 146.

146. What chromosomal abnormality is most likely associated with this second-trimester fetus?
- **a.** triploidy
- **b.** trisomy 13
- **c.** trisomy 18
- **d.** Turner syndrome
- **e.** Arnold-Chiari syndrome

FIG. 40

Using Fig. 40, answer question 147.

147. This sagittal image of the lower fetal spine is most suspicious for which abnormality?
- **a.** encephalocele
- **b.** choriocarcinoma
- **c.** myelomeningocele
- **d.** succenturiate placenta
- **e.** sacrococcygeal teratoma

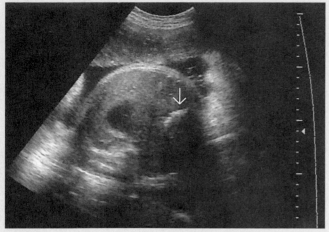

FIG. 41

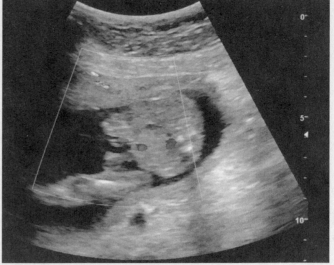

FIG. 42

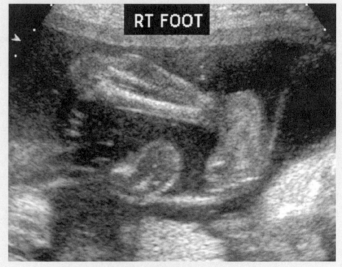

FIG. 43

Using Fig. 41, answer question 148.

148. This cross-sectional image of the fetal abdomen is most suspicious for:
   a. cholelithiasis
   b. nephrolithiasis
   c. meconium ileus
   d. duodenal atresia
   e. umbilical vein varix

Using Fig. 42, answer question 149.

149. This cross-sectional image of the umbilical insertion is most suspicious for which of the following abnormalities?
   a. gastroschisis
   b. omphalocele
   c. umbilical hernia
   d. hyperechoic bowel
   e. meconium peritonitis

Using Fig. 43, answer question 150.

150. This late second-trimester sonogram of the right foot demonstrates:
   a. a clubfoot
   b. polydactyly
   c. a normal foot
   d. a rocker bottom foot
   e. a metatarsal fracture

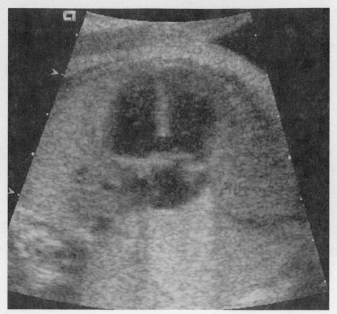

FIG. 44

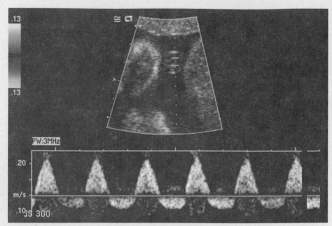

FIG. 45

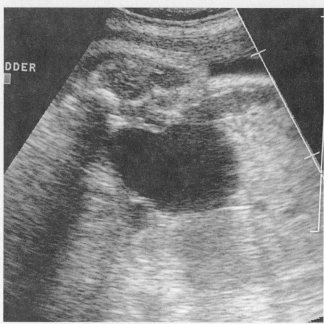

FIG. 46

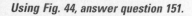

Using Fig. 44, answer question 151.

151. This four-chamber view of the fetal heart is displaying a(n):
   a. normal heart
   b. open mitral valve
   c. open foramen ovale
   d. atrioventricular defect
   e. ventriculoseptal defect

Using Fig. 45, answer question 152.

152. This spectral analysis of the umbilical artery of a 32-week fetus is demonstrating:
   a. absent diastolic flow
   b. a critical spectral waveform
   c. a normal spectral waveform
   d. a slightly abnormal spectral waveform
   e. that spectral analysis is not accurate prior to 36 weeks

Using Fig. 46, answer question 153.

153. This coronal image of the fetal bladder is most suspicious for which of the following abnormalities?
   a. ureterocele
   b. urachal cyst
   c. bladder exstrophy
   d. bladder diverticulum
   e. posterior urethral valve obstruction

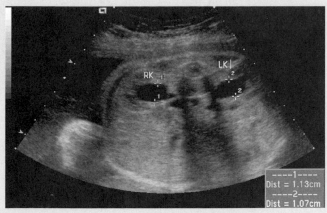

FIG. 47

Using Fig. 47, answer question 154.

154. This cross-sectional image of a third-trimester fetal abdomen is most suspicious for:
    a. prominent renal pelvis
    b. bilateral hydronephrosis
    c. bilateral adrenal hemorrhage
    d. multicystic dysplastic kidneys
    e. infantile polycystic kidney disease

155. A rapid increase in serial human chorionic gonadotropin levels is associated with:
    a. ectopic pregnancy
    b. incomplete abortion
    c. trophoblastic disease
    d. heterotopic pregnancy
    e. anembryonic pregnancy

156. Which pelvic mass is commonly displayed in a normal first-trimester pregnancy?
    a. leiomyoma
    b. cystadenoma
    c. endometrioma
    d. corpus luteal cyst
    e. theca lutein cysts

157. Which portion of the primitive brain displays as a prominent cystic structure?
    a. diencephalon
    b. telencephalon
    c. prosencephalon
    d. mesencephalon
    e. rhombencephalon

158. The maternal side of the developing placenta is termed decidua:
    a. vera
    b. basalis
    c. parietalis
    d. capsularis
    e. frondosum

159. The purpose of the cephalic index is to determine:
    a. fetal weight
    b. gestational age
    c. fetal well-being
    d. mental capacity
    e. normalcy of head shape

160. Normal fetal lung development is dependent on the:
    a. length of the umbilical cord
    b. efficiency of the placental circulation
    c. exchange of amniotic fluid within the lungs
    d. number of placental lakes and fibrin deposits
    e. ability of the fetus to move within the amniotic cavity

161. This term refers to mid-cycle or ovulatory pain:
    a. menorrhea
    b. dyspareunia
    c. dysmenorrhea
    d. mittelschmerz
    e. premenstrual syndrome

162. Which of the following is a sonographic finding associated with trisomy 21?
    a. microcephaly
    b. dolichocephaly
    c. clenched hands
    d. duodenal atresia
    e. rocker-bottom feet

163. All of the following are associated with immune fetal hydrops EXCEPT:
    a. ascites
    b. scalp edema
    c. Rh sensitivity
    d. placentomalacia
    e. pericardial effusion

164. Which of the following abnormalities is LEAST likely associated with polyhydramnios?
    a. facial cleft
    b. omphalocele
    c. duodenal atresia
    d. neural tube defect
    e. intrauterine growth restriction

165. Which of the following is caused by the presence of one defective gene?
    a. triploidy
    b. monosomy X
    c. autosomal recessive
    d. autosomal dominant
    e. Klinefelter syndrome

166. A lemon-shaped cranium is more commonly associated with:
    a. duodenal atresia
    b. ventriculomegaly
    c. myelomeningocele
    d. meconium peritonitis
    e. infantile polycystic disease

167. Visualization of the distal femoral epiphysis documents a fetus with an approximate gestational age of:
    a. 24 weeks
    b. 28 weeks
    c. 32 weeks
    d. 35 weeks
    e. 37 weeks

168. A fixed, small, hyperechoic focus within the left ventricle is most likely the:
    a. mitral valve
    b. foramen ovale
    c. ductus venosus
    d. bicuspid valve
    e. papillary muscle

169. The normal diameter of the lateral ventricle atria should not exceed:
    a. 6 mm
    b. 8 mm
    c. 10 mm
    d. 12 mm
    e. 15 mm

170. The apex of the fetal heart is normally positioned toward the:
    a. left side of the body at 25°
    b. left side of the body at 45°
    c. left side of the body at 65°
    d. right side of the body at 40°
    e. right side of the body at 65°

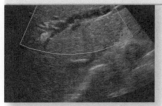

Sonography Principles and Instrumentation Answers

Chapter 1: Patient Care, Safety, and Communication

1. **c.** Transient and stable are the two types of cavitation. Stable cavitation involves microbubbles already present in the tissues. Transient cavitation involves violent expansion and collapsing of bubbles.

2. **d.** Spatial average–temporal average (SATA) has the lowest output intensity.

3. **a.** There are no confirmed significant biological effects in mammalian tissue for exposures below $1 \, W/cm^2$ for focused or $100 \, mW/cm^2$ for unfocused transducers.

4. **c.** SPPA denotes spatial peak pulse average or the peak intensity of the pulse, averaged over the pulse duration.

5. **d.** Pulse Doppler generates the highest output intensity. Continuous wave and color Doppler have slightly lower intensities compared with pulse wave.

6. **a.** Standard precautions apply to blood, all body fluids, secretions, excretions, nonintact skin, and mucous membranes.

7. **e.** Plant studies are useful for understanding cavitation effects on living tissues.

8. **b.** Transient cavitation is dependent on the ultrasound pulse. Cavitational effects from the use of contrast agents have not yet been determined.

9. **b.** Epidemiology studies various factors determining the frequency and distribution of diseases in the human community. Biological effects describe the effect of ultrasound waves on living organisms, including their composition, function, growth, origin, development, and distribution.

10. **a.** Mechanical index indicates the likelihood of cavitation occurring with diagnostic ultrasound, and thermal index relates to the heating of tissue.

11. **b.** Spatial peak–temporal average is used when researching and reporting possible biological effects of diagnostic ultrasound.

12. **b.** Clinical trials and animal testing are forms of in vivo research. In vivo refers to experimentation done in or on the living tissue as a whole. Ex vivo refers to experimentation done in or on living tissue in an artificial environment outside the organism.

13. **c.** Temporal peak is the greatest intensity during the pulse. Spatial peak is the greatest intensity across the beam.

14. **c.** Pulse average is defined as the average intensity over the duration of a pulse (pulse duration).

15. **e.** Cavitation is the interaction of the sound wave with microscopic bubbles found in tissues.

16. **b.** The Food and Drug Administration (FDA) regulates ultrasound equipment according to the application, output intensities, thermal and mechanical indexes. American College of Radiology (ACR) serves patients and society by maximizing the value of radiology. Commission on Accreditation on Allied Health Educational Programs (CAAHEP) is the largest program accreditor in the allied health science fields.

17. **c.** The AIUM recommends prudent use of ultrasound in the clinical environment. Examinations solely for sex determination are discouraged. Biological effects are dependent on the output intensity and duration of exposure.

18. **d.** Cavitation is the result of pressure changes in soft tissue causing the formation of gas bubbles. Contrast agents have a potential for cavitational changes in soft tissue from the introduction of bubbles into the tissues and circulation.

19. **b.** Absorption of the sound beam is highest in bone, especially in the fetus.

20. **c.** Thermal index in soft tissue is proportional to the operating frequency. Increasing the frequency will increase the thermal index.

21. **e.** Washing of hands before and after an examination are examples of standard precautions.

22. **a.** Watts (W) or milliWatts (mW) are the units used for power. Units of pressure are pascals (P) or megapascals (MPa).

23. **b.** The mission of the ALARA principle (as low as reasonable achievable) is to reduce biological effects in humans and the fetus by minimizing the exposure time and intensity.

24. **e.** The mechanical index is used as an indicator of the likelihood cavitation will occur. Thermal index relates to the heating of tissues.

25. **b.** Spatial peak is the greatest intensity across the sound beam.

26. **d.** Research has revealed a rapid increase in the temperature of the cranium when utilizing TCD.

27. **a.** As a form of energy, ultrasound has a small potential to produce a biological effect. Contrast agents may increase the risk of cavitation.

28. **c.** Biological studies of the cytoskeleton have shown ultrasound induced changes are nonspecific and temporary.

29. **b.** The introduction of bubbles into the tissues and circulation from

contrast agents increases the risk of cavitation.

30. **d.** The ALARA principle encourages prudent and conservative use of ultrasound exercised by minimizing exposure time and output intensity. Mechanical index is an indicator of cavitation.

31. **d.** Ex vivo refers to experimentation done on living tissue in an artificial environment outside the organisms. In vitro refers to the technique of performing a given experiment in a controlled environment outside a living organism.

32. **d.** Heat is most dependent on the SATA intensity. SPTA is used when researching and reporting biological effects of diagnostic ultrasound.

33. **a.** Pulses with peak intensity exceeding 10 MPa or 3300 W/cm² can induce cavitation in mammals.

34. **a.** Focused transducers require higher intensities to produce biological effects.

35. **a.** Stable cavitation involves microbubbles already present in tissues. Mechanical index is an indicator of cavitation.

36. **e.** There is no confirmed significant biological effects in mammalian tissue for exposures below 100 mW/cm² for unfocused OR 1 W/cm² for focused transducers.

37. **c.** Temporal average is the average intensity during the PRP. Pulse average is the average intensity over the pulse duration. The average intensity within the beam from the beginning of one pulse to the beginning of the next pulse defines SATA intensity.

38. **c.** Occupational Safety and Health Act (OSHA) are federal standards to increase occupational safety and reduce occupational injury. These standards include wearing gloves during patient contact, proper placement and handling of contaminated needles, employee safety training, and reporting of all needle sticks to OSHA to ensure proper follow-up care. OSHA requires health care facilities to offer hepatitis B vaccinations to employees, an infectious control plan, and expected work practice standards to reduce occupational injury.

39. **e.** In vitro refers to the technique of performing a given experiment

in a test tube or controlled environment outside a living organism.

40. **d.** The force exerted by the sound beam on an absorber or reflector defines radiation force. Registration accuracy is the ability to place echoes in the proper position when imaging from different orientations.

41. **b.** Pulse average is the average (common) intensity over the duration (extent) of a pulse.

42. **e.** In situ, temperatures above 41°C are dangerous to the fetus. Above 39°C, biological effects are determined by the temperature and exposure time.

43. **b.** Epidemiology studies of the bioeffects of diagnostic ultrasound have determined there are no significant biological differences between exposed and unexposed patients.

44. **a.** Cavitation is a result of pressure changes in soft tissue causing formation of gas bubbles.

45. **a.** When pressure is applied, microbubbles will expand and collapse.

46. **b.** Low acoustic output and limited exposure time are consistent with the ALARA principle of achieving information with the least amount of energy exposure to the patient.

47. **d.** Utilization of ultrasound is ONLY recommended when medically indicated.

48. **c.** The rate at which work is performed or the rate at which energy is transmitted into the body defines power.

49. **b.** Animal testing and clinical trials are examples on in vivo research. Test tube research is a form of in vitro testing.

50. **c.** The intensity of M-mode imaging is greater than the intensity of gray scale imaging.

Chapter 2: Physics Principles

1. **e.** In soft tissue propagation speed is influence by the stiffness and density of the medium. A change in frequency will not affect the propagation speed.

2. **b.** Bandwidth is the range of frequencies found within a pulse of ultrasound. Harmonics frequencies are even and odd multiples of the fundamental frequency generated as sound travels through tissues. Duty factor is the fraction of time pulse ultrasound is transmitting.

3. **a.** Sonography generally uses 2 to 3 cycles per pulse while Doppler imaging uses 5 to 30 cycles per pulse.

4. **b.** Audible frequencies range between 20 Hz and 20,000 Hz (20 kHz).

5. **c.** The stiffness and density of a medium determine the propagation speed of the sound wave. The amount of reflection and transmission occurring as a wave propagates through tissue is determined by the impedance differences between the media.

6. **d.** Acoustic variables include pressure, density, and particle motion. (distance, and temperature were previously included).

7. **b.** Spatial pulse length is equal to the number of cycles in a pulse multiplied by the wavelength. Wavelength is equal to propagation speed divided by the frequency:

$$SPL\,(mm) = \frac{2 \times 1.54\,(mm/\mu s)}{7.5\,(MHz)}$$
$$= 2 \times 0.2$$
$$= 0.4\,(mm)$$

8. **b.** Increasing the stiffness of a medium increases the propagation speed (i.e., bone). Increasing the density will decrease the propagation speed.

9. **d.** The length of a pulse from the beginning to end is termed the spatial pulse length. Wavelength is the length of a cycle. Pulse duration and pulse repetition period correlate with the time of a pulse and the time from the start of one pulse to the next, respectively.

10. **c.** Stiff structures (bone) increase the propagation speed of a sound wave.

11. **e.** Frequency is equal to propagation speed divided by wavelength:

$$f = \frac{1.54}{0.1} = 15.4\,MHz$$

12. **b.** The intensity of a sound wave is equal to the amplitude squared. If the amplitude doubles (2×) then the intensity will quadruple (2²×).

13. **c.** Pulse duration is the amount of time for one pulse to occur. Pulse repetition period is the time from the start of one pulse to the beginning of the next pulse. Duty factor defines the amount of time pulse ultrasound is transmitting.

14. **a.** Bandwidth is the range of frequencies contained in a pulse. Widening the bandwidth improves image quality (lower Q-factor) and shortens the spatial pulse length.

15. **d.** Sound waves contain regions of high pressure or density (compressions) and regions of low pressure and density (rarefactions).

16. **b.** Duty factor equals the amount of time the ultrasound transducer is emitting sound. DF = PD / PRP.

17. **d.** Resistance to the propagation of a sound wave through soft tissue describes acoustic impedance. Attenuation is a weakening of sound as it propagates through a medium.

18. **d.** It takes 13 μs round-trip for sound to travel one centimeter in soft tissue.

Round-trip time = 13 μs/cm × 5 cm = 65 μs

19. **e.** Reducing the gain setting by one-half is equal to a 3-dB reduction in amplitude.

New gain setting = 36 dB − 3 dB = 33 dB

20. **a.** Attenuation occurring with each centimeter sound travels through soft tissue defines the attenuation coefficient. Attenuation coefficient is equal to ½ operating frequency (MHz).

21. **c.** Spatial relates to space while temporal relates to time.

22. **b.** Attenuation is measured in decibels (dB). Attenuation coefficient (dB/cm) measures the attenuation occurring with each centimeter traveled. Impedance is measured in rayls while intensity is measured in mW/cm².

23. **c.** If frequency increases, period decreases, reducing the pulse duration.

24. **d.** Giga is the metric prefix designated to represent one billion.

25. **b.** The number of pulses per second defines the pulse repetition frequency (PRF) The unit of measurement for the PRF is kHz.

26. **e.** Density and propagation speed determine the impedance of a medium. Impedance is equal to the density of the medium multiplied by the propagation speed of the medium.

27. **d.** Attenuation is the weakening of a sound wave as it travels through a medium. Acoustic impedance is the resistance to sound traveling through a medium. Scattering and reflection redirect the sound wave.

28. **c.** Specular reflections occur when a sound wave strikes a smooth large surface at a perpendicular angle. Specular reflections are angle dependent, make up the boundaries of organs, and reflect sound in only one direction. Nonspecular reflections (scatter) occur when the reflector is smaller, irregular, or rough.

29. **d.** Ninety-nine percent of the incident beam transmits to the next medium with perpendicular incidence.

30. **e.** Amplitude is the maximum variation occurring in an acoustic variable. Acoustic variables include density, pressure, and particle motion. Units will vary with each acoustic variable.

31. **b.** The duty factor defines the percentage of time pulse ultrasound is transmitting. Increasing the pulse repetition frequency (PRF) will increase the duty factor because there is less "silence" between pulses. PRF is inversely proportional to the penetration depth, spatial pulse length and pulse repetition period.

32. **d.** Propagation speed depends on the stiffness and density of the medium. Increasing the density of the medium will decrease the propagation speed of a wave. Increasing the stiffness of the medium will increase propagation speed.

33. **c.** For short pulses (fewer number of cycles), the Q factor is equal to the number of cycles in a pulse. The lower the Q factor, the better the image quality.

34. **e.** The positive and negative halves of a pressure wave correspond to the compression and rarefaction of the wave, respectively.

35. **a.** Intensity reflection coefficient (IRC) is determined by the following formula:

$$IRC\,(\%) = \frac{(Z_2 - Z_1)}{(Z_2 + Z_1)}$$

$$IRC = \frac{(50 - 40)}{(50 + 40)} = (10/90)^2$$

$$IRC = (0.1)^2 = 0.01 = 1\%$$

36. **c.** Redirection or bending of the transmitting sound beam once it passes through one medium to the next describes refraction. Scattering is a redirection of the sound beam in several directions upon encountering a rough surface. Multiple reflections occurring between the transducer and a strong a reflector describes reverberation.

37. **d.** Attenuation is a result of absorption (most common), reflection, and scattering.

38. **a.** Half value layer is the depth of penetration required to reduce the intensity of the sound beam by one-half. A 3-dB reduction decreases the intensity of the sound beam by one half.

39. **c.** Homogeneous is a term used to describe a regular, uniform, and consistent echo texture. Hyperechoic texture is more commonly used to describe a dense echo pattern.

40. **c.** Impedance is proportional to the propagation speed and density of the medium. Impedance determines how much of the incident beam will reflect and how much will transmit from one medium to the next.

41. **b.** Decibel is a unit used to compare the ratio of amplitudes or intensities of two sound waves or two points along the wave path. Attenuation occurring with each centimeter of travel is measured in dB/cm.

42. **a.** Attenuation is proportional to the frequency of the sound.

43. **d.** A difference in impedance between two media determines how much of the incident beam reflects from the first medium and how much transmits into the second medium.

44. **e.** Attenuation of the sound wave is NOT a result of transmission of the sound wave. Attenuation of the sound wave is a result of absorption (heat), reflection, and scattering.

45. **c.** Attenuation is equal to the attenuation coefficient multiplied by the path length. Using this formula, we can determine the depth.

Attenuation (dB) = ½[Frequency (MHz)]
× path length (cm)

9 dB = ½[3.0] × path length

$$\frac{9}{1.5} = \text{path length}$$

6 cm = path length

46. **c.** Snell's law determines the refraction of the sound wave at an

interface. The difference in acoustic impedance between two structures and the angle of incidence determine the reflection and transmission of a sound wave.

47. **b.** Reflection angle, incidence angle, and angle of incidence are terms used to describe the direction of the incident beam with respect to the media boundary. The transmission angle depends on the propagation speeds of the media.

48. **c.** Specular reflections make up the boundaries of organs and reflect sound in only one direction. Specular reflections are angle dependent.

49. **b.** The penetration depth (half value layer) is the thickness of tissue required to reduce the intensity of the sound beam by one-half. It is equal to six divided by the frequency (MHz):

$$\text{Penetration depth (cm)} = \frac{6}{3.5} = 1.71\,\text{cm}$$

50. **c.** The greater the impedance difference between the media the greater the reflection.

Chapter 3: Ultrasound Transducers

1. **e.** The sound beam diverges (widens) in the Fraunhofer (far) zone. In the Fresnel (near) zone, the sound beam tapers as it nears the focal point.

2. **c.** Grating lobes are secondary weak sound beams emitted from a multi-element transducer. Side lobes are associated with single-element transducers.

3. **e.** The thickness and propagation speed of the active element determines the resonant (operating) frequency of a pulse wave. For continuous wave, the frequency of the sound wave is equal to the electrical frequency of the ultrasound system.

4. **d.** Heat sterilization exceeds the Curie point, resulting in the loss of piezoelectric properties of the crystal.

5. **b.** Continuous wave ultrasound does not employ pulses to transmit the sound beam. Damping reduces duration of the pulse. Two piezoelectric elements are located in one transducer assembly with continuous wave ultrasound. One element operates transmission of the sound source and the other

element receives the returning echo reflections.

6. **a.** The width of the sound beam determines lateral resolution. Spatial pulse length determines axial resolution.

7. **a.** Axial resolution in soft tissue is calculated using the following formula:

$$\text{Axial Resolution (mm)} =$$
$$\frac{0.77 \times \text{number of cycles in a pulse in soft tissue}}{\text{Frequency (MHz)}}$$

$$\text{Axial Resolution (mm)} = \frac{0.77 \times 2\,\text{cycles}}{5}$$
$$= \frac{1.54}{5}$$

$$\text{Axial Resolution} = 0.3\,\text{mm}$$

8. **e.** Operating frequency is calculated using the following formula:

$$\text{Operating frequency (MHz)} =$$
$$\frac{\text{Propagation speed of the Element (mm/µs)}}{2 \times \text{Element Thickness (mm)}}$$
$$= \frac{4}{2 \times 0.2}$$
$$= \frac{4}{0.4}$$

$$\text{Operating frequency} = 10\,\text{MHz}$$

9. **d.** Diagnostic ultrasound transducers operate on the piezoelectric effect or principle. Huygens principle states: ". . . points on a wave front are the point source for the production of secondary wavelets." Snell's law determines the amount of refraction at an interface. ALARA principle refers to using the minimal amount of energy to achieve diagnostic information.

10. **b.** The width of the sound beam at the focal point is equal to one-half of the transducer diameter.

11. **e.** Constructive interference occurs when two waves in phase with each other create a new wave with amplitude greater than the original waves. Destructive interference occurs when two waves out of phase with each other create a new wave with amplitude less than the original waves.

12. **d.** The matching layer reduces the impedance difference between the active element and the skin. Aqueous gel is not a component of the transducer assembly. Damping (backing) layer reduces the number of cycles in each pulse.

13. **a.** The sound beam is more uniform in intensity in the far field

(Fraunhofer zone). Intensity variations are greatest in the near field (Fresnel zone). Maximum intensity of the sound beam occurs at the focal point (focus).

14. **d.** The formula for calculating near zone length is:

$$\text{Near Zone Length (mm)} =$$
$$\frac{[\text{Transducer Diameter (mm)}]^2 \times \text{Frequency (MHz)}}{6}$$
$$= \frac{[6]^2 \times 5}{6}$$
$$= \frac{36 \times 5}{6}$$

$$\text{Near Zone Length} = 30\,\text{mm}$$

15. **e.** Use cleaning agents recommended by the transducer manufacturer not the infectious control department.

16. **e.** Near Zone Length =

$$\frac{(\text{Diameter})^2 \times \text{Frequency}}{6}$$
$$= \frac{(3)^2 \times 10}{6}$$
$$= \frac{90}{6}$$

$$\text{Near Zone Length} = 15\,\text{mm}$$

17. **d.** Operating frequency and the diameter of the element are directly related to the focal length (NZL). Higher frequencies and wider elements increase the near zone length. Using the formula from the previous question, the focal length of a 5-mm 10-MHz transducer is greater than a 3-mm 15-MHz transducer.

18. **c.** The distance from the transducer face to the point of spatial peak intensity (focal point) is termed the focal or near zone length.

19. **c.** The focal point (focus) is the narrowest and most intense portion of the sound beam. The focal zone is the region or area of the focus.

20. **d.** Apodization is a non-uniform driving (excitation) of the elements in an array transducer used to reduce grating lobes.

21. **c.** The diameter at the focal point is equal to one-half of the transducer diameter. Axial resolution is equal to one-half of the spatial pulse length. Thickness and propagation speed of the element determine the operating frequency of the transducer.

22. **c.** The impedance of the damping layer is similar to that of the element. The impedance of the matching

layer is between that of the element and skin.

23. **e.** Backing (damping) reduces the number of cycles in a pulse, pulse duration, and spatial pulse length. Damping increases the bandwidth and axial resolution.

24. **b.** Vector, sequenced, and phased are types of transducer operation. Linear, convex, and annular are types of transducer construction.

25. **b.** Lateral resolution varies with distance and is directly related to the diameter of the sound beam. Focusing (narrowing) the sound beam improves lateral resolution. Axial resolution does not vary with depth and is directly related to the operating frequency.

26. **e.** The ultrasound system alters the electronic excitation of the elements, steering the beam in various directions. Delays in the reflected echoes also occur.

27. **e.** Exceeding the Curie point of a transducer element will result in a loss of all piezoelectric properties (i.e., heat sterilization).

28. **a.** Calculate operating frequency by using the following formula:

Operating frequency (MHz) =

$$\frac{\text{Propagation Speed of the Element (mm/μs)}}{2 \times \text{Element Thickness (mm)}}$$

$$= \frac{4}{2 \times 0.8} = \frac{4}{1.6}$$

Operating frequency = 2.5 MHz

29. **d.** Using the formula from the previous question:

$$5\,\text{MHz} = \frac{4}{2\times}10\times = 4$$

Thickness = 0.4 mm

30. **b.** Temporal resolution is the ability to separate two points in time, and is determined by the frame rate. Beam width determines lateral resolution. Operating frequency relates to axial resolution.

31. **a.** Axial resolution in soft tissue is calculated using the following formula:

Axial resolution (mm) =

$$\frac{0.77 \times \text{number of cycles in a pulse}}{\text{Frequency (MHz)}}$$

$$= \frac{0.77 \times 2}{5}$$

$$= \frac{1.54}{5}$$

Axial resolution = 1 mm

32. **e.** A linear sequenced array transducer applies voltage pulses to groups of linear elements in succession. Phased array transducers operate by applying voltage pulses to most or all of the elements using minor time differences.

33. **d.** Focusing of the sound beam is only accomplished within the near field.

34. **a.** At one near zone length (focal point) the diameter of the sound beam is one-half of the original transducer diameter.

35. **e.** Azimuthal (lateral) resolution is the ability to distinguish two structures in a path perpendicular to the sound beam.

36. **e.** Lead zirconate titanate (PZT) is the most common piezoelectric element used in ultrasound transducers.

37. **a.** Sub-dicing reduces grating lobes by dividing the elements into smaller pieces.

38. **c.** Diagnostic frequencies presently range between 2.0 and 15.0 MHz.

39. **a.** Detail resolution includes both axial (spatial) and lateral resolution.

40. **d.** Diagnostic ultrasound transducers convert electrical energy into acoustic energy during transmission and acoustic energy into electrical energy for reception.

41. **e.** The piezoelectric principle states that some materials produce a voltage when deformed by an applied pressure. Ohm's acoustic law states, "Musical sound is perceived by the ear as the sum of the number of cycles of pure harmonic tones."

42. **b.** Damping reduces the sensitivity of the pulse while increasing the bandwidth and axial resolution. A low quality factor is a good thing.

43. **c.** Doppler imaging utilizes 5 to 30 cycles per pulse while real-time imaging generally uses 2 to 3 cycles per pulse.

44. **c.** Electronic focusing allows the operator to determine the depth and number of focal zones. Internal focus, external focus, and acoustic mirrors are predetermined and out of the operator's control.

45. **d.** The impedance of the matching layer is less than that of the crystal and greater than the impedance of the skin.

46. **b.** Vector array transducers convert the format of a linear array into a trapezoidal image. Vector array transducers combine linear sequential and linear phase array technologies.

47. **c.** The ability to differential similar or dissimilar tissues describes contrast resolution. Contrast resolution is directly related to both axial and lateral resolution (detail resolution).

48. **b.** Section thickness (z-axis) is related to the width of the beam and determined by the transducer.

49. **e.** Operating frequency is directly related to the propagation speed of the element and inversely related to the element thickness.

50. **c.** In a focused transducer, the diameter at the focus is equal to one-half of the diameter of the transducer.

Chapter 4: Pulse-Echo Instrumentation

1. **d.** Real-time imaging is a two-dimensional display demonstrating motion of moving structures. Static imaging does not demonstrate motion. M-mode is a one-dimensional display. Temporal resolution is the ability to precisely position a moving structure.

2. **b.** The vertical or y-axis represents the penetration depth in a B-mode display. The horizontal or x-axis represents the medial and lateral or right and left aspect of the body.

3. **a.** The number of images (frames) per second is termed the frame rate. The pulse repetition frequency determines the number of scan lines per frame.

4. **d.** Increasing or decreasing the imaging depth will change the frame rate. The sonographer can also modify the frame rate by adjusting the number of focal zones.

5. **c.** Line density is the number of scan lines in a single image (frame). Frame rate is the number of images (frames) per second. Pulse repetition frequency determines the number of scan lines per frame.

6. **c.** A-mode (amplitude mode) demonstrates the strength of the echo along the vertical (y) axis. Depth of penetration is displayed on the y-axis in B-mode imaging.

7. **e.** Frame rate is determined by the propagation speed of the medium and penetration depth. Frame rate determines temporal resolution.

8. **a.** Frame rate and temporal resolution are inversely related to the line density. Increasing the line density will decrease the frame rate and temporal resolution. Line density is directly related to the pulse repetition frequency and spatial resolution.

9. **a.** Propagation speed of the medium limits the penetration depth. Harmonic frequencies are determined by the fundamental (operating) frequency. Temporal resolution is determined by the frame rate.

10. **a.** Maximum penetration depth is calculated using the following formula:

Maximum Penetration Depth (cm)

$$= \frac{77}{PRF\ (kHz)}$$

$$= \frac{77}{10} = 7.7\ cm$$

11. **c.** The maximum number of lines per frame is determined using the following formula:

Depth (cm) × Number of focal zones × Lines per frame × Frame rate ≤ 77,000

10×2 focal zones × ? × 30 × frames/sec ≤ 77,000

$600 \times ? \leq 77,000$

Maximum lines per frame

$$= \frac{77,000}{600} = 128$$

12. **a.** Line density is directly related to the pulse repetition frequency (PRF). Imaging depth and operating frequency are inversely related to the PRF.

13. **b.** Signal-to-noise ratio is proportional the output of the ultrasound machine. Increasing the output by 3 dB will increase signal-to-noise ratio and double the acoustic intensity.

14. **d.** The T/R switch protects the receiver components from the large driving voltage of the pulse. The transducer delivers electrical voltages to the memory. The pulser adjusts the PRF with changing imaging depth. Focusing controls the width of the sound beam.

15. **c.** Ultrasound systems employ an output range up to 500 volts.

16. **b.** Suppression is a function of the receiver that eliminates selective low-level echoes. Pulse delays control beam steering and focusing, aperture, and apodization in phased array operation.

17. **e.** Time gain or depth gain compensation offset for attenuation by boosting the amplitudes of deep reflections and suppressing superficial reflections.

18. **c.** The transducer receives returning echo reflections producing an electrical voltage and delivers this voltage to the memory. Memory stores the echo amplitudes and locations of the reflectors.

19. **e.** The knee of the time gain compensation curve is the deepest region attenuation compensation can occur. The area of maximum amplification describes the far zone.

20. **a.** When imaging depth is changed, the pulser will readjust the pulse repetition frequency.

21. **d.** The T/R switch is part of the beam former. It directs the driving voltage from the pulser to the transducer and the returning echo voltage from the transducer to the receiver.

22. **e.** An independent pulse delay and element combination constitutes a transmission channel. Each independent element, amplifier, analog-to-digital converter, and delay path constitutes a reception channel.

23. **d.** Demodulation modifies the shape of the returning signal to a form the system components can process. There are no visible changes in the image with demodulation.

24. **b.** Threshold selectively suppresses or eliminates low-level echoes decreasing acoustic noise. Smoothing levels out the rough edges of the signal.

25. **b.** Code excitation employs a series of pulses and gaps allowing for multiple focal zones and harmonic frequencies. Controlling the characteristics of the sound beam is directly related to the number of channels employed.

26. **a.** Cine loop is a post-processing feature that stores the last several frames of a real-time imaging display. 3-D acquisition is a preprocess-

ing attribute while 3-D presentation is a post-processing function.

27. **c.** Binary number 0110010 is equal to 0 + 32 + 16 + 0 + 0 + 2 + 0 = 50.

28. **d.** A 6-bit memory is equal to 2 to the 6th power = $2 \times 2 \times 2 \times 2 \times 2 \times 2$ = 64.

29. **c.** A pixel is the smallest picture element in a digital image.

30. **c.** Television monitors display 30 images (frames) per second. Rates of 20 frames per second or less demonstrate flickering.

31. **c.** Old data of single emulsion x-ray files are purged from the system. Data stored in picture archiving and communication systems do not deteriorate over time and allows for storage of old data files. PACS electronically communicates images and associated information to workstations external to the ultrasound system using a local area network (LAN).

32. **b.** Read zoom is a post-processing feature that displays only the original data. The number of pixels or scan lines is the same as the original image.

33. **c.** Flickering occurs with frame rates below 20 frames per second. A CRT presents images at a rate of 30 frames per second or 60 fields per second.

34. **b.** Increasing or decreasing the pixel density has a direct relationship to the spatial resolution of the image. The number of gray shades relates to the number of memory bits.

35. **a.** Storage of the last several real-time frames describes a post-processing feature, cine-loop. Freeze frame displays a single real-time frame.

36. **e.** This is the best answer. Matrix denotes the rows and columns of pixels in a digital image. The number of picture elements in a digital image describes pixel density.

37. **b.** Color presents different echo intensities in various color shades improving contrast resolution. Rejection suppresses weak intensities without affecting the intense amplitudes. Persistence reduces noise and smoothes the image.

38. **d.** Write zoom rescans only the area of interest increasing the number of pixels or scan lines in the image.

39. **e.** Improper location of a true reflector is displayed with range ambiguity, propagation speed error, refraction, grating lobes, side lobes, and multipath artifacts. Reverberation, comet tail, and mirror image artifacts display additional false reflectors. Focal banding demonstrates improper brightness in the focal zone(s).

40. **c.** Doppler gain set too high will most likely demonstrate a mirror image artifact. Acoustic speckle is a gray scale interference artifact. Aliasing relates to a pulse repetition frequency set too low. Range ambiguity relates to a pulse repetition frequency set too high.

41. **e.** A pulse repetition frequency set too high results in range ambiguity. Decreasing the PRF will decrease the likelihood of range ambiguity.

42. **c.** The ultrasound system assumes sound travels directly to and from a reflector. Other assumptions include: sound travels in a straight line and at a constant speed in soft tissue, echoes only originate from the central sound beam, intensity of the echo corresponds to the strength of a reflector, the imaging plane is thin, and distance to the reflector is proportional to the time it takes an echo to return.

43. **c.** Shadowing is a reduction (weakening) of echoes distal to a strongly attenuating or reflecting structure. Enhancement describes an increase in echo amplitude distal to a weakly attenuating structure.

44. **b.** Errors in propagation speed will display reflectors at an improper depth.

45. **c.** Enhancement of displayed reflectors occurs posterior to a weakly attenuating structure, resulting in false brightness to distal reflections.

46. **c.** A change in direction of the sound beam is more commonly a result of the sound wave striking a boundary at an oblique angle. Resonance phenomenon is associated with ring-down artifact.

47. **d.** Grating lobes are a result of the spacing between the active elements of an array transducer. They produce minor secondary sound beams that travel in directions different than the primary central beam.

48. **d.** Distance to a reflector is proportional to the time it takes for an echo to return. The ultrasound machine assumes the propagation speed of the medium is a constant 1.54 mm/μs.

49. **c.** Imaging a surgical clip will most likely demonstrate a comet tail reverberation artifact. A surgical clip may cause acoustic speckle.

50. **c.** Shadowing and enhancement are useful artifacts caused by a strong or weakly attenuating structure, respectively.

Chapter 5: Doppler Instrumentaion and Hemodynamics

1. **e.** Red blood cells (erythrocytes) are the major cellular component of blood. The concentration of RBC may directly affect the intensity of the Doppler shift.

2. **a.** Bruits are auscultory consequences or products of turbulent blood flow. Turbulent or disturbed flow is a consequence of arterial narrowing.

3. **e.** Hemodynamics is the science or physical principles concerned with the study of blood circulation. A fluid system produces hydrostatic pressure.

4. **a.** Plug flow, found in large arteries like the aorta, display a constant flow velocity across the entire vessel.

5. **c.** Microcirculation consists of the arterioles, capillaries, and venules.

6. **d.** Capillaries are the smallest portion of the circulatory system, receiving blood from the arterioles and allowing the exchange of vital nutrients with the tissue cells.

7. **e.** Decreasing the depth to the sample volume increases the pulse repetition frequency, allowing for a larger display of Doppler shifts. Increasing the pulse repetition period decreases the pulse repetition frequency. Increasing the operating frequency increases sensitivity of low flow velocities.

8. **c.** A positive Doppler shift occurs when the received frequency is greater than the transmitted frequency. A positive Doppler shift displays above the baseline.

9. **c.** Increasing the operating frequency increases system's sensitivity of the Doppler shifts. Increasing the Doppler angle decreases the Doppler shift and can bring it down below the Nyquist limit.

10. **a.** Doppler shifts do not occur when the received and transmitted frequencies are equal.

11. **d.** The ability to measure high velocities is a major advantage of CW Doppler. Aliasing is not an issue with continuous wave Doppler. Interrogation of multiple vessels simultaneously is a disadvantage. Placement of the sample volume is an advantage of duplex imaging.

12. **e.** The Doppler equation determines the Doppler shift (change in the transmitted and reflected frequencies). Poiseuille's equation determines the volume flow rate.

13. **e.** A Reynolds number greater than 2000 consistently predicts the onset of turbulent flow.

14. **c.** A difference in pressure is necessary for flow to occur. The circulatory system creates hydrostatic pressure.

15. **c.** Blood flow velocity is dependent on left ventricular output, resistance of the arterioles, vessel course, and cross-sectional area.

16. **b.** Venous pressure is lowest when the patient is lying flat (supine or prone). Venous pressure is the highest when the patient is standing.

17. **c.** The greatest portion of circulating blood is located in the venous system. Veins accommodate larger changes in blood volume with little change in pressure.

18. **e.** Parabolic flow is a type of laminar flow where the average flow velocity is equal to one-half the maximum flow speed in the center. Laminar flow demonstrates a maximum flow velocity in the center of the artery and minimum flow velocity near the arterial wall.

19. **a.** Phasic flow describes the normal respiratory variations in venous blood flow. Bi-directional or pulsatile flow is a normal finding in the hepatic veins and proximal inferior vena cava. Unprompted venous flow is termed spontaneous.

20. **a.** Duplex imaging requires a decrease in the imaging frame rate to allow for interlaced acquisition of the Doppler information. Duplex imaging can utilize high operating frequencies.

21. **b.** Clutter is noise within the Doppler signal that is generally a result of high amplitude Doppler shifts. Flash is an extension of color Doppler outside of the vessel wall caused by motion.

22. **c.** Pressure is the driving force of blood flow. Velocity is the speed at which RBCs travel in a vessel. Volume flow rate is the quantity of blood moving through a vessel per unit of time.

23. **d.** Observed frequency changes of moving structures most accurately defines Doppler EFFECT. Doppler shift is the actual change in frequency equal to the reflected intensity minus the transmitted frequency.

24. **e.** The Nyquist limit is equal to one-half of the pulse repetition frequency.

25. **a.** Hue color Doppler maps use any one or combination of primary colors to display the presence of blood flow, blood flow direction, and mean flow velocity. Saturation dilutes colors with various amounts of white.

26. **d.** Thickening of the spectral trace is a result of an increase in the range of Doppler shift frequencies.

27. **d.** Spectral broadening describes a vertical thickening of the spectral trace caused by an increase in the range of Doppler shift frequencies. Clutter is a result of high amplitude Doppler shifts.

28. **d.** The receiver gate length, beam diameter, and length of the ultrasound pulse determine the size of the sample volume (gate).

29. **d.** Spectral analysis utilizes a fast Fourier transfer (FFT) to convert Doppler shift information into a visual spectral display. Autocorrelation is necessary for color flow Doppler.

30. **d.** Packet describes the multiple samples gates positioned in the area of interest in color Doppler imaging. Pixels are the smallest elements of a digital image.

31. **d.** Variance mode calculates the average velocities, placing the colors side-to-side. Velocity mode calculates the average velocities from each color gate, placing the colors up and down.

32. **d.** Blood flows from the higher pressure to the lower pressure. A difference in pressure is required for flow to occur.

33. **e.** Increasing operating frequency will increase the sensitivity to low Doppler shifts. Decreasing operating frequency may overcome aliasing.

34. **a.** Angle correction is not a quandary with spectral ratios. The ability to obtain different information involving blood flow and vascular impedance are not obtained by absolute velocity information alone.

35. **e.** The pressure gradient is proportional to the flow rate (volume of blood flow).

36. **e.** Resistance to blood flow is proportional to the length of the vessel and inversely proportional to the blood flow volume.

37. **d.** During inspiration, abdominal pressure increases and thoracic pressure decreases.

38. **e.** Continuous wave is the simplest form of Doppler.

39. **e.** The vertical axis of a spectral analysis represents the frequency shift or velocity. The horizontal axis represents time.

40. **c.** Velocity is defined as the rate of motion with respect to time. Acceleration is an increase in velocity.

41. **e.** Poiseuille's equation predicts flow volume in a cylindrical vessel. Reynolds number predicts the onset of turbulent flow.

42. **e.** Pulse wave Doppler utilizes a minimum of 5 cycles per pulse and a maximum of 30 cycles per pulse.

43. **d.** Autocorrelation is necessary for rapid obtainment of color Doppler frequency shifts. Fast Fourier transfer converts Doppler shift information into a visual spectral display.

44. **e.** Continuous wave Doppler transmits sound nonstop.

45. **a.** Color Doppler is commonly used to demonstrate nonvascular motion (e.g., ureteral jets).

46. **d.** Power Doppler displays the amplitude or z-axis of the signal. Spectral analysis displays the frequency shift (velocity).

47. **e.** Power Doppler demonstrates an increase in sensitivity to Doppler shifts but is unable to demonstrate flow direction.

48. **c.** Increasing the Doppler angle is a method of overcoming aliasing. Changing the Doppler angle may overcome a mirror image.

49. **b.** Smaller arteries commonly display laminar flow while larger arteries display plug flow.

50. **b.** Increasing the packet size of the color Doppler will decrease the frame rate and temporal resolution. Sensitivity and accuracy are increased.

Chapter 6: Quality Assurance, Quality Control of Equipment

1. **a.** The number of correct test results divided by the total number of tests determines test accuracy. Registration accuracy is the ability to place echoes in proper location when imaging from different orientations.

2. **c.** Specificity is the number of correct negative test results divided by the total number of negative tests. Sensitivity is equal to the number of positive test results divided by the total number of positive tests.

3. **b.** A hydrophone measures acoustic output. A beam profiler measures transducer characteristics. A string phantom is useful for testing characteristics of the Doppler beam.

4. **d.** The most accurate definition of quality assurance. QA is the routine, periodic evaluation of the ultrasound system including transducers.

5. **e.** The beam profiler is a testing device that measures transducer characteristics. A hydrophone measures acoustic output.

6. **c.** Preventive maintenance service is generally scheduled 2 to 3 times per year. It includes internal cleaning and overall evaluation of the ultrasound system.

7. **e.** Registration accuracy is the ability to place echoes in proper position when imaging from different acoustic windows. Accuracy in this chapter pertains to the number of correct test results divided by the total number of tests.

8. **d.** Routine periodic assessment of the ultrasound system is a part of a quality assurance (QA) program. QA ensures image quality and consistency. A periodic internal cleaning and overall evaluation of the ultrasound system describes preventive maintenance service.

9. a. Phantom is the most common term used to illustrate a tissue-equivalent device.

10. e. After each patient, transducers utilized during the examination should be cleaned and disinfected. Cleaning of the keyboard after each patient is encouraged.

11. b. The AIUM 100 test object cannot evaluate compression (dynamic range), gray-scale, or penetration. The test object provides measurement of system performance evaluates dead zone, axial and lateral resolution, vertical, and horizontal calibration, and compensation.

12. c. Record keeping for each ultrasound unit is necessary for hospital and outpatient clinic accreditation. Record keeping aids in detection of gradual or sporadic changes in the system, and scheduling the next preventive maintenance service.

13. e. Accuracy of an examination is equal to the number of correct test results divided by the total number of tests. If 10 tests are misdiagnosed, then 90 tests received the correct diagnosis.

$$Accuracy = \frac{90}{100} \times 100 = 90\%$$

14. c. The number of correct positive test results divided by the total number of tests calculates the positive predictive value.

15. b. AIUM test object evaluates system sensitivity. Contrast resolution, gray scale characteristics, direction of blood flow and sample volume location are evaluated by tissue and Doppler phantoms.

16. a. A hydrophone uses a small transducer element mounted on the end of a hollow needle or a large piezoelectric membrane with small electrodes on each side.

17. a. Quality assurance programs provide assessment of image quality and consistency.

18. e. A tissue-equivalent phantom is utilized in many quality assurance programs.

19. c. A force-balance system measures the power or intensity of the sound beam.

20. d. The hydrophone measures acoustic output, period, pulse repetition period, and pulse duration.

21. c. Test sensitivity is calculated by dividing the number of correct positive test results by the total number of positive tests. Positive predictive value divides the number of correct positive test results by the total number of tests.

22. b. The beam profiler is a testing device that plots 3-D reflection amplitudes received by the transducer.

23. d. The AIUM 100 test object, tissue-equivalent, and Doppler phantoms evaluate the operation of the ultrasound system. Beam former, hydrophone, and force-balance system evaluate the acoustic output of the ultrasound system.

24. c. Acoustic output testing evaluates the safety and biological effects of ultrasound and Doppler imaging.

25. a. Negative predictive value is the ability of a diagnostic test to predict normal findings. Identifying the true absence of disease defines specificity.

26. b. The output of the hydrophone indicates the pressure or intensity of the sound beam. A testing device measures acoustic output. Acoustic exposure is dependent on the acoustic output and exposure time.

27. e. Periodic internal cleaning and overall evaluation of the ultrasound system function describes preventive maintenance service (PMS). Quality assurance is a routine monthly assessment of the ultrasound system and transducers.

28. a. The hydrophone evaluates the relationship between the acoustic pressure and the voltage produced. Hydrophones measure the acoustic output, period, pulse repetition period, and pulse duration of an acoustic wave.

29. e. Assessment of the transducers, cables, and connections is a routine responsibility of all sonographers.

30. c. Doppler phantoms can evaluate flow direction. Tissue mimicking phantom can evaluates penetration, compression, lateral resolution, and system sensitivity.

31. c. Acoustic output testing requires specialized equipment and considers only the pulser and transducer.

32. c. The width of the sound beam determines lateral resolution.

33. b. Quality assurance programs ensure diagnostic image quality and consistency from routine assessment of the ultrasound system. Developing a quality assurance program does not ensure lab accreditation.

34. a. Positive predictive value is equal to the number of correct positive tests (20) divided by the total number of tests (100).

$$Positive\ Predictive\ Value = \frac{20}{100}$$
$$= 0.2 = 20\%$$

35. c. Test sensitivity is equal to the number of correct positive test results (20) divided by the total number of positive tests (25).

$$Sensitivity = \frac{20}{25} = 0.8 = 80\%$$

36. d. Overall test accuracy is equal to the number of correct test results (95) divided by the total number of tests (100).

$$Accuracy = \frac{95}{100} = 0.95 = 95\%$$

37. b. Negative predictive value is equal to the number of correct negative tests (75) divided by the total number of tests (100).

$$Negative\ Predictive\ Value = \frac{75}{100}$$
$$= 0.75 = 75\%$$

38. b. Fan filters should be cleaned and evaluated by the sonographer weekly or bi-weekly.

39. a. Dead zone is the region closest to the transducer face in which imaging cannot be performed.

40. b. Test sensitivity is defined as the ability of a diagnostic technique to identify the presence of disease when disease is actually present.

41. a. A large piezoelectric membrane with small metallic electrodes centered on each side is a type of hydrophone.

42. c. Blood mimicking Doppler phantoms simulate clinical conditions.

43. b. The ability of a diagnostic technique to identify the absence of disease when no disease is present is termed specificity. Registration accuracy is the ability to place echoes in proper position when imaging from different orientations.

44. e. Biomedical engineers employed by a private company or system manufacturer perform preventive maintenance on each ultrasound system approximately twice a year.

45. **d.** Accuracy is the quality of being near to the true value. It is equal to the number of correct test results divided by the total number of tests.

46. **c.** Tissue mimicking phantoms cannot evaluate blood flow.

47. **b.** The beam profiler plots 3-D reflection amplitudes received by the transducer to evaluate the characteristics of the transducer.

48. **d.** Moving string Doppler phantom scatters the sound beam and can produce pulsatile and retrograde flow.

49. **a.** The hydrophone evaluates the relationship between the amount of acoustic pressure and the voltage produced.

50. **d.** Accuracy is equal to the number of correct test results divided by the total number of tests.

$$\text{Accuracy} = \frac{18}{20} = 0.9 = 90\%$$

Sonography Principles and Instrumentation Mock Exam

1. **d.** Prudent utilization of sonographic imaging (as low as reasonably achievable) is the mission of the ALARA principle.

2. **b.** Spatial pulse length is proportional to the number of cycles in a pulse and the wavelength. Operating frequency is proportional to the thickness of the crystal. Pulse repetition frequency is proportional to the duty factor.

3. **d.** The Doppler shift frequency is proportional to the velocity of the reflector and dependent on the Doppler angle and transducer frequency.

4. **a.** The beam width diverges in the Fraunhofer (far) zone and the intensity becomes more uniform.

5. **c.** Reverberation artifact displays as equally spaced reflections of diminishing amplitude with increasing depth. Grating lobes are the result of regular element spacing in an array transducer.

6. **d.** Enhancement describes the increase in reflection amplitude from structures beneath a weakly attenuating structure. Shadowing occurs beneath a strongly attenuating structure.

7. **d.** Dynamic range (compression) describes the ratio of the largest power to the smallest power the ultrasound system can handle. Bandwidth is the range of frequencies found in pulse ultrasound. Amplitude refers to the strength of a reflector.

8. **e.** Axial resolution is directly related to the operating frequency and inversely related to the spatial pulse length and penetration depth.

9. **e.** The crystal will increase or decrease according to the polarity of the applied voltage.

10. **d.** The resistance of the arterioles accounts for about one-half of the total resistance in the systemic system.

11. **d.** Rayleigh scattering occurs when the sound wave encounters a reflector much smaller than the wavelength of the sound beam.

12. **d.** The color black always represents the baseline in color Doppler imaging.

13. **c.** Frequency is equal to the number of complete cycles in a wave occurring in one second. Pulse repetition frequency is the number of pulses occurring in 1 second.

14. **e.** Scan converters make grayscale imaging possible and is not part of an A-mode system.

15. **e.** Grating lobes are additional weak beams caused by the regular periodic space of the elements in array transducers.

16. **a.** Clutter is noise in the Doppler signal caused by high amplitude Doppler shifts. Increasing the wall filter can reduce clutter in the Doppler signal.

17. **e.** Compressions are regions of high pressure or density in a compression wave.

18. **e.** Compression is measured in decibels. Units for amplitude vary with the acoustic variable.

19. **d.** Impedance determines how much of sound wave will transmit to the next medium or reflect back towards the transducer. Impedance is the product of the density and propagation speed of the medium.

20. **b.** Focusing of the sound beam improves lateral resolution and creates a tapering of the near field (Fresnel zone). The focal point exhibits the maximum intensity of the sound beam.

21. **d.** Increasing the diameter of the transducer will increase the near zone length and decrease the divergence of the sound beam in the far field.

22. **e.** Freeze frame holds and displays a single image of sonographic information. Cine loop stores the last several frames of information.

23. **b.** Binary number 0010011 = 0 + 0 + 16 + 0 + 0 + 2 + 1 = 19.

24. **e.** The thickness of the matching layer is equal to one-quarter of the wavelength of the transducer.

25. **e.** Increasing the operating frequency improves both axial and lateral resolution. Decreasing the beam width improves lateral resolution. Increasing the frame will improve temporal resolution.

26. **a.** Vector array transducers convert the format of a linear transducer in to a trapezoidal image.

27. **d.** Heat sterilization of ultrasound transducers will raise the temperature of the element above the Curie point, losing its piezoelectric properties.

28. **d.** Huygens' Principle explains how all points on a wave front are point sources for the production of circular secondary wavelets. Snell's law relates to amount of refraction at an interface.

29. **c.** The Fresnel or near zone is the region between the transducer and focal point.

30. **e.** Volumetric flow rate must remain constant because blood is neither created or destroyed as it flows through a vessel (continuity rule).

31. **b.** The greater the impedance difference between two structures the greater the reflection.

32. **a.** The greatest Doppler shift occurs parallel with the blood flow at a 0° angle.

33. **d.** Increasing transducer frequency, increases image quality, sensitivity to Doppler shifts and attenuation of the sound beam.

34. **d.** Shorter pulse lengths, increasing the operating frequency, and decreasing the beam width will improve image quality.

35. **b.** Damping material reduces the number of cycles in each pulse,

pulse duration, spatial pulse length, and sensitivity. Matching layer diminishes the reflections near the transducer face and improves sound transmission into the body.

36. **a.** The pulser generates the electric pulses to the crystal producing pulsed ultrasound waves. The master synchronizer instructs the pulser to send a pulse to the transducer.

37. **c.** The beam former is a part of the pulser and determines the firing delays for array systems.

38. **c.** Stiffness and density of the medium determines the propagation speed of a tissue or structure.

39. **a.** Shifting the baseline may eliminate aliasing. Other methods include increasing the Doppler angle or pulse repetition frequency and decrease imaging depth or transducer frequency.

40. **d.** Focal banding is a product of horizontal enhancement or increase in intensity at the focal zone.

41. **a.** Duplex imaging permits switching between imaging and Doppler functions several times per second, decreasing the imaging frame rate and temporal resolution. Aliasing may occur for Doppler shifts with high peak velocities.

42. **d.** If the crystal diameter is constant, the highest frequency will display the longer near zone length. With a comparable frequency, unfocused transducers have a longer focal length than focused transducers. Increasing the crystal diameter will also produce a longer focal length.

43. **a.** Duty factor (transmitting time) is proportional to the pulse duration and pulse repetition frequency and inversely proportional to the pulse repetition period and penetration depth.

44. **a.** Depth or time gain compensation offsets attenuation by boosting the amplitudes of deep reflections and suppressing superficial reflections.

45. **b.** The Reynolds number predicts the onset of turbulent flow. A vessel with a Reynolds number of 2000 or greater will demonstrate turbulence. Nyquist limit predicts the onset of aliasing.

46. **a.** Axial resolution depends on the operating frequency and is equal to one-half of the spatial pulse length. Lateral resolution depends on the beam width and temporal resolution depends on the frame rate.

47. **e.** The function of the matching layer is to reduce the impedance difference between the element and skin, improving sound transmission across the tissue boundary. Damping reduces the number of cycles in each pulse, pulse duration, and spatial pulse length.

48. **c.** The number of memory bits is equal to 2^n. 128 shades of gray = $2 \times 2 \times 2 \times 2 \times 2 \times 2 \times 2 = 128$ or 2^7 (to the 7th power).

49. **c.** Read zoom is a postprocessing function that magnifies and displays stored data. Write zoom is a preprocessing function that increases the number of pixels per inch improves spatial resolution, acquires, and magnifies new information.

50. **b.** Persistence is a preprocessing, sonographer adjustable function that changes imaging frame rates.

51. **c.** In areas of stenosis flow speed increases, resulting in a decrease in pressure (Bernoulli effect).

52. **d.** Reducing the gain setting by one-half (−3 dB) would display a new gain setting of 27 dB.

53. **b.** Attenuation is a progressive weakening of the intensity or amplitude of the sound beam as it travels through soft tissue, resulting from absorption, reflection, and scattering of the sound wave.

54. **d.** The sound beam diverges (widens) in the far zone (Fraunhofer) and tapers in the near zone toward the focal point.

55. **b.** Specificity defines the ability of a diagnostic technique to identify correctly the absence of disease (normalcy).

56. **e.** No confirmed significant biological effects in mammalian tissue for exposures below $100 \text{ mW}/\text{cm}^2$ with unfocused and $1 \text{ W}/\text{cm}^2$ with focused transducers.

57. **d.** Intensity ranges from smallest to highest are SATA (smallest), SPTA, SATP, and SPTP (highest).

58. **d.** Diagnostic ultrasound transducers operate on the piezoelectric effect or principle.

59. **a.** The sound beam is more uniform in intensity in the far field. Maximum intensity occurs at the focal point. Intensity variations are greatest in the near field.

60. **d.** Output or power functions control the intensity of both the transmitted and received signals. The amplifier increases small electric voltages received from the transducer to a level suitable for processing.

61. **a.** Threshold suppresses or eliminates smaller amplitude voltages produced by weak reflections. Elimination of weak reflections is not the intended function of compensation.

62. **e.** Line density is directly related to the pulse repetition frequency and spatial resolution and inversely related to temporal resolution and frame rate.

63. **e.** 4, 8, and 12 MHz are even harmonic frequencies of a 2.0 MHz fundamental frequency.

64. **d.** Range ambiguity is most likely a result of a pulse repetition frequency set too high. Aliasing is a result of a pulse repetition frequency set too low. Decreasing amplification can overcome acoustic speckle and flash artifacts.

65. **b.** Mechanical index is an acoustic output-labeling standard used as an indicator for when cavitation is likely will occur.

66. **b.** Mirror image is duplication of a structure on the opposite side of a strong reflector. Impedance difference determines how much of the incident beam will reflect and transmit at a media boundary.

67. **a.** Approximately 1% of the sound beam reflects back to the transducer and 99% of the sound beam transmits from a media boundary with perpendicular incidence, if the impedances are different.

68. **e.** Distance to a reflector (placement of an echo) is dependent on the round-trip time and propagation speed of the medium.

69. **b.** An early gate time denotes a shallow sample volume depth.

70. **d.** The pulse repetition frequency determines the number of scan lines per frame. Contrast resolution is dependent on the number of bits per pixel.

71. **e.** A change in propagation speed as a sound wave travels through a medium does not affect the frequency of the wave.

72. **d.** Arterial diastolic flow reveals the state of downstream arterioles. Diastolic flow reversal indicates high resistance distally.

73. **b.** Focusing of the sound beam is ONLY available in the near field.

74. **e.** Linear phased array transducers contain a compact line of elements about one-quarter of a wavelength wide. Linear sequenced array transducers demonstrate a straight line of rectangular elements about one wavelength wide.

75. **d.** The delay portion of the time gain compensation curve represents the depth at which variable compensation begins.

76. **b.** The scan converter properly locates each series of echoes in individual scan lines for storage, transferring incoming echo data into a suitable format for display.

77. **e.** Specular reflections occur when the sound wave strikes a smooth large surface perpendicularly.

78. **e.** Increasing the number of focal zones and resonant frequency will improve lateral resolution. Decreasing the imaging depth and beam width will also improve lateral resolution.

79. **c.** Contrast resolution is the ability to distinguish between tissues of slightly different intensity (amplitudes).

80. **d.** Propagation speed and thickness of the element determine the operating frequency.

81. **b.** Duty factor is the fraction of time pulse ultrasound is transmitting. Period is the time to complete one cycle.

82. **d.** Duty factor and the number of cycles in a pulse are proportional to the pulse duration. Pulse repetition frequency is inversely proportional to the pulse duration.

83. **e.** Increasing the packet size will decrease the frame rate and temporal resolution.

84. **a.** Multiple focal zones results in a reduction in the frame rate and temporal resolution. Lateral resolution is proportional to the number of focal zones utilized.

85. **b.** Compression is the ratio of the largest to smallest amplitudes the ultrasound system can display.

86. **a.** Imaging depth and propagation speed of the medium determines the frame rate.

87. **b.** Apodization reduces grating lobes by utilizing a varying excitation of the elements in an array. Subdicing divides each element into small pieces to reduce grating lobes.

88. **a.** Thermal index is the ratio of acoustic power and the power required to raise tissue temperature 1°C.

89. **e.** Mechanical index is inversely proportional to the operating frequency and proportional to the acoustic output.

90. **b.** A linear phased array sweeps the ultrasound beam electronically, by delayed activation of the crystals in the array.

91. **b.** Pulse inversion is a harmonic imaging technique utilizing two pulses per scan line with the second pulse an inversion of the first.

92. **e.** Dynamic focusing utilizes a variable receiving focus that follows the changing position of the pulse as it propagates through tissue.

93. **c.** Matrix denotes the rows and columns of pixels in a digital image. Increasing the number of rows and columns increases the spatial resolution.

94. **a.** Nyquist limit is the highest frequency in a sampled signal represented unambiguously and is equal to one-half the pulse repetition frequency.

95. **d.** Compensation provides equal amplitude for all similar structures regardless of the depth. Amplification allows identical amplification despite the depth.

96. **d.** Spatial compounding directs scan lines in multiple directions improving visualization of structures beneath a highly attenuating structure.

97. **a.** Microbubbles from contrast agents increase scatter and emit sound waves at harmonic frequencies.

98. **b.** Frequency is proportional to image quality and attenuation. Wavelength, period, and penetration depth are inversely proportional to frequency.

99. **b.** During reception, ultrasound transducers converts acoustic energy into electrical energy. Conversion of electrical energy to acoustic energy occurs during transmission.

100. **a.** Plug flow is found in larger arteries and demonstrates a constant velocity across the entire vessel. Parabolic flow is a type of laminar flow where the average flow velocity is equal to one-half of the maximum flow speed at the center.

101. **b.** The intensity of a sound wave is equal to the amplitude squared. If the amplitude is doubles, then the intensity will quadruple.

102. **d.** Hypoechoic is a comparative term used to describe a decrease in echogenicity when compared to then surrounding structures or than normally expected for the structure.

103. **c.** Oblique incidence and a change of velocity or propagation speed between the media MUST take place for refraction to occur.

104. **c.** Power Doppler imaging has an increased sensitivity to Doppler shifts (presence of flow), but is unable to display flow direction, velocity, or characteristics.

105. **e.** Line density directly relates to the pulse repetition frequency and spatial resolution. Frame rate and temporal resolution relates inversely to the line density.

106. **c.** A hydrophone measures acoustic output. Beam profiler measures transducer characteristics.

107. **b.** A rise in tissue temperature is significant when it exceeds 2°C.

108. **a.** Two near zone lengths is equal to the diameter of the transducer. One near zone length is equal to one-half of the transducer diameter.

109. **c.** Comet tail artifact displays a series of closely spaced reverberation echoes behind a strong reflector.

110. **c.** Angling the color Doppler box to the right or left changes the Doppler shift and Doppler angle.

111. **a.** Slower propagation speeds will place a reflector deeper than it is actually located.

112. **e.** To overcome range ambiguity the pulse repetition frequency should be reduced.

113. **e.** Altering the electronic excitation of the elements, steering the beam in various directions.

114. **c.** Spectral analysis allows visualization of the Doppler signal providing quantitative data, including peak, mean, and minimum flow velocities, flow direction, and flow characteristics.

115. **b.** Air has the highest attenuation coefficient when compared to fat, liver, kidney, and muscle. Bone has a higher attenuation coefficient compared to air.

116. **b.** Bandwidth is the range of frequencies found within a pulse.

117. **a.** Infrasound is below human hearing with a frequency range below 20 Hz.

118. **e.** Continuous wave (CW) utilizes separate transmit and receiver elements housed in a single transducer assembly.

119. **b.** Assumptions of the ultrasound system is the most likely cause of sonographic artifacts.

120. **d.** Structures within the focal zone may display an improper brightness.

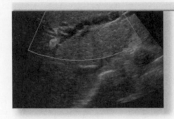

Abdomen Answers

Chapter: 7 Liver

1. **c.** Hepatomegaly is suggested **once** the AP diameter exceeds 15 cm or the length exceeds 18 cm. An AP diameter of 20 to 22 cm is considered enlarged but the keyword in this question is **once**. The normal adult liver measures 15 to 17 cm in length and 10 to 12.5 cm in anterior-posterior (AP) diameter.

2. **d.** Portal hypertension is associated with compression or occlusion of the portal veins. Clinical findings may include: hepatomegaly, splenomegaly, hepatofugal flow in the main portal vein, increased resistance in the hepatic artery, formation of venous collaterals and an increase in diameter of the main portal, splenic and superior mesenteric veins. Echogenicity of the liver parenchyma is generally hyperechoic. Hypoechoic liver parenchyma is more commonly associated with hepatitis.

3. **e.** Polycystic disease is associated with the development of multiple cysts in the parenchyma of the liver, kidneys, pancreas, and spleen. The adrenal glands are not typically involved in polycystic disease.

4. **b.** A smooth circular or oval shaped hyperechoic mass is the **most** common sonographic appearance of a cavernous hemangioma. A complex appearance attributed to necrosis or hemorrhage is less common. An irregular hypoechoic or complex mass is suspicious for malignancy or abscess formation. A smooth hypoechoic mass is suspicious for an adenoma, normal liver tissue with associated fatty infiltration, or malignancy.

5. **c.** The ligamentum of venosum separates the left lobe from the caudate lobe of the liver. The coronary ligament separates the subphrenic space from Morison's pouch. The falciform ligament divides the subphrenic space into right and left compartments. The hepatoduodenal ligament connects the liver to the duodenum. The gastrohepatic ligament connects the lesser curvature of the stomach to the liver.

6. **c.** Cirrhosis is a general term used for chronic and severe insult to the liver cells leading to fibrosis and regenerating nodules. Alcohol abuse is the **most common** cause of cirrhosis. Other etiologies may include: biliary obstruction, viral hepatitis, Budd-Chiari syndrome, nutritional deficiencies, or cardiac disease.

7. **e.** Patients presenting with hepatocellular carcinoma (hepatoma) may demonstrate a decrease in serum albumin, suggesting a decrease in protein synthesis. Clinical findings of a hepatoma may include: abdominal pain, palpable mass, weight loss, hepatomegaly, jaundice, unexplained fever, elevated AST, ALT and alkaline phosphatase, positive alpha-fetoprotein, and a decrease in serum albumin.

8. **c.** In the United States, ascending cholangitis is the most common cause of a hepatic abscess. Additional etiologies may include: recent travel abroad, biliary infection, appendicitis, or diverticulitis. Pseudocyst formation is the most common complication associated with acute pancreatitis. Portal vein thrombosis and Budd-Chiari syndrome are at risk for developing portal hypertension. Biliary obstruction is not directly linked with hepatic abscess formation.

9. **e.** The left lobe of the liver is separated from the right lobe by the middle hepatic vein superiorly and the main lobar fissure inferiorly. The left hepatic vein separates the left lobe into medial and lateral segments and the right hepatic vein separates the right lobe into anterior and posterior segments. The ligamentum venosum separates the caudate and left lobes of the liver.

10. **d.** The right hepatic vein divides the right lobe of the liver into anterior and posterior segments. The middle hepatic vein divides the right lobe from the left medial lobe. Portal veins course within the liver segments (intrasegmental) while the hepatic veins course between the liver segments (intersegmental). Intrahepatic arteries parallel the portal veins and are not generally visualized with ultrasound.

11. **b.** Fever and an increase in white blood count is suspicious for an underlying infection. A complex liver mass in a patient who recently traveled abroad is most suspicious for an abscess. An echinococcal cyst is associated with travel abroad but appears as a cystic mass on ultrasound. These clinical and sonographic findings are inconsistent with an adenoma or cystadenoma. A possible differential consideration is a hepatoma but is **not as likely** as an abscess formation.

12. **c.** Hepatitis B increases a patient's risk for developing cirrhosis or a hepatoma. Focal nodular hyperplasia and cavernous hemangioma are vascular malformations not related to hepatitis B. Adenomas are related to the use of oral contraceptives, while hepatic abscess formation is most commonly caused by ascending cholangitis.

13. **e.** A "daughter cyst" is defined as a cyst containing smaller cysts. This finding is associated with an echinococcal cyst. A cystadenoma appears as a multiloculated cystic mass. Hepatoma and adenoma are solid masses while a fungal abscess demonstrates a complex appearance.

14. **c.** The hepatic veins course **between** the lobes of the liver

(**interlobar**) The portal veins, hepatic arteries, and biliary ducts generally course parallel with one another **within** the lobes of the liver (**intralobar**) The inferior vena cava is not a hepatic structure.

15. **a.** Flow in the main portal vein varies with respiration and is termed phasic flow. Blood courses into the liver (hepatopetal) at a low velocity (10-30 cm/sec). Continuous flow does not vary with respiration. Multiphasic (pulsatile) flow is demonstrated in the hepatic veins. Retrograde is defined as a reversal in the normal flow direction.

16. **d.** An **asymptomatic obese** patient with elevated AST and ALT levels commonly demonstrates an increased amount of fat within the liver. The hypoechoic area represents normal liver tissue surrounded by fatty infiltration. These focal areas of normal parenchyma are most commonly located anterior to the porta hepatis or near the inferior vena cava. An enlarged lymph node is a possible differential but not as likely of a diagnosis. Nodular fibrosis is related to cirrhosis. A hepatic abscess or malignant lesion is an unlikely diagnosis in an asymptomatic patient.

17. **c.** The liver parenchyma appears hyperechoic. The intrahepatic vessel walls are difficult to distinguish but course in a straight pattern. This is most consistent with fatty infiltration. Lymphoma, candidiasis, liver metastasis, or cirrhosis is generally associated with additional clinical symptoms along with elevated liver function tests.

18. **d.** A solitary hyperechoic mass demonstrating smooth wall margins is most suspicious for a cavernous hemangioma. Hemangiomas may cause right upper quadrant pain and typically do not elevate liver function tests. An adenoma and focal nodular hyperplasia are related to oral contraceptive use and hormone levels respectively. These pathologies are unlikely in a non–hormone-replaced postmenopausal patient. Abscess formation is not a likely diagnosis with these sonographic findings and clinical history.

19. **d.** The main portal vein should demonstrate flow into the liver (hepatopetal; above baseline). In this duplex image, the main portal vein is demonstrating flow away from the liver (hepatofugal; below baseline). Hepatofugal flow is **most commonly** associated with portal hypertension. When hepatofugal flow is encountered, the sonographer should evaluate for splenic enlargement and venous collaterals. Budd-Chiari syndrome is associated with thrombosis of the hepatic veins. Hepatitis, fatty infiltration and liver metastasis are not associated with hepatofugal flow in the portal venous system.

20. **c.** The image demonstrates the hepatic veins entering the inferior vena cava. The arrow identifies the hepatic lobe located between the left and middle hepatic veins. The medial left lobe is bordered by the left and middle hepatic veins. The left hepatic vein divides the medial and lateral segments of the left lobe. The middle hepatic vein divides the medial left lobe from the anterior right lobe. The right hepatic vein divides the right lobe into anterior and posterior segments.

21. **d.** Extension of the liver anterior and inferior to the right kidney and a left lobe not extending across the midline is **mostly likely** a nonpathological Reidel lobe. This anatomical variant is an incidental finding with a female prevalence. Postprandial pain is not related to a Reidel lobe. Occasionally a patient's clinical history is not directly related to a specific sonographic finding. This anomaly may be confused with hepatomegaly. Careful evaluation of the left lobe should help to differentiate between these conditions. Hepatitis, cirrhosis, and fatty infiltration are not characterized by a homogeneous extension of the right hepatic lobe.

22. **a.** A **single** anechoic area demonstrating posterior acoustic enhancement is identified in the area in question. In an asymptomatic patient, this finding is most consistent with a simple hepatic cyst. Polycystic disease is associated with multiple cysts. The structure is identified as nonvascular, which rules out a hepatic varix. An echinococcal cyst demonstrates a septated appearance. A resolving hematoma can appear anechoic but is not as likely a diagnosis as a simple cyst.

23. **c.** A hyperechoic focus demonstrating strong posterior acoustic shadowing is identified in the gallbladder. These are characteristic sonographic findings of cholelithiasis. A small echogenic focus demonstrating a comet tail reverberation artifact is identified in the anterior gallbladder wall consistent with adenomyomatosis. The echogenicity of the liver does not appear dense or fatty. Posterior acoustic enhancement is demonstrated posterior to the hepatic cyst, falsely increasing the echogenicity of the liver tissue.

24. **b.** Candidiasis is a rare fungal infection found in immune-compromised patients. Hypoechoic or target lesions may develop in the liver parenchyma. Hepatic adenomas are associated with the usage of oral contraceptives. Echinococcal cysts are associated with recent travel to an underdeveloped country. Immune-suppressed patients are not at an increased risk for developing polycystic disease or cavernous hemangiomas.

25. **c.** Metastatic lesions involving the liver **most commonly** originate from a malignant neoplasm of the colon. Metastatic neoplasms of the pancreas, breast, and lung can also metastasize to the liver.

26. **c.** The right coronary ligament serves as a barrier between the subphrenic and subhepatic spaces (bare area). Fluid cannot directly ascend from Morison's pouch into the right subphrenic space. The falciform ligament separates the subphrenic space into two compartments. The gastrohepatic and hepatoduodenal ligaments attach the liver to the stomach and duodenum, respectively.

27. **b.** Varix is the most common term used to describe a dilated vein. Aneurysm is more commonly used to describe a focal arterial dilatation. Shunt or stent describes a type of passageway between two structures. Perforator veins connect

the superficial and deep venous systems.

28. b. Traditional lobar anatomy divides the liver into the right, left, caudate and quadrate lobes. Functional lobar or segmental anatomy divides the liver into three lobes: left, right, and caudate. Couinaud's anatomy divides the liver into eight segments using an imaginary "H" pattern.

29. a. Cirrhosis is a general term used to describe chronic and severe insult to the liver cells leading to inflammation of the parenchyma and subsequent necrosis. Portal hypertension is generally a secondary pathology caused by underlying liver disease (i.e., cirrhosis). Fatty infiltration is simply an increase in the amount of fat contained within the liver parenchyma. Budd-Chiari syndrome is associated with thrombosis of the hepatic veins. Focal nodular hyperplasia is considered a congenital vascular malformation.

30. e. Von Gierke's disease is the most common type of glycogen storage disease (Type I). Patients have a predisposing factor for developing a hepatic adenoma. Schistosomiasis is caused by a parasite. Polycystic disease or cirrhosis are not related to Von Gierke's disease.

31. b. Prominence of the wall margins of the portal veins or "star effect" is characteristic with hepatitis. In cases of fatty infiltration, cirrhosis, and glycogen storage disease, the liver demonstrates an increase in parenchymal echogenicity decreasing the distinction of the portal veins, hepatic veins, and biliary ducts.

32. a. The TIPS is **commonly** placed between the right portal and right hepatic veins. The purpose of the shunt is to bypass blood from the engorged portal venous system directly into the hepatic venous system.

33. d. The paraumbilical vein courses within the falciform ligament from the umbilicus to the left portal vein. Recanalization of the paraumbilical vein is caused by an increase in venous pressure within the portal circulation.

34. c. A congenital anterior and inferior extension of the right lobe of the liver is termed a Reidel lobe. Congenital variants of the left lobe include: a larger size extending into the left subphrenic space or a smaller size that does not cross midline. Sinus inversus refers to a lateral reversal of the abdominal and/or thoracic structures from their normal position. Hepatomegaly and hyperplasia are not congenital anomalies.

35. d. The subphrenic space is located superior to the liver and inferior to the diaphragm. The pleura are located superior to the diaphragm. Morison's pouch and the subhepatic space are located inferior to the liver. The lesser sac is located anterior to the pancreas and posterior to the stomach.

36. a. The caudate lobe has a unique blood supply that is routinely spared from disease. Enlargement of the caudate lobe is **most commonly** associated with cirrhosis. Candidiasis, fatty infiltration, liver metastasis, and polycystic disease are not predisposing factors for enlargement of the caudate lobe.

37. c. Hepatic veins demonstrate a multiphasic or pulsatile blood flow pattern, coursing away from the liver toward the inferior vena cava (hepatofugal). In laminar flow, the fastest flow is located in the center of the lumen and slowest flow is located near the lumen walls (i.e., common carotid artery). Parabolic or plug flow demonstrates a steady flow pattern with variable speeds across the vessel lumen (i.e., aorta).

38. b. The falciform ligament attaches the liver to the **anterior** abdominal wall and separates the right and left subphrenic spaces. The right coronary ligament attaches the liver to the lateral abdominal wall. The triangular ligament is the most lateral portion of the coronary ligament. The hepatorenal ligament attaches the kidney to the liver.

39. e. The middle hepatic vein is antegrade (blue), flowing toward the inferior vena cava (IVC) while the left hepatic vein is retrograde (red), flowing away from the IVC.

40. c. The caudate lobe is located posterior to the ligamentum venosum and porta hepatis, anterior and medial to the inferior vena cava and lateral to the lesser sac.

41. b. Multiple engorged vessels in the left upper quadrant in a patient with a history of cirrhosis is most suspicious for gastric varices.

42. c. Hepatomegaly is associated with a hepatic inflammatory process (i.e., hepatitis), fatty infiltration, congestive heart failure, polycystic disease, biliary obstruction, Budd-Chiari syndrome, or a neoplasm. Hepatomegaly is not a complication of acute pancreatitis.

43. d. Severe abdominal pain and loss of appetite are the **most common** symptoms associated with portal vein thrombosis. Weight loss is precipitated by a loss of appetite. Tachycardia and lower extremity edema are more commonly associated with pulmonary embolism and deep vein thrombosis of the lower extremity. Jaundice is not typically a symptom of portal vein thrombosis.

44. d. The diameter of a TIPS should measure a minimum of 8 mm and should range between 8 and 12 mm throughout the stent.

45. a. A long history of oral contraceptive use is a predisposing factor for developing a hepatic adenoma. A hypoechoic liver mass demonstrating a hypoechoic halo is identified in the right lobe of the liver. This is characteristic of an adenoma. Focal nodular hyperplasia is influenced by hormones but presents as a well defined isoechoic or hyperechoic mass(es). A hepatoma could be a differential consideration but not a likely diagnosis in this case. Cavernous hemangiomas can undergo degeneration changing the echo pattern but are not associated with a hypoechoic halo. Adenoma is the most likely diagnosis for this liver mass with these sonographic findings and clinical history.

46. d. The liver parenchyma appears heterogeneous, demonstrating multiple hyperechoic masses throughout the right lobe. The patient's clinical history includes pain and an increase in alkaline phosphatase. This is most consistent with liver metastasis. Cirrhosis is associated with a hyperechoic liver parenchyma, ascites, and *an irregular liver contour*. Fatty infiltration may demonstrate *hypoechoic* focal areas of fat sparing but is not associated with elevation in alkaline phosphatase levels. Portal hypertension may demonstrate peritoneal ascites but is not associated with multiple hyperechoic liver masses. Hypoechoic or target lesions are characteristic of candidiasis.

47. **e.**   A small fluid collection is identified inferior to the diaphragm (hyperechoic linear structure) and superior to the liver in the right subphrenic space. The pleura are located superior to the diaphragm. The lesser sac is located anterior to the pancreas. The subhepatic space and right paracolic gutter are located inferior to the liver.

48. **e.**   The transverse sonogram identifies the hepatic veins emptying into the inferior vena cava. Arrow **A** is identifying the inferior vena cava.

49. **d.**   The transverse sonogram identifies the hepatic veins emptying into the inferior vena cava. Arrow **B** is identifying the more lateral right hepatic vein.

50. **c.**   The transverse sonogram identifies the hepatic veins emptying into the inferior vena cava. Arrow **C** is identifying the middle hepatic vein.

Chapter 8: Biliary System

1. **e.**   A malignant neoplasm located at the junction of the right and left hepatic ducts is termed a Klatskin tumor. A biloma is an extrahepatic collection of extravasated bile. A hepatoma is a parenchymal malignancy. Extension of pancreatic inflammation into the peripancreatic tissues describes a phlegmon. Folding of the gallbladder fundus is termed a phyrgian cap.

2. **c.**   Supine, left posterior oblique, and left lateral decubitus positions are routinely used in abdominal imaging. The cystic duct is not routinely visualized in these positions. Trendelenburg or right lateral decubitus positions may aid in visualization of the cystic duct. A prone position helps in visualizing some retroperitoneal structures.

3. **a.**   A fold or septation located between the neck and body of the gallbladder describes a junctional fold. Hartmann pouch is a small posterior pouch located near the neck of the gallbladder. A phyrgian cap describes a fold in the gallbladder fundus. Adenomyomatosis or diverticulosis of the gallbladder are polypoid masses protruding from the gallbladder wall into the lumen.

4. **b.**   Demonstration of a focal hyperechoic gallbladder **wall** with **marked** posterior acoustic shadowing is characteristic of a porcelain gallbladder. Emphysematous cholecystitis appears as an echogenic focus in the gallbladder wall or lumen with **ill-defined** posterior acoustic shadowing. Cholelithiasis is an intraluminal abnormality. Adenomyomatosis demonstrates a comet tail reverberation artifact. Mirrizi syndrome is a condition caused by a lodge stone in the neck of the gallbladder or cystic duct.

5. **d.**   Nonshadowing, low amplitude echoes located in the dependent portion of the gallbladder describes biliary sludge. The keywords in this question are: dependent and nonshadowing. This implies the echoes are mobile and do not demonstrate posterior acoustic shadowing. Mobile echoes rules out adenomyomatosis and polypoid masses. Nonshadowing echoes rules out cholelithiasis. Cholecystitis describes an inflammatory process affecting the gallbladder.

6. **c.**   Cholesterolosis is an accumulation of triglycerides and esterfied sterols in the wall of the gallbladder caused by a local disturbance in cholesterol metabolism. There are two types of cholesterolosis: cholesterosis and cholesterol polyps. Cholesterolosis is NOT associated with serum cholesterol levels.

7. **d.**   The spiral valves of Heister are located in the cystic duct. These valves make visualization difficult on ultrasound.

8. **a.**   Localized thickening of the gallbladder wall in a patient with acute upper abdominal pain and a positive Murphy's sign is most consistent with acute cholecystitis. A porcelain gallbladder demonstrates a localized hyperechoic wall with marked acoustic shadowing. Adenomyomatosis is not associated with a positive Murphy's sign. A non-fasting gallbladder demonstrates symmetrical wall thickening.

9. **b.**   A hyperechoic focus demonstrating posterior acoustic shadowing is identified in the **common bile duct** consistent with choledocholithiasis. Choledocholithiasis is associated with right upper quadrant pain and biliary obstruction (jaundice). Cholangiocarcinoma appears as a **nonshadowing** intraluminal echogenic focus. Thickening of the bile duct walls is consistent with cholangitis.

10. **a.**   Complications associated with choledocholithiasis may include biliary obstruction, cholangitis, and pancreatitis. Cholelithiasis is a predisposing factor for choledocholithiasis but not a complication. Choledocholithiasis is not a precipitating factor of portal hypertension or lymphadenopathy.

11. **b.**   The gallbladder demonstrates a gallstone and thickening of the anterior gallbladder wall. A hypoechoic area is also demonstrated between the anterior gallbladder wall and liver suspicious for pericholecystic fluid. These findings are most suspicious for acute cholecystitis. Emphysetamous cholecystitis demonstrates shadowing within the thickened wall. The sonographic findings are inconsistent with adenomyomatosis or metastatic gallbladder disease.

12. **a.**   The arrows identify an anechoic structure contiguous with the gallbladder fundus. This is most likely a fold in the gallbladder fundus, termed a phyrgian cap. Gallbladder duplication exhibits as two distinct anechoic structures lying adjacent to one another in the gallbladder fossa. A junctional fold is located between the neck and body of the gallbladder. Gallbladder diverticulum and adenomyomatosis are masses protruding from the gallbladder wall into the lumen.

13. **b.**   A refractive artifact is demonstrating a "shadow" posterior and medial to the phyrgian cap of the gallbladder. Sound is refracted in a lateral direction from the projected path, leaving weak echoes to return from the expected path. This causes a shadow appearance. Refraction occurs at the edge of generally round or oval-shaped structures and is commonly termed an edge artifact. Grating lobes are addi-

tional, weaker sound beams traveling in different directions from the primary beam. Reverberation demonstrates multiple equally spaced echoes. Mirror image is a form of reverberation artifact where structures that exist on one side of a strong reflector are also identified on the opposite side. Slice thickness artifact decreases detail resolution.

14. **e.**   The biliary system has three main functions: 1. transport bile to the gallbladder through the biliary ducts; 2. store and concentrate bile in the gallbladder; and 3. transport bile through the bile ducts from the gallbladder to the duodenum to aid in the digestion of fats.

15. **b.**   Biliary sludge is not necessarily a pathological condition. It may be demonstrated in patients with abnormal eating patterns or prolonged fasting. Cholelithiasis and cholangitis are related to biliary stasis but are not as likely to occur as biliary sludge. Polypoid or malignant lesions are unrelated to episodes of fasting.

16. **d.**   The gallbladder wall is composed of four layers: **1.** outer serosal, **2.** subserosal, **3.** muscular, **4.** inner epithelial.

17. **d.**   The CBD courses inferiorly through the head of the pancreas terminating in the descending portion of the duodenum at the ampulla of Vater. The superior portion of the common bile duct is located near the hepatic hilum and neck of the gallbladder.

18. **b.**   The common hepatic duct lies anterior to the main portal vein and lateral to the proper hepatic artery in the region of the porta hepatis.

19. **c.**   Tenderness over McBurney's point is a clinical sign of appendicitis. Abdominal pain, postprandial pain, elevated liver function tests, fatty food intolerance, or a positive Murphy's sign are common indications for a biliary sonogram.

20. **d.**   The release of cholecystokinin stimulates gallbladder contraction and secretion of pancreatic enzymes. Cholecystokinin is released when food reaches the duodenum. Gastrin stimulates the secretion of gastric acids. Amylase, lipase, and bilirubin are not hormones.

21. **b.**   The normal fasting adult gallbladder measures 8-10 cm in length and 3-5 cm in diameter. Diameters exceeding 5 cm are considered enlarged or hydropic.

22. **e.**   The sonogram is demonstrating a fluid/fluid layer within the gallbladder lumen. The fluids consist of echogenic biliary sludge in the dependent portion of the gallbladder and the less dense anechoic bile. Empyema and abscess formation are most likely associated with a fever. The layering effect of the two types of fluid rules out an intraluminal mass.

23. **c.**   The hyperechoic linear structure extends from the right portal vein (echogenic walls) to the gallbladder fossa. This is most consistent with the main lobar fissure. The main lobar fissure is an **inter**segmental boundary between the right and left lobes of the liver. The ligamentum of venosum separates the caudate and left lobes of the liver. The ligamentum Teres and falciform ligament are located in the left lobe.

24. **c.**   The main lobar fissure is a boundary between the left and right lobes of the liver and is routinely used as a sonographic landmark for locating the gallbladder fossa. The ligamentum venosum is a sonographic landmark used to locate the caudate lobe. The falciform ligament and ligamentum Teres are sonographic landmarks used for locating the superior portion of the paraumbilical vein.

25. **a.**   Multiple small echogenic foci are located in the dependent portion of the gallbladder. Acoustic shadowing is demonstrated posteriorly. These sonographic findings are most consistent with cholelithiasis. The gallbladder wall appears thin and smooth, ruling out adenomyomatosis, porcelain gallbladder, and acute cholecystitis as differential considerations. Tumefactive sludge is generally irregular in shape, slow moving, and nonshadowing.

26. **e.**   Changing the patient position will document mobility of the echogenic foci consistent with cholelithiasis. An intercostal approach or deep inspiration may increase resolution of the foci, but would not demonstrate mobility. Ingestion of water aids in visualization of the pancreas.

27. **e.**   Complications in biliary atresia include: death, cirrhosis, portal hypertension, cholangitis and a **small or absent gallbladder.**

28. **b.**   Alkaline phosphatase is an enzyme produced primarily by the liver, bone and placenta and excreted via the bile ducts. Marked elevation is associated with obstructive jaundice. ALT is an enzyme found in high concentrations in the liver and lower concentrations in the heart, muscle, and kidneys. AST is an enzyme present in many types of tissue. Bilirubin and prothrombin are not enzymes.

29. **a.**   Under normal conditions, the common bile duct will decrease in size or remain unchanged after ingestion of a fatty meal. Enlargement is associated with biliary disease.

30. **b.**   In the fasting state, the gallbladder wall usually measures 1-2 mm in thickness and should not exceed 3 mm.

31. **c.**   Dilatation of only the intrahepatic ducts suggests obstruction within the liver (intrahepatic) A Klatskin tumor is an intrahepatic tumor located at the junction of the left and right hepatic ducts. Cholangitis, choledocholithiasis, and choledochal cysts are generally extrahepatic pathologies.

32. **b.**   Cholelithiasis is a predisposing factor of acute cholecystitis, not a complication. Complications of acute cholecystitis may include: perforation of the gallbladder, liver abscess, empyema, septicemia, gangrenous cholecystitis, emphysematous cholecystitis, ascending cholangitis, or pericholecystic abscess.

33. **d.**   The intrahepatic biliary tree, hepatic arteries, and portal venous system course adjacent with one another. Progressive dilatation of the bile ducts compresses and flattens the portal veins. A beaded appearance to the intrahepatic biliary ducts is characteristic of Caroli's disease.

34. **d.**   In the hepatic hilum, the hepatic artery lies anterior to the main portal vein and medial to the common duct.

35. **a.**   The inferior vena cava lies immediately anterior to the spine.

36. **e.**   The main portal vein lies posterior to the common duct and hepatic

artery in the hepatic hilum (aka: porta hepatis; portal triad).

37. b. Hyperechoic foci demonstrating posterior acoustic shadowing in a patient with a previous history of biliary surgery is most suspicious for pneumobilia. Ascariasis and abscess formation are generally associated with symptoms of an infection. Calculus within a bile duct and arterial calcifications are not as likely a diagnosis as pneumobilia.

38. d. Multiple hyperechoic foci are identified in the anterior gallbladder **wall**. Comet-tail reverberation artifact is demonstrated posterior to the foci. These sonographic findings are characteristic of adenomyomatosis. Chronic or acute cases of cholecystitis generally demonstrate a thicken gallbladder wall. Malignant neoplasms typically demonstrate irregular wall margins. Gallstones are typically gravitationally dependent.

39. a. A form of reverberation, the comet-tail artifact occurs with marked impedance changes. It appears as a dense, tapering trail of echoes just distal to a strongly reflecting structure. This type of artifact is characteristic in adenomyomatosis. Refraction occurs at the edge of generally round or oval shaped structures and is commonly termed an edge artifact. Mirror image is a form of reverberation artifact where structures that exist on one side of a strong reflector are also identified on the opposite side. Posterior acoustic enhancement is an increase in echo strength behind weakly attenuating structures.

40. c. A small posterior pouch near the neck of the gallbladder describes Hartmann pouch. A junctional fold is defined as a septation or fold near the gallbladder neck. Morison's pouch is located in the lateral subhepatic space. Fetal lobulation describes a lobulated contour to the kidney. Choledochal cysts do not involve the neck of the gallbladder.

41. a. Imaging of dilated intrahepatic ducts parallel with the associated portal vein is termed parallel channeling, double channel sign, or shotgun sign. Prominence of the portal veins is seen in hepatitis and termed the star effect. Mouse sign is

used to describe the cross-sectional plane of the portal triad.

42. c. Bilirubin is a product of the breakdown of hemoglobin in old red blood cells. AST, ALT, and alkaline phosphatase are liver enzymes. Alpha-fetoprotein is a protein normally synthesized by the fetus.

43. d. Risk factors include: family history of gallstones, female gender, fertility, pregnancy, diabetes mellitus, and obesity. Hepatitis is not a predisposing factor associated with the development of cholelithiasis.

44. a. Increasing the transducer frequency increases the axial resolution necessary to demonstrate shadowing posterior to small gallstones. Decreases in the image depth, overall gain, and number of focal zones will not increase the image's axial resolution. Increasing the dynamic range increases the gray scale of the image.

45. e. Intraductal pressure differences are affected by the flow rate of bile from the liver, resorption and filling of bile in the gallbladder, and activity of the sphincter of Oddi. The location of the bile duct is not related to intraductal pressure.

46. b. Pneumobilia generally demonstrates as a hyperechoic focus with posterior acoustic shadowing. A surgical clip, stent, calculus, or vascular calcification can appear on ultrasound as a hyperechoic focus with or without posterior acoustic shadowing. A hemangioma appears as a nonshadowing, hyperechoic, or complex mass.

47. d. The patient is placed in the left decubitus position. The masses do not demonstrate gravitational dependency (mobility). Polypoid masses, adenomas, and malignant neoplasms are nonmobile structures. Tumefactive sludge, while slow moving, is generally mobile.

48. c. Sonographic and clinical findings are most consistent with metastatic gallbladder disease. Metastasis to the gallbladder is a likely diagnosis with the following criteria: 1. focal intraluminal masses, 2. history of pancreas neoplasm, 3. no associated cholelithiasis. The patient has a history of pancreatic cancer. The gallbladder demonstrates immobile echogenic masses without associated gallstones.

49. c. Two nonconnecting sonolucencies are identified in the **gallbladder fossa**. This is most suspicious for gallbladder duplication. The gallbladders are located in the gallbladder fossa. Strawberry gallbladder is not a congenital anomaly.

50. c. Acute cholecystitis is the most likely diagnosis with a history of a positive Murphy sign and a thickened gallbladder wall.

Chapter 9: Pancreas

1. d. Annular pancreas is a congenital anomaly in which the head of the pancreas surrounds the duodenum. This may result in obstruction of the biliary tree or duodenum. Pancreas divisum is an anomaly of the pancreatic ducts. Phlegmon is a complication of acute pancreatitis. The uncinate process is a normal portion of the pancreatic head.

2. a. Indications may include: biliary disease, weight loss, abdominal pain, sudden onset of diabetes mellitus, or elevation of pancreatic enzymes. Flank pain is commonly associated with abnormalities of the kidneys. Even though the pancreas is a retroperitoneal organ, it is generally evaluated in an abdominal ultrasound examination.

3. d. Trypsin is a highly digestive enzyme that breaks down proteins into amino acids. Amylase breaks down carbohydrates and lipase breaks down fats. Gastrin and cholecystokinin are hormones.

4. c. The uncinate process, a medial portion of the pancreatic head, is located directly posterior to the superior mesenteric vein and anterior to the inferior vena cava. The uncinate process is located posterior and medial to the gastroduodenal artery and main portal vein.

5. d. Pseudocyst formation is the most common complication of acute pancreatitis. Additional complications may include: phlegmon, hemorrhage, abscess formation or duodenal obstruction.

6. c. Islet cells of Langerhans secrete hormones directly into the bloodstream. These hormones include: glucagon (alpha cells), insulin (beta cells), and somatostatin (delta cells).

7. c. In a Whipple procedure (pancreatoduodenectomy) normal pancreatic tissue is attached to the duodenum. The gallbladder is removed, if present. The common bile duct is anastomosed to the duodenum distal to the pancreas and the stomach is anastomosed to the duodenum distal to the common bile duct.

8. c. A phlegmon is an extension of pancreatic inflammation into the peripancreatic tissues. A pseudocyst is a collection of fluid caused by a leakage of pancreatic enzymes. Annular pancreas and pancreas divisum are congenital anomalies. An abscess is a collection of a purulent substance.

9. e. Biliary disease is the most common cause of acute pancreatitis followed by alcohol abuse. Additional etiologies may include: trauma, peptic ulcer disease, and hyperlipidemia.

10. c. The sonogram demonstrates a complex mass near the lesser sac and anterior pararenal space. The complex appearance may be related to hemorrhage or necrosis. Pseudocyst formation is the most common complication in acute pancreatitis and the **most likely** diagnosis with this clinical history. A phlegmon is an extension of the inflammation into the peripancreatic tissues and generally appears as a solid hypoechoic mass. An islet cell tumor, while typically located in the body or tail of the pancreas, is not the most likely diagnosis. A biloma is typically located in the region of the porta hepatis. The mass identified in the sonogram is located in the left upper quadrant more consistent with the stomach not duodenal region.

11. e. An anechoic tubular structure is located anterior to the splenic vein within the body of the pancreas. This is most consistent with the main pancreatic duct (duct of Wirsung). The splenic artery courses superior to the body of the pancreas. The common bile duct courses through the posterior lateral portion of the pancreatic head. The gastroduodenal artery is located in the anterior lateral portion of the head of the pancreas. The superior mesenteric vein courses in a sagittal plane.

12. a. The arrow is identifying an anechoic structure located anterior

to the spine, lateral to the inferior vena cava and posterior to the pancreas, left lobe of the liver, superior mesenteric artery, and portosplenic confluence. This is most consistent with the abdominal aorta.

13. c. A hypoechoic mass is identified in the head of the pancreas. An enlarged pancreatic duct anterior to the splenic vein is also identified. Based on this clinical history, the sonographic findings are most suspicious for a malignant neoplasm.

14. c. An anechoic tubular structure is identified anterior to the splenic vein within the body of the pancreas. This is **most likely** a dilated pancreatic duct secondary to compression from the neoplasm. A tortuous splenic artery is a **possible** consideration. Doppler imaging would help differentiate between a vascular or nonvascular structure. Prior to color Doppler imaging, anatomical landmarks and real-time imaging were used to differentiate between a vascular and nonvascular structure.

15. a. A pseudocyst is **most often** located in the lesser sac followed by the anterior pararenal space. Since it does not contain a lining membrane, it will conform to the surrounding space(s).

16. c. Lipase is an enzyme responsible for changing fats into fatty acids and glycerol. Amylase is an enzyme that breaks down carbohydrates. Tryspin is an enzyme that breaks down proteins into amino acids. Gastrin and secretin are hormones.

17. d. The pancreas lies in a transverse oblique plane with the tail portion located most superiorly and the uncinate process most inferiorly. The body is considered the most anterior portion of the pancreas.

18. c. A congenital anomaly, ectopic pancreatic tissue may be located in the stomach, duodenum, or small or large intestines.

19. a. The pancreas and surrounding vascular landmarks should be examined from the level of the celiac axis (superior to the pancreas) to below the renal veins (inferior to the pancreas).

20. e. Microcystic cystadenomas account for 50% of cystic neoplasms involving the pancreas with the

majority located in the body or tail. It generally appears as a echogenic or complex mass due to multiple small cystic structures.

21. a. Pancreatic enzymes, amylase and lipase, are associated with acute pancreatitis. Amylase and lipase rise a similar rate, but the elevation in lipase persists for a longer period of time. Alkaline phosphatase and bilirubin are associated with biliary obstruction.

22. b. The pancreatic duct is routinely visualized in the body of the pancreas. A tortuous splenic artery may be mistaken as the pancreatic duct. The common bile duct is visualized in the posterior lateral portion of the pancreatic head.

23. a. Ninety percent of nonfunctioning islet cell tumors are malignant and appear as a small, well-defined hypoechoic mass. Islet cell tumors are most commonly located in the tail or body of the pancreas. A nonfunctioning tumor would not be related to insulin levels.

24. e. Sonographic findings associated with chronic pancreatitis include: atrophy, hyperechoic parenchyma, calcifications, irregular borders, and/or pseudocyst formation.

25. d. Clinical findings associated with pancreatic carcinoma may include: weight loss, severe back pain, abdominal pain, painless jaundice, or new onset of diabetes. Abdominal bloating, lower extremity edema, and chest pain are not commonly associated with pancreatic carcinoma.

26. d. The sonogram demonstrates a small, well-defined mass in the tail of the pancreas. History of elevating insulin levels and a solid tumor in the tail of the pancreas is most suspicious for a functioning islet cell tumor (insulinoma). Adenocarcinoma and focal pancreatitis are differential considerations but not as likely a diagnosis with a clinical history of elevating insulin levels.

27. c. Arrow **A** is identifying a circular anechoic structure in the anterior lateral portion of the pancreatic head. This is most likely the gastroduodenal artery, a branch of the common hepatic artery. Pancreatic cysts are not a common finding.

28. a. Arrow **B** is identifying a circular anechoic structure in the posterior lateral portion of the pancreatic head. This is most likely the common bile duct.

29. **c.** Endocrine functions of the pancreas include secretion of insulin, glucagon, and somatostatin. Exocrine functions include: secretion of enzymes (amylase, lipase, and tryspin) and the release of hormones (cholecystokinin, gastrin, and secretin).

30. **b.** The celiac axis is the first branch of the abdominal aorta located superior to the pancreas. The splenic vein and superior mesenteric artery are used as landmarks for locating the body of the pancreas. The pancreas should be evaluated from the celiac axis (superior to the pancreas) to below the renal veins (inferior to the pancreas).

31. **c.** The tail of the pancreas **generally** extends toward the splenic hilum and **occasionally** extends toward the left renal hilum.

32. **d.** The splenic vein is a vascular landmark used for locating the tail of the pancreas. The tail of the pancreas courses parallel with the splenic vein.

33. **b.** The diameter of a normal pancreatic duct in the head/neck region should not exceed 3 mm. The normal diameter in the body should not exceed 2 mm. The hyperechoic walls should also appear smooth coursing parallel with each other.

34. **b.** Acinar cells are responsible for the secretion of highly digestive pancreatic enzymes via the pancreatic duct. Alpha and beta cells are hormones secreted by the islet cells of Langerhans directly into the bloodstream.

35. **c.** The neck is located between the body and head of the pancreas directly anterior to the superior mesenteric vein and porto-splenic confluence. The celiac axis is located superior to the pancreas. The uncinate process lies directly posterior to the superior mesenteric vein.

36. **a.** The head is involved in 75% of cases of malignant neoplasms involving the pancreas, while 20% involve the body.

37. **a.** Islet cell tumors are more commonly located in the body and tail of the pancreas. Adenocarcinoma most commonly involves the pancreatic head.

38. **c.** The duct of Santorini is the secondary secretory duct of the pancreas. The duct of Wirsung is the primary secretory duct of the pancreas.

39. **c.** Elevation in serum lipase may be reported in cases of pancreatitis, cirrhosis, obstruction of the pancreatic duct, acute cholecystitis, or severe renal disease.

40. **d.** The superior mesenteric vein (SMV) is identified by the letter **D**. The SMV courses parallel with the superior mesenteric artery (B) and the aorta (A).

41. **e.** The body of the pancreas is identified by the letter **E**. The body of the pancreas lies anterior to the SMV and posterior to the left lobe of the liver (C).

42. **c.** The left lobe of the liver is identified by the letter **C**. The left lobe of the liver lies anterior and lateral to the pancreas (E) and SMV (D).

43. **e.** The vascular structure is a common sonographic landmark used in locating the pancreas. The hyperechoic echoes surrounding this vessel and location are characteristic of the superior mesenteric artery.

44. **c.** The vascular structure is located in the hepatic hilum consistent with the main portal vein. The hepatic veins converge on the inferior vena cava.

45. **a.** The majority of cystadenomas involving the pancreas are located in the body and tail.

46. **c.** The body is the largest and most anterior section of the pancreas. The tail lies most superior.

47. **d.** Lack of gallstones is not among preoperative criteria in a pancreatoduodenectomy. The gallbladder, if present, is removed during surgery. Preoperative criteria include absence of extra pancreatic metastasis, patency of the portal, splenic, and superior mesenteric veins, and patency of the celiac axis and superior mesenteric artery.

48. **d.** Rapid progression of pancreatic inflammation describes a phlegmon. A phlegmon may cause necrosis or hemorrhage and is considered a complication of acute pancreatitis.

49. **c.** The sphincter of Oddi is a sheath of muscle fibers surrounding the distal common bile and pancre-

atic ducts as they cross the wall of the duodenum through the ampulla of Vater.

50. **c.** Leakage of pancreatic enzymes into the surrounding peritoneal space describes a pseudocyst. Phlegmon is an extension of pancreatic inflammation into the surrounding tissues. Seromas contain serous fluid while bilomas contain bile. Abscess is a collection of a purulent substance.

Chapter 10: Urinary System

1. **a.** The medullary pyramids commonly appear anechoic in the neonate. The renal cortex generally appears moderate to highly echogenic. A sparse amount of perinephric fat makes it difficult to distinguish the renal capsule or the renal sinus.

2. **c.** A decrease in BUN is associated with liver failure, overhydration, pregnancy, smoking, and decreases in protein intake.

3. **b.** The renal arteries arise from the posterior lateral aspect of the abdominal aorta. The celiac axis and gonadal, superior, and inferior mesenteric arteries arise from the anterior aspect of the abdominal aorta.

4. **b.** The basic functional unit of the kidney is the nephron. The glomerulus is a structure composed of blood vessels or nerve filters. Loop of Henle is the "U"-shaped portion of a renal tubule. Collecting tubules funnel urine into the renal pelvis.

5. **e.** The quadratus lumborum is a muscle of the posterior abdominal wall located posterior and medial to each kidney. The transversus abdominus muscle is located in the anterolateral wall.

6. **b.** A variant of the horseshoe kidney, a cake or lump kidney demonstrates fusion of the medial aspects of both kidneys. Fusion of the both kidneys within the same quadrant in the body describes crossed fused ectopia. Fusion of the superior pole of one kidney to the inferior pole of the contralateral kidney is termed a sigmoid or "S"-shaped kidney.

7. **e.** A hypertrophied column of Bertin extends from the cortex into the medullary pyramids. This anatomical variant may mimic a renal

duplication. Fetal lobulation and dromedary hump are variants associated with the outer renal contour. Congenital variation in the fusion of the superior and inferior poles of the kidney is termed a junctional fold defect. It is identified on sonography as a triangular hyperechoic focus in the anterior aspect of the kidney.

8. d. Synthesis of amino acids is considered a function of the liver. Renal functions include: the production of urine and erythroprotein; influences blood pressure; regulate serum electrolytes and regulate the acid/base balance.

9. a. Fifty percent of patients over 55 years of age demonstrate a simple renal cyst.

10. c. A resistive index (RI) of 0.7 or less is considered within normal limits. Rejection of a renal transplant is suggested once the RI reaches 0.9.

11. d. A circular anechoic structure is identified in the urinary bladder. In a catheterized patient this structure most likely represents the balloon of the catheter surrounded by a thick bladder wall. A ureterocele is a possible differential consideration but not as likely as a catheter balloon. Residual urine is not typically circular in shape or demonstrated in catheterized patients. A bladder diverticulum is defined as an out-pouching of the bladder wall. A urachal sinus connects the apex of the urinary bladder with the umbilicus.

12. c. Anechoic appearance of the medullary pyramids is a normal sonographic finding in a neonatal kidney and may be mistaken for hydronephrosis. Arcuate vessels are peripherally located. A hyperechoic appearance to the kidneys is typically seen with infantile polycystic disease.

13. e. Dilatation of the renal calyces is identified. This is most suspicious for moderate hydronephrosis. Pyelonephritis may demonstrate prominent medullary pyramids. Nephrolithiasis is a possible cause for the hydronephrosis but would appear as a hyperechoic focus. Medullary sponge kidney demonstrates hyperechoic foci in the region of the renal papillae. Polycystic disease consists of multiple parenchymal cysts.

14. c. Obstruction of the urinary tract is the most common cause of hydronephrosis. The cause of the obstruction will vary (i.e., congenital anomaly). Urinary stasis is a predisposing factor for developing a urinary tract infection.

15. d. The sonogram demonstrates an irregular contour to the urinary bladder. An anechoic outward pedunculation in the wall is identified. This is most consistent with a bladder diverticulum. An ovarian cyst may be mistaken as a bladder diverticulum. A dilated ureter is a possible differential, but one would expect to visualize a tapered and longer dilated segment. The urethra is a midline structure and the sonogram is imaged to the right of midline. Ureterocele is a bladder abnormality within the bladder at the ureteric orifice.

16. e. The glomerulus is composed of blood vessels or nerve fibers. The nephron is the basic functional unit of the kidney. Loop of Henle is a portion of the renal tubule. The renal pyramids contain tubules and loops of Henle.

17. a. Renal colic describes sharp, severe flank pain that radiates to the groin. It is considered a clinical symptom of nephrolithiasis. Dysuria and dyspareunia describe painful urination and intercourse, respectively. A positive McBurney's sign describes rebound pain in the area of the appendix. Mittelsmirtz is a termed used to describe pain during ovulation.

18. d. Contained within the renal **sinus** is the major and minor calyces, peripelvic fat, fibrous tissues, segmental arteries, segmental veins, lymphatics, and part of the renal pelvis. The renal artery, renal vein, and ureter are located in the renal **hilum**. **Perinephric** fat surrounds the kidney.

19. e. The transversus abdominus muscle is located lateral to each kidney. The psoas muscle lies posterior to the inferior pole of the kidney. The quadratus lumborum muscle lies posterior and medial to the kidney. The rectus abdominus and internal oblique muscle are portions of the anterior abdominal wall.

20. d. A hyperechoic focus located in the **anterior** renal cortex **most likely** represents a junction parenchymal defect. Renal calculus is a possible differential **but not the most likely** consideration. Ischemic necrosis and renal carcinoma may appear hyperechoic but would likely produce symptoms. An adenoma generally appears as a well-defined hypoechoic mass.

21. b. Postvoid urine volume will vary from case to case but should not exceed 20 cc to be considered within normal limits.

22. d. Generalized swelling of the kidney characterized by well-defined (prominent) renal pyramids is most consistent with pyelonephritis.

23. b. Renal biopsy procedures are generally performed with patients lying on their stomachs in the prone position. A pillow, sponge, or towels may be placed under the abdomen.

24. b. Ureteric orifices appear as small echogenic protuberances located on the posterior aspect of the urinary bladder on ultrasound. Hydroureters, bladder diverticulums, and arcuate vessels generally appear anechoic on ultrasound.

25. a. Clinical findings associated with acute glomerulonephritis may include: proteinuria, hematuria, fatigue, edema, and decreased urine output.

26. e. An isoechoic mass extends from the renal cortex into the medullary pyramids. This is most consistent with a hypertrophied column of Bertin. This anatomical variant may be mistaken for a renal duplication or neoplasm. Dromedary hump and fetal lobulation affect the outer contour of the kidney. Junctional parenchymal defect appears as a small triangular hyperechoic mass on ultrasound. Cross fused ectopia is a congenital anomaly.

27. b. Perinephric fat varies with each patient. Morbidly obese patients commonly demonstrate an increased amount of perinephric fat. The area in question is separate from the liver and kidney. An adrenal adenoma appears as a hypoechoic mass.

28. d. A mass is identified in the lateral aspect of the right kidney. A clinical history of painless hematuria and uncontrolled hypertension combined with a renal mass is **most** suspicious for renal carcinoma. Dromedary hump is a possible differential but not the most likely diagnosis with this clinical history, Angiomyolipoma may demonstrate gross hematuria but appears on ultrasound as a hyperechoic mass. A hematoma or hemorrhagic cyst would not demonstrate internal blood flow.

29. **d.** The hyperechoic septation seen within the bladder in located in the region of the ureteric orifice. This is most consistent with an ureterocele. Ureteral jets are intermittent and demonstrate linear motion into the bladder at the ureteric orifices. Catheter balloon is not intermittent. Urachal cyst is located near the apex of the bladder. A diverticulum is an outward pedunculation of the urinary bladder.

30. **d.** Parapelvic cysts are located **beside** the renal pelvis. A parapelvic cyst may obstruct the kidney. Peripelvic cysts are located **around** the renal pelvis. The renal pelvis **extrudes** from the renal hilum with an extrarenal pelvis. Neither a hydroureter nor hydronephrosis is identified in this sonogram.

31. **d.** Predisposing factors for developing a Wilm's tumor include: hemihypertrophy, sporadic aniridia, omphalocele, male prevalence, 5 years of age or less, and Beckwith-Weidemann syndrome.

32. **e.** Angiomyolipoma is a benign tumor composed of blood vessels **(angio)**, muscle **(myo)**, and fat **(lipoma).**

33. **a.** Fibromuscular hyperplasia is associated with stenosis in the mid to distal portion of the main renal artery. The abdominal aorta is not a renal artery.

34. **c.** A peak systolic velocity exceeding 180 cm/sec suggests the possibility of renal artery stenosis.

35. **d.** Painless hematuria is **most** likely associated with renal cell carcinoma or transitional cell carcinoma of the urinary bladder. Careful evaluation of the urinary tract is warranted with this finding. An angiomyolipoma may cause hematuria but is not the **most likely** condition associated with painless hematuria.

36. **b.** Nephrolithiasis is a condition most frequently associated with urinary stasis. Chronic renal failure is more frequently associated with an inflammatory or vascular condition than urinary stasis from chronic hydronephrosis. **Peri**pelvic cysts may develop from an obstruction. Medullary sponge kidney is a congenital condition.

37. **d.** Sigmoid kidney or S-shaped kidney is a variant of the horseshoe kidney. This congenital anomaly presents as a fusion of the superior pole of one kidney with the inferior pole of the contralateral kidney. Fusion of the medial surfaces of both kidneys describes a cake kidney. Crossed fused ectopia demonstrates fused kidneys located in the same body quadrant.

38. **d.** Aneurysms involving the renal artery are at an increased risk of rupturing once the diameter exceeds 2.0 cm. An aneurysm is identified once the diameter of the artery reaches 1.5 cm or doubles in size.

39. **c.** Renal failure is defined as the complete inability of the kidneys to excrete waste, concentrate urine, and conserve electrolytes. Renal insufficiency is defined as partial kidney function failure characterized by less than normal urine output. Renal colic is a clinical symptom associated with passage of a renal calculus. Renal pstosis describes an unusually mobile kidney. Renal obstruction may be a predisposing factor of renal failure.

40. **b.** Evenly spaced hyperechoic foci are identified in the papillary region of the medullary pyramids. This is most characteristic of a medullary sponge kidney. Metastatic disease is more likely to demonstrate hyper- and hypoechoic mass(es) within the renal parenchyma. Angiomyolipomas are located in the renal cortex. Chronic renal failure is characterized by small hyperechoic kidneys with thinning of the renal cortex. Glomerulonephritis is characterized by enlarged kidney(s) demonstrating a hyperechoic renal cortex.

41. **d.** The superior pole of the left kidney is fused to the inferior pole of the right kidney consistent with a sigmoid or S-shaped kidney. Fusion of the medial aspect of both kidneys is termed a cake or lump kidney. Duplication involves two distinct collecting systems within one kidney. Dromedary hump is an anatomical variant of the lateral cortex.

42. **d.** A tubular structure extends from the apex of the bladder to the umbilicus. The sonographic and clinical findings in this case are most consistent with an urachal sinus. The patient denies a history of fever or abdominal trauma to substantiate an umbilical abscess or rectus abdominus hematoma as the most likely diagnosis. Meckel's diverticulum is an anomalous sac protruding from the ileum. An umbilical hernia demonstrates a disruption in the peritoneal cavity into the umbilicus.

43. **c.** A hyperechoic enlarged kidney with a history of proteinuria is most suspicious for glomerulonephritis. Enlargement of the kidney(s) is not a typical finding in chronic renal failure or renal sinus lipomatosis. Pyelonephritis may demonstrate renal enlargement but does not increase the echogenicity of the renal parenchyma. Medullary sponge kidney is characterized by hyperechoic foci in the region of the renal papillae.

44. **d.** Multiple small cysts are located throughout the right kidney, decreasing identification of the renal parenchyma. These findings are most suspicious for polycystic renal disease. Multiple simple renal cysts are not commonly visualized in a 40-year-old patient. The cystic areas demonstrated in this sonogram do not appear to involve the renal calyces or renal pelvis found with hydronephrosis. A nephroblastoma demonstrates as a solid, well-defined renal mass on ultrasound. Renal sinus lipomatosis demonstrates an increase in the echogenicity of the renal sinus.

45. **c.** A solid mass demonstrating internal blood flow is demonstrated in an elderly patient's urinary bladder. This is most suspicious for bladder malignancy.

46. **c.** When encountering a mass within the urinary bladder, the sonographer should ask the patient whether he or she has noticed any blood in the urine (hematuria).

Painless hematuria is a common clinical indication in bladder carcinoma.

47. **b.** Motion in the area of the right ureteric orifice is most suspicious for a ureteral jet.

48. **e.** Complications following a renal transplant may include abscess formation, lymphocele, hematoma, urioma, renal artery stenosis, and renal vein thrombosis. Formation of a parapelvic cyst is not considered a complication following renal transplant surgery.

49. **d.** Vessels located near the corical periphery are most likely arcuate vessels. Without spectral analysis it is difficult to evaluate whether these are arcuate arteries or veins or both.

50. **c.** The normal renal cortex measures a minimum of 1.0 cm. Thinning of the renal cortex raises suspicion of chronic renal disease.

Chapter 11: Spleen

1. **d.** Accessory spleens are commonly located medial to the splenic hilum. The tail of the pancreas may extend toward the splenic or left renal hilum.

2. **e.** The spleen is responsible for the destruction of old red blood cells. Red blood cells are removed and hemoglobin is recycled. Other functions include: storage and filtering of the blood along with production of antibodies and lymphocytes.

3. **b.** Splenomegaly may be associated with **hyper**tension, diabetes mellitus, cirrhosis, portal hypertension, congestive heart failure, portal vein thrombosis, hepatitis, trauma, or hemolytic anemia.

4. **d.** The cavernous hemangioma is the **most common benign neoplasm** of the spleen. Cysts and cystadenomas involving the spleen are uncommon findings. An accessory spleen is considered a congenital anomaly. Hematomas are not considered neoplasms.

5. **c.** Hematocrit is the percentage of red blood cells in the blood. Hemoglobin is the oxygen-carrying pigment of the red blood cell. Platelets are formed in the bone marrow and some are stored in the spleen.

6. **a.** Anemia is the **most** common clinical finding associated with a hemangiosarcoma involving the spleen. Other symptoms may include: left upper quadrant pain, weight loss, and leukocystosis.

7. **c.** Metastasis to the spleen is rare. Metastatic disease involving the spleen most commonly originates from melanoma. Other primary neoplasms metastasizing to the spleen may arise from the pancreas, breast, or lung.

8. **b.** Patients with a history of multiple splenic infections is at an increased risk for developing candidiasis. This condition is most commonly found in auto-immune–compromised patients. An embolism originating from the heart is the most common cause of splenic infarction. Calcifications in the spleen are more commonly caused by granulomatosis or infarction. Formation of an arterial aneurysm is not a complication of multiple infections.

9. **c.** The normal adult spleen measures approximately 10-12 cm in length; 7 cm in width; 3-4 cm in height (AP).

10. **a.** Hemangiosarcoma is a rare primary malignant neoplasm of the spleen that frequently metastasizes to the liver.

11. **b.** Alcohol abuse is associated with cirrhosis. Chronic insult to the liver cells leads to a decrease in liver function leading to splenomegaly. This sonogram demonstrates an enlarged spleen measuring 19.4 cm in length (normal ≤13 cm in length). Lymphoma may demonstrate splenomegaly but is **not the most likely** differential in this case.

12. **b.** Splenomegaly in a patient with **a long history of alcohol abuse** should be evaluated for liver disease.

13. **d.** A smooth, solid mass is identified medial to the spleen and left kidney. This mass demonstrates an echo pattern similar to the spleen (isoechoic). These sonographic findings are most consistent with an accessory spleen. An enlarged lymph node appears as an oval-shaped hypoechoic mass with a prominent hyperechoic fatty center.

14. **a.** A round anechoic mass is located in the superior medial portion of the spleen. Smooth, thin wall margins are identified along with posterior acoustic enhancement. This is most consistent with a splenic cyst. Hematoma or abscess formation is an unlikely consideration for an incidental finding in an asymptomatic patient. Cystic lymphangioma demonstrates a multilocular cystic mass appearance. Cavernous hemangiomas most commonly appear as hyperechoic or complex masses.

15. **b.** Formation of a splenic abscess is most commonly associated with infective endocarditis. Infarction of the spleen may be caused by emboli from the heart, subacute bacterial endocarditis, leukemia, sickle cell anemia, metastasis, or pancreatitis. Parenchymal calcifications may be related to granulomatosis or infarction. Hematomas are generally associated with trauma. Harmartomas are composed of lymphatic tissue.

16. **d.** The spleen is an intraperitoneal structure located lateral to the pancreas, anterior to the left kidney, inferior to the left hemidiaphragm, and lateral to the stomach and left adrenal gland.

17. **d.** Factors associated with an increase risk for developing an aneurysm of the splenic artery include: female prevalence, trauma, atherosclerosis, infection, and portal hypertension.

18. **d.** Polysplenia is associated with multiple small spleens, two left lungs, and congenital anomalies of the gastrointestinal tract, cardiovascular and biliary systems. Aplasia is described as the failure of the spleen to develop. Asplenia syndrome is associated with two right lungs, gastrointestinal and urinary anomalies, and a midline placement of the liver. Accessory spleen and wandering spleen are not associated with additional anomalies.

19. **b.** The celiac axis (trunk) is the first branch of the abdominal aorta. The celiac axis trifurcates into the splenic, left gastric, and common hepatic arteries. Branches of the superior mesenteric artery supply the head of the pancreas and portions of the small and large intestine.

20. **d.** Normal splenic tissue may appear hypoechoic or isoechoic when compared with the normal liver parenchyma.

21. **c.** Hyperechoic foci within the parenchyma are **most** suspicious for splenic calcifications. Calcifications are generally an incidental finding commonly associated with granulomatosis. Other etiologies may include splenic infarction, calcified cyst, or abscesses. Pneumobilia is associated with air in the biliary tree.

22. **b.** Splenic calcifications are generally an incidental finding. Follow-up is typically recommended only if clinically indicated. Splenic calcifications are most commonly associated with granulomatosis or in response to infection.

23. **b.** A cystic mass in a patient with a history of abdominal trauma most likely represents a intraparenchymal hematoma. Pseudocyst formation is a complication of acute pancreatitis. A loculated abscess is an unlikely diagnosis in an afebrile patient. Lymphoma and polycystic disease are unlikely considerations in a 13-year-old patient.

24. **d.** Cavernous hemangiomas are common benign masses that may develop in the splenic parenchyma. Hemangiomas are the most common benign solid mass and the most likely diagnosis of this hyperechoic intraparenchymal mass. Lipoma is a differential consideration but not a common finding within the splenic parenchyma. Calcification of a splenic vessel in a middle-age patient is an unlikely consideration. Primary malignancy of the spleen and abscess formation are unlikely considerations in an asymptomatic patient.

25. **c.** In a patient with a history of leukemia, the parenchymal nodules most likely represent primary malignant tumors. Leukemia may demonstrate hypoechoic or hyperechoic splenic masses on ultrasound. The nodules are within the splenic parenchyma inconsistent with lymphadenopathy. Metastatic disease to the spleen most commonly originates from melanoma or malignancy of the breast, lung, or pancreas. Candidiasis and multiple splenic abscesses is unlikely in an afebrile patient.

26. **d.** Hemoglobin carries carbon dioxide from the cells back to the lungs. Platelets are essential for the coagulation of blood and the maintenance of hemostasis. Hematocrit is the percentage of red blood cells in the blood. Lymphocytes and leukocytes are associated with infection.

27. **c.** Leukemia is associated with a proliferation of white blood cell (leukocytosis) Other symptoms may include: lymphadenopathy, palpable spleen, joint pain, weakness, and fever.

28. **d.** Elevation in the serum amylase is an indication for an ultrasound of the pancreas or biliary system. Indications for an ultrasound of the spleen may include: chronic liver disease, infection, leukocytosis, leukopenia, abdominal or left upper quadrant mass, fatigue, leukemia, lymphoma, or trauma.

29. **b.** Granulomatosis is defined as an abnormal increase in the total number of granulocytes in the blood. Granulomatosis occurs in response to infection. Calcifications within the splenic parenchyma are associated with granulomatosis.

30. **c.** Splenomegaly is the most common sonographic finding associated with portal hypertension. Other findings may include hepatomegaly, diameter enlargement of the main portal, splenic, and/or superior mesenteric veins, development of portosplenic collaterals, and changes in the flow or direction pattern of the portal circulation.

31. **e.** Leukocytosis is **defined** as a white blood count **above** 20,000. Normal serum levels range between 4,500 and 11,000 mm^3.

32. **d.** A subcapsular hematoma is located between the splenic capsule and parenchyma. It most commonly appears on ultrasound as a crescent-shaped fluid collection inferior to the diaphragm.

33. **a.** Splenic candidiasis and metastatic lesions most commonly demonstrate a "wheel within a wheel" or target pattern on ultrasound. A cavernous hemangioma or hemangiosarcoma generally appears on ultrasound as a hyperechoic or complex mass. Infarction may appear hypoechoic when acute or hyperechoic in chronic cases. Cystic lymphangiomatosis demonstrates as a multiloculated cystic mass.

34. **a.** An embolism originating in the heart is the most common source of a splenic infarction. Thrombus extending from the lower extremity is the most common etiology of a pulmonary embolism.

35. **b.** Elevation in hematocrit may be related to infection, dehydration, shock, and polycythemia vera. Decreases are associated with hemorrhage, anemia, and leukemia.

36. **a.** Arrow **A** is identifying the superior medial portion of the spleen.

37. **c.** Arrow **B** is identifying the mid portion of the spleen known as the splenic hilum.

38. **b.** Arrow **C** is identifying the inferior lateral portion of the spleen.

39. **e.** The sonogram demonstrates the length of the left kidney. The spleen and kidney lie closest to the transducer footprint, and the spinous processes lie furthest from the transducer footprint. These findings are most consistent with a coronal plane. There are three basic scanning **planes:** sagittal, transverse, and coronal.

40. **a.** Anechoic free fluid is identified inferior to the diaphragm and superior to the spleen as well as inferior to the spleen. These sonographic findings are most suspicious for ascites.

41. **d.** The possibility of internal hemorrhage is a concern for the emergency department physician in cases involving trauma. Ultrasound is a portable imaging tool used to quickly evaluate the abdominal and pelvic cavity for hemoperitoneum.

42. **b.** To decrease venous pressure in portal hypertension, the splenic vein will **most** likely shunt blood directly into the left renal vein. The gastric vein is also considered a porto-splenic collateral but is not the most likely bypass for an engorged splenic vein.

43. **d.** The main portal vein is formed at the junction of the splenic and superior mesenteric veins.

44. **a.** Leukopenia is defined as a white blood count below 4,000 mm^3. Normal serum levels range between 4,500 and 11,000 mm^3.

45. **d.** The spleen is a major destruction site of old red blood cells. The red blood cells are removed and the hemoglobin is recycled into iron.

46. **b.** A decrease in leukocytes may be associated with lymphoma, viral infections, and diabetes mellitus.

Leukemia is usually related to a proliferation in white blood cells. Anemia is defined as a decrease in hemoglobin levels.

47. **c.** Normal hemoglobin levels vary between males and females but should not exceed 20 g/dL. Hemoglobin is developed in the bone marrow and is the oxygen-carrying pigment in the blood.

48. **c.** In adults, splenomegaly is suggested once the length of the spleen exceeds 13 cm. The normal spleen measures approximately 10 to 12 cm in length, 7 cm in width, and 4 cm in height.

49. **b.** Accessory spleens are rarely a source of a patient's clinical symptoms. They are considered an incidental finding.

50. **d.** A harmatoma is a benign neoplasm composed of lymphoid tissue. A lipoma is composed of fatty tissue. An adenoma is an epithelial neoplasm. A seroma is composed of serous fluid and a cavernous hemangioma is a benign tumor consisting of a mass of blood vessels.

Chapter 12: Retroperitoneum

1. **d.** Glucocorticoids (cortisol) modify the body's response to inflammation. Androgens are gonadal hormones. Aldosterone helps maintain the body's fluid and electrolyte balance. Norepinephrine modifies blood pressure. Epinephrine increases in times of excitement or emotional stress.

2. **d.** Rhabdomyosarcoma is a highly malignant neoplasm derived from striated muscle. Leiomyosarcoma contains smooth muscle. Pheochromocytoma is a rare vascular tumor of the adrenal medulla. Myxoma and mesothelioma are benign retroperitoneal neoplasms.

3. **d.** The inferior vena cava is located within the perirenal space. The anterior pararenal space is located between the posterior peritoneum and Gerota's fascia. Structures located within the anterior pararenal space include: pancreas, descending portion of the duodenum, ascending and descending colon, superior mesenteric vessels, and inferior portion of the common bile duct.

4. **a.** Hyperplasia of both adrenal glands is associated with hyperaldosteronism. Conn's syndrome involves a benign tumor of a single adrenal gland. Adrenal hemorrhage or surgical removal of both adrenal glands is associated with Addison's syndrome. Cushing's disease may be caused by an adrenal mass. Bouvenet's syndrome involves paroxysmal tachycardia.

5. **d.** Lymph nodes filter the lymph of debris and organisms. Lymphocytes and antibodies are produced in response to an infection. Glucocorticoids modify the body's response to inflammation. Aldosterone regulates sodium and water levels, which affects blood volume and pressure.

6. **b.** Severe anxiety is a symptom associated with pheochromocytoma (vascular tumor of the adrenal medulla). Symptoms associated with adrenocortical carcinoma include: hypertension, weakness, weight loss, abdominal pain, and weakening of the bones.

7. **d.** Renal function is an indication for an ultrasound of the genitourinary system. Indications for an ultrasound of the adrenal glands include: tachycardia, severe anxiety, hypertension, abdominal distention, sweating, weight loss, diabetes mellitus, and evaluation of a mass demonstrated on a previous medical imaging study.

8. **b.** Liposarcomas and fibrosarcomas are malignant neoplasms likely to infiltrate surrounding structures and tissues.

9. **c.** An urinoma is most likely to develop in the perinephric space. An urinoma is defined as a urine-filled cystic mass adjacent to or within the urinary tract.

10. **a.** Liposarcoma is the most common neoplasm located in the retroperitoneum.

11. **e.** The superior suprarenal artery arises from the inferior phrenic artery. The middle suprarenal artery arises from the aorta, and the inferior suprarenal artery arises from the renal artery. The medulla comprises 10% of the gland. The right suprarenal vein drains directly into the IVC. Gonadal hormones are secreted by the cortex, and norepinephrine is secreted by the medulla.

12. **b.** The anterior pararenal space is located between the posterior peritoneum and Gerota's fascia. While the anterior pararenal space does lie between the anterior abdominal wall and the psoas muscle, this is **not the best** choice in defining the most accurate location.

13. **d.** Neuroblastoma is an adrenal neoplasm most commonly found in young children. Wilms' tumor (nephroblastoma) is a malignant tumor of the kidney. Liposarcoma is the most common retroperitoneal neoplasm. Pheochromocytoma is a vascular tumor of the adrenal medulla.

14. **c.** The posterior parietal peritoneum forms the anterior border of the retroperitoneum. The diaphragm and pelvic rim form the superior and inferior borders of the retroperitoneum respectively. The posterior abdominal wall muscles form the posterior border and the transversalis fascia defines the lateral border of the retroperitoneum.

15. **d.** Structures located within the perirenal space include: kidneys, adrenal glands, perinephric fat, ureters, renal vessels, aorta, and inferior vena cava. The psoas muscles are located in the posterior pararenal space.

16. **e.** Etiologies of a retroperitoneal hemorrhage may include: aneurysm rupture, trauma, neoplasm, and infarction. Internal hemorrhage is not generally related to the formation of a retroperitoneal abscess.

17. **b.** Pheochromocytoma is a rare vascular tumor of the adrenal medulla. It is associated with hypertension, sweating, tachycardia, chest or epigastric pain, headache, palpitations, severe anxiety, and elevation in epinephrine and norepinephrine levels.

18. **d.** Visceral lymph nodes are located in the peritoneum and course along the vessels supplying the major organs. Parietal nodes are located in the retroperitoneum and course along the prevertebral vessels. The perineum supports and surrounds the urogenital area of the body. The adrenal glands are retroperitoneal structures.

19. **b.** The adrenal glands are located anterior, medial, and superior to the

kidneys. The **right adrenal gland** is located posterior and lateral to the IVC.

20. **d.** Clinical findings in Addison's disease may include: elevation in serum potassium, decrease in serum sodium and glucose, anorexia, chronic fatigue, dehydration, bronze skin pigmentation, hypotension, gastrointestinal disorders and emotional changes. Cushing's disease and hyperaldosteronism may demonstrate a decrease in serum potassium.

21. **c.** Risk factors associated with development of an adrenal adenoma include diabetes mellitus, obesity, hypertension and the elderly population.

22. **d.** Lymphadenopathy surrounding the aorta gives the appearance the aorta is "floating." This is termed the "floating aorta sign."

23. **a.** An adrenal cyst is a rare, benign, and generally unilateral condition. Patients may present with hypertension but are generally asymptomatic. Proliferation of adrenal cells is demonstrated in cases of adrenal hyperplasia.

24. **b.** The adrenal medulla secretes epinephrine and norepinephrine hormones. The adrenal cortex secretes cortisol, androgens, estrogens, progesterone, and aldosterone.

25. **b.** Addison disease is caused by complete or partial failure of the adrenocortical function. Also known as adrenocortical insufficiency. Overproduction of cortisol is found in Cushing disease. Conn syndrome may cause hyperaldosteronism. Budd-Chiari syndrome and Graves disease involve the liver and thyroid gland, respectively.

26. **d.** The adrenal glands are prominent in the neonate demonstrating a hypoechoic outer cortex and a central hyperechoic medulla. The arrow is identifying the normal medulla. An adrenal hemorrhage may occur following a traumatic or hypoxic birth. Hemorrhage general appears as a cystic adrenal mass.

27. **a.** Based on the clinical history, the anechoic structure is most suspicious for an adrenal cyst. An adrenal cyst may cause hypertension. A pheochromocytoma may cause hypertension but generally pre-

sents as a solid homogenous mass. Liver cysts are not linked to hypertension. A retroperitoneal hemorrhage generally demonstrates as a hypoechoic mass on ultrasound and is not likely to cause hypertension. An adenoma is a solid neoplasm.

28. **c.** An adrenal cyst is considered a rare finding. A cyst in the liver is generally an incidental finding. Hemorrhage may result from trauma. An adrenal adenoma is a benign cortical neoplasm. Pheochromocytoma is considered a rare vascular tumor of the adrenal medulla.

29. **c.** Hypoechoic masses are identified in the para-aortic region. Clinical history includes a history of weight loss, back pain, and elevated alkaline phosphatase. These symptoms are suspicious for a malignancy of the pancreas. Lymphadenopathy is the most likely consideration for the hypoechoic masses. Retroperitoneal fibrosis could be a differential consideration, although not as likely with this clinical history. Liposarcoma is the most common neoplasm of the retroperitoneum but demonstrates as a hyperechoic lesion. Lymphoceles are generally related to a recent surgery. Pseudomyxoma peritonei is found in the peritoneum.

30. **c.** Hydronephrosis is the most likely complication of retroperitoneal fibrosis. Fibrotic masses may place pressure on the ureter(s), ultimately causing an obstruction. Aneurysms are caused by a weakening in the arterial walls.

31. **c.** A enlarged lymph node demonstrating a normal oval shape and smooth wall margins is most consistent with an underlying infection. A round shape or irregular margins is suspicious for an underlying malignancy.

32. **d.** An urinoma develops in the first few weeks after renal transplant surgery. It demonstrates a rapid increase in size on serial examinations.

33. **e.** Mesotheliomas are caused by an abnormal growth of epithelial cells. A myxoma consists of connective tissue, a lipoma consists of fat, a teratoma consists of different

types of tissue, and leiomyosarcoma is a malignant tumor of the smooth muscle.

34. **c.** Leiomyosarcoma is a malignant neoplasm containing large spindle cells of smooth muscle. Rhabdomyosarcoma is derived from striated muscle. Fibrosarcomas contain fibrous connective tissue and a liposarcoma is a malignant growth of fat cells.

35. **b.** A liposarcoma is a malignant growth of fat. A hyperechoic mass with thick wall margins is the most common sonographic appearance.

36. **d.** Identification of a complex adrenal mass in a neonatal patient, with decreased hematocrit levels, is highly suspicious for an adrenal hemorrhage. There is no mention in the clinical history of a fever or leukocytosis expected with an abscess. Adrenal cysts are rare findings. Adrenal adenomas are more commonly identified in the elderly patient. Adrenocortical carcinoma is an unlikely finding in the neonate.

37. **d.** A complex mass inferior to the spleen and medial to the superior pole of the kidney is suspicious for an adrenal mass. Based on the clinical history, a solid mass of the adrenal gland in a toddler is most suspicious for a neuroblastoma. Nephroblastoma is a renal neoplasm. Adrenal hemorrhage is a possible differential but not the most likely consideration with this clinical history. Splenic rupture and intussusception are unlikely considerations.

38. **d.** An oval-shaped hypoechoic mass with a hyperechoic center is identified in the left groin. This is most likely a prominent lymph node. Lymph nodes are common incidental findings in the groin region. The echo pattern is well defined, which is uncharacteristic of a complex hematoma. A well-defined hyperechoic mass is the most common appearance of both a fibroma and a lipoma. Connection to the femoral artery is not demonstrated in this sonogram, characteristic of a pseudoaneurysm.

39. **e.** The cortex is the outer portion of the adrenal gland, which comprises 90% of the total gland. The medulla, or inner portion, comprises the other 10%.

40. c. The suprarenal glands is another term used to describe the adrenal glands.

41. c. The right suprarenal vein empties directly into the inferior vena cava. The left suprarenal vein drains into the left renal vein.

42. d. Epinephrine is secreted by the adrenal medulla during times of excitement or emotional stress. Also known as adrenaline and "fight or flight" hormone. Norepinephrine and renin affect blood pressure. Cortisol modifies the body's response to infection, surgery, or trauma. Aldosterone helps to maintain the body's fluid and electrolyte balance.

43. a. Sodium is a major component in determining blood volume. Potassium is essential to the normal function of every organ. Vitamin K is related to normal clotting times. Calcium aids in the transportation of nutrients through the cell membranes.

44. c. Predisposing factors of developing an adenoma of the adrenal gland include: obesity, hypertension, diabetes mellitus, and the elderly population.

45. e. Adrenocorticotrophic hormone is produced by the pituitary gland. Insulin is a hormone secreted by the Islet cells of Langerhans. Tryspin is an enzyme produced by the pancreas. Epinephrine and aldosterone are produced by the adrenal glands.

46. a. Producing hormones is a function of the adrenal glands. The release of secretin hormones is an exocrine function of the pancreas. Regulation of serum electrolytes is a function of the kidneys. The release of glycogen as glucose is a function of the liver. The parathyroid glands maintain homeostasis of blood calcium concentrations.

47. e. Pheochromocytoma is a rare vascular tumor of the adrenal gland. Rhabdomyosarcoma is a neoplasm derived from striated muscle.

48. d. The medulla is the inner portion and the cortex is the outer portion of the adrenal glands. The inner lining of a blood vessel composed of a single layer of cells describes the tunica intima. A hilum is described as a recess at the portion of an organ where vessels and nerves enter. A cavity or channel defines a sinus.

49. d. The left adrenal gland is located posterior and medial to the splenic artery. The adrenal glands lie anterior and medial to the superior border of the each kidney. The adrenal glands are located lateral to the aorta. The right adrenal gland lies posterior to the inferior vena cava.

50. b. The **most common** etiology of Cushing's disease is a pituitary mass. Other causes may include: an adrenal mass, polycystic ovarian disease, and an excessive amount of glucocorticoid hormone.

Chapter 13: Abdominal Vasculature

1. b. The diameter of the abdominal aorta must reach a minimum diameter of 3.0 cm to be considered a true abdominal aortic aneurysm. An ectatic aneurysm describes an arterial dilatation that measures larger than a more proximal segment but less than 3.0 cm in diameter.

2. c. A fusiform aneurysm is characterized by a uniform dilatation of the arterial walls. An arterial dilatation characterized by a focal out-pouching of one arterial wall describes a saccular aneurysm. Dilatation of an artery due to damage to one or more layers of the arterial wall defines a pseudoaneurysm. Dilatation of an artery when compared to a more proximal segment describes an ectatic aneurysm.

3. b. The celiac axis is the first **visceral** branch of the abdominal aorta. The celiac artery courses approximately 1 to 3 cm before trifurcating into the splenic, left gastric, and common hepatic arteries. Inferior phrenic arteries are the first parietal branches of the abdominal aorta.

4. e. The left renal vein receives the left suprarenal vein superiorly and the left gonadal vein inferiorly. The coronary vein enters the superior portion of the porto-splenic confluence and the inferior mesenteric vein enters the inferior portion of the porto-splenic confluence.

5. d. The main portal vein bifurcates at the hepatic hilum into the right and left portal veins. The left portal vein subdivides into the medial and lateral left portal veins. The right portal vein subdivides into the anterior and posterior right portal veins.

6. d. Normal compression from the mesentery may cause dilatation of the left renal vein. Renal veins demonstrate a spontaneous phasic flow pattern. The left renal artery is located posterior to the left renal vein. The superior mesenteric artery courses anterior to the left renal vein. The right renal artery courses posterior to the inferior vena cava.

7. e. The head of the pancreas lies anterior to the inferior vena cava. The spine, psoas muscles, right adrenal gland, and diaphragmatic crura are located posterior to the inferior vena cava.

8. c. The abdominal aorta bifurcates into the right and left common iliac arteries at the level of the fourth lumbar vertebra (umbilicus). The inferior vena cava is formed at the level of the fifth lumbar vertebra.

9. e. The celiac axis branches into the common hepatic, left gastric, and splenic arteries.

10. e. A palpable vibration ("thrill") within an artery is highly suspicious for an arteriovenous fistula.

11. b. Saccular-shaped aneurysms are most often caused by an infection or trauma. A mycotic aneurysm generally demonstrates a focal out-pouching of one arterial wall. Small saccular aneurysms primarily affecting the cerebral arteries are termed berry aneurysm. Fusiform aneurysms are the most common type of abdominal aortic aneurysms.

12. b. The gonadal arteries arise from the anterior aspect of the abdominal aorta inferior to the renal arteries and superior to the lumbar arteries.

13. c. The gastroepiploic artery is a branch of the splenic artery.

14. d. Hepatic veins course between the segments of the liver towards the inferior vena cava. The middle hepatic vein divides the liver into right and left segments.

15. c. The diameter of the main portal vein should not exceed 1.3 cm to be considered within normal limits.

16. b. Based on a history of pulmonary embolism, the echogenic mass is most suspicious for a thrombus. The majority of pulmonary embolisms propagate from the lower extremities through the IVC to the lungs.

17. **d.** A cross sectional image of a vascular structure is identified posterior to the inferior vena cava. This most likely represents the right renal artery.

18. **b.** An **anechoic** structure is identified posterior to the liver in the region of the gallbladder fossa.

19. **b.** Arrow **A** is identifying a proximal anterior branch of the aorta. The celiac axis is the first visceral branch of the abdominal aorta. The inferior phrenic artery is the first parietal branch of the abdominal aorta.

20. **d.** An anechoic tubular structure is branching from the anterior aspect of the abdominal aorta. Arrow **B** is identifying the superior mesenteric artery, a common sonographic landmark. The renal arteries arise from the lateral aspect of the abdominal aorta.

21. **d.** Twenty-five percent of patients with a popliteal aneurysm demonstrate a coexisting abdominal aortic aneurysm.

22. **d.** Arteriosclerosis is the most common predisposing factor for developing an abdominal aortic aneurysm. Pathological thickening, hardening, and loss of wall elasticity allow the weakened arterial walls to stretch.

23. **c.** Dissecting aneurysms of the abdominal aorta may be idiopathic or linked to hypertension, pregnancy, Marfan's syndrome, extension of a thoracic dissection, or trauma.

24. **e.** The inferior vena cava usually measures less than 2.5 cm and is considered enlarged once the diameter exceeds 3.7 cm.

25. **d.** Hypertension is not considered a predisposing factor in the development of an arteriovenous fistula. Development of an arteriovenous fistula may be congenital or caused by trauma, surgery, inflammation, or a neoplasm.

26. **c.** Neoplasms from the kidney extend into the renal vein and may infiltrate the inferior vena cava. The liver and adrenal gland are possible differentials but not the most likely origin of an IVC neoplasm. The portosplenic venous system does not directly empty into the inferior vena cava.

27. **d.** **Direct** extension of thrombus into the inferior vena cava may originate from the femoral, iliac, renal, hepatic or right gonadal veins. The splenic vein terminates at the portosplenic junction.

28. **c.** Berry aneurysms are small saccular aneurysms (1.0-1.5 cm) primarily affecting the cerebral arteries. The carotid and vertebral arteries are considered extracranial structures.

29. **b.** Approximately 10% to 20% of the population will demonstrate duplication of the main renal arteries (1 or 2 out of 10).

30. **c.** Hemodynamics in the hepatic artery is not generally linked to cholecystitis. Abnormal blood flow patterns (i.e., velocity, resistance) in the hepatic artery are linked with jaundice, cirrhosis, lymphoma, and metastases.

31. **d.** The clinical history includes: leukocytosis and an enlarging pulsatile abdominal mass. The distal aorta measures 5 cm in height and 6 cm in width. Complex intraluminal echoes are also identified. Based on the clinical history, the sonographic findings are most suspicious for a mycotic abdominal aortic aneurysm.

32. **c.** The vascular structure identified by arrow **A** courses in a transverse plane, anterior to the superior mesenteric artery and posterior to the body of the pancreas. This is most consistent with the splenic vein.

33. **e.** Arrow **B** identifies a vascular structure located posterior to the body of the pancreas and is surrounded by a thick hyperechoic rim. These findings are most consistent with the superior mesenteric artery.

34. **d.** A complex aortic aneurysm demonstrating smooth wall margins is identified in an asymptomatic patient. The anechoic area represents the lumen of the aorta, and the complex area represents chronic changes in intraluminal thrombus. Chronic thrombus within an aneurysm may demonstrate a complex appearance mimicking a dissection or rupture.

35. **e.** Vessel **A** is located in the upper abdomen and courses in a transverse plane, posterior to the liver. If arrow **B** is the inferior vena cava and arrow **C** is the aorta, then arrow **A** most likely represents the right renal vein.

36. **c.** Vessel **B** courses in a sagittal plane directly posterior to the liver. This is most consistent with the inferior vena cava. The superior mesenteric artery lies directly posterior to the body of the pancreas.

37. **d.** A pseudoaneurysm is defined as a dilatation of an artery caused by damage to one or more layers of the arterial wall. Trauma and aneurysm rupture are the most common etiologies.

38. **c.** The common iliac artery is considered enlarged once the diameter exceeds 2.0 cm in diameter.

39. **c.** The right renal artery is a common sonographic landmark coursing posterior to the inferior vena cava.

40. **d.** The gastroduodenal artery lies between the superior portion of the duodenum and the anterior aspect of the pancreatic head.

41. **b.** The diameter of the IVC generally measures less than 2.5 cm and is considered enlarged once the diameter exceeds 3.7 cm.

42. **e.** The inferior mesenteric artery supplies the left transverse colon, descending colon, upper rectum, and sigmoid.

43. **c.** Marfan syndrome is a musculoskeletal condition that affects the elastic fibers in the media of the aorta, increasing the risk for developing an aneurysm.

44. **b.** 15% of abdominal aortic aneurysms measuring 6.0 cm in diameter will rupture within 5 years.

45. **e.** Approximately 70% of the blood supplied to the liver is from the portal venous system, while 30% is supplied by the hepatic artery.

46. **c.** The left renal vein courses anterior to the aorta and left renal artery and posterior to the superior mesenteric artery (SMA). The splenic vein courses anterior to the SMA.

47. **b.** The normal diameter of the splenic vein should not exceed 1.0 cm.

48. **c.** The splenic artery is a tortuous branch of the celiac axis and is most commonly mistaken as a dilated pancreatic duct.

49. **d.** An ectatic aneurysm is a dilatation of an artery when compared

with a more proximal segment. In cases of abdominal aortic aneurysms, the ectatic dilatation does not exceed 3.0 cm in diameter.

50. a. Venous walls are thinner and less elastic when compared with the arterial walls.

Chapter 14: Gastrointestinal Tract

1. b. The esophagus begins at the pharynx, courses through the esophageal hiatus of the diaphragm, and terminates at the cardiac orifice of the stomach.

2. e. Male infants have an increased risk for developing infantile pyloric stenosis.

3. c. Heartburn is not a clinical symptom of acute appendicitis. Clinical symptoms may include: fever, nausea/vomiting, periumbilical or right lower quadrant pain, and a positive McBurney sign.

4. b. Rugae describe the ridges and folds found in the mucosal layer of the stomach. The recesses found in the walls of the transverse and ascending colon are termed haustra.

5. d. Pepsin is a protein digesting enzyme produced by the stomach. Gastrin, lipase, amylase, and secretin are produced by the pancreas.

6. d. The duodenum secretes large quantities of mucus to protect the small intestines from the strong stomach acids. The stomach secretes pepsin and hydrochloric acid. Bacteria in the colon produce vitamin K and some B complex vitamins.

7. c. Crohn's disease is a chronic inflammation of the intestines most commonly occurring in the ileum.

8. d. Intussusception occurs when one section of bowel has prolapsed into the lumen of an adjacent section of bowel. An ileus may be a complication of intussusception. Meckel's diverticulum describes a congenital anomalous sac protruding from the ileum.

9. d. The jejunum and ileum demonstrate small folds in the intestinal wall similar in appearance to a keyboard. WES sign describes the appearance of a stone filled gallbladder. Olive sign describes a palpable abdominal mass associated with pyloric stenosis. Doughnut

sign correlates to the telescoping appearance in intussusception.

10. b. The ileum is a division of the small intestines. The regions of the large intestines includes: cecum, appendix, ascending colon, transverse colon, descending colon, sigmoid, rectum, and anal canal.

11. d. The right margin of the esophagus is contiguous with the lesser curvature of the stomach. The left margin of the esophagus is contiguous with the greater curvature of the stomach.

12. e. The ascending and transverse colon demonstrate haustral wall markings.

13. e. The small intestines extend from the pyloric opening of the stomach to the junction of the ileum and cecum (ileocecal valve).

14. d. To be considered within normal limits, the pyloric canal should not exceed 18 mm in length or 15 mm (1.5 cm) in diameter.

15. c. The normal adult appendix should not exceed 6 mm in diameter or 2 mm in wall thickness.

16. c. Extreme pain or tenderness over McBurney's point is most commonly associated with acute appendicitis. Murphy's sign correlates to extreme pain over the gallbladder fossa consistent with acute cholecystitis.

17. b. Fifty percent of cases of carcinoma involving the colon are located in the rectum.

18. b. The descending portion (second portion) of the duodenum receives bile from the common bile duct. The duodenum is divided into the superior, descending, horizontal, and ascending portions.

19. c. Patients may experience gastritis following an episode of excessive alcohol consumption. Symptoms may include: upper abdominal discomfort, decrease in appetite, belching, nausea/vomiting, fatigue, and fever. Ileus is more likely related to acute pancreatitis.

20. d. The stomach is considered the principal organ of digestion. The majority of food absorption occurs in the small intestines. The mouth, pharynx, and esophagus allow ingestion of food.

21. b. The walls of the stomach contain two individual layers of muscle. The five individual layers include

the serosal, muscularis propria, submucosal, muscular, and mucosal layers.

22. c. McBurney's point is located between the umbilicus and the right iliac crest.

23. d. The duodenum is divided into the superior, descending, horizontal, and ascending portions.

24. e. Gastroparesis is a failure of the stomach to empty caused by a decrease in the gastric mobility. Distention of the small bowel with fluid or air describes an ileus. An ileus may be caused by a bowel obstruction, peritonitis, renal colic, acute pancreatitis, bowel ischemia, or neoplasm.

25. c. The sonogram demonstrates an out-pouching in the wall of the colon. The patient's clinical symptoms include lower abdominal pain and occasional rectal bleeding. Based on the clinical history, the sonographic finding is most suspicious for a diverticulum.

26. d. The length of the pyloric canal and thickness of the pyloric wall exceed the normal limits. Based on the clinical history, the sonographic findings are most consistent with hypertrophied pyloric stenosis.

27. b. Clinical findings in this case include a negative pregnancy test, leukocytosis, and severe pelvic pain. A noncompressible mass is identified lateral to the ovary in a nonpregnant patient. Based on the clinical suspicion of infection, the mass most likely represents acute appendicitis.

28. c. Gastric dilatation is associated with gastric obstruction, gastroparesis, duodenal ulcer, inflammation, pylorospasm, neurological disease, neoplasm, and side affects of medication. This patient was diagnosed with gastroparesis.

29. d. A target mass is demonstrated in this sonogram of the upper abdomen. This is most suspicious for the gastroesophageal junction. The pyloric canal is a possibility but not as likely a diagnosis.

30. c. Crohn's disease is a chronic disease affecting the small intestines. Clinical symptoms may include: abdominal cramping, blood in stool, diarrhea, fever, decreased appetite, and weight loss. This sonogram of the small intestines demonstrates a thick, matted loop of bowel. Based on the clinical history, the sonographic findings are most suspicious for Crohn's disease.

31. e. The recesses demonstrated in the walls of the **ascending** colon are most suspicious for normal haustral wall markings in a fecal-filled colon. Transducer pressure on a fecal-filled section of intestines may cause abdominal or pelvic discomfort.

32. d. The mucosal layer is the layer of the duodenum nearest the lumen, demonstrating a thin, hyperechoic, linear appearance.

33. e. The clinical symptoms in this case include a history of rectal bleeding and a change in normal bowel habits. A complex mass is identified in the most common site for malignancy (rectum). Based on the clinical history, the sonographic finding is most suspicious for a malignant neoplasm.

34. b. Wall thickness of the pyloric canal should not exceed 3 to 4 mm to be considered within normal limits.

35. d. Releasing glycogen as glucose is a function of the liver. Functions of the gastrointestinal tract include: ingest food, digest food, secrete mucous and digestive enzymes, absorb and break down food, resorb fluids in the intestinal walls, form and release solid waste.

36. d. The lesser curvature of the stomach is the most common location for gastric ulcers to develop.

37. a. Fluid- or air-filled loops of small intestines describes an ileus. Crohn's disease generally demonstrates as **thick or matted** loops of small bowel.

38. a. Wall thickness of an adult appendix should not exceed 2 mm to be considered within normal limits.

39. c. Chyme is a semi-liquid composed of food and gastric juices. The duodenum secretes a large amount of mucus, protecting the small intestines from the acidic chyme. Pepsin is secreted by the stomach. Bile is formed in the liver and transported through the biliary ducts. Cholecystokinin and sodium bicarbonate are released by the pancreas.

40. e. The ileum is the distal portion of the small intestines, extending from the jejunum to the junction with the cecum (ileocecal junction).

41. c. The small intestines are responsible for the majority of food absorption. The stomach is responsible for digestion.

42. e. The descending colon terminates at the junction with the sigmoid colon. The transverse colon terminates at the junction with the descending colon. The sigmoid colon terminates at the rectum.

43. d. Peristalsis is the forward movement of intestinal contents through the digestive tract through serial rhythmic contractions of the intestinal walls. Pylorospasm is associated with pyloric stenosis. Ridges or folds in the stomach lining are termed rugae.

44. b. Clinical symptoms in this non-pregnant patient include right lower quadrant pain and vomiting. Possible etiologies may include: appendicitis, ovarian torsion, ovarian cyst, or tubo-ovarian abscess. Right **upper** quadrant pain with vomiting might be suspicious for pancreatitis.

45. c. A large cystic mass is not typically associated with malignancy. Gastric carcinoma may appear as a target lesion, gastric wall thickening, or as a hypervascular left upper quadrant mass.

46. c. Seventy-five percent of gastric ulcers are caused by a bacterial infection.

47. d. Diffuse thickening of the gastric walls and prominence of the rugae are the most common sonographic findings in cases of gastritis. A fluid-filled mass in the left upper quadrant is generally associated with gastroparesis. Gastric masses are not typically linked to an inflammation of the stomach lining.

48. d. Gastritis is not associated with the formation of a mucocele. Mucoceles are distensions of the appendix or cecum with mucous fluid. Inflammatory scarring involving the large intestines is the most common cause of a mucocele. Other etiologies may include neoplasm, fecalith, or polyp.

49. c. The colon demonstrates the largest lumen diameter in the cecum and gradually decreases in size as it nears the rectum.

50. a. A polyp is the most common tumor of the stomach. It appears on ultrasound as a hypoechoic mass protruding from of stomach wall. Cases of gastric polyps are generally asymptomatic.

Chapter 15: Superficial Structures: Breast, Abdominal Wall, and Musculoskeletal Sonography

1. b. The acini is the smallest functional unit in the breast parenchyma. The lobule is considered the simplest functional unit in the breast parenchyma.

2. e. The muscles and joints of the shoulder allow a full range of motion (360°) in the sagittal plane. The shoulder can abduct and adduct, extend in front, behind, above the torso, as well as rotate. This remarkable range of motion makes the shoulder the most mobile joint in the body. The hip is a multiaxial joint, producing motion in more than one axis.

3. d. The support or skeletal framework in the breast parenchyma is provided by strands of connective tissue. These strands are termed Cooper's ligaments. They appear as hyperechoic linear structures on ultrasound.

4. e. Polythelia (accessory nipple) is the most common congenital breast anomaly. Amastia describes the complete absence of one or both breasts. The presence of a nipple without breast tissue describes amazia. Athelia is a complete absence of the nipple. An accessory or supernumerary breast describes polymastia.

5. c. The transversus abdominus muscle is located posterior to both the internal and the external oblique muscles.

6. b. A galactocele describes a palpable retroareolar mass developing shortly after childbirth. This is most likely caused by an obstruction of a lactating duct. Fibroadenomas are influenced by estrogen levels and composed of dense epithelial and fibrotic tissues. A harmartoma is mass caused by the proliferation of normal breast tissues. Cystosarcoma phylloides is an uncommon benign neoplasm composed of fibroepithelial tissues. Invasive ductal carcinoma is an unlikely differential consideration.

7. **d.** Anisotropy can be a problem in musculoskeletal imaging. It is associated with a false hypoechoic area within the tendon. This occurs when the ultrasound beam is not perpendicular with a tendon's fibers.

8. **b.** In breast imaging, the standoff pad should not exceed 1.0 cm in thickness due to the fixed focus in the elevation plane (short axis) of the transducer.

9. **e.** Cystosarcoma phylloides is an uncommon benign breast neoplasm that may undergo malignant transformation.

10. **d.** Amastia is defined as the complete absence of one or both breasts. Amazia demonstrates a nipple without corresponding breast parenchyma. Athelia describes the complete absence of the nipple. A lack of vision not caused from damage to the eye defines amaurosis. The absence of a spinal cord defines amyelia.

11. **e.** Fatty enlargement of one or both breasts in a male patient is a clinical finding of gynecomastia. Development of a harmartoma is a possible differential for an abnormal enlargement of the breast parenchyma, but is not the best answer. Galactoceles are found in lactating (female) patients. Mastitis is an inflammatory condition found in both males and females. An accessory or additional breast defines polymastia.

12. **d.** Lymph vessels generally course along with the venous system. Superficial veins lie deep to the superficial fascia. Deep veins may drain into the internal mammary, axillary, subclavian, and intercostal veins. Superficial veins of the right and left breast can communicate.

13. **d.** Fatty breast lobules most commonly demonstrate a medium-gray echo pattern (moderately hypoechoic).

14. **e.** Terminal ductal lobular units (TDLU) are formed by the acini and terminal ducts. Nearly all breast pathology originates in the TDLU.

15. **d.** The deep layer of the superficial fascia (deep fascia) is located **within** the retromammary space. The mammary zone is located between the subcutaneous fat and the retromammary space. Cooper's ligaments are located within the subcutaneous layer of the breast.

16. **d.** Glandular tissue appears moderately hyperechoic when compared with the normal fatty tissue of the breast. Fatty breast lobules demonstrate a medium-level gray echogenicity.

17. **e.** The lactiferous ducts normally enlarge near the areola but should not exceed 3.0 mm in diameter.

18. **c.** Painful or tender breasts 7 to 10 days prior to the onset of menses is mostly likely a symptom of fibrocystic disease. Mastitis and gynecomastia are not related to menstrual cycles. Metastatic breast disease demonstrates superficial breast masses.

19. **d.** Invasive ductal carcinoma is the most common malignant breast neoplasm. An irregular heterogeneous breast mass demonstrating posterior acoustic shadowing is suspicious for invasive ductal carcinoma.

20. **c.** An abdominal wall **defect** allows extension of the intestines and/or omentum.

21. **d.** The Thompson test (pointing the toes while squeezing the calf) is used to check the integrity of the Achilles tendon. A positive Thompson test is suspicious for a ruptured Achilles tendon.

22. **a.** A simple cyst is the most common benign breast lesion in middle-age women. Fibroadenomas are more common in young females.

23. **d.** Fibroadenomas are frequently influenced by estrogen levels. Mastitis is generally caused by a bacterial infection. Galactoceles are linked to an obstruction of a lactating duct.

24. **a.** Tendons attach muscles to bone with bands of dense fibrous connective tissue. A flexible band of fibrous tissue binding joints together defines a ligament. A fibril is a small filamentous fiber. A fibrous sac found between a tendon and bone defines a bursa.

25. **c.** The shape and support of the breast parenchyma is provided by the Cooper's ligaments. The pectoralis muscles surround the muscles of the chest.

26. **d.** A hypoechoic mass within the rectus sheath is identified in the left lower quadrant. A rectus sheath hematoma may develop with severe or chronic coughing. A urachal sinus connects the apex of the bladder with the umbilicus. An abdominal wall abscess in a non-susrgical, **afebrile** patient is a possible differential but less likely.

27. **b.** A nonvascular anechoic fluid collection is identified in the medial portion of the popliteal fossa or knee joint. This is most suspicious for a synovial (Baker's) cyst.

28. **a.** A well-defined anechoic mass demonstrating posterior acoustic shadowing is identified in a middle-age female. This is most suspicious for a simple cyst.

29. **c.** A defect is identified in the anterior abdominal wall allowing extension of the omentum and intestines. This is most consistent with a hernia. An urachal sinus connects the apex of the bladder with the umbilicus.

30. **c.** An oval-shaped, well-defined hypoechoic mass is identified in a child-bearing patient. This is most suspicious for a fibroadenoma. The mass appears to compress the surrounding tissues without breaching the fascial plane. Lymph nodes demonstrate a hyperechoic center.

31. **d.** An ill-defined mass demonstrating posterior acoustic shadowing is identified in the upper outer quadrant of the right breast. A possible breach of the superficial fascial plane is also identified. These sonographic findings are most suspicious for invasive ductal carcinoma. Invasive ductal carcinoma is the most common breast malignancy. Well-defined mass(es) are demonstrated in papillary carcinoma, metastatic breast disease, and cystosarcoma phylloides. Fibrocystic disease demonstrates multiple breast cysts.

32. **c.** A hyperechoic linear structure is identified in the subcutaneous fat layer of the right breast. This is most consistent with a Cooper's ligament. Cooper's ligaments provide a "skeletal" framework for the breast.

33. **a.** The anterior recess of the left hip joint is 2.3 mm thicker in diameter when compared to the contralateral right hip. Asymmetry exceeding 2 mm in diameter is considered abnormal. This is most sus-

picious for a septic left hip. Septic hip can be a complication of a recent infection. Clinical findings include limping or a change in gait.

34. **d.** The hyperechoic structure is most suspicious for a foreign body. Fascial planes appear as a continuous hyperechoic line. Ligaments bind joints together. Calcified vessel and lipoma are unlikely considerations.

35. **a.** Sonographic findings include a homogeneous Achilles tendon demonstrating smooth margins. The thickness of the tendon does not exceed 5 mm. These findings are most consistent with a normal Achilles tendon. Focal disruption is generally identified in a complete or incomplete tear of the tendon. Tendonitis demonstrates a thickening in the tendon.

36. **c.** Approximately 15 to 20 individual lobes form the parenchyma of each breast.

37. **c.** Thickness of a normal Achilles' tendon should not exceed 7 mm. Tendonitis is suggested once the thickness exceeds 7 mm in diameter.

38. **d.** Possible etiologies of a rectus sheath hematoma may include trauma, pregnancy, long-term steroid use, severe or chronic coughing, sneezing, heavy exercise, and anticoagulant therapy. Hernias are possible complications of an abdominal wall defect.

39. **b.** The linea alba is a midline tendon extending from the xiphoid process to the symphysis pubis. The rectus abdominus muscles are located lateral to the linea alba and extend the entire length of the anterior abdominal wall.

40. **b.** The fascial interface of the anterior abdominal wall is located **directly** anterior to the peritoneum. The linea alba, rectus abdominus muscles, and the subcutaneous fat are located anterior to the fascial plane.

41. **d.** The Valsalva maneuver is a common technique used when evaluating the anterior abdominal wall, groin or lower extremity venous system.

42. **c.** A **nonvascular** hypoechoic mass following a recent **injury** is most suspicious for a hematoma. Baker's cysts are caused by chronic conditions of the knee joint.

43. **a.** Lactiferous ducts are channels that carry milk from the breast lobes to the nipple. The sinus is as enlargement of the duct near the areola.

44. **b.** The mass is located in the upper outer quadrant of the right breast (10:00) near the axilla (3) and chest wall (C).

45. **d.** A malignant mass generally has a larger height than width. Sonographic findings of invasive ductal carcinoma may also include: hypoechoic mass, heterogeneous mass, irregular or ill-defined margins, posterior acoustic shadowing, breaching of the adjacent fascial plane(s), or thick straight Cooper's ligament(s).

46. **b.** The Achilles tendon should be measured in the transverse plane. The position of the patient is irrelevant.

47. **e.** A complete tear of the Achilles tendon is most commonly located in the distal portion of the tendon approximately 2 to 6 cm from the calcaneus (inferior insertion).

48. **d.** The rectus abdominus **muscles** extend the entire length of the anterior abdominal wall. The linea alba is a tendon not a muscle.

49. **a.** Lymph vessels in the breast generally course parallel with the venous system.

50. **e.** Bloody nipple discharge is associated with a benign papilloma or papillary carcinoma. Symptoms of mastitis may include painful or tender breast(s), erythema, fever, thick nipple discharge, swelling, malaise, and lymphadenopathy.

Chapter 16: Scrotum and Prostate

1. **c.** A hydrocele is defined as an abnormal fluid collection between the two layers of the tunica vaginalis. The tunica vaginalis covers the anterior and lateral portions of the testis and epididymis. The tunica albuginea is a fibrous sheath enclosing each testis. The spermatic cord is located on the posterior border of the testes.

2. **d.** "Bell clapper" is another term used to describe testicular torsion. Twisting of the spermatic cord upon itself gives the appearance the testis is dangling, similar to the clapper in a bell.

3. **a.** The testes generally descend into the scrotal sac during the third trimester of pregnancy. Normal testes will descend into the scrotal sac by 6 months of age.

4. **b.** The peripheral zone comprises approximately 70% of the glandular tissue of the prostate gland and is the most common site of prostatic carcinoma.

5. **d.** Slightly inferior to the main renal arteries, the gonadal arteries (testicular) arise from the anterior aspect of the abdominal aorta.

6. **c.** The tunica albuginea is a fibrous sheath enclosing each testis. The tunica vaginalis is a two-layered serous membrane covering, the anterior and lateral borders of the testis and epididymis.

7. **d.** Functions of the prostate gland include: secretion of an alkaline fluid to aid in the transport of sperm, production of ejaculation fluid, and production of prostate-specific antigen.

8. **e.** The mediastinum testis is the thickened portion of the tunica albuginea. The mediastinum testis appears as a hyperechoic linear structure in the medial and posterior aspect of the testis.

9. **c.** The spermatic cord supports the posterior border of the testes and courses superiorly through the inguinal canal. The rete testis connects the epididymis with the superior portion of the testis. The epididymis carries sperm from the testis to the vas deferens.

10. **e.** A decrease in urine output is an indication for a prostate or retroperitoneal ultrasound. Indications for a scrotal ultrasound may include: scrotal trauma or pain, scrotal swelling, palpable scrotal mass, infertility, undescended testis, and evaluation of a mass demonstrated on a previous medical imaging study.

11. **d.** A cystic structure arising from the rete testis describes a spermatocele. Dilatation of an epididymal tubule describes an epididymal cyst.

12. **c.** Vas deferens are small tubes responsible for transporting sperm from the testes to the prostatic urethra. The spermatic cord is a support structure located on the posterior border of the testes.

13. **b.** The spermatic vein generally measures 1 to 2 mm in diameter. It

is considered dilated once the diameter exceeds 4 mm.

14. **a.** The scrotum is divided into two separate compartments by a medium raphe or septum.

15. **c.** A complex mass is identified within the inferior portion of the left testis. This is most suspicious for a malignant neoplasm. Testicular torsion, epididymitis, and acute orchitis frequently cause scrotal pain. Scrotal herniation is an extra-testicular abnormality.

16. **d.** An echogenic mass is identified superior to the epididymis. This is most suspicious for herniation of the bowel into the scrotal sac. This would explain why the "swelling" is intermittent.

17. **c.** Midline hyperechoic foci are identified at the base of the prostate gland consistent with the central zone. The peripheral zone occupies the posterior, lateral, and apical regions of the prostate gland. Seminal vesicles lie superior to the prostate gland.

18. **d.** Dilated anechoic tubular structures are identified inferior to the testis. This is most suspicious for a varicocele (enlarged spermatic veins). Veins will increase in size with the Valsalva maneuver.

19. **a.** Varicoceles are the most common cause of male infertility.

20. **a.** An anechoic fluid collection is identified superior and anterior to the testis in a patient without a history of trauma. This is most consistent with a hydrocele. A hypoechoic fluid collection is more commonly identified with a hematocele.

21. **e.** The solid structure superior to the testis most likely represents the head of the epididymis or possibly a testicular appendix.

22. **c.** A lower urinary tract infection is the most common cause of epididymitis.

23. **c.** Benign prostatic hypertrophy (BPH) is a noninflammatory enlargement of the prostate usually occurring in the transitional zone of the gland. The majority of carcinoma occurs in the peripheral zone.

24. **e.** Twisting of the spermatic cord leads to obstruction of the blood vessels supplying the testis and epididymis leading to torsion of the testis. Spermatocele is a retention cyst arising from the rete testis.

25. **a.** A hypervascular enlarged hypoechoic testis is most suspicious for orchitis. Symptoms of orchitis may include fever, scrotal pain or swelling, and nausea/vomiting. Epididymitis is an inflammation of the epididymis, not testis.

26. **e.** A sudden onset of severe scrotal pain in an **adolescent** patient is most suspicious for testicular torsion. Adolescents are at an increased risk for developing testicular torsion.

27. **c.** The rete testis is a network of ducts formed in the mediastinum testis connecting the epididymis to the superior portion of the testis. Vas deferens transport sperm from the testis to the prostatic urethra.

28. **c.** The seminal vesicles are responsible for storing sperm. Ducts of the seminal vesicles enter the central zone and join the vas deferens to form the ejaculatory ducts.

29. **b.** Two thirds of the blood supplied to the prostate gland is through the capsular artery. The urethral artery supplies one third of the blood into the prostate gland.

30. **c.** An enlarged hypoechoic epididymis is identified posterior and inferior to the left testis. This is most suspicious for epididymitis. Epididymitis is the most common cause of acute scrotal pain.

31. **d.** The structure is contiguous with the body of the epididymis and superior to the testis most consistent with the head of the epididymis.

32. **e.** A nonvascular cystic mass is identified in the region of the mediastinum testis. This most likely represents tubular ectasia of the rete testis. **Chronic** orchitis may demonstrate complex areas of necrosis. **Acute** orchitis most commonly demonstrates as an enlarged hypoechoic testis.

33. **e.** Tubular ectasia of the rete testis is usually a bilateral condition.

34. **d.** A cystic structure superior to the testis is most consistent with a spermatocele or epididymal cyst. Spermatoceles arise in the rete testis and do not compress the testicle. An epididymal cyst may compress the testicle.

35. **d.** A small hypoechoic mass is identified by the calipers in the peripheral zone. The peripheral zone comprises approximately 70% of the glandular tissue and occupies the posterior, lateral, and apical regions of the prostate gland.

36. **d.** The verumontanum divides the urethra into proximal and distal segments.

37. **b.** Normal monoclonal levels of PSA should not exceed 4 ng/mL. Elevation of 20% or an increase of 0.75 ng/mL within 1 year is indicative of carcinoma.

38. **d.** Decreased urinary output is most commonly associated with benign hypertrophy of the prostate gland (BPH).

39. **d.** The epididymis lies posterior and lateral to the testis.

40. **c.** The cremasteric and deferential arteries supply blood to the epididymis, scrotal tissue and testis. Two thirds of the blood supply to the prostate gland is through the capsular artery. The testicular artery courses along the periphery of the testicle. Inferior vesical artery supplies the base of the bladder, seminal vesicles, and distal ureter.

41. **a.** The left testicular vein empties into the left renal vein. The inferior vena cava receives the right testicular vein.

42. **d.** All of the conditions may cause scrotal pain. Epididymitis is the **most** common cause of **acute** scrotal pain.

43. **d.** The seminal vesicles appear hypoechoic on ultrasound and are located superior to the prostate gland, posterior to the urinary bladder, and lateral to the vas deferens. The ducts of the seminal vesicles enter the central zone of the prostate gland.

44. **a.** The cremasteric and deferential arteries are contained in the spermatic cord.

45. **e.** Clinical symptoms of BPH include urinary frequency, decrease in urinary output, dysuria, and urinary tract infection.

46. **d.** Patients with an undescended testis are at an increased risk for developing testicular torsion, malignancy, and infertility.

47. **c.** The transitional zone comprises only 5% of the glandular tissue of

the prostate gland. The periurethral glands comprise approximately 1% of the glandular tissue.

48. **d.** The tissue of the prostatic urethra is lined by the periurethral glands. The verumontanum divides the urethra into proximal and distal segments.

49. **e.** The prostate gland consists of five lobes: the anterior, middle, posterior, and two lateral **lobes**. It is also divided into the central, peripheral, and transitional **zones.**

50. **a.** The mediastinum testis appears as a hyperechoic linear structure located in the posterior medial aspect of each testis.

Chapter 17: Neck

1. **d.** The superior and middle thyroid veins empty directly into the internal jugular vein. The external jugular empties into the subclavian vein. The vertebral vein empties into the brachiocephalic (innominate) vein.

2. **c.** Thyroid stimulating hormone (TSH) controls the secretion of thyroid hormones. TSH is produced by the anterior pituitary gland. Coordination of volunteer muscle activity is a function of the cerebellum. The hypothalamus activates, controls, and integrates the peripheral autonomic nervous system, endocrine processes, and many somatic functions.

3. **d.** Muscle cramps are a symptom of **hypo**thyroidism. Symptoms associated with **hyper**thyroidism may include: nervousness, weight loss, exophthalmos, increased heart rate, heat intolerance, palpitations, and diarrhea.

4. **d.** Hashimoto's disease is often painless and considered the most common cause of hypothyroidism. Graves' disease is most commonly associated with hyperthyroidism.

5. **e.** The parathyroid glands maintain homeostasis of blood calcium concentrations. The thyroid glands secrete calcitonin. The kidneys regulate serum electrolytes. The spleen initiates an immune reaction resulting in the production of antibodies and lymphocytes. Producing hormones is a function of the adrenal glands.

6. **b.** The right and left vertebral arteries ascend through the vertebral processes and join at the base of the skull, forming the basilar artery.

7. **c.** A superficial cystic structure lying directly below the angle of the jaw is most likely a brachial cleft cyst. Cystic structures may contain internal debris. A thyroglossal cyst is located between the isthmus of the thyroid gland and the tongue.

8. **b.** A pyramidal lobe is a congenital anomaly associated with a third thyroid lobe arising from the superior portion of the isthmus and ascending to the level of the hyoid bone.

9. **b.** The vertebral vein receives blood from the **posterior** brain, descending the neck and emptying into the brachiocephalic (innominate) vein. The subclavian vein receives blood from posterior cranium and deep facial structures through the external jugular vein. The subclavian joins the internal jugular vein to form the brachiocephalic vein.

10. **c.** A decrease in the thyrotropin (TSH) level is the **first** indication of thyroid gland failure. A decrease in thyroxine is an indication of thyroid disease or a nonfunctioning pituitary gland. Hashimoto's thyroiditis is associated with a decrease in triiodothyrone (T_3).

11. **b.** A homogeneous thyroid mass demonstrating a prominent hypoechoic peripheral "halo" is most consistent with an adenoma. A thick incomplete peripheral "halo" is demonstrated with papillary carcinoma.

12. **d.** Triiodothyrone (T_3) regulates tissue metabolism. Parathyroid hormone (PTH) regulates calcium metabolism in conjunction with calcitonin.

13. **b.** Clinical findings associated with thyroiditis may include hyperthyroidism followed by hypothyroidism, fever, leukocytosis, neck pain, and dysphagia. The thyroid gland generally demonstrates diffuse enlargement with an increase in vascular blood flood within the gland. Goiters and hyperplasia generally demonstrate multiple solid nodules within an enlarged thyroid gland.

14. **c.** A thyroglossal cyst is located between the isthmus of the thyroid gland and tongue.

15. **d.** The main blood supply to the eyes and brain is through the internal carotid artery. The internal carotid artery may remain patent with occlusion of the ipsilateral common carotid artery by collateral flow through the ipsilateral external carotid artery or through the circle of Willis.

16. **b.** An anechoic structure is identified posterior and slightly lateral to the thyroid lobe. A symmetrical structure is identified on the contralateral side. This most likely represents the carotid artery.

17. **d.** An isoechoic echogenic "bridge" is identified between the left and right thyroid lobes consistent with the isthmus.

18. **b.** The strap muscles are a group of muscles located anterior and lateral to the thyroid lobes. The strap muscles appear hypoechoic compared to the adjacent thyroid parenchyma. The superficial sternocleidomastoid muscle lies lateral to the strap muscles. The longus colli muscle is located posterior to the thyroid lobe. The trachea is located posterior to the isthmus of the thyroid gland.

19. **d.** The thyroid lobe appears slightly enlarged and hypoechoic without any evidence of a focal or discrete mass. Hypervascular flow is identified within the thyroid lobe on color Doppler imaging. Thyroiditis (Hashimoto's disease or DeQuervain's syndrome) is the most likely diagnosis with these sonographic findings and a clinical history of fatigue following an infection. Patients with Graves' disease more commonly complain of palpitations, nervousness, and an increase in heart rate. The thyroid gland generally enlarges and demonstrates multiple solid nodules in Graves' disease.

20. **b.** Hashimoto's disease is the most common cause of **hypo**thyroidism. Fatigue, sore throat, dyspnea, and dysphagia are symptoms associated with hypothyroidism. Graves' disease is associated with hyperthyroidism. Increases in calcium may be related to an underlying malignancy, hyperthyroidism, or hyperparathyroidism.

21. **b.** A smooth heterogeneous mass is identified within the thyroid lobe. A prominent hypoechoic peripheral "halo" is demonstrated around the majority of the mass. In an asymptomatic patient, these sonographic findings are most suspicious for an adenoma. Chronic adenomas may undergo degeneration and demonstrate a heterogeneous echo pattern.

22. **c.** A complex mass is identified in the anterior neck extending from the isthmus of the thyroid gland to the tongue. This is most suspicious for a thyroglossal cyst. Cystic hygromas are generally located in the posterior neck. A brachial cleft cyst is located directly below the angle of the mandible. Chronic cysts may contain internal debris.

23. **c.** Approximately 80% of the population has two **paired** (4), bean-shaped parathyroid glands located posterior to the thyroid glands.

24. **c.** The ophthalmic artery is the first branch of the internal carotid artery. The vertebral arteries arise from the subclavian arteries. The superior thyroid artery arises from the external carotid artery. The internal carotid artery terminates at the circle of Willis.

25. **e.** Clinical symptoms of hypercalcemia may include: abdominal pain, formation of stones, weight loss, anorexia, confusion, gout, arthritis, bone demineralization, muscle pain, and weakness. Hyperparesthia of the hands, feet, lips, and tongue are symptoms of hypocalcemia. Fatigue and weight gain are symptoms of hypothyroidism. Palpitations is a symptom of hyperthyroidism.

26. **c.** Clinical symptoms of pancreatitis, hypertension **and** hypercalcemia, are related to the development of an adenoma of a parathyroid gland. Other symptoms may include formation of calculi or a decrease in serum phosphorus levels.

27. **d.** Clinical findings associated with Graves' disease may include **hyper**thyroidism, dyspnea, dysphagia, exophthalmos, and a palpable neck mass.

28. **d.** An inadequate drainage of lymph fluid into the jugular vein or an increase in secretion from the epithelial lining of the neck are the most common causes of a cystic hygroma. An impaired synthesis of thyroid hormones is related to development of a goiter. Hyperparathyroidism is most commonly caused by an adenoma of a parathyroid gland.

29. **c.** The internal carotid artery terminates at the circle of Willis. The left common carotid generally arises directly from the aortic arch. The ECA courses medial to the ICA. The common carotid artery typically does not demonstrate any branches. The ICA generally courses posterior to the ECA.

30. **e.** Subacute thyroiditis secondary to a viral infection defines DeQuervain's syndrome. Graves' disease is a multisystemic autoimmune disorder characterized by pronounced hyperthyroidism. Addison syndrome involves the adrenal glands. Caroli's and Mirrizi syndromes involve the biliary tree.

31. **d.** The longus colli muscles are located posterior to the thyroid lobes. The platysma and sternocleidomastoid muscles are located lateral to the thyroid lobes. The strap muscles (omohyoid, sternothyroid, and sternohyoid) are located anterior and lateral to the thyroid lobes.

32. **d.** An audible bruit is an indication for a carotid duplex examination. Indications for a thyroid sonogram may include: fatigue, dysphagia, palpitations, palpable neck mass, abnormal thyroid function tests, dyspnea, serial evaluation of thyroid nodules, or evaluation of a thyroid mass identified on a previous medical imaging study.

33. **e.** Exposure to ionizing radiation is a predisposing factor for development of a **para**thyroid adenoma.

34. **d.** Primary thyroid carcinoma is **known** to extend to the cervical lymph nodes, lung, bone, and larynx. The majority of metastatic lesions in the liver are extensions of primary carcinoma in the colon, pancreas, breast, and lung.

35. **b.** Hashimoto's disease is associated with an increase risk for developing a malignancy of the thyroid gland.

36. **d.** A normal adult thyroid lobe measures approximately 4.0 cm in length, 2.0 cm in height (AP), and 3.0 cm in width.

37. **b.** 100 to 200 mg of iodide must be ingested per week for normal thyroxine production.

38. **c.** Dynamic range should be increased when imaging the thyroid gland. Increasing dynamic range increases the shades of gray demonstrated in the sonographic image.

39. **b.** Tremors are associated with **hyper**thyroidism. Clinical symptoms related to hypothyroidism may include: arthritis, muscle cramps, weight gain, skin dryness, fatigue, constipation, slow metabolic rate, and a decrease in heart rate.

40. **c.** The superior thyroid artery is the first branch of the external carotid artery. The ascending pharyngeal is the second branch followed by the lingual and facial arteries.

41. **b.** Serial imaging of a multinodular goiter should include the overall measurements of the thyroid lobe along with measurements of the **largest** nodules.

42. **a.** Sixty percent of thyroid nodules identified on ultrasound are benign lesions.

43. **b.** Graves' disease typically demonstrates multilocular nodules within the thyroid gland. DeQuervain's syndrome and Hashimoto's disease demonstrate a generalized enlargement of the thyroid gland without specific evidence of a nodule(s).

44. **c.** Hyperthyroidism is a precipitating factor in the development of osteoporosis and nephrolithiasis.

45. **b.** Sonographic findings associated with thyroid carcinoma include: hypoechoic mass, irregular borders, microcalcifications and a thick incomplete peripheral "halo."

46. **c.** The parathyroid glands lie posterior to the thyroid lobes and anterior to the longus colli muscles.

47. **c.** The platysma muscles are located in the lateral neck just beneath the subcutaneous tissues. The strap muscles consisting of the sternohyoid, omohyoid, and sternothyroid muscles are located posterior to the platysma muscles.

48. d. The longus colli muscles are most often affected by a whiplash injury.

49. c. Pronounced swelling of the neck is **most** commonly caused by an enlarging thyroid gland.

50. c. In 80% of cases, hyperparathyroidism is caused by an adenoma of a parathyroid gland. Other etiologies may include: renal disease or a deficiency in calcium or vitamin D.

Chapter 18: Peritoneum, Noncardiac Chest, and Invasive Procedures

1. d. An intra-abdominal fluid collection (subphrenic) following a recent trauma, most likely represents blood within the peritoneal cavity (hemoperitoneum).

2. e. Infectious or inflammatory conditions of the lungs and cardiovascular disease are predisposing factors for developing a pleural effusion.

3. e. The subhepatic space is the most common site for ascites to collect followed by Morison's pouch.

4. b. The peritoneum is an extensive serous membrane lining the abdominal cavity. The lesser and greater omentum are part of the peritoneum. The mesentery is a double layer of peritoneum suspending the intestines from the posterior abdominal wall. The retroperitoneum is the space behind the peritoneum and the posterior abdominal wall.

5. c. The patient is generally placed in a sitting position, bent slightly forward at the waist during a thoracentesis procedure.

6. d. The lesser sac communicates with the subhepatic space through the foramen of Winslow. Foramen of Monro is located between the third and lateral ventricles in the brain. Cerebral spinal fluid travels from the fourth ventricle to subarachnoid space through the foramen of Magendie and foramen of Luschka. Foramen ovale is located between the atrium of the heart. The common bile duct enters the descending portion of the duodenum through the *ampulla* of Vater.

7. c. The pancreas is located in the retroperitoneum. Organs contained within the peritoneum include the liver, spleen, stomach, gallbladder, uterine body, and portions of the small and large intestines.

8. d. A collection of chyle and emulsified fats in the peritoneal cavity (chylons ascites) is most commonly associated with an abdominal neoplasm. Cirrhosis, acute cholecystitis, and congestive heart failure demonstrate benign ascites. Ectopic pregnancy is more commonly related to hemoperitoneum.

9. d. The paracolic gutters are located lateral to the intestines. The retrovesical pouch is located posterior to the urinary bladder and anterior to the rectum.

10. d. A lymphocele is an accumulation of lymphatic fluid more commonly occurring following a renal transplant. Lymphoceles are usually located medial to a renal transplant.

11. e. Paracentesis is an invasive procedure where fluid is withdrawn from the abdominal cavity for diagnostic or therapeutic purposes. Biopsies remove a small portion of living tissue.

12. c. Polycystic disease is not associated with free fluid within the peritoneum. Peritoneal ascites is associated with malignancy, postsurgery, postovulation, chronic liver disease, cardiovascular disease, infection, and inflammation.

13. d. A decrease in hematocrit is suspicious for hemorrhage.

14. e. The greater omentum is a double fold of peritoneum that spreads like an apron over the transverse colon and small intestines. The mesentery suspends the intestines from the posterior abdominal wall. The perineum supports and surrounds the distal portions of the urogenital and gastrointestinal tracts of the body.

15. d. The peritoneum extends from the diaphragm to the deep pelvic spaces and from the anterior abdominal wall to the retroperitoneum and paraspinal tissues.

16. c. The vesicouterine pouch or anterior cul de sac is located anterior to the uterus and posterior to the urinary bladder. The retrouterine space is located posterior to the uterus and anterior to the rectum. The retropubic and prevesical spaces are located anterior to the urinary bladder and posterior to the symphysis pubis.

17. a. The pleura is a fine, delicate, serous membrane composed of a visceral and parietal layers.

18. b. On ultrasound, visualization of the biopsy needle is obtained in a plane **parallel with the needle path.**

19. b. The bare area (lacking peritoneum) is a triangular space located between the two layers of the right coronary ligament.

20. e. Fine needle aspiration (FNA) uses a thin needle and gentle suction to obtain tissue samples for pathological testing. A large core needle is used in core biopsy procedures.

21. d. The arrow is identifying a space posterior to the right lobe of the liver and superior and lateral to the right kidney. This is most consistent with Morison's pouch. Pouch of Douglas is located anterior to the rectum in the posterior pelvis.

22. b. The liver is located in the peritoneal cavity. The pancreas, kidneys, and great vessels are located within the retroperitoneum.

23. d. A hyperechoic linear structure is extending from the liver to the undersurface of the diaphragm is identified by Arrow **A**. This is most consistent with the coronary ligament. The right coronary ligament serves as a barrier between the right subphrenic space and Morison's pouch.

24. c. Arrow **B** is identifying an anechoic area posterior to the diaphragm and anterolateral to the liver. This is most consistent with free fluid (ascites) in the right subphrenic space. Blood typically demonstrates internal echoes.

25. d. Arrow **C** identifies a peritoneal space posterior to the liver and lateral to the gallbladder. This is most consistent with the subhepatic space.

26. d. Ascites is identified adjacent to hyperechoic bowel in the right paracolic gutter. The retrovesicle pouch is located posterior to the urinary bladder and anterior the rectum. Space of Retzius is located anterior to the urinary bladder and posterior to the symphysis pubis.

27. b. A fluid collection is identified anterior to the diaphragm consistent with a pleural effusion. Sub-phrenic ascites would be located posterior to the diaphragm.

28. c. Free fluid is identified posterior to the uterus and anterior to the rectum consistent with the pouch of Douglas posterior cul de sac, or retrouterine pouch.

29. a. The pancreas is identified in this transverse sonogram of the upper abdomen. The lesser sac separates the pancreas from the stomach.

30. c. A **large** core needle is identified consistent with a core needle biopsy. A slender needle is used in fine needle aspiration procedures.

31. d. The peritoneum secretes serous fluid to reduce friction between organs. It also enfolds and suspends peritoneal organs. The coronary ligament serves as a barrier between the subphrenic and subhepatic spaces.

32. d. The lesser omentum extends from the lower end of the esophagus to the liver and is also known as the gastrohepatic omentum. The lesser sac is also known as the omental bursa.

33. c. The falciform ligament divides the subphrenic space into right and left sides. The crura of the diaphragm extend from the diaphragm to the vertebral column.

34. e. The lungs are **separated** into right and left hemispheres by the pleural membrane. The heart is located between the inferior borders of the lungs. The pleural cavity is a space within the thorax that contains the lungs. The sternum is the middle portion of the anterior thorax.

35. b. An intercostal (between the ribs) approach is typically used in noncardiac imaging of the chest. Intracostal pertains to the inner surface of the rib. Subcostal and suprasternal are utilized in cardiac imaging.

36. b. Omental cysts are small cystic structures developing adjacent to the stomach or lesser sac (pancreas).

37. b. Patients are typically placed in the supine position for a paracentesis procedure. Renal biopsies are generally performed with the patient in a prone position. The

patient is placed in a sitting position for a thoracentesis.

38. a. The prevesical space is located in the pelvis, lying anterior to the urinary bladder and posterior to the symphysis pubis. It is also known as the retropubic space.

39. a. An abnormal collection of **free** fluid in the peritoneal cavity describes abdominal ascites. Seroma, abscess, hematoma, and lymphocele are restricted fluid collections.

40. a. The greater omentum has the potential to seal off infections or hernias within the peritoneal cavity. The greater omentum spreads like an apron covering most of the abdominopelvic cavity.

41. a. The pouch of Douglas (retro-uterine pouch) is located in the most posterior portion of the pelvis. It is formed by the inferior portion of the parietal layer of the peritoneum.

42. c. The paracolic gutters are located in the lateral portions of the abdominopelvic cavity and serve as conduits between the upper abdomen and the deep pelvis.

43. b. Cirrhosis generally demonstrates benign intraperitoneal ascites. Blood in the peritoneal cavity (hemoperitoneum) can be associated with trauma, rupture of an abdominal blood vessel, postsurgical complication, ectopic pregnancy, fistulas, and necrotic neoplasms.

44. b. Congenital failure of the mesentery to fuse is a congenital anomaly associated with development of an omental cyst. Mesentery cysts are related to the Wolffian or lymph ducts.

45. c. The "sandwich sign" (anechoic mass with a hyperechoic center) is the most common term used to describe the sonographic appearance of mesenteric lymphomatous.

46. d. The inferior end of the esophagus is enclosed by the lesser omentum. The lesser omentum extends from the portal fissure of the liver to the diaphragm.

47. d. An accumulation of blood and fluid in the **pleural cavity** describes a hemothorax.

48. c. Exudative ascites is defined as an accumulation of fluid, pus or

serous fluid in the peritoneal cavity. Transudative ascites contains small protein cells. Chylous ascites contains chyle and emulsified fats. Peritonitis is an inflammation of the peritoneal cavity.

49. a. A biopsy removes a small piece of living tissue for microscopic analysis. Surgical incision of a tumor without removal of surrounding tissue describes a lumpectomy. Fine needle aspiration utilizes a thin needle and suction to obtain tissue sampling for pathological testing.

50. d. When localizing a fluid collection for a paracentesis procedure, the sonographer must align the transducer perpendicular to the table or floor. Care should be taken to use minimal transducer pressure for accurate depth measurement.

Abdomen Mock Exam

1. c. The main lobar fissure is a sonographic landmark used to locate the gallbladder fossa. It extends from the right portal vein to the gallbladder fossa. It is also considered a boundary between the left and right lobes of the liver.

2. b. Biliary disease is the most common cause of acute pancreatitis followed by alcohol abuse. Other etiologies may include trauma, peptic ulcer disease, and hyperlipidemia. Occasionally acute pancreatitis is idiopathic.

3. c. Gerota's fascia provides a protective covering around the kidneys. The liver is covered by Glisson's capsule and the spleen is covered by the peritoneum.

4. d. Increased pressure within the porto-splenic venous system will most likely lead to portal hypertension. Fatty infiltration and hepatitis may compress or occlude the portal veins causing an increase in venous pressure.

5. c. The diameter of the main portal vein varies with respiration and fasting state but should not exceed 1.3 cm to be considered within normal limits.

6. c. The Thompson test (pointing the toes while squeezing the calf muscles) checks the integrity of the Achilles tendon.

7. **d.** Chronic pancreatitis is associated with atrophy of the pancreas and hyperechoic parenchyma.

8. **d.** Endocrine glands release hormones and include the pituitary gland, thyroid gland, parathyroid glands, adrenal glands, pancreas, ovaries, and testes.

9. **e.** A septated cystic (honeycomb) mass is a sonographic finding of an echinococcal cyst. The five patterns of liver metastasis include: 1. bull's eye or target lesions, 2. hyperechoic masses, 3. cystic masses, 4. complex masses, and 5. diffuse pattern.

10. **e.** Cholecystitis is not associated with an increase risk in developing gallbladder carcinoma. Risk factors for developing cholangiocarcinoma include a history of cholangitis, ulcerative colitis or choledochal cyst, and male gender.

11. **b.** A Baker's cyst is a synovial cyst located in the posterior medial portion of the popliteal fossa.

12. **b.** The superior mesenteric vein should not exceed 1.0 cm in diameter to be considered within normal limits.

13. **a.** Budd-Chiari syndrome is a life-threatening condition associated with thrombosis of the hepatic veins. The sonographer should thoroughly evaluate the liver.

14. **d.** The left lobe of the liver is divided into medial and lateral segments by the left hepatic vein and the ligamentum of Teres. Ligamentum of venosum separates the caudate lobe from the left lobe of the liver.

15. **e.** Cholecystokinin is stimulated once food reaches the duodenum causing the secretion of pancreatic enzymes and contraction of the gallbladder.

16. **d.** The gallbladder lies anterior and medial to the right kidney, lateral to the IVC, and inferior to the main lobar fissure.

17. **C.** Destruction of red blood cells is a function of the liver. Functions of the pancreas include breaking down fats (lipase), carbohydrates (amylase), and proteins (trypsin), regulating sugar metabolism (islet cells of Langerhans), and stimulating the secretion of cholecystokinin, gastric acids, and bicarbonate.

18. **d.** Clinical symptoms of severe back pain, weight loss and painless jaundice are most suspicious for a malignant neoplasm in the pancreas.

19. **b.** A popliteal artery is considered dilated once the diameter exceeds 1.0 cm. Approximately 25% of patients with a popliteal aneurysm will have a coexisting abdominal aortic aneurysm.

20. **e.** Glisson's capsule surrounds the liver. Gerota's fascia surrounds each kidney.

21. **e.** Mirrizi syndrome results in jaundice caused by compression of the common hepatic duct from an impacted stone in the cystic duct or neck of the gallbladder. Courvoisier's sign results in painless jaundice and a hydropic gallbladder secondary to an obstruction of the distal common bile duct by an external mass (i.e. pancreatic neoplasm).

22. **b.** Nonshadowing spaghetti-like echogenic structure(s) within a bile duct describe sonographic findings in ascariasis. Schistosomiasis demonstrates thick hyperechoic portal veins on ultrasound. Clonochiasis demonstrates dilated intrahepatic ducts.

23. **d.** Gallbladder wall thickening is not a sonographic finding in hyperalbuminema. Gallbladder wall thickening is a sonographic finding in nonfasting patients, patients with benign ascites, cirrhosis, congestive heart failure, hypoalbuminemia, and acute hepatitis.

24. **e.** Multiple echogenic intraluminal foci are demonstrated in cases of cholesterosis, similar in appearance to a strawberry.

25. **b.** A fluid collection caused by extravasated bile is termed a biloma. Seroma is a collection of serous fluid.

26. **c.** Renal artery stenosis is suggested once the renal artery to aorta ratio exceeds 3.5.

27. **a.** The spleen is located within the peritoneal cavity. The kidneys, pancreas, adrenal glands, inferior vena cava, and aorta are located in the retroperitoneum.

28. **d.** The pancreas, descending duodenum, ascending and descending colon, superior mesenteric vessels, and the inferior portion of the common bile duct lie within the anterior pararenal space.

29. **d.** The crura of the diaphragm are tendinous structures extending from the diaphragm to the vertebral column. They lie superior to the celiac axis, posterior to the inferior vena cava, and anterior to the abdominal aorta.

30. **c.** Splenomegaly is a consistent finding in cases of portal hypertension. Hepatocellular carcinoma and Budd-Chiari syndrome (thrombosed hepatic veins) may demonstrate splenomegaly secondary to liver congestion (i.e., portal hypertension).

31. **d.** Direct extension of carcinoma into the gallbladder may originate in the pancreas, stomach, or bile duct. Indirect extension may originate in the lung, kidney, esophagus, or skin (melanoma) via the lymphatic system or bloodstream.

32. **d.** Obstruction of the common bile duct by a distal external neoplasm instigating enlargement of the gallbladder is termed Courvoisier's sign.

33. **a.** The superior and inferior borders of the retroperitoneum are defined by the diaphragm and pelvic rim respectively.

34. **d.** Elevation in prostatic-specific antigen is a clinical finding suspicious for carcinoma of the prostate gland.

35. **d.** Budd-Chiari syndrome is a rare life-threatening condition associated with thrombosis of the hepatic veins. Couinaud's anatomy divides the liver into eight segments in an imaginary "H" pattern. Caroli's disease involves the biliary tree.

36. **c.** Left untreated, obstruction of the cystic duct eventually initiates an episode of acute cholecystitis.

37. **a.** A dilated renal vein, hydroureter, or parapelvic cyst may be mistaken as an extrarenal pelvis.

38. **c.** A febrile patient demonstrating a complex liver mass following a recent trip abroad is most suspicious for a hepatic abscess. A "honeycomb" cystic mass is generally identified with echinococcal cysts.

39. **a.** Varix or varicose vein is a common term to describe an

abnormally enlarged or dilated vein.

40. e. Ascending cholangitis is the most common cause of a hepatic abscess. Other etiologies may include: recent travel abroad, biliary infection, appendicitis, and diverticulitis.

41. c. The gastroduodenal artery lies in the anterolateral portion of the pancreatic head. The common bile duct lies in the posterolateral portion and the portosplenic confluence is located in the mid portion of the pancreatic head. The superior mesenteric artery and splenic vein lie posterior to the body of the pancreas.

42. c. An echogenic mass demonstrating a prominent hypoechoic halo is most consistent with an adenoma of the thyroid gland. Carcinoma demonstrates an irregular peripheral halo surrounding a hypoechoic mass.

43. a. The liver manufactures heparin and glycogen, releases glycogen as glucose, breaks down red blood cell–producing bile pigments, secretes bile into the duodenum, and converts amino acids into urea and glucose. Production of antibodies and lymphocytes is a function of the spleen.

44. c. A normal adult spleen measures approximately 10 to 12 cm in length and should not exceed 13 cm in length to be considered within normal limits.

45. b. Mycotic aneurysms develop secondary to an underlying bacterial infection. A dissecting aneurysm is the result of a tear in the intimal lining. Damage to one or more layers of the arterial wall is the most common cause of a pseudoaneurysm.

46. c. Pepsin is a protein–digesting enzyme produced by the stomach. Amylase and lipase are enzymes produced by the pancreas. Gastric and cholecystokinin are related to the pancreas.

47. c. McBurney's point is located between the umbilicus and right iliac crest. Rebound pain at McBurney's point (McBurney's sign) is most commonly associated with an appendicitis.

48. e. An anechoic mass (cyst) located alongside the renal pelvis is most

suspicious for a parapelvic cyst. Peripelvic cysts lie around the renal pelvis.

49. e. Severe abdominal pain is the most common symptom associated with portal vein thrombosis.

50. c. TIPS should measure 8 to 12 mm throughout the entire length of the shunt.

51. e. A nonshadowing, smooth hyperechoic neoplasm located in the renal cortex is most suspicious for an angiomyolipoma. Angiomyolipomas are generally asymptomatic but may cause flank pain or gross hematuria.

52. e. The prominence of the collecting system may signify mild hydronephrosis or residual dilatation of the calyces from the previous episode of hydronephrosis. This would likely depend on the severity of the original obstruction.

53. b. The distal abdominal aorta demonstrates an abnormal increase in diameter compared to a more proximal portion. A measurement of 2.7 cm is consistent with an ectatic abdominal aortic aneurysm. A true abdominal aortic aneurysm measures a minimum of 3.0 cm in diameter.

54. d. The right renal artery courses posterior to the inferior vena cava and is a common sonographic landmark utilized in abdominal and retroperitoneal scanning.

55. d. The gallbladder demonstrates a smooth, thick edematous wall with a coexisting gallstone most consistent with acute cholecystitis. Carcinoma of the gallbladder demonstrates gallstone(s) and a thick, irregular gallbladder wall in the majority of cases.

56. a. An anechoic fluid collection is identified anterior and lateral to the right testis. This is most consistent with a hydrocele.

57. d. The anechoic structure measures 2.7 mm and is located in the body of the pancreas. This is most consistent with a prominent pancreatic duct. To be considered within normal limits, the diameter of the pancreatic duct should not exceed 3.0 mm and demonstrate smooth margins.

58. c. A diffuse increase in liver echogenicity is identified in an obese

patient. The hepatic vessels appear within normal limits. Based on the clinical history, these sonographic findings are most suspicious for fatty infiltration of the liver parenchyma. Elevation of liver function tests is a clinical finding in many liver abnormalities, including fatty infiltration.

59. b. Comma-like recesses are identified by the arrows in the walls of the transverse colon. These saccular indentations are consistent with haustral wall markings found in the ascending and transverse colon. Haustra are located approximately 3 to 5 cm apart.

60. e. A cavernous hemangioma is the most common benign neoplasm of the spleen and appears as a well-defined hyperechoic mass on ultrasound.

61. e. The spleen measures approximately 16.0 cm in AP diameter (height) in a patient with a history of alcohol abuse. Based on the clinical history, the sonogram is most consistent with splenomegaly.

62. e. Splenomegaly in a patient with a history of alcohol abuse is suspicious for portal hypertension. The sonographer should document the flow direction of the main portal vein and evaluate for venous collaterals.

63. d. A calculus is identified in the common bile duct (the sonographer is most likely measuring the common duct, NOT the neck of the gallbladder). This is most consistent with choledocholithiasis (calculus within a bile duct).

64. e. An out-pouching of the bladder wall is most consistent with a bladder diverticulum. A ureterocele is related to the prolapse of the distal ureter into the ureteric orifice on the posterior aspect of the urinary bladder.

65. e. Symptoms of renal cell carcinoma include uncontrolled hypertension, painless hematuria, and headaches. An angiomyolipoma may demonstrate hematuria but does not affect blood pressure. A cortical bulge on the lateral aspect of the kidney describes a dromedary hump. A renal abscess does not demonstrate internal blood flow.

66. **d.** Mild dilatation of the renal calyces is identified consistent with mild hydronephrosis.

67. **c.** Multiple lobulations are identified in the renal contour. This is consistent with fetal lobulation. A solitary cortical bulge on the lateral aspect of the kidney describes a dromedary hump. A triangular echogenic area in the anterior aspect of the kidney defines a junctional parenchymal defect.

68. **e.** A complex lesion demonstrated in the region of the mediastinum testis is suspicious for tubular ectasia of the rete testis. This lesion is typically bilateral and asymptomatic. It may vary in size and is associated with a previous history of scrotal trauma or inflammation.

69. **e.** An extratesticular anechoic structure is identified superior to the testis in the region of the epididymal head. This is most suspicious for an epididymal cyst or possibly a spermatocele.

70. **d.** Two distinct collecting systems are demonstrated in this elongated kidney most consistent with a renal duplication.

71. **c.** Based on the cortical thickness, thinning of the renal cortex in this sonogram is most likely associated with chronic renal disease.

72. **d.** The inferior pole of the right kidney is fused with the superior pole of the left kidney. This is most consistent with a sigmoid kidney. Fusion of the medial aspect of both kidneys is consistent with a cake kidney.

73. **d.** Epididymitis is the most common cause of acute scrotal pain. The left epididymis appears enlarged and slightly hypoechoic when compared with the contralateral side. This is most suspicious for inflammation of the left epididymis (epididymitis).

74. **c.** Ascites is identified superior to the liver and inferior to the diaphragm consistent with the right subphrenic space. Fluid is also demonstrated inferior to the gallbladder in the subhepatic space.

75. **e.** The presence of a thick hyperechoic gallbladder wall surrounded by benign free fluid is most consistent with a noninflammatory condition of the gallbladder. A nonfunctioning gallbladder is a possible differential but not as likely.

76. **e.** The ligamentum venosum separates the caudate lobe from the left lobe of the liver. The falciform ligament divides the subphrenic space. The main lobar fissure is considered a boundary between the left and right hepatic lobes.

77. **d.** The anterior right hepatic lobe is bordered by the middle and right hepatic veins. The middle hepatic vein separates the left medial lobe from the right anterior lobe. The right hepatic vein separates the anterior and posterior right lobes.

78. **b.** A smooth anechoic renal mass is most likely a simple cyst. An extrarenal pelvis would not displace the renal calyces. A chronic hematoma may appear anechoic but is unlikely to demonstrate a smooth circular contour.

79. **c.** The urinary bladder should be evaluated for evidence of a ureter or bladder outlet obstruction when hydronephrosis is identified. A neoplasm, calculus, or stricture of the distal ureter or urethra may cause the obstruction.

80. **a.** The renal sinus is barely visible in the neonate.

81. **d.** Increasing axial resolution by increasing the transducer frequency may aid in the demonstration of posterior acoustic shadowing.

82. **c.** A prone position would not be helpful in visualizing the abdominal aorta due to the vertebral column.

83. **d.** A phlegmon is associated with acute pancreatitis and is defined as an extension of pancreatic inflammation into the peripancreatic tissues.

84. **e.** Fatty infiltration is not associated with an elevation in conjugated bilirubin levels. Elevation is associated with obstruction, hepatitis, cirrhosis, and liver metastasis.

85. **e.** Levels of aldosterone are most commonly associated with abnormalities of the adrenal gland(s).

86. **e.** A hypertrophied column of Bertin is an inward extension of the renal cortex located between the medullary (renal) pyramids.

87. **a.** The small and tortuous splenic artery is the most common vascular structure mistaken as the pancreatic duct. The larger caliber splenic vein is a sonographic landmark utilized in identifying the body of the pancreas.

88. **c.** Cortical thickness of the normal adult kidney will vary but should measure a minimum of 1.0 cm.

89. **b.** Addison's disease is associated with a partial or complete failure of the adrenocortical function. Cushing's disease is a metabolic disorder resulting from chronic and excessive production of cortisol. Caroli's disease is associated with the biliary tree.

90. **d.** The main renal arteries arise from the lateral aspect of the aorta approximately 1.0 to 1.5 cm below the inferior margin of the superior mesenteric artery.

91. **c.** Cholelithiasis is not associated with splenomegaly. Splenomegaly can be associated with cirrhosis, hepatitis, mononucleosis, congestive heart failure, portal hypertension, diabetes mellitus, hypertension, trauma, or hemolytic anemia.

92. **b.** Hepatic veins course away from the liver toward the inferior vena cava, termed hepatofugal flow. Hepatic veins demonstrate spontaneous multiphasic (pulsatile) flow.

93. **c.** The "olive sign" is a clinical finding associated with hypertrophied pyloric stenosis.

94. **c.** Appendicitis is shown as a noncompressible tubular structure demonstrating a diameter exceeding 6 mm and wall thickness exceeding 2 mm.

95. **e.** Hypertrophied column of Bertin is the most common structure frequently mistaken as a renal neoplasm. A junctional parenchymal defect is less frequently mistaken as a lipoma or angiomyolipoma.

96. **b.** Elevation in indirect or nonconjugated bilirubin is associated with nonobstructive conditions.

97. **b.** The neck is the most superior portion of the gallbladder.

98. **c.** Hashimoto's disease is an inflammatory condition of the

thyroid gland(s) associated with an increased risk in developing a thyroid malignancy.

99. **a.**   A core biopsy uses a large-core needle to remove a small piece of living tissue for microscopic analysis.

100. **a.**   A pancreatic pseudocyst most commonly develops in the lesser sac followed by the anterior pararenal space.

101. **d.**   Elevated serum lipase in a patient with severe left upper quadrant pain is suspicious for acute pancreatitis. Biliary disease is the most common cause of acute pancreatitis.

102. **b.**   A cortical bulge on the lateral aspect of the kidney describes a dromedary hump. Fetal lobulation demonstrates multiple indentations in the contour of the renal cortex. Hypertrophied column of Bertin extends from the cortex into the medullary pyramids.

103. **e.**   Fusion of both kidneys within the same body quadrant describes a congenital anomaly termed cross fused ectopia.

104. **c.**   Doppler imaging demonstrates turbulent or swirling arterial blood flow within a fluid collection adjacent to the common femoral artery. A pseudoaneurysm is associated with trauma to the arterial wall, permitting the escape of blood into the surrounding tissues (angioplasty).

105. **d.**   Fibroadenomas are the most common breast neoplasm in young women. An oval-shaped hypoechoic mass is a common sonographic finding in this benign neoplasm.

106. **c.**   Removal of foreign material from the blood is a function of the spleen. Other functions include initiating an immune reaction resulting in production of antibodies and lymphocytes, reservoir for blood, destruction site of old red blood cells, and recycling hemoglobin.

107. **b.**   "Comet tail" reverberation artifact is characteristic sonographic finding of adenomyomatosis. Pneumobilia may demonstrate an imprecise posterior acoustic shadow but is not an abnormality of the gallbladder wall.

108. **d.**   Lymphadenopathy is generally associated with inflammation or an infection. Thickening of the circular pyloric muscle fibers results in stenosis of the pyloric canal. Clinical symptoms generally include weight loss, dehydration, projectile vomiting, and a palpable upper abdominal mass (olive sign).

109. **c.**   Meckel's diverticulum is a congenital anomaly of the yolk stalk. On ultrasound, the diverticulum appears as an anechoic or complex mass, slightly to the right of the umbilicus.

110. **e.**   Tendonosis is a termed used to describe non-inflammatory degenerative changes in a tendon. Pain referred to a tendon describes tenalgia and tenodyna. Tenesmus is related to spasms of the rectum or urinary bladder.

111. **a.**   There is a 5% risk that an abdominal aortic aneurysm measuring 5 cm in diameter will rupture within 5 years.

112. **e.**   The inferior mesenteric artery is the last major visceral branch of the abdominal aorta prior to the bifurcation into the right and left common iliac arteries. The median sacral artery is the last main parietal branch of the abdominal aorta.

113. **e.**   Twenty-five percent of popliteal aneurysm cases demonstrate a coexisting abdominal aortic aneurysm. Deep vein thrombosis is a possible complication of popliteal aneurysm.

114. **c.**   The subphrenic space is located superior to the liver and inferior to the diaphragm.

115. **e.**   Hepatitis B carriers have a predisposing risk for developing hepatocellular carcinoma (hepatoma). Hepatitis C carriers may develop portal hypertension due to an increased risk for developing cirrhosis.

116. **c.**   The majority of metastatic lesions in the liver originate from colon carcinoma. Pancreas, breasts, and lungs are additional primary sites commonly metastasizing to the liver.

117. **d.**   The common bile duct joins the duct of Wirsung before passing through the ampulla of Vater to enter the duodenum. The sphinc-

ter of Oddi is a sheath of muscle fibers surrounding the distal common bile and pancreatic ducts as they cross the wall of the duodenum.

118. **c.**   Hashimoto's disease is the most common cause of hypothyroidism. Hyperthyroidism is a common symptom in Graves' disease.

119. **b.**   The pyramidal or third lobe arises from the superior aspect of the isthmus and ascends the neck to the level of the hyoid bone.

120. **a.**   The renal sinus contains the major and minor calyces, peripelvic fat, fibrous tissues, arteries, veins, lymphatics, and part of the renal pelvis. The ureter is an extrarenal structure.

121. **b.**   An ureterocele is defined as a prolapse of the distal ureter into the urinary bladder caused by a congenital obstruction of the ureteric orifice.

122. **b.**   Postvoid residual in an adult urinary bladder should not exceed 20 mL to be considered within normal limits.

123. **b.**   Acute pancreatitis is not directly associated with portal hypertension. Splenomegaly is a consistent finding in cases of portal hypertension. Other findings may include intrinsic liver disease, dilated main portal vein, or portosystemic collaterals.

124. **c.**   The left renal vein courses posterior to the superior mesenteric artery (SMA) and anterior to the abdominal aorta. The splenic vein, gastroduodenal artery, and splenic artery course anterior to the SMA. The superior mesenteric vein courses parallel with the SMA.

125. **a.**   On ultrasound, visualization of a biopsy needle is obtained at a plane parallel to the needle path. Perpendicular incidence is utilized in gray-scale imaging.

126. **b.**   A diffuse heterogeneous parenchyma containing multiple echogenic foci is identified in this transverse sonogram of the liver. This is most suspicious for metastatic liver lesions.

127. **c.**   A round anechoic structure demonstrating posterior acoustic enhancement is visualized within the hepatic parenchyma. This most

likely represents a simple hepatic cyst.

128. b. A large gallstone within a contracted gallbladder demonstrating strong posterior acoustic shadowing is an excellent example of the Wall Echo Shadow (WES) sign.

129. e. A hyperechoic linear structure is identified posterior to the left lobe and anterior to the caudate lobe of the liver. This is most consistent with the ligamentum venosum.

130. b. Patients with a history of hepatitis B are at an increased risk for developing hepatocellular carcinoma (HCC; hepatoma). Variable echogenicity in a solid hepatic mass surrounded by a hypoechoic halo are common sonographic findings for a hepatoma.

131. b. Caroli's disease is characterized by a segmental, saccular, or beaded appearance to the intrahepatic ducts. Intermittent jaundice and abdominal cramping or pain are clinical symptoms of Caroli's disease.

132. b. Renal cysts are frequent incidental findings in middle-age and elderly patients. The mass is identified in the kidney (stated in the question). The sonographic findings are characteristic of a cystic structure. The clinical history is not suspicious for a renal abscess or hematom.

133. d. Chronic intraluminal thrombus commonly appears complex secondary to degenerative changes. In this sonogram, the lumen of the distal aorta is surrounded by complex intraluminal thrombus. In many cases, rupture of an aortic aneurysm will demonstrate blood within the peritoneum and a normal caliber aorta.

134. b. An oval hypoechoic mass demonstrating a prominent hyperechoic center and hilum are common sonographic findings of a normal lymph node. Lymph nodes are commonly located in the axilla but may be found throughout the body.

135. e. In the neonate, the renal sinus is barely visible and is surrounded by prominent anechoic medullary (renal) pyramids and a moderately echogenic renal cortex. This image demonstrates the typical appearance of a normal neonatal kidney.

136. b. A hyperechoic septation identified within the urinary bladder is identified at the ureteric orifice. This most likely represents a ureterocele.

137. e. Carcinoma of the gallbladder is the 5th most common malignancy. Ninety percent of cases are associated with cholelithiasis and may demonstrate on ultrasound as an irregular, immobile intraluminal mass(es). Absence of cholelithiasis is more commonly associated with metastatic lesions involving the gallbladder Comet-tail reverberation artifact is a characteristic sonographic finding in adenomyomatosis.

138. d. A smooth, hyperechoic hepatic mass is identified in an asymptomatic thin female patient is most suspicious for a cavernous hemangioma. Hepatic adenomas generally demonstrate as solid, slightly hypoechoic masses. Abnormal laboratory values are typically identified in cases of malignancy. Fatty infiltration is unlikely in a thin patient with normal laboratory values.

139. e. Visualization of intrahepatic vascular and biliary structures is difficult, giving the impression of dense liver parenchyma. Excessive deposition of fat within the parenchymal cells increases the density of the liver and may increase liver function tests. Fatty infiltration is associated with hypoechoic focal area(s) of fat sparing. Fat sparing is commonly located anterior to the portal vein and adjacent to the IVC.

140. a. Hyperechoic echogenic foci demonstrating posterior acoustic shadowing are demonstrated in the neck of the gallbladder. This is most consistent with cholelithiasis.

141. e. Calculi appear to be lodged within the neck of the gallbladder. This finding increases the risk for the patient to develop acute cholecystitis.

142. b. A hyperechoic focus demonstrating posterior acoustic shadowing is identified near the corticomedullary junction of the left kidney. This is most suspicious for a renal calculus.

143. a. The gallbladder demonstrates multiple intraluminal, hyperechoic, nonshadowing, immobile foci most consistent with gallbladder polyps (adenomas).

144. b. Changes in the patient position will demonstrate mobility of the intraluminal foci, narrowing down the differential considerations.

145. b. Dilated tortuous vascular structures are identified in the inferior portion of the left scrotal sac most consistent with a varicocele.

146. b. Development of a varicocele has been linked to male infertility.

147. d. The pyloric wall exceeds 3 mm in thickness and the stomach is still distended with fluid three hours after the infants last feeding. This is most consistent with stenosis of the pyloric canal.

148. e. The head/neck regions of the pancreas appear hypoechoic and enlarged, suspicious for a solid mass. A mass in the head of the pancreas, in a patient with elevated direct bilirubin and severe upper back pain, is most suspicious for a malignant neoplasm.

149. d. A complex intratesticular mass is identified in the left testis. Based on the clinical history, the mass most likely represents a malignant neoplasm.

150. a. Fluid collections are identified superior to the diaphragm bilaterally, consistent with bilateral pleural effusions.

151. d. The pyloric canal should not exceed 18 mm in length or 15 mm in diameter to be considered within normal limits. The thickness of the pyloric wall should not exceed 3 mm to maintain normal limits.

152. d. The Whipple procedure (pancreatoduodenectomy) is a surgical resection of the pancreatic head or periampullary region area. Resection will relieve a biliary obstruction often caused by a malignant tumor of the pancreas.

153. e. Free fluid most commonly accumulates in the subhepatic space.

154. a. Omental cysts generally develop adjacent to the stomach or lesser sac.

155. a. Portal veins are intralobar or intrasegmental in location.

156. d. A superficial cystic mass located just beneath the angle of the mandible is most likely a brachial cleft cyst.

157. d. The normal inferior vena cava generally measures less than 2.5 cm in diameter. The inferior vena cava is considered dilated once the diameter exceeds 3.7 cm.

158. b. A round, solid, homogeneous mass is located near the splenic hilum. The echogenicity of the mass is isoechoic to the adjacent splenic parenchyma. This is most likely an accessory spleen.

159. c. A decrease in hematocrit is associated with hemorrhage. Hemoglobin carries oxygen from the lungs to the cells and returns carbon dioxide back to the lungs.

160. c. A thoracentesis is typically performed with the patient in a sitting position, slightly bent forward at the waist, with the arms leaning on a table.

161. c. Transplant kidneys are more commonly placed superficially in the right lower quadrant.

162. A. Pneumonia may accumulate fluid within the pleural cavity (pleural effusion). Recent surgery, chronic liver disease, congestive heart failure, or obstruction of the portal venous system may cause fluid to accumulate in the peritoneal cavity.

163. d. Under normal conditions, the internal carotid arteries supply the majority of blood to the brain and eye. The subclavian arteries supply the vertebral column, spinal cord, ear, and brain. Blood to the neck, scalp, and face is supplied through the external carotid arteries.

164. c. Fifty percent of all malignant neoplasms involving the colon are located in the rectum and 25% in the sigmoid colon.

165. d. Annular pancreas describes a congenital anomaly where the head of the pancreas surrounds the duodenum. This anomaly may result in obstruction of the biliary tree or duodenum. In pancreas divisum, there is abnormal fusion of the pancreatic ducts.

166. c. Biliary sludge appears on ultrasound as nonshadowing, low amplitude internal echoes that layer in the dependent portion of the gallbladder. Tumefactive sludge resembles a polypoid mass (sludge ball).

167. a. The tail of the pancreas is the most superior portion of the pancreas lying anterior and parallel with the splenic vein. The body is the most anterior portion, and the uncinate process is the most inferior portion of the pancreas.

168. d. Polycystic disease is an inherited disorder, and multicystic dysplasia is a noninherited disorder of the kidney.

169. e. Renal dialysis patients have an increased risk for developing a renal cyst, adenoma or carcinoma.

170. d. The common iliac arteries should not exceed 2.0 cm in diameter to be considered within normal limits.

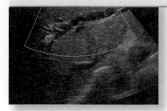# Obstetrics and Gynecology Answers

Chapter 19: Pelvic Anatomy

1. **d.** The ovarian ligament extends from the cornua of the uterus to the medial aspect of the ovary. The round ligament arises in the cornua of the uterus and extends to the pelvic sidewalls.
2. **b.** Arcuate vessels are commonly visualized near the periphery of the uterus as anechoic circular structures. Nabothian cysts are located in the cervix.
3. **e.** The obturator internus muscles abut the lateral walls of the urinary bladder. The iliopsoas muscles are lateral landmarks of the true pelvis lying lateral and anterior to the obturator internus muscles.
4. **b.** Adnexa is the term used to describe the region of the ovary and fallopian tube. Space of Retzius is located anterior to the urinary bladder and posterior to the symphysis pubis. The one fimbriae attached to the ovary is termed the fimbriae ovarica.
5. **c.** The interstitial segment of the fallopian tube passes through the cornua of the uterus. The infundibulum is the most lateral segment of the oviduct.
6. **e.** The flanged portions of the iliac bones and the base of the sacrum form the posterior boundary of the false pelvis.
7. **c.** With anteflexion, the fundus of the uterus bends on top of the cervix. The uterus bends behind the cervix in retroflexion.
8. **c.** Only the functional layer (echogenic) is included when measuring endometrial thickness. The hypoechoic basal layer or fluid within the endometrial cavity is NOT included when measuring the thickness of the endometrium.
9. **e.** The suspensory ligaments extend from the lateral aspect of the ovary to the pelvic sidewalls.

The broad ligaments extend from the lateral aspect of the uterus to the pelvic sidewalls.

10. **d.** **Failure** of the müllerian ducts to fuse will result in uterine didelphys. **Partial** failure of these ducts to fuse will result in a bicornuate uterus. Failure of the müllerian ducts to develop results in uterine agenesis.
11. **c.** The anterior-posterior dimension of the endometrium is ONLY measured in the sagittal plane.
12. **c.** The external or serosal layer of the uterus is termed the perimetrium. The myometrium is the thickest layer of the uterus and composed of smooth muscle.
13. **b.** The ovaries receive blood primarily from the ovarian arteries and secondarily through the uterine arteries. The uterine arteries arise from the hypogastric arteries.
14. **b.** The vesicouterine pouch (anterior cul de sac) is located anterior to the uterus and posterior to the urinary bladder. The retrouterine space (posterior cul de sac) is located posterior to the uterus and anterior to the rectum.
15. **c.** The cervix is twice as large as the corpus during premenarche. The cervix to corpus ratio is 2:1.
16. **e.** The cervix and corpus appear equal in size (1:1) This is most consistent with a postmenopausal uterus. The cervix is twice the size of the corpus in a premenarche patient (2:1).
17. **a.** The uterus bends slightly anterior (forward), characteristic of anteversion. With anteflexion, the uterus bends upon the cervix. Dextroflexion displaces the uterus to the left of the cervix.
18. **b.** The levator ani and piriformis muscles form the pelvic floor and lie posterior to the vagina. Obturator internus and iliopsoas muscles

are located in the lateral true pelvis. Suspensory and uterosacral are pelvic ligaments.

19. **d.** Fluid is demonstrated posterior to the uterus in the pouch of Douglas. The vesicouterine pouch is located anterior to the uterus.
20. **a.** The uterus is lying in the anteverted position. In retroflexion, the fundus and body curve backward upon the cervix.
21. **d.** A L-shaped homogeneous ovarian contour is a normal anatomical variant.
22. **d.** The uterus displays myometrial tissue between two individual endometrial cavities. This is **most** consistent with a bicornuate uterus.
23. **c.** Evenly spaced, hypoechoic or anechoic, circular structures identified in the outer portion of the myometrium **most** likely represent arcuate veins. Uterine arteries are located in the broad ligament lateral to the uterus.
24. **b.** The hyperechoic linear structure extends from the uterus to the **pelvic sidewall**. This is **most** consistent with the broad ligaments. The fallopian tubes are tortuous and do not attach to the pelvic sidewall.
25. **e.** The obturator internus muscles abut the lateral walls of the urinary bladder. Iliopsoas muscles demonstrate a classic hyperechoic central echo.
26. **c.** The arrows identify two individual endometrial cavities most consistent with a bicornuate uterus. Note: fundal notch.
27. **d.** Free fluid is identified anterior and posterior to the uterus in the vesicouterine and retrouterine spaces. The small anechoic area represents a small amount of urine in an otherwise empty bladder.
28. **e.** The uterus displays a posterior tilt and the cervix forms an angle

less than 90° to the vaginal canal, characteristic of retroversion.

29. **e.** An anechoic pedunculation of the urinary bladder describes a diverticulum.

30. **b.** An anechoic tubular structure terminates in the posterior lateral wall of the urinary bladder. This is most consistent with a hydroureter.

31. **c.** The ovaries attach to the mesovarian portion of the broad ligament. The cervix anchors to the angle of the bladder by the parametrium. The tunica albuginea is an outer covering of the ovary.

32. **a.** Ovarian volume is lowest during the luteal phase and highest during the periovulatory phase.

33. **e.** The segments of the fallopian tube include the interstitial, isthmus, ampulla, and infundibulum.

34. **b.** Pelvic ligaments are not routinely visualized. With the presence of intraperitoneal fluid, pelvic ligaments appear as thin, hyperechoic linear structures.

35. **d.** The cornua are the lateral funnel-shaped horns of the uterus located between the uterine fundus and fallopian tube.

36. **d.** The spiral artery arises from the radial arteries (a branch of arcuate artery) and is the primary blood supply to the endometrium.

37. **b.** Coexisting renal anomalies occur in 20%-30 % of patients with a congenital uterine anomaly.

38. **b.** The arcuate or heart-shaped uterus is **most** likely to display a **shallow** fundal notch. A bicornuate uterus generally displays a **deep** fundal notch.

39. **d.** It is common to visualize a small amount of free fluid in the retrouterine space (posterior cul de sac).

40. **c.** Premenarche is the portion of time prior to the onset of menstruation. Puberty is the physical process of changing into an adult body capable of reproduction.

41. **c.** Situated between the symphysis pubis and coccyx, the perineum is located below the pelvic floor. The mesentery, omentum, peritoneum, and retroperitoneum are located within the abdominopelvic cavity.

42. **a.** Septate uterus displays a normal uterine contour with a fibrous or myometrial separation in the endometrial cavity. Arcuate, bicornuate, unicornuate, and didelphys are congenital uterine anomalies demonstrating an abnormal contour to the fundus.

43. **b.** The uterus is derived from the fused caudal portion of the paired müllerian ducts. Partial fusion will most likely result in a uterine anomaly.

44. **d.** The iliopectineal line is a bony ridge on the inner surface of the ilium and pubic bones that divides the true from the false pelvis. The iliopsoas muscles are lateral landmarks of the true pelvis, coursing anterior and lateral through the false pelvis.

45. **d.** The pelvic floor is formed by pelvic ligaments and muscles.

46. **b.** The uterosacral ligament extends from the superior cervix to the lateral margins of the sacrum. The round ligaments arise in the uterine cornua, extending from the fundus to the pelvic sidewalls.

47. **c.** The junctional zone is the innermost layer of the myometrium. The functional and basal layers are the inner and outer layers of the endometrium respectively. The tunica albuginea covers the cortex of each ovary.

48. **c.** In the **menarche** patient, the endometrial thickness should not exceed 14 mm. Without hormone replacement therapy, the endometrium should not exceed 8 mm in the postmenopausal patient.

49. **c.** The ovaries are the only abdominopelvic organ **not** lined by peritoneum. A thin layer of germinal epithelium covers each ovary.

50. **e.** Ovarian volume varies with age and menstrual status. Periovulatory phase exhibits the highest ovarian volume, and the luteal phase reveals the lowest volumes.

Chapter 20: Physiology of the Female Pelvis

1. **a.** Progesterone levels increase in the endometrial secretory phase and the ovarian luteal phase.

2. **e.** During the early proliferation or late menstrual phases, the endometrial lining is thin, typically measuring 2 to 3 mm.

3. **b.** Estradiol levels reflect the activity of the ovaries. Luteinizing hormone reflects ovulation. Progesterone levels increase after ovulation. Follicular stimulating hormone initiates follicular growth.

4. **b.** Postmenopausal patients may display simple ovarian cysts. Simple cysts <5.0 cm are most likely benign. Visualization of a simple cyst in postmenopausal or premenarche patients is not a rare finding.

5. **d.** If fertilization does not occur, the corpus luteum will regress and progesterone levels will decrease. When anticipating fertilization, the corpus luteum may increase in size, and secrete some estrogen and an increasing amount of progesterone.

6. **b.** The endometrium is thinnest in the late menstrual/early proliferative phases. During this overlapping phase, the endometrium appears as a thin, hyperechoic line measuring around 2 to 3 mm.

7. **c.** The cumulus oophorus appears as a hyperechoic focus within a mature follicle. Ovulation generally will occur within the next 36 hours.

8. **b.** A corpus luteum originates from a ruptured graafian follicle. Corpus luteal cysts are common in early pregnancy but do not indicate fertilization has occurred.

9. **a.** The ovarian luteal phase has a consistent 14-day lifespan. The time from the start of menstruation to ovulation can vary from cycle to cycle (follicular phase).

10. **e.** The anterior pituitary gland secretes luteinizing hormone. The hypothalamus produces luteinizing hormone releasing factor.

11. **e.** Adrenal glands, liver, and the breasts produce small amounts of estrogen.

12. **d.** Luteinizing hormone stimulates ovulation. Follicular stimulating hormone initiates follicular growth and stimulates maturation of the graafian follicle.

13. **d.** Fluid within the endometrial cavity is not included when measuring the endometrial thickness. Granulosa cells produce fluid in the follicular cyst.

14. **b.** Mittelschmerz (middle pain) is a local effect of the enlarging graafian follicle prior to ovulation.

15. **a.** Theca lutein cysts are a result of elevated levels of hCG. Polycystic ovarian disease is an endocrine imbalance causing chronic anovulation.

16. **c.** During the late menstrual and early proliferative phases, anechoic areas within the ovary **most** likely represent functional, follicular, or physiological cysts.

17. **c.** Scarring from a previous corpus luteal cyst (corpus albicans) displays as a hyperechoic focus within the ovary and is the **most** likely diagnosis for these hyperechoic foci. An early cystic teratoma (dermoid) is a possible differential consideration.

18. **b.** Secretory phase demonstrates the greatest endometrial thickness. The functional layer appears thick and hyperechoic. The ovarian luteal phase coincides with the secretory phase of the endometrium.

19. **a.** In a patient in the late menstrual phase, an anechoic 2.9-cm ovarian mass demonstrating smooth, thin walls and posterior enhancement **most** likely represents a simple cyst. In a menarche patient, a simple cyst is the failure of a dominant follicle to rupture.

20. **e.** The ovaries display multiple small follicles **most** consistent with the early proliferation phase. Five to eleven follicles typically begin to develop in the early proliferation phase.

21. **e.** A thin endometrial cavity is **most** likely demonstrated in the late menstrual or early proliferative phases.

22. **e.** Strong hyperechoic linear echoes within the endometrial cavity **most** likely represent an IUD.

23. **d.** A hypoechoic ovarian mass associated with severe pelvic pain is **most** suspicious for a hemorrhagic cyst. Endometrioma is a possible differential consideration, although this patient does not have a known history of endometriosis.

24. **c.** An 18-mm anechoic structure with an intraluminal echogenic focus, in a menarche patient, is **most** consistent with a graafian follicle.

25. **e.** An echogenic focus projected within a follicle is most consistent with a cumulus oophorus.

26. **e.** Thick, hypoechoic functional layers between the endometrial cavity echo with a hyperechoic basal layer is characteristic of the late proliferation phase. Endometrial phases include menstrual, proliferation, and secretory.

27. **d.** Triple line or trilaminar echo pattern describes a characteristic sonographic finding during the late proliferative phase.

28. **d.** A hypoechoic ovarian mass in the luteal stage of the cycle (LMP 3 weeks ago) is **most** likely a corpus luteal cyst. Ectopic pregnancies are generally adnexal in location. A graafian follicle is a physiological cyst prior to ovulation. Nondominant follicles generally appear as small anechoic ovarian cysts.

29. **b.** A thin, hyperechoic endometrial cavity is **most** consistent with the late menstrual or early proliferation phases. The adjacent left ovary displays small physiological cysts.

30. **e.** The endometrium is thick, demonstrating a hyperechoic functional layer and a hypoechoic basal layer, most consistent with the secretory phase. The secretory phase of the endometrium coincides with the luteal phase of the ovary. Normal, small, regressing follicles or a corpus luteal cyst is the most likely ovarian mass demonstrated during the secretory or luteal phase.

31. **d.** Menorrhagia defines abnormally heavy or long menses. Dysmenorrhea defines painful menses. Menoxenia defines any abnormality relating to menstruation.

32. **c.** Levels of follicular stimulating hormone begin declining in the late follicular phase and demonstrate a slight increase in the late luteal phase.

33. **e.** Estradiol levels normally range between 200 and 400 pg/mL in the ovulatory phase. Follicular phase ranges between 30 and 100 pg/mL and luteal phase ranges between 50 and 140 pg/mL. These levels are important when monitoring ovulation induction therapy.

34. **c.** The follicular phase of the ovary coincides with the proliferation phase of the endometrium.

35. **b.** The endometrium in patients using hormone contraceptive therapy appears on ultrasound as a thin echogenic line.

36. **c.** In postmenopausal patients **without** hormone replacement therapy, the endometrium should not exceed 8 mm to be considered within normal limits.

37. **e.** Follicular stimulating hormones can be slightly higher after menopause. Progesterone and estrogen levels decrease after menopause.

38. **e.** During the late proliferation phase, the endometrium demonstrates a triple line appearance or a thick, **hypoechoic functional** layer and a **hyperechoic basal** layer. During the secretory phase, the functional layer becomes hyperechoic and the basal layer becomes hypoechoic.

39. **c.** Mittelschmerz (middle pain) is a term used to describe acute pelvic pain prior to ovulation. It is thought to be a result of the increasing size of the graafian follicle.

40. **d.** Preparing and maintaining the endometrium for possible implantation of a blastocyst is a function of progesterone. Estrogen promotes endometrial growth.

41. **e.** Estrogen is secreted by developing graafian follicles. The corpus luteum produces progesterone. The anterior portion of the pituitary gland produces luteinizing and follicular stimulating hormones.

42. **c.** The typical length of a menstrual cycle is 28 days but can normally range between 21 and 35 days.

43. **c.** A rise in hormone levels associated with precocious puberty may be a result of a neoplasm of the hypothalamus, gonads, or adrenal glands.

44. **a.** Increasing levels of estrogen regenerate and promote growth of the functional layer of the endometrium.

45. **b.** During the secretory phase, the endometrium measures 7 to 14 mm, 6 to 10 mm in the late proliferation phase, and 4 to 8 mm during the early menstrual phase.

46. **e.** A hypoechoic ovarian mass in a patient with a history of **acute** lower quadrant pain is **most** suspicious for a hemorrhagic cyst. A graafian follicle may present with acute

lower pain but should appear anechoic.

47. c. The corpus luteum will continue to secrete progesterone if fertilization occurs. The trophoblastic tissue of the blastocyst secretes human chorionic gondadotropin (hCG).

48. a. A thin echogenic line is the most common endometrial appearance with oral contraceptive use.

49. d. Approximately 15% of postmenopause patients will demonstrate a simple ovarian cyst. These cysts are typically follicular in origin.

50. a. Decreases in estrogen in postmenopause patients can shorten the vagina and decrease cervical mucus.

Chapter 21: Uterine and Ovarian Pathology

1. d. Abnormal accumulation of blood within the vagina is termed hematocolpos. Hematometra defines an abnormal accumulation of blood in the endometrial cavity

2. b. Postmenopausal women are at risk for developing endometrial carcinoma. Other risk factors include obesity, diabetes mellitus, and nulliparity.

3. a. Inflammation of the endometrium (endometritis) will likely demonstrate an increase in internal blood flow. Hyperplasia is a noninflammatory process not likely to increase internal vascular flow.

4. c. Dysgerminoma is the most common ovarian malignancy in childhood and is a possible cause for precocious puberty. Fibroma, thecoma, Brenner's tumor, and granulosa cell tumor are benign neoplasms.

5. e. Uterine tenderness during a physical exam, especially during menstruation, is a classic symptom of adenomyosis. Other symptoms include pelvic pain, menorrhagia, dysmenorrhea, uterine enlargement, pelvic pain, or cramping.

6. a. A large multilocular adnexal mass **most** likely represents a serous or mucinous cystadenoma. A less likely differential, theca lutein cysts, can demonstrate a multilocular appearance.

7. c. Uterine fibroids are commonly located within the myometrium (intramural).

8. d. Scarring from a previous endometrial infection or invasive procedure adheres and ablates the endometrial cavity (Asherman syndrome). Ovulatory disorders are the most common cause of female infertility. An endometrial thickness not exceeding 8 mm is associated with a decrease in fertility.

9. c. A coexisting adnexal mass is **commonly associated** with torsion of the ovary. Ectopic pregnancies are generally located in the adnexa, but not typically associated with ovarian torsion.

10. d. A side effect of tamoxifen therapy is an increase in endometrial thickness. This increase can be a result of hyperplasia, polyp formation, or malignancy. Special attention to the endometrial thickness is necessary in tamoxifen patients.

11. b. A complex adnexal mass with diffusely bright internal echoes with or without posterior shadowing is most suspicious for a cystic teratoma (dermoid).

12. d. Cystic teratomas (dermoids) are commonly located superior to the uterine fundus. They arise from the wall of a follicle and may contain fat, hair, skin, and teeth.

13. a. Nabothian cysts can result from obstruction of an inclusion cyst. Serous cystadenomas are epithelial neoplasms.

14. d. A submucosal fibroid distorts the endometrium and will most likely cause bleeding irregularities. The location of cervical fibroid in relation to the endometrial canal will determine clinical symptoms.

15. c. Polycystic ovary disease can result from an endocrine imbalance causing chronic anovulation. Theca lutein cysts can result from follicular hyperstimulation and high levels of hCG. Endometrial abnormalities can result from unopposed estrogen.

16. e. Tamoxifen therapy is an antiestrogen medication used in treating breast cancer. Endometrial abnormalities are side effects of tamoxifen. These may include endometrial polyps, carcinoma, or hyperplasia. Adenomyosis generally demonstrates a normal endometrial cavity with poorly defined anechoic and hypoechoic myometrial masses.

17. b. A homogeneous hypoechoic uterine mass in a **premenarche** 13-year-old patient is most suspicious for hematometra. An accumulation of blood in the vagina defines hematocolpos.

18. b. A subserosal or possible pedunculated fibroid is the most likely diagnosis for the anterior hypoechoic mass with this clinical history.

19. d. A small amount of free fluid is demonstrated posterior to the uterus in the retrouterine space.

20. b. A dense, hypoechoic, ovarian mass with diffusely bright internal echoes is identified in a menarche patient. Based on this clinical history, the mass is **most** suspicious for a cystic teratoma (dermoid). Severe acute pelvic pain is generally associated with hemorrhagic cysts. This patient is expressing a history of **chronic** pelvic pain.

21. a. A hypoechoic mass is identified in the inferior portion of the cervix. Pathological testing revealed a cervical carcinoma. The endometrial thickness is within normal limits.

22. c. Pelvic fullness is the most likely symptom associated with this inferior cervical mass. The mass does not compress or encroach the endometrial lining.

23. a. Leiomyomas are the most common uterine mass. This isoechoic mass is compressing the endometrial cavity.

24. b. A submucosal leiomyoma is **most** likely associated with menorrhagia. Dysmenorrhea is a possible clinical finding, but not the most likely.

25. c. Two contiguous masses are distorting the outer portion of the uterus. In an asymptomatic patient, this is most consistent with two adjacent subserosal fibroids.

26. b. The uterine and cervix display a posterior tilt consistent with a **retroverted** position. The subserosal fibroids are located on the anterior surface of a retroverted uterus.

27. c. Presence of more than 11 small follicles around the periphery of the ovary is **most** suspicious for polycystic ovarian disease. Theca lutein cysts typically appear as a multilocular ovarian mass on ultrasound.

28. c. Clinical findings in polycystic ovary disease include irregular menses, hirsutism, obesity, and infertility.

29. b. A small cystic structure in the cervix demonstrating posterior acoustic enhancement is most likely a nabothian cyst.

30. c. A multilocular anechoic mass demonstrating smooth, thick wall margins is **most** suspicious for a mucinous cystadenoma. Cystadenocarcinoma is a differential consideration. Small clusters of cysts are the typical sonographic finding in surface epithelial cysts.

31. d. The hyperechoic mass within functional layer of the endometrium is most suspicious for an endometrial polyp. The small indentation in the fundal endometrium is suspicious for an arcuate uterus.

32. d. Asherman syndrome is a result of adhesions within the endometrial cavity making it difficult to distinguish the endometrium on ultrasound. Bright endometrial echoes within the endometrium are also associated with Asherman syndrome.

33. d. A coexisting adnexal or ovarian mass is commonly associated with ovarian torsion. Other sonographic findings include decreased or absent blood flow to the ovary and a large heterogeneous ovarian mass.

34. d. Polycystic ovarian disease is a result of an endocrine imbalance causing chronic anovulation. Clinical findings include hirsutism, irregular menses, infertility, and obesity.

35. b. Serous and mucinous cystadenomas are a common cause of a rapid increasing pelvic mass. A rapid increase in a leiomyoma is highly suspicious for malignancy.

36. d. Surface epithelial cysts arise from the cortex of the ovary, appearing on ultrasound as a small cluster of ovarian cysts.

37. d. Submucosal fibroids distort the endometrium and most likely to cause menstrual abnormalities and infertility.

38. e. Ovulation is **regulated** by the hypothalamus. The anterior portion of the pituitary gland **secretes** follicular stimulating hormone and luteinizing hormone.

39. b. During the secretory phase the thick functional layer of the endometrium may demonstrate posterior acoustic enhancement.

40. a. Ovarian carcinoma generally appears as an irregular hypoechoic ovarian mass on ultrasound.

41. d. An endometrial thickness of 2 cm is abnormal regardless of the menstrual status and suspicious for proliferation of the endometrium.

42. c. Cystic teratomas (dermoids) arise from the wall of a follicle and may contain fat, hair, skin, and bone.

43. a. Multiparity, elevated estrogen, and aggressive curettage are risk factors associated with development of adenomyosis. Polycystic ovary disease is a result of an endocrine imbalance causing chronic anovulation.

44. b. A benign stromal mass, the thecoma appears as a hyperechoic ovarian mass with prominent posterior acoustic shadowing. Fibromas **may** demonstrate posterior shadowing.

45. c. An intramural fibroid distorts the myometrium, and a submucosal fibroid distorts the endometrium.

46. d. A small cyst within the vagina is termed a Garner's duct cyst. Nabothian cysts are cervical in location.

47. c. A heterogeneous intrauterine mass in a patient with postmenopausal bleeding is suspicious for an uterine malignancy.

48. d. Tamoxifen can affect the endometrial lining of the uterus. Additional evaluation of the endometrium is required in patients on tamoxifen therapy.

49. d. An **ill-defined**, multilocular, complex ovarian mass is **most** suspicious for a cystadenocarcinoma. Cystadenomas generally demonstrate smooth wall margins.

50. a. Meigs' syndrome is a term used to describe a combination of a pleural effusion, ascites, and an ovarian mass, which resolve after surgical removal of the mass. Stein-Leventhal syndrome is a polycystic ovarian disease.

Chapter 22: Adnexal Pathology and Infertility

1. c. Krukenberg tumors are metastatic lesions most commonly resulting from primary gastric carcinoma. Other primary structures may include breast, large intestine, and appendix.

2. c. Parovarian cysts are typically located in the broad ligament. The fallopian tube is contained within the superior portion of the broad ligament.

3. e. Endometriosis is a condition occurring when active endometrial tissue invades the peritoneal cavity. Endometriomas are collections of extravasated endometrial tissue.

4. d. Infertility is suggested when conception does not occur within 1 year.

5. c. Multiple embryos are transferred to the endometrial cavity, increasing the likelihood of multiple gestations and decreasing the likelihood of ectopic pregnancy.

6. e. An **ill-defined,** complex adnexal mass in a patient with symptoms of an infection is most suspicious for a tubo-ovarian abscess.

7. e. Peritoneal inclusion cysts are caused by adhesions trapping normal secretions produced by the ovary. Clinical symptoms include lower abdominal pain and a palpable pelvic mass. Septated fluid collections **surrounding** a normal-appearing ovary is a common sonographic finding of a peritoneal inclusion cyst.

8. d. The GIFT technique transfers oocytes and sperm into the fallopian tube. ZIFT transfers a zygote to the fallopian tube. In vitro fertilization transfers embryos to the endometrial cavity.

9. b. Estradiol levels reflect the maturity of the stimulated follicles. The size and number of follicles, along with the estradiol level, determines when ovulation is induced.

10. d. Metastatic lesions in the adnexa (Krukenberg tumors) are more commonly associated with a primary malignancy of the gastrointestinal tract.

11. b. Hydrosalpinx is a common consequence of pelvic inflammatory disease. Parovarian cysts are typically located in the broad ligament and are mesothelial in origin.

12. c. Endometrial thickness not exceeding 8 mm during the menstrual cycle is associated with a decrease in fertility. Note: In reproductive patients, the endometrial thickness should exceed 8 mm during the late proliferative and secretory phases. The endometrium in a postmenopausal patient without hormone replacement therapy should not exceed 8 mm.

13. d. GIFT or gamete intrafallopian transfer mixes oocytes with sperm to the fallopian tube. ZIFT places a zygote in the fallopian tube. IVF places embryos in the endometrium.

14. e. Ovarian hyperstimulation syndrome is the **most** likely complication associated with ovulation induction therapy. Ultrasound examinations monitor the size and number of maturing follicles to prevent hyperstimulation and aid in timing of ovulatory medication.

15. b. Hydrosalpinx is a common complication of pelvic inflammatory disease (PID). Parovarian cyst is a possible differential consideration, but it is not related to PID.

16. b. A circular anechoic mass is identified contiguous with the right ovary located between the uterus and ovary. This is most suspicious for a simple ovarian cyst vs. parovarian cyst.

17. d. Repeating the pelvic sonogram in 6 to 8 weeks is the **most** likely follow-up care on this patient. This will allow enough time for regression of a simple cyst. The size of a parovarian cyst would remain unchanged. This cystic structure regressed and was no longer apparent in a follow-up sonogram eight weeks later.

18. a. A complex mass located in the adnexa **adjacent to a normal ovary** is **most** suspicious for an endometrioma. Cystic teratomas involve the ovary.

19. b. A tubular anechoic structure courses directly to the left ovary. In a patient with a **previous** history of pelvic infection, this sonographic finding is most suspicious for a hydrosalpinx.

20. d. An "L-shaped" ovary is a normal anatomic ovarian variant. This irregular contour can be misdiagnosed as an isoechoic ovarian or adnexal mass.

21. e. The presence of five similar sized follicles (16 mm) increases the likelihood of medical stimulation. At this point, the stimulated follicles are within normal limits. Con-

tinual monitoring to evaluate for **hyper**stimulation syndrome is likely.

22. d. Endometriosis is the ectopic location of the endometrium within the peritoneal cavity. Adenomyosis describes the invasion of endometrial tissue within the myometrium. An accumulation of ectopic endometrial tissue describes an endometrioma.

23. a. A hypoechoic adnexal mass in a patient with a history of endometriosis is **most** likely an endometrioma.

24. d. Massive, **bilateral** enlargement of the ovaries or adnexae should raise the suspicion of Krukenberg tumors (metastatic lesions). Primary ovarian malignancies are rarely solid.

25. c. A round anechoic structure is identified between the left and right ovaries. There is a separation between the mass and left ovary. These sonographic findings are **most** suspicious for a parovarian cyst. A simple ovarian cyst is a possible differential consideration.

26. e. Adhesions can trap fluid normally produced by the ovary. A septated fluid collection (arrowheads) surrounding an ovary is most suspicious for a peritoneal inclusion cyst. Parovarian cysts are not associated with previous pelvic surgery, appearing as a round anechoic mass between the uterus and ovary.

27. c. An ill-defined adnexal mass in a patient with severe pelvic pain and fever is **most** suspicious for a tubo-ovarian abscess. The patient has a negative pregnancy test, making an ectopic pregnancy an unlikely differential consideration.

28. b. An arcuate uterus can be thought of as a uterine variant. This anomaly is not typically the source of infertility. The fundal contour of the uterus appears smooth and regular, ruling out a submucosal fibroid.

29. b. An anechoic tubular structure contiguous with the left ovary in a patient with a history of prior pelvic infection is most suspicious for a hydrosalpinx.

30. a. Ascites and pleural effusion are additional findings associated with ovarian hyperstimulation syndrome.

31. d. Pelvic inflammatory disease (PID) is a general classification for inflammatory conditions of the cervix, uterus, ovaries, fallopian tubes, and peritoneal surfaces. It can be a result of a bacterial infection, diverticulitis, or appendicitis. Tubo-ovarian abscess is commonly a result of sexually transmitted diseases and pelvic infections.

32. b. During ovarian induction therapy, only follicles greater than 1 cm are measured.

33. c. Nabothian cysts are a common finding in the uterine cervix and would NOT likely cause infertility. A submucosal fibroid could cause infertility.

34. b. Parovarian cysts are not affected by cyclic changes in hormone levels and will generally remain the same size on serial examinations.

35. c. Dysmenorrhea is a **common** symptom associated with endometriosis. Other symptoms may include pelvic pain, irregular menses, dyspareunia, and infertility.

36. e. A peritoneal inclusion cyst is a result of adhesions trapping fluid normally secreted by the ovary, creating a septated fluid collection around the ovary.

37. e. A hypoechoic, homogeneous adnexal mass is the most common sonographic appearance associated with an endometrioma. Other findings may include fluid/fluid levels and internal solid components.

38. b. Salpingitis is a result of a pelvic infection causing inflammation within the fallopian tube.

39. e. Under normal circumstances, a surge in luteinizing hormone stimulates ovulation. With ovarian induction therapy, intramuscular injection of human chorionic gondadotropin (hCG) triggers ovulation.

40. b. Scarring within the endometrium caused by a previous dilation and curettage or spontaneous abortion is termed synechiae.

41. c. Fixation of the ovaries posterior to the uterus is a sonographic finding in cases of endometriosis.

42. e. Depending on the severity of the infection, a tubo-ovarian abscess may present as a total breakdown of normal adnexal anatomy.

43. a. Inflammation of the endometrium is an **acquired** cause of infertility. Other acquired conditions include, endometriosis, pelvic inflammatory disease, and Asherman syndrome. Congenital uterine anomalies are not acquired conditions.

44. e. Synechiae are a result of scarring caused by previous D&C or spontaneous abortion and demonstrate as a bright band of echoes within the endometrium.

45. e. A baseline study prior to starting ovarian induction therapy is performed to assess the ovaries for an ovarian cyst or dominant follicle and the uterus for anomalies or abnormalities.

46. c. A **focal** hypoechoic adnexal mass describes the sonographic appearance of an endometrioma. Sonographic findings in pelvic inflammatory disease can vary from a normal-appearing pelvis to an ill-defined multilocular adnexal mass.

47. b. Endometriomas are collections of ectopic endometrial tissue. Endometriosis is an acquired condition occurring when active endometrial tissue invades the peritoneal cavity (ectopic location of functional endometrial tissue). Endometrial tissue will attach to the fallopian tubes, ovaries, colon, and urinary bladder. Adenomyosis is ectopic endometrial tissue within the myometrium.

48. d. A submucosal fibroid distorts the endometrial cavity and is a possible cause of female infertility.

49. a. Sonographic findings in salpingitis include a thick wall and a nodular tubular adnexal mass demonstrating posterior acoustic enhancement. Pyosalpinx attenuates the sound wave.

50. e. Ovarian hyperstimulation syndrome demonstrates as a multicystic ovarian mass generally measuring greater than 5 cm in diameter.

Chapter 23: Assessment of the First Trimester

1. c. Ninety-five percent of ectopic pregnancies are located in the fallopian tube with the majority in the ampullary portion. Approximately 3% are located in the ovary and 2% in the cornua of the uterus.

2. d. Within the fallopian tube, cells of the zygote multiply, forming a cluster of cells termed the morula. Fluid rapidly fills the morula, forming a blastocyst. The **blastocyst** implants into the endometrium.

3. e. Trophoblastic tissue secretes human chorionic gondadotropin (hCG). Decidua basalis and decidua parietalis describe portions of the endometrium in relation to the implanting blastocyst.

4. a. Measurement of nuchal translucency is most accurate from gestational age of 11 weeks 0 days to 13 weeks 6 days. Measurements exceeding 3 mm are abnormal and suspicious for fetal chromosomal abnormalities. The larger the measurement the higher the probability an abnormality exists.

5. d. The amnion attaches to the embryo at the umbilical cord insertion.

6. b. Measurement of gestational age begins with the mean sac diameter. Once an embryo is evident, crown–rump length is the measurement of choice for determining gestational age. Cardiac activity helps to visualize the embryo but does not determine the measuring method. The yolk sac is the first structure visualized within the gestational sac.

7. d. Gestational weeks 6 to 10 constitute the embryonic phase or period. Weeks 11 and 12 are part of the fetal phase. The first trimester extends through the twelfth week of pregnancy.

8. d. The double decidua sign is composed of the decidua capsularis and decidua parietalis giving the appearance of a thick, hyperechoic rim surrounding an intrauterine pregnancy.

9. b. A **rapid** decline in serial hCG levels is most likely associated with a spontaneous abortion (miscarriage). The gestational sac will continue to expand in a blighted ovum, keeping hormone levels elevated.

10. b. Visualization of the amnion without a coexisting embryo is an abnormal finding. The rhombencephalon displays as a prominent cystic structure in the posterior portion of the brain during the first trimester. Take care not to mistake this normal finding for a cystic mass. Physiological herniation of the bowel into the umbilical cord is a normal finding through the twelfth week.

11. b. Implantation of the blastocyst into the endometrium may result in a low-grade hemorrhage between the uterine wall and chorionic cavity. This may result in a miscarriage but more likely will resolve over time. Vaginal spotting is the most common clinical finding.

12. b. Pseudocyesis is a psychological condition where a patient believes she is pregnant when she actually is not. The patient will demonstrate clinical symptoms of early pregnancy, including amenorrhea, nausea, vomiting, abdominal distention, and a negative pregnancy test.

13. d. Mean sac diameter (MSD) is calculated by adding the length, height, and width of the gestational sac and dividing this total by three.

14. c. The amnion expands with the growth of the fetus and accumulation of fluid. **By the** 16th gestational week, the amnion should obliterate the chorionic cavity.

15. c. Hyperemesis is a common clinical finding associated with trophoblastic disease (molar pregnancy). Multifetal gestations (i.e., twins) is another consideration for hyperemesis.

16. b. A solid-appearing adnexal mass in a patient with a positive pregnancy test is most suspicious for an ectopic pregnancy.

17. e. Hemoperitoneum is the most likely diagnosis for echogenic free fluid in the peritoneal cavity. Notice how the fluid conforms to the peritoneal space.

18. e. A small yolk sac is demonstrated in an early intrauterine pregnancy.

19. e. A cystic midline uterine mass in a patient with dramatic elevation in hCG levels is most suspicious for gestational trophoblastic disease (hydatitiform mole).

20. a. Theca lutein cysts are associated with rapidly increasing hormone levels. Approximately 40% of molar pregnancies demonstrate theca lutein cysts.

21. a. Hyperemesis is a common clinical symptom of rapidly increasing hormone levels associated with molar pregnancies, multiple gestation, and ovarian hyperstimulation.

22. **d.** A midline, echogenic fluid collection is identified inferior to an intrauterine pregnancy. This is most suspicious for a subchorionic hemorrhage.

23. **c.** The double decidual sign is characteristic of an intrauterine pregnancy. Myometrium surrounds the entire gestational sac, ruling out a possible cornual pregnancy.

24. **b.** The amnion displays as a thin, hyperechoic linear structure surrounding the developing embryo. This is a normal sonographic finding for an 8-week gestation. Note: LMP (lower left) of 10/17/07 and a sonogram date of 12/18/07 (upper left).

25. **c.** An extrauterine gestational sac (double decidua sign) demonstrated in the right adnexa is most suspicious for an ectopic pregnancy.

26. **d.** Ectopic pregnancies demonstrate an abnormal rise in hCG levels. Decreasing hCG levels are more likely associated with an incomplete abortion.

27. **c.** The sonogram demonstrates a large intrauterine gestational sac without evidence of a yolk sac or embryo. An anembryonic pregnancy, or blighted ovum, occurs when a blastocyst implants into the endometrium, and the inner cell mass does not develop into an embryo. Pseudogestational sacs are typically much smaller.

28. **e.** A complex endometrial cavity following a therapeutic abortion is most suspicious for retained products of conception.

29. **e.** A cystic structure in the posterior cranium between 7 and 10 gestational weeks is most likely the developing rhombencephalon. This structure will ultimately contribute to the fourth ventricle, brain stem, and cerebellum. It can be confused with a Dandy-Walker cyst, hydrocephalus, or subarachnoid cyst.

30. **b.** The amnion obliterates the chorionic cavity by the 16th gestational week. The hyperechoic structure is most likely the normal amnion. An abnormal nuchal translucency is a differential consideration. Uterine synechiae is a

differential consideration but not as likely.

31. **a.** Nuchal translucency measuring 3 mm is a normal finding between 11 weeks 0 days and 13 weeks 6 days. Measurements exceeding 3 mm in thickness are abnormal, suggesting additional testing.

32. **b.** An hCG level of 1000 mIU/ml normally demonstrates a small gestational sac on transvaginal imaging. Levels as low as 500 mIU/ml have demonstrated evidence of a small gestational sac with the transvaginal approach.

33. **b.** **Normal** hCG levels should double every 30 to 48 hours. Normal and abnormal levels can increase every 24 hours. Levels peak at the 10th gestational week and then begin to decline until the 18th week, where they level out for the duration of the pregnancy.

34. **c.** Transvaginally, failure to identify cardiac activity in a gestational sac with a mean sac diameter ≥16 mm is an abnormal finding. Under normal circumstances, cardiac activity should be evident with a maximum mean sac diameter of 16 mm with transvaginal imaging. Failure to identify cardiac activity in a gestational sac with an MSD of 25 mm is an abnormal finding in transabdominal imaging.

35. **a.** Failure to visualize the amnion surrounding an embryo is a normal finding. Visualizing an amnion without identifying an embryo is an abnormal finding.

36. **c.** When utilizing a transvaginal approach, failure to demonstrate a yolk sac within a mean sac diameter of ≥8 mm is an abnormal sonographic finding and suspicious for anembryonic pregnancy.

37. **d.** Gender determination is not an indication for a first trimester sonogram and rarely an indication for second or third trimester sonograms.

38. **b.** The secondary yolk sac is located in chorionic cavity and provides nutrition to the developing embryo. Trophoblastic tissue secretes hCG.

39. **c.** **Initial** visualization of the hyperechoic choroid plexuses is expected near the 10th gestational week.

40. **d.** Vascular flow near the junction of the interstitial portion of the fallopian tube and the cornua of the uterus is increased when compared to other areas in the female pelvis. An ectopic pregnancy in this location can become life threatening.

41. **b.** Trophoblastic disease (molar pregnancy) can be attributed to trophoblastic changes in retained placental tissue or hydatid swelling in an anembryonic pregnancy (blighted ovum).

42. **e.** A heterotopic pregnancy describes the coexistence of both an extrauterine and intrauterine pregnancy. This is a dizygotic pregnancy occurring in 1:30,000 pregnancies. An increase in the size of an adnexal mass on serial sonograms with a co-existing intrauterine pregnancy should raise suspicion of a heterotopic pregnancy.

43. **a.** The amnion is an extra-embryonic membrane that lines the chorion and contains the fetus and amniotic fluid.

44. **c.** The term embryo is used to describe a developing zygote through the tenth gestational week (Callen) and fetus beginning in the 11th gestational week.

45. **b.** A solid mass of cells formed by the cleavage of a fertilized ovum (zygote) is termed the morula. Fluid rapidly enters the morula, forming a blastocyst. The blastocyst implants into the endometrium approximately 5 to 7 days after fertilization.

46. **d.** The chorionic villi become more prolific near the implantation site and areas away from implantation become smooth. The chorionic villi and decidua basalis form the placenta.

47. **d.** The cardiovascular system is the first to function in the developing embryo. Fluid in the fetal stomach is identified around the 12th gestational week.

48. **d.** A hypervascular peripheral rim is displayed in both the trophoblastic tissue of an ectopic pregnancy and a corpus luteal cyst termed "ring of fire"

49. **a.** Human chorionic gondadotropin peaks at the 10th gestational week (100,000 mIU/ml) and then declines, leveling off around the

18th gestational week (5,000 mIU/ml). A gestational sac is routinely visualized transvaginally with hCG levels of 1,000 mIU/ml and as early as 500 mIU/ml.

50. c. The crown–rump length is the most accurate measurement for determining gestational age.

Chapter 24: Assessment of the Second Trimester

1. a. The left atrium lies most posterior closest to the fetal spine. The right ventricle lies most anterior closest to the chest wall.

2. a. Abdominal circumference is measured slightly superior to the cord insertion at the junction of the left and right portal veins of the liver.

3. a. Cavum septum pellucidi is located in the midline portion of the anterior fetal brain, slightly inferior to the anterior horns of the lateral ventricles. It resolves approximately 2 years after birth.

4. b. Prior to 33 weeks' gestation, anterior-posterior diameter of the renal pelvis should not exceed 4 mm. After 33 weeks, normal diameter increases to 7 mm.

5. c. The third ventricle is visualized in the biparietal diameter along with the falx cerebri, thalamic nuclei, cavum septum pellucidi, and the atrium of the lateral ventricle.

6. c. The umbilical arteries arise from the internal iliac (hypogastric) arteries. The placenta receives blood from the umbilical arteries.

7. e. Visualization of the gallbladder peaks around 20 to 32 gestational weeks and signifies the presence of a biliary tree. Normal liver function is not the sole responsibility of the biliary tree.

8. e. The cephalic index was devised to determine the normalcy of the shape of the fetal head. Biparietal diameter and head circumference do not account for changes in vertical cranial diameter. A normal cephalic index averages just under 80%.

9. c. The biparietal diameter is an accurate predictor of gestational age prior to 20 weeks. It is the most widely used biometric parameter for determining gestational age

starting in the second trimester of pregnancy. The abdominal circumference is difficult to obtain and a great predictor of fetal **growth**, not gestational age.

10. c. Choroid plexus cysts can be a normal finding and generally resolve by 23 weeks. They can be associated with trisomy 18.

11. c. In the coronal plane, the normal fetal spine displays three parallel hyperechoic lines. Two curvilinear hyperechoic lines are demonstrated in the sagittal plane.

12. b. The normal cervical length ranges from 2.5 to 4.0 cm. In the second trimester, a cervical length below 2.5 cm is worrisome for early cervical incompetence. Multiple measurements and imaging techniques should be used when evaluating cervical competence.

13. b. The cisterna magna is a fluid-filled space located between the undersurface of the cerebellum and the medulla oblongata. Normal anterior-posterior diameter of the cisterna magna should not exceed 10 mm.

14. c. Measurement of the nuchal thickness is accurate up to 20 gestational weeks. Thickening of the nuchal fold is associated with aneuploidy.

15. b. Ventricular enlargement is evaluated by measuring the atrium of the lateral ventricle. Measurements exceeding 10 mm raise suspicions of mild ventriculomegaly.

16. e. The arrow is pointing to a small midline "box" in the anterior portion of the fetal brain at the level of the thalami. This most likely represents the cavum septum pellucidi.

17. b. The sonogram displays a normal chest, abdomen, and diaphragm in a late second trimester fetus. The image is off midline displaying only a portion of the fetal heart.

18. b. An elongated anechoic structure is located in the right upper quadrant, posterior to the fetal liver and lateral to the umbilical vein. This is most consistent with a normal fetal gallbladder.

19. b. Arrow A points to one side of a dumb-bell–shaped solid structure located in the posterior fossa. This

is most consistent with a lateral horn of the cerebellum. The vermis is located between the cellebellar hemispheres.

20. c. Arrow **B** points to a fluid space between the cerebellum and calvarium. This is most consistent with the cisterna magna.

21. b. The arrow identifies a smooth, elongated solid structure inferior to the fetal stomach. This is most likely a normal left kidney.

22. b. A round anechoic structure is identified in the pelvic midline. This is **most likely** the urinary bladder.

23. a. Echogenic foci within the fetal stomach are normal incidental findings, thought to be a result of the fetus swallowing vernix in the amniotic fluid. It is associated in 30% of Down syndrome cases.

24. e. The sonogram displays a normal right ventricular outflow tract.

25. b. The calipers are measuring a dumb-bell–shaped structure in the posterior fossa. This is most consistent with the normal cerebellum.

26. b. A low-lying placenta is located within 2 cm of the internal os. This placenta margin exceeds 2 cm.

27. b. The placenta is located on the anterior wall of the amniotic cavity and clear of the internal cervical os. A lateral placenta or anterior fundal placenta is possible, but the question states, "**This image** displays the location of the placenta as . . ."

28. a. The arrow identifies a **round** anechoic structure in the upper fetal abdomen. This is most suspicious for the fetal stomach. Gallbladder displays an elongated shape.

29. c. The image displays three parallel hyperechoic lines in the lumbar portion of the spine consistent with a coronal imaging plane. The arrows identify the normal tapering of the vertebral ossification centers between the sacroiliac joints.

30. e. The normal fetal spine imaged in the transverse plane displays three equidistant ossification centers surrounding the spinal (neural) canal.

31. e. The abdominal circumference is measured slightly superior to the cord insertion at the junction of the left and right portal veins (hockey stick).

32. **b.** Elevation in maternal alpha-fetoprotein levels can be a result of an abdominal wall defect, underestimation of gestational age, multifetal gestations, open neural tube defect, cystic hygroma, and fetal death.

33. **c.** The biparietal diameter (BPD) is measured in a plane that passes through the third ventricle and thalamic cerebri.

34. **b.** The left ventricular outflow tract denotes the ascending aorta, and the right ventricular outflow tract denotes the pulmonary artery.

35. **e.** The fetus becomes the major producer of amniotic fluid by 16 weeks through swallowing and urine production. Amniotic fluid volume provides information of renal and placental function.

36. **c.** The atrium of the lateral ventricle normally measures 6 to 10 mm throughout the pregnancy and will be the first area to demonstrate ventricular enlargement.

37. **c.** Low maternal AFP levels are associated with chromosomal abnormalities. Increases in AFP are suspicious for neural tube and abdominal wall defects.

38. **e.** The papillary muscle is commonly displayed in the left ventricle of the fetal heart as a small echogenic focus within the ventricle.

39. **c.** The umbilical cord inserts into the fetal abdomen at a level superior to the bladder and inferior to the liver and adrenal glands.

40. **d.** The tangential view, similar to the Water's view in radiology, is the best imaging plane to evaluate the upper lip and nostrils to rule out cleft lip/palate.

41. **c.** Crown–rump length measures gestational age during the first trimester. Biparietal diameter, head circumference, abdominal circumference, and femur length are routine second trimester biometric measurements.

42. **b.** Oxygenated blood leaves the placenta and **enters the fetus** through the umbilical vein. After entering the fetal abdomen, blood courses through the ductus venosum to the right atrium of the heart.

43. **b.** Nuchal thickness is measured in the axial plane at a level to include the cerebellum, cisterna magna, and cavum septum pellucidi. Thickening is associated with aneuploidy and is accurate up to 20 weeks' gestation.

44. **b.** During the second trimester the normal small bowel is moderately echogenic and hyperechoic compared to the normal liver and large intestines and hypoechoic compared to fetal bone.

45. **b.** Swirling echogenic debris within the amniotic cavity (vernix) is a normal sonographic finding. Vernix can collect in the fetal stomach and demonstrate as a focal echogenic mass within the stomach.

46. **b.** The fetus **becomes** the major producer of amniotic fluid through swallowing and urine production after 16 weeks (early second trimester).

47. **e.** Presence of the cavum septum pellucidi excludes almost every subtle midline brain abnormality.

48. **e.** Meconium is a material that collects in the intestines of the fetus, forming the first stool of a newborn.

49. **c.** The head circumference is measured in a plane that must include the cavum septum pellucidi and the tentorium.

50. **e.** Abdominal circumference is a better predictor of fetal **growth** than gestational age. Up to 20 weeks, biparietal diameter is a good predictor of gestational age.

Chapter 25: Assessment of the Third Trimester

1. **b.** Maternal hypertension increases the risk of intrauterine growth restriction by 25%. The fetus has major control over the amniotic fluid volume through swallowing and urine production.

2. **d.** An amniotic fluid index (AFI) exceeding 20 cm is termed polyhydramnios. AFI above 24 cm is consistently associated with coexisting fetal anomalies.

3. **c.** By 32 weeks' gestation, the distal femoral epiphysis is consistently visualized. A few weeks later, the proximal tibial epiphysis can be visualized.

4. **d.** By the third trimester the fetus is the major producer of amniotic fluid. Decrease in urine production from renal abnormalities is the most likely fetal contributor to oligohydramnios.

5. **d.** Maternal obesity and diabetes are common causes of macrosomia. Maternal hypertension and cigarette smoking can contribute to a reduction in normal fetal growth.

6. **d.** Amniotic fluid volume is a chronic marker of fetal hypoxia. Acute markers of fetal hypoxia include fetal breathing movement, fetal tone, non-stress test, and fetal movement.

7. **d.** When measuring amniotic fluid volume, the transducer must remain **perpendicular** to the maternal **coronal** plane and **parallel** to the maternal **sagittal** plane.

8. **d.** A gestation greater than 42 weeks is considered post term. The third trimester covers weeks 27 to 42.

9. **b.** **Symmetrical** IUGR is a result of **embryologic** disturbance. Asymmetrical IUGR is associated with maternal hypertension and placental insufficiency.

10. **e.** The systolic to diastolic ratio of the umbilical artery can evaluate fetal well-being after 30 weeks' gestation. A ratio greater than 3.0 is abnormal. Absent or reversal of the diastolic component is also abnormal.

11. **c.** Macrosomia is a condition in which accelerated fetal growth results in an infant with a birth weight greater than 4000 grams or a fetal weight above the 90th percentile for gestational age.

12. **e.** Fetal tone is one of five parameters included in a biophysical profile. One complete episode of flexion to extension and back to flexion documents fetal tone. Three separate fetal movements document fetal movement.

13. **d.** Frank breech describes a fetal position where both the head and feet are located in the uterine fundus with the buttocks as the presenting part. Footling or incomplete breech demonstrate one or both feet as the presenting part. With a complete breech position, the knees are bent with the feet down near the buttocks.

14. **c.** Maternal hypertension is defined as a systolic pressure above 140 mm Hg or a diastolic pressure above 90 mm Hg.

15. **b.** An amniotic fluid index (AFI) below 5 cm or a single largest pocket below 1 cm defines oligohydramnios.

16. **b.** This single image displays an excessive amount of amniotic fluid in relation to the fetus. This is most suspicious for polyhydramnios.

17. **a.** The image is taken in the maternal transverse plane. The fetus displays a cross-section image in this plane. Therefore, the fetus is laying spine down, parallel with the maternal sagittal plane. Breech versus cephalic presentation can be determined by the fetal heart. The apex of the fetal heart points to the left side of the body. The left side of the fetus is lying on the left side of the mother. In order for the fetus to lie supine with the left side of the body on the maternal left, the head must be located in the superior portion of the uterus.

18. **b.** Severe oligohydramnios is present in this third trimester gestation.

19. **d.** In the third trimester premature rupture of membranes is a probable cause of severe oligohydramnios. Genitourinary abnormalities can cause oligohydramnios, but multicystic renal dysplasia is a unilateral disease that does not generally affect amniotic fluid production.

20. **a.** The placenta is located on the anterior surface of the gestational sac.

21. **a.** A slight increase in amniotic fluid is present in this one image. The sonographer needs to evaluate and document the amniotic fluid index to rule out polyhydramnios.

22. **e.** Overall accuracy falls within 18% of the actual weight in 95% of the cases.

23. **c.** During the late second trimester and early third trimester, the circumference of the fetal head is slightly larger than the circumference of the abdomen. During the late third trimester, with the increase of fetal body fat, the abdominal circumference is typically equal to or slightly larger than the head circumference.

24. **e.** Placental insufficiency is the most **common** cause of intrauterine growth restriction (IUGR). Other factors associated with IUGR include maternal hypertension, chromosomal abnormalities, and uterine infection.

25. **c.** Biparietal diameter, abdominal circumference, and femur length are the most common biometric measurements used to calculate estimated fetal weight.

26. **b.** The liver is one of the most severely affected fetal organs. Decrease in liver size results in a decrease in abdominal circumference.

27. **c.** The amniotic fluid **index** (AFI) is a technique for assessing amniotic fluid volume by using the sum of four equal quadrants.

28. **d.** The abdominal circumference is the **single** most sensitive indicator of intrauterine growth restriction (IUGR).

29. **a.** Fetuses with macrosomia have an increase incidence of morbidity and mortality resulting from head injuries and cord compression during delivery.

30. **b.** Of all the techniques to assess amniotic fluid volume, the amniotic fluid index (AFI) is both valid and reproducible.

31. **d.** Maternal diabetes can result in macrosomia and polyhydramnios. Preclampsia describes pregnancy-induced hypertension.

32. **c.** Complete extension and flexion of both lower extremities (2 points). Minimum of three separate fetal movements (2 points). Amniotic fluid volume above 5 cm (2 points). Normal non-stress test (2 points). No fetal breathing movement (0 points).

33. **b.** Placenta previa is the most common cause of **painless** vaginal bleeding during the third trimester of pregnancy. Placenta abruption is generally associated with severe pelvic pain.

34. **c.** A decrease in the growth of the abdominal circumference with appropriate growth of the fetal head circumference and femur length on serial examinations is the expected sonographic finding in asymmetrical IUGR cases.

35. **d.** A fetal weight at or below the 10th percentile for gestational age defines IUGR.

36. **e.** Evaluation of the amniotic fluid volume, estimated fetal weight, and maternal blood pressure has the best diagnostic accuracy in determining intrauterine growth restriction.

37. **c.** Placenta previa is a possible cause of a transverse fetal lie in the late third trimester. Polyhydramnios typically allows free fetal movement.

38. **e.** Incomplete or footling breech places the fetal foot as the presenting part and places the greatest risk for cord prolapse.

39. **d.** A biophysical profile is a sonographic method of evaluating fetal well being by displaying specific movements, responses, and amount of amniotic fluid.

40. **e.** Multicystic dysplastic kidney disease is a unilateral disease. The normal contralateral kidney will continue urinary function, allowing the amniotic fluid volume to remain normal.

41. **c.** Maternal risk factors for developing intrauterine growth restricted fetus include hypertension, poor nutrition, and drug or alcohol abuse.

42. **b.** A minimum of 3 weeks between sonographic evaluations is necessary to determine interval fetal growth.

43. **c.** Proteins, calcium, iron, and carbohydrates are stored in the placenta and released into the fetal circulation. The amniotic fluid protects the fetus from injury, allows the fetus free movement within the amniotic cavity, allows symmetrical fetal growth, maintains intrauterine temperature, and prevents adherence of the amnion to the fetus.

44. **d.** The biparietal diameter continues appropriate growth while the abdominal circumference demonstrates a decrease in growth in cases of asymmetrical intrauterine growth restriction (IUGR). A small placenta, oligohydramnios, and normal femur growth are additional sonographic findings associated with asymmetrical IUGR.

45. **b.** The systolic-to-diastolic (S/D) ratio of the umbilical artery evaluates fetal well-being after 30 weeks' gestation. A ratio of greater than 3.0 after 30 weeks' gestation is abnormal.

46. **e.** The abdominal circumference is probably the single most useful parameter of assess fetal **growth.**

47. b. Presentation of the fetal head in the uterine fundus and the lower extremities or buttocks in the lower uterine segment describes a breech presentation.

48. c. Breech presentation in the third trimester may increase cranial pressure, resulting in an elongated appearance to the pliable fetal cranium (dolicocephalic).

49. e. A transverse fetal presentation is perpendicular to the maternal sagittal plane.

50. d. The proximal tibial epiphysis is first visualized around 35 gestational weeks. Visualization of the distal femoral epiphysis first occurs near 32 gestational weeks.

Chapter 26: Fetal Abnormalities

1. c. Echogenic debris within the fetal stomach is a normal finding with fetal swallowing. The debris is likely vernix or possibly blood from a recent amniocentesis. In approximately 30% of the cases, duodenal atresia is associated with Down syndrome.

2. c. **Unilateral demonstration** of multiple renal cysts is most suspicious for a multicystic dysplastic kidney. With infantile polycystic disease, multiple cysts are too small to visualize, giving the kidneys an enlarged hyperechoic appearance.

3. c. The dilated stomach and proximal duodenum found in duodenal atresia produces a sonographic sign termed the "double bubble" sign.

4. b. Both Dandy-Walker syndrome and arachnoid cysts will splay the hemispheres of the cerebellum. Dandy-Walker syndrome additionally displays a complete or partial absence of the vermis while an arachnoid cyst demonstrates a normal cerebellar vermis.

5. e. Agenesis of the corpus callosum (midline structure) demonstrates a dilation of the third ventricle and outward angling of the frontal and lateral horns on ultrasound. Holoprosencephaly displays a large, single central ventricle with an absence of the midline structures including the third ventricle.

6. a. Marked increases in maternal alpha-fetoprotein levels are expected in cases of gastroschisis.

7. e. Thanatophoric dysplasia is a lethal skeletal dysplasia demon-

strating severe rhizomelia, bell shaped chest, and a cloverleaf skull.

8. c. A crescent-shaped cerebellum (banana sign) raises suspicion of spina bifida and signals the sonographer to give additional evaluation and documentation of the fetal spine.

9. e. Abdominal calcifications with associated dilated bowel and polyhydramnios are suspicious for meconium peritonitis.

10. b. Anencephaly is **the most common** neural tube defect.

11. c. Protrusion of the forehead (frontal bossing) is most likely associated with hydrocephalus. The forehead is absent in anencephaly and an encephlocele is more commonly located in the occipital region of the head. Caudal regression affects the lower spine, pelvis, and lower extremities.

12. a. An encephlocele is defined as the extension of a brain filled sac through a bony calvarium defect.

13. b. Facial abnormalities frequently affect the ability of the fetus to swallow, resulting in polyhydramnios.

14. d. Osteogenesis imperfecta is a collagen disorder leading to brittle bones and bone fractures.

15. d. A large central single ventricle is most suspicious for alobar holoprosencephaly. Hydranencephaly is an abnormality of the brain tissue.

16. b. The lateral ventricle measures 1.1 cm, consistent with mild ventricular enlargement. The occipital horn is generally the first portion to dilate.

17. e. A solid mass is extending from the posterior buttock. The sacrum and skin line appears normal. This is most suspicious for a sacrococcygeal teratoma.

18. c. A sacrococcygeal teratoma demonstrates a normal spine and may extend into the pelvis and abdomen, displacing the urinary bladder and resulting in hydronephrosis.

19. c. An enlarged hyperechoic kidney is present, most suspicious for infantile polycystic kidney disease.

20. d. Infantile polycystic disease demonstrates severe oligohydramnios and the absence of urine in the fetal bladder.

21. b. An anechoic renal pelvis is **most** suspicious for hydronephrosis, likely a result of ureteropelvic junction obstruction. Renal cysts are uncommon findings.

22. a. The fetal forehead is present. Fetal brain is present above the orbits but the calvarium does not appear calcified. This is most suspicious for acrania.

23. a. An open spinal defect is displayed in the sacral portion of the fetal spine. An anechoic mass extending from the defect is most likely a myelocele.

24. c. A multilocular cystic cervical mass is contiguous with the posterior surface of the fetal head and neck. This is most suspicious for a cystic hygroma.

25. d. A cystic hygroma is a classic sonographic finding in Turner syndrome (chromosomal abnormality).

26. b. The cerebrum and skull are absent with the presence of orbits and brainstem most suspicious for anencephaly. Microcephaly relates to the overall size of the cranium. Acrania will eventually result in anencephaly from exposure of the brain tissue to the amniotic fluid.

27. e. Anencephaly is the most common neural tube defect and typically demonstrates elevation in maternal alpha-fetoprotein levels.

28. e. An abnormal formation of the bronchial tree replaces normal pulmonary tissue with cysts. On ultrasound, a cystic mass identified in the fetal chest is most suspicious for cystic adenomatoid malformation.

29. d. A large single ventricle with fused thalami is most suspicious for holoprosencephaly. Hydranencephaly is a destruction of brain tissue, not a congenital malformation.

30. e. Demonstration of multiple **unilateral** renal cysts is most suspicious for a multicystic dysplastic kidney. Hydronephrosis is a differential consideration but not the most likely diagnosis. Additional congenital renal anomalies occur in up to 40% of cases.

31. d. Lateral ventricular enlargement exceeding 10 mm defines ventriculomegaly (hydrocephalus).

32. e. Caudal regression syndrome is a neural tube defect seen almost exclusively in diabetic patients.

Fetuses demonstrate fusion of the pelvis with short legs.

33. d. Cystic hygroma is the most common fetal neck mass caused by an obstruction of the lymphatic system.

34. d. Holoprosencephaly is the most likely abnormality to demonstrate a proboscis or cyclopia.

35. b. Pulmonary hypoplasia is a lethal condition associated in cases of oligohydramnios, genitourinary abnormalities, diaphragmatic hernia, skeletal dysplasia, and chromosomal abnormalities.

36. e. Diagnosis of clubfoot (talipes) is made with persistent abnormal inversion of the foot at an angle perpendicular to the lower leg.

37. a. Gastroschisis is a defect involving all layers of the anterior abdominal wall. Small bowel herniates through the defect, floating freely within the amniotic cavity. Gastroschisis is not typically associated with other fetal anomalies.

38. a. Achondroplasia is a nonlethal skeletal dysplasia with abnormal cartilage deposits at the long bone epiphysis. Diastrophic dysplasia is a very rare autosomal-recessive disorder characterized by micromelia, talipes, cleft palate, and hand abnormalities.

39. e. An obstruction at the ureteropelvic junction (UPJ) is the most common cause for hydronephrosis in utero and the neonate.

40. b. The contents of an omphalocele are covered by a membrane consisting of the amnion and peritoneum.

41. d. Presence of a posterior fossa cyst and **agenesis of the cerebellar vermis** is characteristic of Dandy-Walker malformation.

42. d. Common causes of hydrocephalus include spina bifida, encephlocele, Dandy-Walker malformation, agenesis of the corpus callosum, holoprosencephaly, and aqueduct stenosis.

43. c. Replacement of **brain tissue** with anechoic masses is most suspicious for hydranencephaly. Hydranencephaly results from vascular compromise or congenital infection.

44. e. Failure of the callosal fibers to form a normal connection results in agenesis of the corpus callosum. Outward angling of the frontal and

lateral horns of the lateral ventricles (steer sign) is a characteristic sonographic finding associated with agenesis of the corpus callosum.

45. c. Pelviectasis greater than or equal to 10 mm is consistent with mild hydronephrosis. An anterior-posterior diameter of less than 4 mm prior to 33 weeks' gestation and less than or equal to 7 mm after 33 weeks is within the limits of normal.

46. c. The fetus is the major producer of amniotic fluid after 16 weeks' gestation. Renal agenesis is generally bilateral and results in severe oligohydramnios.

47. a. Multicystic renal dysplasia is generally a unilateral disease presenting as multiple renal cysts of varying size.

48. c. Demineralization of the bone or abnormal limb length or shape may not be apparent before 24 weeks' gestation.

49. b. Type II is most severe, demonstrating hypomineralization, a thin cranium, bell-shaped chest, significant bone shortening, and multiple fractures involving the long bones, ribs, and spine.

50. d. Esophageal atresia is difficult to diagnose with sonography. Absence of the fetal stomach or a consistently small fetal stomach on serial sonograms is suspicious for esophageal atresia especially when accompanied by polyhydramnios.

Chapter 27: Complications in Pregnancy

1. c. Eighty percent of Edward syndrome cases (trisomy 18) are associated with a clenched fetal fist. Clinodactyly is associated with Down syndrome.

2. c. Generalized massive edema (anasarca) is often seen in cases of fetal hydrops.

3. d. Sonographic findings associated with Beckwith-Weidemann syndrome include macroglossia, omphalocele, and hemihypertrophy.

4. c. Eagle-Barrett syndrome (prune belly) is associated with hydronephrosis, megaureter, and oligohydramnios.

5. d. A fetal weight discordance of ≥20% defines twin-twin transfusion. The donor twin may display oligohydramnios and IUGR while

the receiving twin may display polyhydramnios and fetal hydrops.

6. b. Duodenal atresia is associated in approximately 30% of Down syndrome cases.

7. e. Fetal papyraceous is a term used to describe a twin pregnancy in which one twin has died and is too large to reabsorb.

8. d. In twin-twin transfusion, **arterial** blood from the **donor** twin pumps into the **venous** system of the **receiving** twin.

9. b. Syndactyly describes a fusion of the fingers or toes. The prefix *syn* defines the joining or union of structures.

10. b. Meckel-Gruber syndrome is associated with infantile polycystic disease, nonvisualization of the fetal bladder, **encephlocele**, and polydactyly.

11. e. Sonography **cannot differentiate** immune from nonimmune fetal hydrops. Antibodies in the maternal circulation destroy fetal red blood cells resulting in immune fetal hydrops.

12. e. Approximately 70% of twin gestations will end up delivering a singleton pregnancy.

13. b. Inward curving of the fifth finger (clinodactyly) is associated with Down syndrome. Polydactyly is associated with Patau (trisomy 13) and Meckel-Gruber syndromes.

14. d. Amniocentesis for genetic testing can be performed as early as 12 weeks but is generally scheduled between 15 and 18 gestational weeks.

15. b. Trisomy 13 is also known as Patau syndrome. Edward syndrome is also known as trisomy 18. Triploidy demonstrates three complete sets of chromosomes.

16. b. Overlapping of the cranial bones is a common sonographic sign of fetal demise termed Spalding sign. A decrease in amniotic fluid leads to compression and overlapping of the calvarial bones.

17. b. Separation of the big toe from the other digits is a sonographic finding termed sandal toe.

18. c. "Sandal toe" is a sonographic finding associated with trisomy 21 (Down syndrome).

19. e. A single anechoic cyst is located within each choroid plexus.

20. **b.** Choroid plexus cysts are generally incidental findings that resolve by 23 gestational weeks. Occasionally, these cysts are associated with trisomy 18.

21. **e.** A multilocular cervical mass demonstrating a thin membrane extends from the posterior neck of the fetus. This most likely represents a cystic hygroma.

22. **c.** Cystic hygroma is a common sonographic finding in Turner syndrome. Turner syndrome can elevate the maternal alpha-fetoprotein levels. Meckel-Gruber syndrome is associated with an encephlocele and infantile polycystic renal disease.

23. **d.** Identification of intra-abdominal fluid (ascites) is a sonographic finding in fetal hydrops.

24. **c.** The anterior abdominal walls of this twin pregnancy are conjoined. Since **this** image is at the abdominal level, diagnosis of acardiac twin is not possible.

25. **b.** A membrane is present between the two fetuses (di**amniotic**). It is too early to determine placenta number and location (dichorionic).

26. **d.** Nuchal thickness greater than 6 mm is abnormal and suspicious for Down syndrome (trisomy 21). Measurement of nuchal thickness is accurate up to 20 weeks' gestation.

27. **d.** Approximately 30% of trisomy 21 cases are associated with duodenal atresia.

28. **b.** Holoprosencephaly and polydactyly are findings associated with trisomy 13. Other abnormalities include microcephaly, enlarged cistern magna, agenesis of the corpus callosum, omphalocele, bladder exstrophy, and echogenic bowel

29. **b.** Clubfoot or rocker bottom feet is associated with trisomy 13.

30. **b.** Preeclampsia is an abnormal condition of pregnancy characterized by the onset of acute hypertension after the 24th week of gestation. The classic triad of symptoms includes maternal hypertension, proteinuria, and edema. The cause of the condition is unknown.

31. **e.** Preterm labor is the onset of labor prior to the 37th gestational week. A full-term pregnancy ranges between 37 and 42 gestational weeks.

32. **e.** Division of the zygote 4 to 8 days after fertilization will demonstrate two amnions (two gestational sacs) and one chorion (one shared placenta).

33. **d.** In twin-twin transfusion the arterial blood of the donor twin shunts into the venous system of the recipient twin.

34. **b.** The recipient twin receives too much blood and may acquire hydrops fetalis, placentomegaly, and polyhydramnios. The donor twin may display IUGR and oligohydramnios.

35. **e.** Two individual amnions will demonstrate two separate gestational sacs. Monoamniotic pregnancies can demonstrate two allantoic ducts, yolk sacs, and embryos. Dichorionic pregnancies will demonstrate two individual placentas.

36. **e.** Fetal hydrops is an abnormal accumulation of fluid in the body cavities and soft tissue of the fetus. This can result in anasarca, scalp edema, pleural effusion, abdominal ascites, and pericardial effusion. Additional findings include placenta edema and polyhydramnios.

37. **d.** Fetal hydrops resulting from fetal **tachycardia** will commonly demonstrate a fetal heart rate of 200 to 240 beats per minute. Normal fetal cardiac rhythm ranges from 120 to 160 beats per minute.

38. **c.** Fraternal or dizygotic twins arise from separate ova that are individually fertilized.

39. **b.** Amniotic bands are fibrous strands of sticky amnion that may entangle fetal parts causing amputations or malformations of the fetus.

40. **e.** The ruptured sticky amnion entangles fetal parts resulting in amputation.

41. **e.** Beckwith-Weidemann syndrome demonstrates a normal karyotype and is associated with hemihypertrophy, macroglossia, and omphalocele.

42. **a.** Two zygotes will always demonstrate dichorionic/diamniotic gestational sacs.

43. **c.** Eclampsia is the gravest form of pregnancy-induced maternal hypertension, characterized by seizures, proteinuria, edema, and coma.

44. **c.** Sonographic findings of fetal hydrops in Rh sensitization (immune) include placentomegaly, scalp edema, pleural effusion, pericardial effusion, and polyhydramnios. Ultrasound cannot differentiate between immune and non-immune hydrops fetalis.

45. **a.** Acardiac twin is a rare anomaly of a monozygotic pregnancy. The acardiac twin demonstrates a poorly developed upper body and an absent or rudimentary heart and receives blood through the normal twin gestation.

46. **d.** Eagle-Barrett syndrome (prune-belly) is manifested by dilatation of the renal collecting system. Sonographic findings include hydronephrosis, megaureter, oligohydramnios, small thorax, large abdomen, scoliosis, hip subluxation or dislocation, and cryptorchidism.

47. **a.** Acardiac twins shunt blood from the vein of one twin to the other or from one artery to the other. Twin-twin transfusion demonstrates an arteriovenous anastomoses.

48. **d.** Holoprosencephaly is a common abnormality associated with trisomy 13. Other associated abnormalities include microcephaly, polydactyly, echogenic kidneys, facial anomalies, cardiac defects, intrauterine growth restriction, abnormal cisterna magna, and echogenic cardiac focus.

49. **c.** Congenital disorder characterized by two major defects—ectopia cordis and an abdominal wall defect.

50. **b.** Inward curving of the fifth finger (clinodactyly) is associated with Down syndrome.

Chapter 28: Placenta and Umbilical Cord

1. **c.** Placenta accreta describes a condition where the chorionic villi of the placenta are in direct contact with the superficial myometrium.

2. **a.** In a low-lying placenta, the edge of the placental margin lies within 2 cm of the internal os. With a marginal placenta previa, the edge of the placenta abuts the cervical os.

3. **d.** Focal dilatation of the umbilical **vein** is commonly located in an **extrahepatic** portion of the fetal abdomen.

4. **a.** The umbilical cord is **covered** by the amnion and Wharton's jelly

surrounds the vessels within the umbilical cord.

5. a. Battledore placenta is a term used to describe an umbilical cord insertion into the end margin of the placenta.

6. c. Placenta accreta is a condition where the chorionic villi growth invades the superficial layer of the myometrium, disrupting the normal uteroplacental vessels and myometrial border (retroplacental complex).

7. b. A single umbilical artery typically measures greater than 4 mm and appears similar in size to the adjacent umbilical vein.

8. c. The length of the umbilical cord during the first trimester is equal to the crown–rump length of the fetus.

9. b. Clinical findings associated with placental abruption include severe pelvic pain and vaginal bleeding. Painless vaginal bleeding is a classic symptom of placenta previa.

10. b. The umbilical arteries arise from the hypogastric arteries of the fetus. Each hypogastric artery courses alongside the fetal bladder and returns venous blood from the fetus back to the placenta.

11. e. Placenta percreta is a condition where the chorionic villi of the placenta encroach through the myometrial and serosal layer of the uterus into the adjacent maternal urinary bladder.

12. e. The chorion frondosum develops into the fetal side of the placenta. Chorionic villi are the vascular projections of the chorion at the placental site.

13. e. Circumvallate placenta is a condition in which the chorionic plate is smaller than the basal plate, resulting in attachment of the placental membrane to the fetal surface of the placenta.

14. d. A true nuchal cord demonstrates **two or more** complete loops of umbilical cord **around** the fetal neck. This is can be a significant finding during the late third trimester or in cases of oligohydramnios.

15. d. A marginal placenta previa abuts but does not cross the internal cervical os. A low-lying placenta lies close to but does not border the cervix.

16. b. The placenta is completely covering the internal cervical os. The hypoechoic area is the retroplacental complex, not infiltration of the placenta into the myometrium demonstrated with placenta accreta.

17. d. Painless vaginal bleeding is the most common clinical finding associated with placenta previa, especially during the third trimester. A transverse fetal presentation can be associated with placenta previa.

18. a. The image is sagittal and the placenta is located within the most superior portion of the uterine fundus.

19. a. A circular homogeneous hypoechoic placental mass is most likely a chorioangioma arising from the amnion surface of the placenta.

20. c. A small piece of solid tissue, similar in echogenicity to the placenta, lies adjacent to the primary anterior placenta. This is most suspicious for a succenturiate placenta.

21. d. Two vessels of similar size are contained within the umbilical cord. This is consistent with a single umbilical artery.

22. d. Cases of single umbilical arteries are more common in multifetal gestations. In this case, the umbilical cord demonstrated both two umbilical arteries and one umbilical artery within the same cord. A single umbilical artery is associated with malformations of all major organ systems and chromosomal abnormalities.

23. e. A shortening of the cervical length is consistent with an incompetent cervix. A small amount of amniotic fluid is funneling within the dilated cervix.

24. c. Placenta abruption often presents with severe pelvic pain and bleeding. The hemorrhage is located between the uterine wall and retroplacental complex (retroplacental hemorrhage).

25. b. The distance from the end margin of the placenta to the internal cervical os is 2.55 cm. A low-lying placenta lies **within** 2 cm of the internal os.

26. b. The placenta is completely covering the internal cervical os, consistent with a complete placenta previa.

27. e. Painless vaginal spotting or bleeding is the most common clinical symptom associated with placenta previa.

28. b. An abnormal increase in placental thickness is present in this sonogram, consistent with placentomegaly. Placentomegaly in this case is a result of Rh sensitivity.

29. b. Placentomegaly is associated with maternal diabetes mellitus, anemia, and intrauterine infection.

30. d. Velamentous umbilical cord inserts into the amniochorionic membrane of the gestational sac adjacent to the placenta.

31. c. By 16 gestational weeks, the amnion and chorion have completely fused together.

32. d. A battledore placenta refers to the insertion of the umbilical cord into the end margin of the placenta. Circumvallete placenta demonstrates an abnormal placental shape.

33. b. In a marginal placenta previa, the end margin of the placenta abuts or encroaches upon the internal cervical os. A complete previa will completely cover the internal cervical os.

34. b. Chorionic villi are the vascular projections at the implantation site and the major functioning unit of the placenta.

35. d. Chorionic villus in direct contact with the maternal urinary bladder is consistent with placenta **percreta**. Placenta increta demonstrates chorionic villi extension into the uterine myometrium.

36. c. Coiling of the cord is a normal finding. Noncoiling is associated with fetal or cord abnormalities.

37. b. Fibrin deposits are found throughout the placenta but more commonly beneath the chorionic plate.

38. d. Primary causes of placentomegaly include maternal diabetes mellitus and Rh sensitivity. Placentomegaly is associated with maternal anemia, twin-twin transfusion, fetal anomalies, and intrauterine infection.

39. b. Complication of placenta previa includes increased risk of intrauterine growth restriction, premature delivery, and life-threatening maternal hemorrhage, stillbirth, and placenta accreta.

40. b. Additional placental tissue adjacent to the main placenta is termed an accessory or succenturiate placenta. This accessory is a result of the lack of the chorionic villi to atrophy.

41. e. A circumvallete placenta demonstrates an abnormal shape presenting with a irregular rolled up placenta edge. The upturned placenta may contain fluid or hemorrhage.

42. e. An abnormal increase in placental size is not associated with intrauterine growth restriction (IUGR). IUGR is more likely to demonstrate a small placenta. Placentomegaly is associated with maternal diabetes and anemia, Rh sensitivity, twin-twin transfusion, fetal anomalies, and intrauterine infection.

43. c. The decidua basalis (maternal side) and the decidua frondosum (fetal side) form the placenta.

44. b. Placenta thickness will vary with gestational age but generally measures around 2-3 cm in greatest thickness and should not exceed 4 cm.

45. e. Placentomalacia (small placenta) is associated with chromosomal abnormalities, intrauterine growth restriction, and intrauterine infection.

46. a. Vasa previa occurs when large fetal vessels coursing in the fetal membranes cross the internal cervical os, placing the patient and fetus at risk.

47. a. An increase in the length of the umbilical cord increases the risk of nuchal cord.

48. b. The presence of the umbilical cord before the presenting fetal part during the birthing process describes a prolapsed cord. Focal dilatation of an umbilical vessels describes an umbilical varix. A nuchal cord surrounds the fetal neck with more than one loop.

49. b. A succenturiate placenta is at an increased risk for a velamentous cord insertion and possible cause of a vasa previa.

50. a. Coiling of the umbilical cord is generally toward the left.

Chapter 29: Patient Care and Technique

1. b. An advance directive is a legal document describing a patient's health care wishes, if he or she is unable to communicate them.

2. e. The sonographer should introduce himself or herself to the patient and explain the requested sonogram prior to beginning the examination. Many patients are not sure why their doctor sent them for an ultrasound. Obtaining patient history and explaining the examination are important parts of the sonographers' health care role.

3. d. HIPAA oversees many health care functions, the primary being confidentiality. Breach in a patient's confidentiality can result in large federal fines to the health care facility and/or employee.

4. b. A technical report is a private communication of the real-time examination between the sonographer and the interpreting physician. This is NOT an official report and never shared with the patient.

5. c. Suppressing or inhibiting (subjugation) a patient's self-sufficiency (autonomy) is against the patient care partnership.

6. e. Upon completion of the examination, the sonographer should inform the patient of the expected timeframe for examination results. Cleaning the transducers, keyboards, and exam table, and writing the technical impression of the real-time examination are duties generally occurring upon completion of the examination. Reviewing examination protocols generally occurs prior to the examination. Clinical information is more commonly obtained prior to and sometimes during the examination.

7. b. Clean and sterilize medical imaging transducers after each use according to the manufacturer's recommendation. Supervising sonographers and infectious control departments are generally involved in the decision, but typically follow the manufacturer's recommendation (warranty).

8. e. The transabdominal technique should be the first imaging approach for pelvic examinations. It allows a wider field of view and can visualize both deep and superficial pelvic structures. Transvaginal and translabial techniques are complementary approaches to the standard transabdominal technique.

9. b. The uterus and iliac vessels are common landmarks utilized in transvaginal imaging. The vagina is a landmark with translabial imaging.

10. c. Translabial imaging is an excellent approach for evaluating the vagina and cervix.

11. d. Overdistention of the bladder may result in a misdiagnosis of placenta previa. Increasing bladder volume compresses and distorts pelvic structures.

12. d. Transvaginal imaging is contraindicated in premenarche or virgin patients.

13. b. Body habitus can limit the detail of a transabdominal image but does not generally affect the detail of transvaginal imaging.

14. e. The superior portion of the uterus determines optimal bladder distention. Some patients find it difficult to tolerate an optimally full bladder.

15. b. The transperineal (translabial) approach is an excellent method for imaging the vagina and cervix.

16. e. The transabdominal approach displays a larger field of view and the ability to evaluate both superficial and deep structures.

17. a. The image is produced using the endovaginal or transvaginal approach. The position of the uterus is anteverted.

18. b. With a transvaginal approach in the sagittal plane, Label A identifies the anterior surface of the uterus.

19. e. With a transvaginal approach in the **sagittal** plane, Label B identifies the superior border of the uterus.

20. e. Label C identifies the posterior aspect of the uterus.

21. b. Label D identifies the inferior portion of the uterus.

22. c. A transperineal or labial approach is imaging the lower uterine segment of a pregnant uterus.

23. e. Partial emptying of the urinary bladder is the most likely technique to aid in visualizing a posterior placenta.

24. e. The quality of this sonogram is good; additional focal zones may increase overall fetal detail.

25. b. The sonogram is in a sagittal plane with the right side of the **screen** representing the inferior portion of the patient.

26. d. The sonogram is in a sagittal plane with the left side of the **screen** representing the superior (cephalic) portion of the patient.

27. e. The arrow is identifying the posterior surface of an anteverted uterus.

28. e. The sonogram demonstrates an incompetent cervix using the transperineal approach in a sagittal imaging plane.

29. d. The sonographer is responsible for explaining the ultrasound examination to the patient prior to beginning. The referring physician provides examination results to the patient.

30. d. Knowledge of the patient's menstrual cycle is important when evaluating and monitoring the uterus and ovaries. Cyclic changes in hormones vary endometrial thickness and ovarian follicles.

31. b. Measuring the anterior posterior diameter of the endometrium is part of a normal gynecological ultrasound.

32. c. Translabial imaging is an excellent approach for evaluating placental location.

33. a. Ethics is a system of valued behaviors and beliefs that govern proper conduct to ensure protection of an individual's rights.

34. b. Autonomy is the self-governing or self-directing freedom to choose and have one's choices respected.

35. b. The SDMS has adopted a code of ethics for medical sonographers. JRC-DMS and CAAHEP are organizations working together for accreditation of diagnostic medical sonography programs.

36. e. In utero, the foramen ovale opens and closes between the right and left atrium of the fetal heart. After birth, the foramen ovale closes and remains closed, forming a competent atrial septum.

37. d. Overdistending the urinary bladder may give a false impression of an increased cervical length. Emptying the urinary bladder and translabial imaging are methods of evaluating for cervical incompetence.

38. e. The purpose of certification in diagnostic medical sonography is to assure the public and medical community the sonographer possesses the necessary knowledge, education, skills, and experience to perform diagnostic ultrasound examinations.

39. c. Transvaginal is the best method for measuring cervical length. Transperineal (translabial) can foreshorten the cervical length.

40. c. Translabial or transvaginal with an empty or partially full maternal bladder.

41. d. A transverse scanning plane best demonstrates the splaying of the posterior ossification centers.

42. e. Protecting the patient's medical and personal privacy (confidentiality) is a duty of all health care professionals.

43. e. Thermal effects are major biological effects of ultrasound and can be minimized by the sonographer by extending the focus as deep into the body as possible, not scanning in one spot (especially over fetal bone), and decreasing acoustic output and examination time.

44. e. The posterior cul de sac must be included in a pelvic sonogram.

45. a. Due to the minimal invasiveness of transvaginal imaging, patient consent is a **mandatory** requirement prior to performing a transvaginal examination. Starting a gynecological examination with transabdominal imaging is encouraged but not mandatory.

46. d. When a pelvic mass is encountered, the kidneys should be evaluated for evidence of hydronephrosis.

47. b. The patient is placed supine with the hips and knees flexed and the thighs abducted and rotated externally (lithotomy position).

48. e. Transvaginal imaging is advantageous with obese patients and uterine retroflexion and retroversion.

49. e. Assessment of fetal growth can be determined with examinations a minimum of 3 weeks apart.

50. d. Bladder preparation for a pelvic sonogram is adjusted for children according to their menstrual age and body weight.

Obstetrics and Gynecology Mock Exam

1. e. A cloverleaf shape to the skull is characteristic of skeletal dysplasia (thanatophoric dwarf). Overlapping of the calvarium bones is present with long-standing fetal demise termed Spalding's sign.

2. e. The presence of valves within the **male** urethra results in a urinary obstruction demonstrating a dilated bladder and posterior urethra (keyhole sign).

3. b. The broad ligament provides a small amount of support for the uterus and contains the **uterine blood vessels and nerves**. The suspensory ligaments contain the ovarian vessels.

4. b. Placenta accreta is a condition where the chorionic villi invade the superficial layer of the uterine myometrium, obliterating the retroplacental complex.

5. e. Identification of the falx does not indicate the proper level for the biparietal diameter (BPD). Measurement of the BPD is at a level passing through the third ventricle and thalamic cerebri. Other landmarks include the cavum septum pellucidi and the atrium of the lateral ventricle.

6. d. Crown–rump length during the first trimester is generally the best and most accurate method for measuring gestational age.

7. b. **Symmetric bilateral** pelvic masses are **most** likely pelvic muscles. Bilateral follicular cysts, theca lutein cysts, or uterine fibroids are unlikely symmetrical.

8. b. A **hypoechoic** adnexal mass separate from the ovaries is most suspicious for an endometrioma. A complicated parovarian cyst is a differential consideration, but unlikely the diagnosis.

9. d. HIPAA is a federal agency overseeing may health care functions, the primary being patient confidentiality.

10. c. The biophysical profile is a sonographic evaluation of fetal well-being. It includes a specific time or number of fetal movements, breathing movements, fetal tone, amniotic fluid volume, and a non-stress test.

11. b. During the secretory phase, the functional layer of the endometrium continues to thicken and may demonstrate posterior acoustic enhancement. The luteal phase of the ovary corresponds with the secretory phase of the endometrium.

12. **d.** Normal serum maternal alpha-fetoprotein levels will vary with gestational age and number. Abnormal levels can be a result of improper estimation of gestational age.

13. **c.** A diamniotic/monochorionic twin pregnancy will demonstrate two gestational sacs (diamniotic) and one placenta (monoamniotic).

14. **a.** **Symmetrical** intrauterine growth restriction (IUGR) is generally a result of first trimester insult. **Asymmetrical** IUGR may be a result of placental insufficiency, chromosomal abnormality, uterine infection, or maternal hypertension.

15. **e.** The ductus arteriosus carries oxygenated blood from the pulmonary artery to the descending aorta (shunts blood away from the fetal lungs). The ductus venosus carries oxygenated blood from the umbilical vein to the inferior vena cava.

16. **c.** Twin-twin transfusion demonstrates an arteriovenous anastamoses. The arterial blood of the donor twin pumps into the venous system of the recipient twin. Acardiac twinning demonstrates a venous-to-venous or arterial-to-arterial anastomosis.

17. **b.** Thecomas are usually benign and unilateral, comprising 1% of ovarian neoplasms with 70% occurring in postmenopausal women. Dysgerminoma is a malignant neoplasm in childhood. Fibromas also occur in postmenopausal women.

18. **c.** Hydranencephaly is a replacement of normal cerebral cortex with cerebrospinal fluid, resulting from vascular compromise or congenital infection of the fetal brain tissue.

19. **e.** Dandy-Walker syndrome is a malformation of the cerebellum and fourth ventricle. Sonographic findings include an enlarged posterior fossa, splaying of the cerebellar hemispheres, and complete or partial absence of the vermis.

20. **b.** Clinical findings associated with adenomyosis include dysmenorrhea and uterine tenderness **during a physical examination**. Sonographic findings of adenomyosis include an inhomogeneous myometrium, diffuse uterine enlargement, poorly defined anechoic areas within the myometrium, and a normal endometrial canal.

21. **c.** The arrow is identifying an artifactual decrease in echogenicity of the uterine fundus. This is a refraction artifact (edge shadow) resulting from underdistention of the urinary bladder. Proper bladder distention extends slightly beyond the most superior portion of the uterus.

22. **a.** Hypoechoic ill-defined uterine masses are present in this sagittal sonogram of the uterus. Differential considerations would include uterine fibroids, leiomyosarcomas, adenomyosis, and peritoneal mass secondary to endometriosis.

23. **c.** A solid, predominately hypoechoic mass containing hyperechoic foci with acoustic shadowing is most suspicious for a cystic teratoma (dermoid). An endometrioma or hemorrhagic cyst generally does not demonstrate calcifications. Ectopic pregnancy is unlikely with a history of normal menstrual cycles and a last menstrual period of 3 weeks ago.

24. **b.** Absence of the cranial vault and underlying cerebral hemispheres is present in this sonogram. Anencephaly may be diagnosed in the late first trimester and is associated with bulging eyes, polyhydramnios, elevated maternal alpha-fetoprotein, and other spinal defects.

25. **c.** This image is documenting a "T-shaped" hyperechoic linear structure within the endometrium of the uterus. This is most consistent with an intrauterine contraceptive device (IUD).

26. **d.** Tamoxifen is an anti-estrogen medication used in treatment of primary breast carcinoma. Side effects of tamoxifen therapy include an endometrial neoplasm (polyp or carcinoma) or endometrial hyperplasia. Complex appearance to the endometrial cavity is a sonographic finding of the tamoxifen effect.

27. **b.** A large, hypoechoic midline mass in a patient with amenorrhea is most suspicious for hematometra (blood accumulation in the uterus). The anechoic area contiguous with the superior uterus is most likely dilatation of the uterine cornua.

28. **e.** A slightly irregular cystic structure is demonstrated on the left ovary in a mid cycle menarche patient. Prominent echogenic walls are also present. This is most suspicious for a corpus luteal cyst.

29. **c.** One fluid filled and one brain-filled sac is extending through calvarial defects, most consistent with encephloceles. This abnormality would demonstrate a normal maternal alpha-fetoprotein levels. This fetus also demonstrates caudal regression.

30. **d.** The sonogram demonstrates fluid dilation of the fetal bowel. This is most consistent with meconium peritonitis. It can be a result of bowel atresia or meconium ileus.

31. **c.** During the late menstrual phase, the endometrium lining demonstrates a thin 2 to 3 mm diameter.

32. **e.** Physiological herniation of the fetal bowel into the umbilical cord permits development of the abdominal organs. Bowel herniation resolves by the 11th gestational week and is abnormal if it persists after 12 gestational weeks.

33. **b.** Type II is the most lethal classification of osteogenesis imperfecta demonstrating hypomineralization, bell-shaped chest, and significant bone shortening.

34. **d.** A submucosal fibroid displaces and distorts the endometrial canal resulting in irregular or heavy uterine bleeding.

35. **e.** Cross-section measurement of the abdominal circumference is made slightly superior to the cord insertion at the junction of the left and right portal veins.

36. **d.** The right ventricle lies most anterior, closest to the chest wall, while the left atrium lies most posterior, closest to the spine.

37. **b.** Normal nuchal translucency does not exceed 3 mm. Measurement of nuchal translucency is made between 11 weeks 0 days and 13 weeks 6 days.

38. **d.** Premature detachment of the placenta is a critical condition and an indication for immediate deliv-

ery. Placenta previa, vasa previa, and placenta accreta are conditions that will require a cesarean section but are not indications for immediate delivery.

39. **c.** Chorionic villus sampling is commonly performed between 10 and 12 gestational weeks. Scheduling of a genetic amniocentesis is generally between 15 and 18 gestational weeks and as early as 12 weeks.

40. **c.** A Gartner's duct cyst is located within the vagina. This is the most common cystic lesion of the vagina and is usually an incidental finding.

41. **c.** Hyperechoic bowel is associated with Down syndrome, cystic fibrosis, chromosomal abnormalities, and intrauterine growth restriction. When isolated, echogenic bowel is associated with a normal fetal outcome.

42. **e.** Clinodactyly is a congenital characterized by abnormal curvature of one or more digits.

43. **a.** Thickness of the postmenopausal endometrium is consistently benign when measuring 5 mm or less and should not exceed 8 mm.

44. **d.** Fluid within the endometrium is not included in the endometrial measurement. Fluid within the endometrial cavity is not always pathological in origin.

45. **d.** The premenarche cervix is twice the size of the uterine body (2:1). During the menarche phase, the cervix is one half the size of the corpus (1:2). The cervix and corpus are equal in size after menopause (1:1).

46. **d.** The failure of the corpus callosum to develop results in dilation of the third ventricle and outward angling of the frontal and lateral horns of the lateral ventricles.

47. **d.** The narrowest portion of the fallopian tube, the interstitial segment passes through the highly vascular uterine cornua. Rupture in this area can cause severe internal hemorrhaging.

48. **c.** Esophageal atresia results from a congenital malformation of the foregut. Absence of the stomach or small stomach size in serial sonograms with associated polyhydramnios is the most common

sonographic findings in esophageal atresia.

49. **b.** The normal yolk sac should not exceed 6 mm in diameter. A yolk sac diameter exceeding 8 mm is abnormal.

50. **b.** The external iliac vessels lie lateral to the ovaries. The internal iliac vessels lie posterior to the ovaries.

51. **e.** Dandy-Walker syndrome consists of variable degrees of cerebellar vermis agenesis, dilatation of the fourth ventricle, and enlargement of the posterior fossa. The cerebellar vermis is open in early gestation and closes by 18 weeks' gestation. Approximately 75% of cases are associated with chromosomal abnormalities. Coexisting anomalies may include microcephaly, encephlocele, facial malformations, and polydactyly.

52. **e.** An enlarged stomach and proximal duodenum (double bubble) are present in this sonogram, resulting from a duodenal obstruction. Duodenal atresia is associated with Down syndrome and cardiac and urinary anomalies.

53. **c.** Polyhydramnios is a common finding in cases of duodenal atresia.

54. **b.** Central **umbilical cord insertion** into a midline anterior abdominal wall mass is most suspicious for an omphalocele. The defect will contain varying amounts of abdominal contents and is covered by a membrane of peritoneum.

55. **c.** Normal or slightly elevated maternal serum alpha-fetoprotein (MSAFP) levels are typically observed in cases of omphalocele. Gastroschisis demonstrates a marked elevation in MSAFP levels.

56. **d.** Multiple small peripherally located follicles and an enlarged or round ovary are common features of polycystic ovarian disease. Polycystic ovaries generally demonstrate 10 or more small follicles.

57. **c.** A small amount of fluid is identified in the pericardial sac consistent with a small pericardial effusion. A small amount of pericardial fluid (≤2 mm) can be a normal finding in the second trimester or associated with chromosomal abnormalities.

58. **b.** An avascular tubular adnexal mass demonstrating thin wall margins is identified in an **asymptomatic** patient with a **previous** history of pelvic inflammatory disease. This is most suspicious for a hydrosalpinx. Demonstration of low-level internal echoes may occur in some cases.

59. **a.** A hypoechoic homogenous **adnexal** mass demonstrating well-defined margins is most suspicious for an endometrioma.

60. **e.** Bilateral enlarged multicystic ovaries in a patient undergoing ovulation induction therapy is most suspicious for ovarian hyperstimulation syndrome.

61. **b.** Evaluation of Morison's pouch and right paracolic gutter for ascites.

62. **d.** The graafian follicle typically ruptures with a diameter between 20 and 25 mm.

63. **c.** Approximately 40% of trophoblastic disease cases will demonstrate theca lutein cysts.

64. **c.** When the edge of the placenta is a minimum of 2.0 cm from the internal cervical os, placenta previa is ruled out. A low-lying placental edge is located within 2.0 cm of the cervix.

65. **c.** Dangling of the choroid plexus from gravitational forces is a sonographic finding in severe ventriculomegaly.

66. **d.** Developmental defect of the lymphatic system typically results in a cystic hygroma. In the early stages, nuchal thickness may appear increased.

67. **d.** Demonstration of a triple line appearance to the endometrial cavity occurs in the **late proliferation** phase. A thin echogenic endometrium occurs during the early proliferation phase.

68. **a.** The **internal** iliac arteries course posterior to the ovaries and uterus and provide an imaging landmark for imaging of the ovaries.

69. **b.** The piriformis muscles form part of the pelvic floor and course posterior to the ovaries. The obturator internus muscles are located in the lateral portion of the true pelvis.

70. **a.** **Estrogen stimulates** proliferation of the endometrium, develop-

ing an environment for possible implantation.

71. **d.** Benign endometrial hyperplasia is the most common cause of postmenopausal bleeding. Endometrial carcinoma is a differential consideration but not as likely.

72. **e.** Extrauterine masses are most likely to develop on the broad ligament. The broad ligament is a wing-like fold of peritoneum draping over the fallopian tubes, uterus, ovaries, and blood vessels.

73. **b.** Graafian follicle describes a mature physiological cyst containing a cumulus oophorus.

74. **a.** The levator ani muscles along with the piriformis muscles form the pelvic floor supporting and positioning the pelvic organs. They are located posteriorly at the level of the vagina and cervix.

75. **b.** Nabothian cysts are a result of an obstructed inclusion cyst or a result of chronic cervicitis. Corpus albicans is a scar from a previous corpus luteal cyst. Theca lutein cysts are a result of ovarian hyperstimulation.

76. **d.** Encephloceles are midline cranial defects that more commonly arise in the occipital portion of the fetal cranium.

77. **a.** Acrania is a condition where the brain tissue develops with a complete or partial absence of the cranial bones. Acrania may ultimately develop into anencephaly.

78. **a.** Anencephaly is the most common neural tube defect.

79. **a.** Holoprosencephaly is most often associated with trisomy 13 (Patau syndrome). Noonan syndrome is sometimes termed the male Turner syndrome due to their similarities but can occur in both genders.

80. **c.** An encephlocele is a spherical fluid-filled or brain-filled sac extending from a bony calvarial defect. Omphalocele is a result of an anterior abdominal wall defect.

81. **b.** MSAFP levels generally remain normal in isolated cases of encephlocele. Cases of anencephaly, spina bifida aperta, multifetal gestation, and trophoblastic disease are likely to demonstrate elevated MSAFP levels.

82. **a.** Ectopia cordis is complete or partial displacement of the heart outside the chest cavity. It is most commonly located adjacent to the chest wall, but can exist outside the body cavity in other locations (abdominal or cervical). Ectopia cordis is one of the malformations that constitute the pentalogy of Cantrell.

83. **d.** The arrow identifies an accessory or succenturiate placental lobe. The chorionic villi adjacent to the implantation site do not atrophy, resulting in additional placental tissue.

84. **d.** A hypoechoic, well-defined uterine mass is distorting the endometrial cavity. This is most consistent with a submucosal fibroid. Intramural fibroids distort the myometrium.

85. **c.** Menorrhagia is a common clinical finding with submucosal fibroids.

86. **d.** A well-defined hypoechoic ovarian mass displayed in the late proliferative and early secretory phases is most suspicious for a hemorrhagic corpus luteal cyst.

87. **e.** One vascular structure coursing alongside the normal fetal bladder is most suspicious for a single umbilical artery.

88. **d.** A large unilocular cystic structure in the right adnexa is most suspicious for a cystadenoma. Debris has accumulated in the inferior dependent portion of the mass.

89. **e.** A translabial image of the cervix demonstrates funneling of the amniotic fluid into the cervical canal, consistent with an incompetent cervix.

90. **a.** A thin, hyperechoic linear structure surrounds and extends past the posterior aspect of the fetus, most consistent with a normal amnion. The amnion and chorion are fused by 16 gestational weeks.

91. **b.** The placenta extends from the anterior wall completely across the internal cervical os consistent with a complete placenta previa.

92. **c.** Maximum placental thickness normally does not exceed 4 cm. Placentomegaly demonstrates a maximum thickness greater than 5 cm.

93. **e.** Intrauterine growth restriction (IUGR) is **least likely** associated with polyhydramnios. Facial cleft, anencephaly, duodenal atresia, and diaphragmatic hernia are conditions commonly associated with polyhydramnios.

94. **b.** The ureter and iliac vessels lie posterior to the ovary. The external iliac vessels lie lateral to the ovary.

95. **c.** Caudal regression is most commonly associated with maternal diabetes mellitus.

96. **d.** A surge of luteinizing hormone levels triggers ovulation and initiates the residual follicle into a corpus luteal cyst.

97. **e.** A cystic hygroma is often associated with chromosomal abnormalities (Turner syndrome) and does not demonstrate a cranial defect.

98. **a.** Nabothian cysts are common benign cystic structures located in the cervix.

99. **d.** The occipital horn of the lateral ventricle is the first to dilate in the majority of ventriculomegaly cases.

100. **c.** Theca lutein cysts are associated with marked increases in hormone levels, a clinical finding in trophoblastic disease.

101. **e.** The luteal phase has a constant 14-day life span and occurs after the rupture of the graafian follicle.

102. **a.** Thin or wide separation **within the endometrial cavity** is consistent with a septate uterus. A bicornuate uterus demonstrates two separate endometrial cavities.

103. **a.** Thickness of the endometrium is directly related to hormone levels. Increasing estrogen levels regenerate and thickening the functional layer of the endometrium.

104. **b.** A focal collection of ectopic endometrial tissue is termed an endometrioma or "chocolate cyst."

105. **b.** Sonographic findings consistent with adenomyosis include an enlarged uterus demonstrating anechoic areas within the myometrium and a normal endometrial cavity.

106. **d.** The urinary bladder should display on the upper left por-

tion of the **screen** in the sagittal plane.

107. b. Estradiol is an estrogen hormone that primarily reflects the **activity** of the ovary. Luteinizing hormone **triggers** ovulation and initiates the conversion of the residual follicle into a corpus luteum cyst.

108. c. During the late proliferative phase (day 10), the endometrium demonstrates as a "triple-line." The functional layer is thick and hypoechoic with a hyperechoic basal layer.

109. d. Decreases in estrogen can shorten the vagina and decrease cervical mucus. Ovaries atrophy and may be difficult to visualize. Thickness of the endometrium should not exceed 8 mm and is consistently benign when measuring 5 mm or less.

110. e. The isthmus is the "narrow waist" of the uterus located between the cervix and corpus. The isthmus is termed the lower uterine segment during pregnancy. The isthmus is located near the angle of the urinary bladder.

111. b. The suspensory ligaments extend from the lateral aspect of the ovary to the pelvic sidewalls. The broad ligament extends from the lateral aspect of the uterus to the pelvic sidewalls.

112. a. An anechoic tubular mass in an asymptomatic patient is most likely a hydrosalpinx. Questioning the patient about prior history of pelvic surgeries, appendectomy, or pelvic infections may aid in the diagnosis.

113. a. A widening of the posterior ossification centers with an anechoic protrusion is most likely a sacral spina bifida.

114. c. A patient with a history of tamoxifen therapy demonstrating multiple small cystic structures within the endometrium is most suspicious for an endometrial polyp.

115. a. The endometrial cavity displays a hypervascular appearance. With a recent history of an endometrial invasive procedure, the sonogram is most likely demonstrating endometritis from retained products of conception.

116. d. A complex adnexal mass contiguous with the right ovary is present in a pregnant patient. This is most suspicious for an ectopic pregnancy.

117. d. A large empty gestational sac is present in the endometrial cavity, consistent with an anembryonic pregnancy (blighted ovum).

118. d. An anechoic structure is located superior and posterior to the cervix in the pouch of Douglas (retrouterine pouch).

119. c. Three normal-appearing functional cysts are present in this image of the left ovary.

120. b. The arrow identifies a single ventricle with fused thalamic cerebri, consistent with alobar holoprosencephaly.

121. c. Holoprosencephaly is commonly associated with Patau syndrome. Trisomy 13 is a fatal chromosomal abnormality associated with multiple severe malformations including holoprosencephaly, cardiac defects, omphalocele, and infantile polycystic disease.

122. a. Small cystic structures are present in the endometrium of an early pregnancy. These sonographic findings in a patient with hyperemesis are most suspicious for a molar pregnancy (trophoblastic disease).

123. a. The sonogram is demonstrating anechoic brain tissue, falx cerebri, nonfused thalami (large arrow) and choroid plexus (small arrows), most consistent with hydranencephaly. Holoprosencephaly demonstrates an absence of the falx cerebri and fused thalami. Aqueductal stenosis is the cause of 20% of hydrocephalus cases.

124. e. Cystic teratomas (dermoid cysts) are commonly located superior to the uterine fundus. They arise from the wall of the follicle and may contain fat, hair, skin, and teeth.

125. a. Maternal diabetes mellitus and obesity are risk factors for a fetus developing macrosomia. Caudal regression is almost solely associated with maternal diabetes.

126. d. An intrauterine with coexisting extrauterine pregnancy (heterotopic) occurs in 1 out of 30,000

pregnancies. An intrauterine pregnancy with an enlarging adnexal mass is suspicious for a heterotopic pregnancy.

127. d. In cases of triploidy, three complete sets of chromosomes are present. Most cases will abort spontaneously and occurs in 1 out of 5,000 cases. Arnold-Chiari syndrome is an autosomal recessive condition affecting the posterior fossa and associated with ventriculomegaly and a myelomenigocele.

128. d. Osteogenesis imperfecta is a disorder of collagen production resulting in brittle bones to intrauterine fracture. Diastrophic dysplasia is a rare disorder characterized by micromelia, talipes, cleft palate, and hand abnormalities.

129. d. Hypomenorrhea (decrease in menstruation) is not a symptom of uterine fibroids. Asherman syndrome and hematometra are conditions that may present with hypomenorrhea.

130. d. Second trimester ultrasound examinations are best in determining fetal anatomy. Determination of gestational age is most accurate in the first trimester and fetal weight in the third trimester.

131. c. The foramen ovale allows communication between the right and left atria in utero and closes after birth. The ductus arteriosus communicates between the pulmonary artery and the descending aorta, also closing after birth. The ductus venosus connects the umbilical vein to the inferior vena cava. The mitral valve is an atrioventricular valve between the left atrium and left ventricle.

132. d. An early onset of puberty (precocious puberty) may be the result of a mass involving the hypothalamus, gonads (ovaries or testes), or adrenal glands.

133. e. A **unilocular, thin-walled** cystic structure is identified adjacent to a **normal ovary**. This is **most** consistent with a parovarian cyst. Differential consideration may include a cystadenoma, hydrosalpinx, or peritoneal cyst.

134. d. Endometrial carcinoma is the most common malignancy of the female pelvis.

135. **c.** A bicornuate uterus results from a partial fusion of the müllerian ducts. Complete failure of the müllerian ducts to fuse is associated with uterine didelphys.

136. **c.** Ectopic pregnancies demonstrate an abnormal rise in serial hCG levels.

137. **c.** Ovulation typically occurs within 36 hours of visualizing a cumulus oophorus.

138. **a.** The endometrium demonstrates the greatest thickness in the secretory phase, measuring between 7 to 14 mm.

139. **d.** Fertilization of the ovum occurs in the distal portion of the fallopian tube. Fertilization to endometrial implantation occurs in 5 to 7 days.

140. **e.** The anterior pituitary gland secretes follicular stimulating and luteinizing hormones. The hypothalamus produces follicular stimulating hormone releasing factor and luteinizing hormone.

141. **c.** In postmenopausal patients not receiving hormone replacement therapy, the normal endometrium is expected to appear as a thin echogenic line.

142. **d.** Choroid plexus cysts can be a normal finding and normally resolve by 23 weeks gestation. They can be associated with trisomy 18.

143. **c.** The biparietal diameter is an accurate predictor of gestational age prior to 20 weeks. The crown–rump length is the most accurate parameter for measuring gestational age in the first trimester.

144. **a.** Meigs' syndrome is a combination of a pleural effusion, ascites, and ovarian neoplasm that resolve after surgical removal of the ovarian mass.

145. **a.** Bilateral pleural effusions are present in this sonogram of the fetal chest. Pleural effusion can present throughout pregnancy with 10% of small effusions resolving spontaneously.

146. **d.** Demonstration of a cystic hygroma is a characteristic sonographic finding associated with Turner syndrome.

147. **e.** A solid and cystic mass is seen in the region of the fetal sacrum. The fetal skin line shows no evidence of a defect. This is most suspicious for a sacrococcygeal teratoma.

148. **a.** A hyperechoic focus is present in the right upper quadrant in the area of the gallbladder fossa.

149. **a.** An anterior abdominal wall defect is present adjacent to a normal cord insertion characteristic of gastroschisis.

150. **a.** Persistent abnormal inversion of the fetal foot at an angle perpendicular to the lower leg is most suspicious for a clubfoot.

151. **e.** A ventriculoseptal defect (VSD) is the most common isolated congenital cardiac defect. It is essential to visualize the septum perpendicular to the sound beam.

152. **b.** Umbilical artery analysis is evaluated after 30 weeks' gestation. A reversal of diastolic flow in the umbilical artery is a critical finding.

153. **e.** Dilatation of the bladder and proximal urethra (keyhole sign) are most likely demonstrated in this image of the fetal bladder, consistent with posterior urethral valve obstruction.

154. **b.** Hydronephrosis demonstrates pelviectasis ≥10 mm (1.0 cm). The right renal pelvis measures 1.1 cm and the left renal pelvis is 1.0 cm in diameter. Normal pelviectasis in a third trimester should not exceed 0.7 cm.

155. **c.** Proliferation of the trophoblastic tissue results in dramatic increases in hCG levels. Vaginal bleeding and hyperemesis are additional clinical findings associated with gestational trophoblastic disease.

156. **d.** The corpus luteum is a physiological cyst that secretes progesterone early in pregnancy until the placenta develops.

157. **e.** The primitive hindbrain (rhombencephalon) demonstrates as a prominent cystic space in the posterior portion of the brain.

158. **b.** The decidua basalis forms the maternal side of the placenta, and the decidua frondosum forms the fetal side of the placenta. Decidua capsularis covers the surface of the implanted conceptus.

159. **e.** The cephalic index is devised to determine the normalcy of the fetal head shape.

160. **c.** Normal lung development depends on the exchange of amniotic fluid within the lungs.

161. **d.** Mittelschmerz is a term describing pelvic pain preceding ovulation.

162. **d.** Duodenal atresia is a sonographic finding associated in approximately 30% of Down syndrome cases. Other findings include macrocephaly, brachycephaly, sandal toe deformity, and clinodactyly.

163. **d.** Immune fetal hydrops is a result of Rh sensitivity demonstrating fetal ascites, pericardial and pleural effusion, scalp edema, placentomegaly, and polyhydramnios.

164. **e.** Intrauterine growth restriction (IUGR) is the **least likely choice** to result in polyhydramnios. A decrease in amniotic fluid is more commonly associated with IUGR.

165. **d.** Autosomal dominant is a disorder caused by the presence of **one defective gene**.

166. **c.** A lemon-shaped cranium and banana-shaped cerebellum are associated with a coexisting open neural tube defect (myelomenigocele).

167. **c.** The distal femoral epiphysis is visualized around 32 weeks and the proximal tibial epiphysis around 35 weeks' gestation.

168. **e.** A nonmobile hyperechoic focus within a ventricle is most likely the papillary muscle.

169. **c.** The atrium of the lateral ventricle normally measures between 6 and 10 mm throughout pregnancy and should not exceed 10 mm to remain within normal limits.

170. **b.** The apex of the fetal heart is normally positioned toward the left side of the body at about 45°.

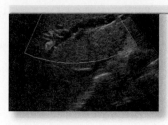

Bibliography

Anderhub B: *General sonography: a clinical guide*, St Louis, 1995, Mosby.

Callen PW: *Ultrasonography in obstetrics and gynecology*, ed 4, Philadelphia, 2004, Saunders.

Cartensen EL: Biological effects of low-temporal, average-intensity, pulse ultrasound, http://www.doi.wiley.com, October 2005.

Curry RA, Tempkin BB: *Sonography introduction to normal structure and function*, ed 2, Philadelphia, 2004, Saunders.

Glossary of Terms; Society of Vascular Ultrasound; 2005.

Gould BE: *Pathophysiology for the health profession*, ed 3, St Louis, 2006, Mosby.

Hagen-Ansert SL: *Textbook of diagnostic medical sonography*, ed 6, St Louis, 2006, Mosby.

Hedrick W, Hykes D, Starchman D: *Ultrasound physics and instrumentation*, ed 4, St Louis, 2005, Mosby.

Henningsen C: *Clinical guide to ultrasonography*, St Louis, 2004, Mosby.

Hrazdira I, Skorpíková J, Dolníková M: Ultrasonically induced alterations of cultured tumour cells, *Eur J Ultrasound* 8(1):43-49, 1998.

Kremkau FW: *Diagnostic ultrasound: principles and instruments*, ed 7, Philadelphia, 2006, Saunders.

Mosby's medical dictionary of medicine, nursing and health professions, St Louis, 2007, Mosby.

Rumack CM, Wilson SR, Charboneau JW et al: *Diagnostic ultrasound*, ed 3, St Louis, 2005, Mosby.

Society of Thoracic Surgeons; http://www.sts.org/aorticaneurysm

SonoWorld; http://www.sonoworld.com

Tempkin BB: *Pocket protocols for ultrasound scanning*, ed 2, Philadelphia, 2007, Saunders.

Ultrasound Diagnosis of Hypertrophied Pyloric Stenosis; Thomas Ball, MD; http://www.radiology.rsnajn/s.org

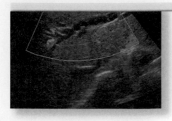

Illustration Credits

Anderhub B: *General sonography: a clinical guide*, St Louis, 1995, Mosby. Figs. 8-4, 8-6, 8-8, 8-9, 11-3, 11-6, 12-2, 12-3, 12-6, 19-9, 19-15, 24-8, 24-10, 24-11, 27-1

Callen PW: *Ultrasonography in obstetrics and gynecology*, ed 5, Philadelphia, 2008, Saunders. Figs. 19-13, 19-18, 20-2 to 20-10, 20-20, 22-8, 23-1, 23-2, 23-12, 28-1, 29-3

Curry RA, Tempkin BB: *Sonography: introduction to normal structure and function*, ed 2, Philadelphia, 2004, Saunders. Figs. 11-1, 12-1, 13-1, 13-2, 16-1, 29-1, 29-2

Hagen-Ansert SL: *Textbook of diagnostic ultrasonography*, ed 6, St Louis, 2006, Mosby. Figs. 7-1, 7-2, 9-1, 12-5, 14-1, 15-1, 15-2, 17-1, 18-1, 19-1, 19-2, 19-4, 19-5, 19-6, 22-9, 22-12, 26-10

Kremkau FW: *Diagnostic ultrasound: principles and instruments*, ed 7, Philadelphia, 2006, Saunders. Figs. 3-1, 3-2, 3-3, 3-4

Perry AG, Potter PA: *Clinical nursing skills and techniques*, ed 6, 2006, Mosby. Originally modified from Centers for Disease Control and Prevention, Hospital Infection Control Practice Advisory Committee: Guidelines for isolation precautions in hospitals, *Am J Infect Control* 24:24, 1996. Standard Precautions Boxes from Chapter 1

Perry AG, Potter PA: *Clinical nursing skills and techniques*, ed 6, 2006, Mosby. Originally modified from Occupational Safety and Health Act: Bloodborne pathogens, Federal Register 56(235):64, 175, 1991. OSHA Standards for Reducing Occupational Exposure to Bloodborne Pathogens Box from Chapter 1

Reuter KL, Babagbemi TK: *Obstetric and gynecologic ultrasound*, ed 2, St Louis, 2007, Mosby. Figs. 25-3, 25-5, 26-8, 26-9, 26-11, 27-8, 27-9, Obstetrics/Gynecology mock exam Figs. 11, 12, 13, 14, 15, 16, 17, 18, 19, 20, 25, 26, 35, 36, 37, 38, 39, 40, 43-47, Color Plate 10

Rumack CM et al: *Diagnostic ultrasound*, ed 3, St Louis, 2005, Mosby. Figs. 7-9, 7-10, 8-13, 10-17, 10-18, 11-7, 14-2, 28-6, Color Plates 1, 2, 3, 4, 5, 9

Tempkin BB: *Pocket protocols for ultrasound scanning*, ed 3, Philadelphia, 2007, Saunders. Fig. 19-3

Courtesies

Paul Aks, BS, RDMS, RVT. Figs. 7-10, 8-12, 10-11, 16-10, 17-5, 18-4, 18-5, 19-10, 19-11, 19-16, 19-17, 21-3, 21-5, 21-7, 23-3, 29-4, 29-9, Abdomen mock exam: Figs. 5, 6, 15, 25, 34, Obstetrics/Gynecology mock exam Figs. 3, 31, 34, 40

Sharon Ballestero, RT, RDMS. Figs. 15-6, 16-9, 27-3, Obstetrics/Gynecology mock exam Figs. 30, 42

Carrie Bensen, RDMS. Figs. 12-4, 13-4, 15-3

Diasonics. Figs. 7-5, 8-5, 8-7, 13-7, 16-7, 18-6, 19-20, 20-1, 20-7, 20-12, 20-13, 20-14, 21-10, 22-21, 23-4, 23-5, 25-1, 27-6

Diane Dlugos, BS, RDMS. Fig. 20-22, Obstetrics/Gynecology mock exam Fig. 27

GE Healthcare. Figs. 11-11, 12-7, 18-9, 23-9

Thomas Hoffman and Jack D. Weiler, Albert Einstein Medical Center, New York. Fig. 12-5

Amy Ly, BS, RDMS, RVT. Obstetrics/Gynecology mock exam Fig. 5

Jackie Menor, BS, RDMS. Fig. 7-3. Abdomen mock exam Fig. 32

Jean Orpin, RT, RDMS. Fig. 28-6

Lynne Ruddell, BS, RDMS. Figs. 10-15, 16-3, 16-8

Diane Short, RT, RDMS. Fig. 24-7

Siemens Medical Solutions, Ultrasound Division. Figs. 8-1, 8-11, 10-3, 10-4, 14-3, 14-7, 16-4, 16-5, 16-6, 16-11, 20-21, 21-8, 22-4, 24-2, 25-2, 27-5, 28-2, 28-4, 29-5, Abdomen mock exam Figs. 20, 26, 35, 36, 37, 38, 39, 40, Obstetrics/Gynecology mock exam Fig. 10

B. Alex Stewart, RT, RDMS. Fig. 26-2

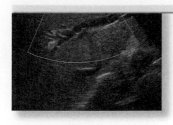

CD Illustration Credits

Anderhub B: *General sonography: a clinical guide,* St Louis, 1995, Mosby. Scrotum question 3; Biliary question 8

Hagen SJ: *Diagnostic ultrasonography,* ed 6, St Louis, 2006, Mosby. Liver questions 31, 32; GI Tract question 6

Middleton WD: *General and vascular ultrasound: case review series,* ed 2, St Louis, 2007, Mosby. Liver questions 22, 23, 26, 30, 33, 34, 35; Neck questions 5, 6; Pancreas questions 13, 14, 22; Urinary questions 18, 19, 24, 25, 28, 29; Spleen question 6; Biliary questions 20, 21, 22, 23; GI Tract question 5

Courtesies

Paul Aks, BS, RDMS, RVT. Liver question 27; Pelvic Anatomy questions 10, 11; First Trimester question 12; Uterine and Ovarian Pathology questions 17, 18, 19; Physiology of the Female Pelvis question 6; Fetal Abnormalities questions 3, 7, 12; OB Complications question 6; Pancreas question 16; Urinary questions 8, 22, 26; Abdominal Vasculature question 22; Superficial Structures question 8; Biliary question 19; Retroperitoneum question 12; GI Tract question 4

Hadish Asfaha, BS, RDMS, RVT. Abdominal Vasculature question 3

Sharon Ballestero, RT, RDMS. Uterine and Ovarian Pathology question 15; Assessment of the Second Trimester question 3

Carrie Bensen, RT, RDMS. Spleen question 2

Diasonics. Liver question 9; Physiology of the Female Pelvis questions 11, 12; Adnexal Pathology and Infertility question 5; Abdominal Vasculature question 5

GE Healthcare. Liver question 10

M. Josh Hall, MS, RDMS. Placenta, Cord question 1; Fetal Abnormalities question 5

Amy Ly, BS, RDMS, RVT. Pelvic Anatomy questions 12, 14; First Trimester question 14; Physiology of the Female Pelvis question 13; Assessment of the Second Trimester questions 4, 7; Fetal Abnormalities question 13

Jackie Menor, BS, RDMS. Liver question 25

Ginger Rose, RT, RDMS. Pancreas question 15

Diane Sharp, RT, RDMS. Liver question 29

Siemens Medical Solutions, Ultrasound Division. Biliary question 6

Kimberly Smith, RDMS. Urinary Question 27

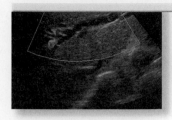

Index

A

A-mode. *See* Amplitude mode
Abdomen. *See also* Abdominal wall
  arteries in, 181-183
  circumference of, 365
  fetal, in second trimester of pregnancy, 366
  measurement of
    in second trimester of pregnancy, 364-365
    in third trimester of pregnancy, 376
  vasculature of, 180-188
  veins in, 183-185
Abdominal aorta
  aneurysm of, 187-188
  location of, 185
  size of, 186
  sonographic examination of, 186
Abdominal circumference, 365
Abdominal hernia, 208
Abdominal wall, 208-224. *See also* Abdomen
  anatomy of, 214-215
  in first trimester of pregnancy, 351
  pathology of, 217
  physiology of, 209
  sonographic examination of, 216
Abortion
  complete, in first trimester of pregnancy, 354
  incomplete, in first trimester of pregnancy, 355
Abruptio placentae, definition of, 410
Abscess
  abdominal wall, etiology and findings associated with, 217
  appendiceal, etiology and findings associated with, 201
  diverticular, etiology and findings associated with, 201
  hepatic, etiology and findings associated with, 91
  pancreatitis associated with, 123
  peritoneal, etiology and findings associated with, 258
  renal, description of, 143
  retroperitoneal, description of, 172
  splenic, 157
AC. *See* Abdominal circumference
Acardiac twin, description of, 403
Accessory spleen, 154, 155
Accountability, definition of, 423
Accuracy, definition of, 66
Achilles tendon
  description of, 208, 215
  tear of, etiology and findings associated with, 217
Achilles tendonitis, etiology and findings associated with, 217
Achondrogenesis, description of, 391
Achondroplasia, description of, 391

Acini
  definition of, 208
  location of, 209f
Acoustic, definition of, 14
Acoustic exposure, definition of, 2, 6
Acoustic impedance, definition of, 14
Acoustic mirror, 31
Acoustic output
  evaluation of, 67
  indexes for, 9
Acoustic output labeling standards, 8-9
Acoustic output quantities, 6
Acoustic output testing, 67
Acoustic speckle, description of, 49
Acoustic variable, definition of, 14
ACR. *See* American College of Radiology
Acrania, description of, 386
Acromelia, definition of, 386
ACTH. *See* Adrenocorticotropic hormone
Acute cholecystitis
  definition of, 103
  etiology and findings associated with, 112
Acute pancreatitis, definition of, 119
Acute tubular necrosis, 132, 140
Addison disease, description of, 166, 170
Adenoma
  definition of, 103
  etiology and findings associated with, 110, 141
  etiology and findings of, 169
  hepatic, 92
  parathyroid, etiology and findings associated with, 247
  thyroid, etiology and findings associated with, 245
Adenomyomatosis, 103, 110
Adenomyosis, 326, 327
Adnexa, definition of, 292
Adrenal cyst, etiology and findings of, 169
Adrenal gland, 166
  anatomy of, 167
  benign pathology of, 169
  function of, 166
  malignant pathology of, 170
  sonography of, 168
  vascular anatomy of, 167
Adrenal hemorrhage, 169
Adrenal hyperplasia, 169
Adrenaline, secretion of, 166
Adrenocortical carcinoma, 170
Adrenocorticotropic hormone, laboratory values for, 168
Adult polycystic kidney disease, etiology and findings associated with, 139
Advance directive, definition of, 423
AFI. *See* Amniotic fluid index
Agency for Healthcare Research and Quality, 423

Agenesis
  description of, 135
  uterine, 299
Agenesis of corpus callosum, description of, 386
AHRQ. *See* Agency for Healthcare Research and Quality
Airborne precautions, 3
AIUM 100 test object, 67
Alanine aminotransferase, laboratory values for, 89, 108
ALARA principle, 2, 6
Aldosterone, laboratory values for, 168
Aliasing
  definition of, 55
  as Doppler artifact, 50, 60
Alimentary tract, definition of, 194
Alkaline phosphatase
  laboratory values for, 89, 107
  prostate gland secretions and, 226
Allantoic duct, definition of, 410
Alpha-fetoprotein
  laboratory values for, 89, 365
  maternal, definition of, 364
Amastia, definition of, 211
Amazia, definition of, 211
Amenorrhea, definition of, 311
American College of Radiology, archiving standards from, 48
Amniocentesis, genetic testing with, 403
Amniochorionic separation, description of, 413
Amnion
  blastocyst development and, 349
  description of, 348
  diagram of, 350f
  sonographic findings of, in first trimester, 353
Amniotic band syndrome, description of, 401
Amniotic fluid
  abnormal, 379
  description of, 378
  function of, in third trimester of pregnancy, 378
  measurement of, in third trimester of pregnancy, 376, 378
  sonographic appearance of, in second trimester of pregnancy, 369
  surveillance of, in second trimester of pregnancy, 366
  volume of, in third trimester of pregnancy, 378
Amniotic fluid index, description of, 378
Amplification, pulse-echo instrumentation and, 43
Amplitude
  definition of, 14
  ultrasound and, 16

Parathyroid gland (*Continued*)
  laboratory values for, 244-245
  location of, 243
  pathology of, 247
  physiology of, 240
  sonographic examination of, 243-244
Paraumbilical vein, collateral of, 95
Parovarian cyst, 338
Patau syndrome, description of, 400
Pathogen, bloodborne, 4
Patient
  communication with, 2-13
  position of, for sonographic examination, 138
  safety and, 2-13
  sonographer interaction with, 5
Patient care, 2-13
  sonography and, 423-434
Patient care partnership, definition of, 423
Patient communication, 2-13
Patient history, sonography and, 424-425
Peak velocity, definition of, 55
Pectoralis muscle, description of, 210
Peliosis hepatitis, etiology and findings associated with, 91
Pelvic, masses in, during early pregnancy, 356
Pelvic inflammatory disease, 337, 338
Pelvic kidney, description of, 136
Pelvic spaces, 256, 295
Pelvis, 292-310
  anatomy of, 292-295
  extrarenal, description of, 135
  false, 292
  female
    anatomy of, 293
    physiology of, 311-325
  ligaments in, 293
  muscles in, 293
  pain in
    patient gynecologic history and, 424
    patient obstetric history and, 425
  pathology of, descriptive terms for, 326
  surgery on, patient gynecologic history and, 424
  surveillance of, in second trimester of pregnancy, 366
  true, 292
    definition of, 292
  vasculature of, 294
Pentalogy of Cantrell, description of, 401
Pepsin, 194
  secretion of, 195
Perflexane lipid microsphere, 19
Perflutren lipid microsphere, 19
Perflutren protein-type A microsphere, 19
Perimetrium, description of, 296
Perinephric fat, 134
Perineum, definition of, 292
Period
  definition of, 14
  formula for, 22
  sound waves and, 16
Peripelvic cyst, 139
Peripheral zone
  definition of, 225
  prostate gland, 227
Peristalsis, definition of, 194
Peritoneal inclusion cyst, etiology and findings associated with, 338
Peritoneal spaces, 256
Peritoneum, 254-266
  anatomy of, 255
  definition of, 254

Peritoneum (*Continued*)
  fluid in, 258
  location of, 256
  masses in, 259
  physiology of, 254
  sonographic examination of, 257
Periurethral gland, 225, 228
Perpendicular incidence, 14, 18
Phantom, definition of, 66
Phased, definition of, 27
Pheochromocytoma, 166, 169
Phlegmon, 119
  pancreatitis associated with, 124
Phrygian cap, 103
  gallbladder anatomy and, 106
Physics, principles of, 14-26
Picture archiving and communication system, pulse-echo instrumentation and, 48
PID. *See* Pelvic inflammatory disease
Piezoelectric effect, 28
Piezoelectric element, description of, 28
Piezoelectricity, 27, 28
Piriformis muscle, description of, 293
Pituitary gland, follicle-stimulating hormone secreted by, 312
Pixel, 38
  pulse-echo instrumentation and, 45, 46
Pixel density, 38
  pulse-echo instrumentation and, 46
Pixel interpolation, 38
  real-time imaging and, 41
Placenta, 410-422
  abnormalities of, 413-414
  anatomy of, 410-411
  blastocyst development and, 349
  diagram of, 350f
  fetal circulation and, 366
  formation of, 348
  functions of, 410-411
  neoplasms in, 414
  sonographic appearance of, in second trimester of pregnancy, 369
  sonographic examination of, 411-414
  surveillance of, in second trimester of pregnancy, 366
Placenta accreta, 410, 413
Placenta increta, definition of, 410
Placenta percreta, definition of, 410
Placenta previa, 410, 412
Placental abruption, 410, 413
Placental infarct, description of, 413
Placental lakes, description of, 413
Placental migration, definition of, 410
Placentomalacia, 414
Placentomegaly, 414
Plants, ultrasound bioeffects on, 8
Platysma muscle, 241
Pleura, anatomy of, 257
Pleural cavity
  description of, 254
  sonographic examination of, 257
Pleural effusion
  description of, 254
  etiology and findings associated with, 259
  fetal, description of, 389
Plug flow, definition of, 55
PM. *See* Preventive maintenance
Pneumobilia, 103, 108
Poiseuille's equation, 55, 57
Polycystic disease, 90, 124
Polycystic kidney disease, 139
Polycystic ovarian disease, 329

Polydactyly, definition of, 399
Polyhydramnios, 376, 379
Polymastia, 211
Polymenorrhea, 311
Polyorchidism, 225, 229
Polyp
  bladder, 303
  colon, 201
  definition of, 103
  endometrial, 328
  stomach, 199
Polysplenia, 154, 155
Polythelia, 211
Porcelain gallbladder, 103, 111
Porta hepatis, definition of, 84
Portal caval shunt, 95
Portal hypertension, 84, 94
Portal hypertension collaterals, 95
Portal vein, 87, 184
  sonographic appearance of, 88
Portal vein thrombosis, etiology and findings associated with, 94
Portosplenic confluence, definition of, 119
Positive predictive value, definition of, 66
Posterior urethral valve obstruction, description of, 390
Postmenopause
  description of, 317-318
  uterine size and, 298
Postpartum thyroiditis, definition of, 240
Postprocessing, pulse-echo instrumentation and, 46
Postterm pregnancy, definition of, 376
Potassium, laboratory values for, 168
Pouch of Douglas, 254, 295
Pourcelot index, 61
Power
  definition of, 6
  Doppler instrumentation and, 60
  pulse-echo instrumentation and, 41
  ultrasound and, 16
Precocious puberty, 311, 313
Preeclampsia, description of, 399
Pregnancy
  complications in, 399-409
  early, pelvic masses during, 356
  ectopic, 339
  first trimester of
    abnormalities in, 354-355
    assessment of, 348-363
    measurements during, 351-352
    pelvic masses during, 356
    sonographic evaluation during, 352-356
    weekly findings during, 354
  heterotopic, in first trimester of pregnancy, 355
  intrauterine, definition of, 348
  molar, definition of, 410
  postterm, definition of, 376
  prior
    patient gynecologic history and, 424
    patient obstetric history and, 425
  second trimester of
    assessment of, 364-375
    measurements during, 364-365
  third trimester of
    assessment of, 376-385
    measurements during, 376
Premenarche
  definition of, 292
  description of, 313
  uterine size and, 298